CEPHALOSPORINS AND PENICILLINS

CHEMISTRY AND BIOLOGY

To

PROFESSOR EDWARD P. ABRAHAM

of the University of Oxford

His fundamental contributions have increased our understanding of the chemistry of natural products and have provided a foundation for advances in the control of infectious diseases.

CEPHALOSPORINS AND PENICILLINS

CHEMISTRY AND BIOLOGY

Edited by EDWIN H. FLYNN

Eli Lilly and Company
Indianapolis, Indiana

ACADEMIC PRESS   New York and London   1972

ACADEMIC PRESS, INC.
111 Fifth Avenue, New York, New York 10003

United Kingdom Edition published by
ACADEMIC PRESS, INC. (LONDON) LTD.
24/28 Oval Road, London NW1

LIBRARY OF CONGRESS CATALOG CARD NUMBER: 75-182626

PRINTED IN THE UNITED STATES OF AMERICA

CONTENTS

Chapter 15   β-Lactam Antibiotics from *Streptomyces*

R. Nagarajan

Chapter 16   **Appendix**

Compiled by E. H. Flynn from data supplied
by contributors

LIST OF CONTRIBUTORS

Numbers in parentheses indicate the pages on which the authors' contributions begin.

E. P. ABRAHAM, Sir William Dunn School of Pathology, University of Oxford, England (1)

DONALD R. BRANNON, The Lilly Research Laboratories, Eli Lilly and Company, Indianapolis, Indiana (370)

ROBERT R. CHAUVETTE, The Lilly Research Laboratories, Eli Lilly and Company, Indianapolis, Indiana (27)

R. D. G. COOPER, The Lilly Research Laboratories, Eli Lilly and Company, Indianapolis, Indiana (183)

P. V. DEMARCO, The Lilly Research Laboratories, Eli Lilly and Company, Indianapolis, Indiana (311)

E. H. FLYNN, The Lilly Research Laboratories, Eli Lilly and Company, Indianapolis, Indiana (662)

MARVIN GORMAN, The Lilly Research Laboratories, Indianapolis, Indiana (532)

KARL HEUSLER, Ciba-Geigy Ltd., Basle, Switzerland (255)

FLOYD M. HUBER, Antibiotic Development Department, Eli Lilly and Company, Indianapolis, Indiana (27)

BILL G. JACKSON, Process Research Division, Eli Lilly and Company, Indianapolis, Indiana (27)

GARY V. KAISER, The Lilly Research Laboratories, Eli Lilly and Company, Indianapolis, Indiana (74)

STJEPAN KUKOLJA, The Lilly Research Laboratories, Eli Lilly and Company, Indianapolis, Indiana (74)

PAUL A. LEMKE, The Lilly Research Laboratories, Eli Lilly and Company, Indianapolis, Indiana (370)

P. B. LODER, Sir William Dunn School of Pathology, University of Oxford, Oxford, England (1)

LOUIS P. MARRELLI, Analytical Chemistry Development, Eli Lilly and Company, Indianapolis, Indiana (609)

P. W. MUGGLETON, Glaxo Research Ltd., Greenford, Middlesex, England (438)

CHARLES F. MURPHY, The Lilly Research Laboratories, Eli Lilly and Company, Indianapolis, Indiana (134)

R. NAGARAJAN, The Lilly Research Laboratories, Eli Lilly and Company, Indianapolis, Indiana (311, 636)

CYNTHIA H. O'CALLAGHAN, Glaxo Research Ltd., Greenford, Middlesex, England (438)

CHARLES W. RYAN, The Lilly Research Laboratories, Eli Lilly and Company, Indianapolis, Indiana (532)

D. O. SPRY, The Lilly Research Laboratories, Eli Lilly and Company, Indianapolis, Indiana (183)

ROBERT M. SWEET, Medical Research Council Laboratory of Molecular Biology, Cambridge, England (280)

J. ALAN WEBBER, The Lilly Research Laboratories, Eli Lilly and Company, Indianapolis, Indiana (134)

JOHN S. WELLES, The Lilly Research Laboratories, Eli Lilly and Company, Indianapolis, Indiana (583)

WARREN E. WICK, The Lilly Research Laboratories, Eli Lilly and Company, Indianapolis, Indiana (496)

PREFACE

The history of medicinal chemistry contains examples of achievements that had their genesis in the singular biological properties of a single compound or a small number of intimate congeners. These achievements were further characterized by a requirement for an intensive but wide-ranging effort which involved many investigators. A major impetus for undertaking such comprehensive studies resides in the promise of possible disease control or elimination. An added fillip has frequently been the association with new and unique chemical knowledge. Studies of the steroid hormones and of penicillin are two instances familiar to all chemists. The prostaglandin effort represents a very recent example of such a research area, still in the process of maturation. The cephalosporins, though perhaps still lacking some of the patina possessed by the first two examples, are an obvious member of this select group.

This treatise is an attempt to assemble and describe those facets of the cephalosporin studies that are germane to our desire to obtain maximum scientific and medicinal benefit from the discovery of cephalosporin C. The timing is such that additional impetus and application of still more scientific expertise may result if this book achieves its purpose.

An examination of the contents will reveal that attention has been devoted to the contributions of every scientific discipline involved, save one. Clinical studies in human medicine have been omitted for practical reasons. The interested reader can find adequate coverage of this subject elsewhere.

A perceptive reader, especially if he is one who has been engaged in research, will be able to identify the application of new techniques and the revelation of new knowledge in each chapter. This is evident in Chapter 8 where nuclear magnetic resonance and mass spectrometry have contributed more insight to our understanding of interactions between component atoms of the molecules being studied. Supplementing and complementing these data are the X-ray structure methods described in Chapter 7. The elegant total synthesis of a cephalosporin by Woodward and co-workers, as detailed in Chapter 6, has contributed new synthetic reactions to organic chemistry and made feasible the preparation of otherwise inaccessible structures. A variety of potentially useful compounds are on the horizon as a result of detailed studies of the chemistry of the β-lactam-dihydrothiazine ring system. These accomplishments are to be found in Chapters 3 and 4. Conversion of the β-lactam-thiazolidine structure to the β-lactam-dihydrothiazine, iterated in Chapter 5, is a *tour de force* as ultimately developed. Methods applicable to the preparation of two compounds having central importance are described in Chapter 2. New organic and biochemical knowledge resulted from work on the preparation of 7-aminocephalosporanic acid and 6-aminopenicillanic acid. Acquisition of cephalosporin C itself, as reported by Professor Abraham in Chapter 1, would have been highly unlikely without the use of modern isolation methods. Structure work also benefited from the application of contemporary physical techniques mentioned earlier. Worthy of note is the felicitous melding of academic and industrial research also described in this chapter.

Those chapters concerned primarily with the biological and biochemical aspects of the cephalsporin relate the benefits of (relatively) recent advances in science. Enzymology occupies a prominent place in our understanding of the mode of action of cephalosporins and in appreciating some of the bases for bacterial resistance. These studies are related in Chapter 10, as is our somewhat circumscribed perception of immunological interactions associated with penicillins and cephalosporins. Laboratory experiments which yield a precognition of clinical experience are invaluable where human medicinal studies must be done. A high degree of success is evident from the studies described in Chapter 11. Chapter 9 is a comprehensive discussion of our knowledge of the biosynthesis of penicillins and cephalosporins. One of the greatest gaps in our overall knowledge resides in this story. No one has been able to demonstrate the facts of actual construction of the 4 : 5 and 4 : 6 ring systems in penicillin and cephalosporin in spite of intensive effort. All of the foregoing is of little value in the medical context unless effects on, and the fate of, these compounds in animals are known and understood. These facets are discussed in Chapter 13 in a comprehensive way; such sophistication was lacking with similar compounds twenty years ago. Correlation of changes in biological properties with change in chemical structure is fundamental to our efforts to design better therapeutic agents from a rational base. Such correlations are described in Chapter 12, relying heavily on data derived from most other segments of cephalosporin research.

Without suitable analytical methods, nearly all of the reported studies would be impossible. Chapter 14 updates and summarizes our knowledge in this important area. Again, modern methodology, such as vapor phase and thin-layer chromatography, and physical chemical techniques proved to be indispensable. The Appendix represents an effort to assemble some of the more generally useful numerical data and experimental procedures with the hope that further research will be facilitated.

It has been my good fortune to be closely associated with nearly all of the contributors to this treatise. Each of them has demonstrated a high level of talent and knowledge in the specific area he was asked to describe. A combination of proficiency and complete willingness to cooperate, evidenced by all of those involved, has made my contribution a superficial but enjoyable one. An example of such cooperation is provided by the Appendix of data which was obtained through the special efforts of Dr. R. D. G. Cooper, Mr. L. P. Marrelli, Dr. C. F. Murphy, Dr. R. Nagarajan, Mr. D. O. Spry, and Dr. J. A. Webber.

This work represents the intellectual and physical efforts of many people. In addition to the authors, thanks are due to Dr. F. R. Van Abeele who supported and encouraged the endeavor as well as provided the initial impetus. Concurrence and support of Eli Lilly and Company was an important factor.

Contributing their own unselfish efforts and unique abilities were Mrs. Phylis Hager, Mrs. Penny Krodel, and Mrs. Doris Coleman. These pleasant co-workers were largely responsible for final manuscript preparation. Academic Press gave invaluable aid in the crucial area of scientific publications technology.

EDWIN H. FLYNN

Chapter 1

CEPHALOSPORIN C

E. P. ABRAHAM and P. B. LODER

Cephalosporin C is the parent substance from which the first cephalosporins to find clinical use were derived. This chapter is concerned mainly with the history of this antibiotic and with work which led to the determination of its chemical structure.

I. Occurrence of the Cephalosporins

Cephalosporin C is produced in very small amounts by a wild strain of a species of *Cephalosporium* [Commonwealth Mycological Institute Kew (C.M.I.) no. 49137], similar to *Cephalosporium acremonium*, which was isolated by Brotzu in 1945. Mutants of this strain have been obtained which produce cephalosporin C in much higher yield. Certain strains of *Emericellopsis terricola* var. *glabra* may also produce small quantities of this antibiotic (Elander *et al.*, 1960).

In addition to cephalosporin C, the *Cephalosporium* sp. C.M.I. 49137 produces cephalosporin N, which is related chemically to cephalosporin C, and an entirely different antibiotic, cephalosporin P (Crawford *et al.*, 1952; Abraham *et al.*, 1953; Abraham, 1962). Cephalosporin N, now known as penicillin N, is identical with an antibiotic which was formerly named synnematin B (Abraham *et al.*, 1955). Work which began with the study of the latter product has shown that the ability to produce penicillin N is shared by a number of different fungi.

In 1943 certain members of the *Fusarium–Cephalosporium* group were found by Waksman and Horning to be antagonistic to the growth of bacteria on a solid medium. Eight years later Gottshall *et al.* (1951) reported that an antibiotic was produced by a member of the genus *Tilachlidium* and by *Cephalosporium charticola*. The *Tilachlidium* was then found to be a new species of *Cephalosporium* and it was named *C. salmosynnematum* (Roberts, 1952). The name synnematin, later changed to synnematin B, was thus given to the antibiotic concerned, whose chemical nature was not then known (Olson *et al.*, 1953).

The perfect stage of *C. salmosynnematum* was observed in 1957 by Grosklags and Swift and this organism was then classified as a new species of the genus *Emericellopsis* Van Beyma (*E. salmosynnematum*). Several species of *Emericellopsis* were shown to produce penicillin N (synnematin) (Grosklags and Swift, 1957; Kavanagh *et al.*, 1958), and the latter was isolated later from the culture fluid of *C. chrysogenum* Thirum. and Sukapure (Sukapure *et al.*, 1965; Pisano, 1970). Only cephalosporin P was found in culture fluids of *E. humicola*, and none of these species was reported to produce cephalosporin C. Penicillin N has also been reported to be formed by a member of the genus

Streptomyces (Miller *et al.*, 1962) and by *Paecilomyces persicinus* (Pisano *et al.*, 1960). However, the configuration of the α-aminoadipic acid residue in the products from these organisms does not appear to have been determined.

It has been suggested by Mangallam *et al.* (1968) that the organism isolated by Brotzu should be classified as a strain of *C. chrysogenum* and by Gams (1971) that it should be described as a strain of *Acremonium chrysogenum*.

II. History of Development

A. Isolation of the Cephalosporium *sp.* in Sardinia

Following the demonstration at Oxford of the chemotherapeutic properties of penicillin, a search for antibiotic-producing organisms was made by Giuseppe Brotzu in Sardinia. Brotzu began this work in July of 1945, soon after he had relinquished the Rectorship of the University of Cagliari, and published an account of it in 1948, a year before he became a member of the Sardinian Regional Council (of which he was later President) and Commissioner for Hygiene, Health and Public Education. The publication, entitled "Ricerche Su di un Nuovo Antibiotico," formed a unique issue of "The Works of the Institute of Hygiene of Cagliari" and had only a small circulation.

Brotzu examined the microbial flora of seawater near a sewage outlet at Cagliari, supposing that the process of self-purification of the water might be due in part to bacterial antagonism. From a spot which is now reclaimed land he isolated a fungus which he concluded was similar to *C. acremonium*. When grown on agar this organism secreted material that inhibited the growth of a variety of gram-positive and gram-negative bacteria (Fig. 1). Selection of colonies from hundreds of serial cultures on agar plates led to the isolation of a strain which produced significant amounts of antibiotic material when grown in glucose–starch broth. From the filtrates of such cultures a crude active concentrate was obtained after precipitation of inactive products with ethanol.

Both culture filtrates and crude active concentrates from the *Cephalosporium* sp. were tested clinically in Sardinia. The filtrates were injected directly into staphylococcal and streptococcal lesions, particularly boils and abscesses, with results that were reported to be good. The concentrates were given intravenously and intramuscularly to patients with typhoid fever, paratyphoid A and B infections, and brucellosis. Although the treatment was complicated by pain and by pyrogenic effects, it usually appeared to produce marked improvement, particularly in cases of typhoid fever. Brotzu believed that his results offered hopeful prospects, but he concluded that the isolation of the active principle would be beyond his resources and expressed the hope, at the end of his publication, that the work would be taken up elsewhere.

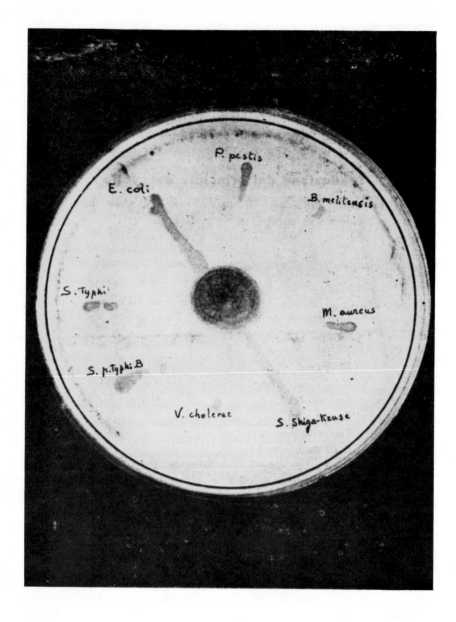

Fig. 1. Three-day-old colony of the Sardinian *Cephalosporium* sp. The different species of bacteria were streaked with a loop to the end of the colony (from Brotzu, 1948).

Attempts by Brotzu to arouse active interest in Italy in his work were unsuccessful. He then wrote to Dr. Blyth Brooke, whom he had met when the latter was a British Public Health Officer in Italy at the end of the war, enclosing a reprint of his paper and suggesting that English research workers should take up the problem. At the suggestion of the Medical Research Council in London, Brooke wrote, in July 1948, to Sir Howard Florey, who replied that he would be glad to arrange for further investigation to be made in the Sir William Dunn School of Pathology at Oxford. Brotzu sent a culture of his organism to Oxford in September 1948, but it was not until nearly 20 years later, when he had become Mayor of Cagliari, that the extensive developments which followed had led to products of established use in medicine.

B. Early Studies in Oxford

The initial experiments at Oxford with the Sardinian *Cephalosporium* sp. (C.M.I. 49137) were carried out by N. G. Heatley, who found that culture fluids contained an acidic antibiotic which was readily extractable into organic solvents. After July 1949 the production of culture fluids was carried out, initially with the help of Kathleen Crawford, by B. K. Kelly and his associates in the Medical Research Council's Antibiotics Research Station at Clevedon, Somerset. At the same time the study of the active material was undertaken by H. S. Burton and E. P. Abraham. Attention was first concentrated on the antibiotic extractable into organic solvents, but it became clear that this substance, which was called cephalosporin P because it showed activity only against certain gram-positive bacteria, was not the antibiotic described by Brotzu.

In August 1949 a second antibiotic was found in Oxford to be present in the culture fluid of the *Cephalosporium* sp. This substance remained in the aqueous phase after the extraction of cephalosporin P and was discovered independently at Clevedon in the following October. It was active against gram-negative as well as gram-positive bacteria and was named cephalosporin N (Burton and Abraham, 1951; Crawford et al., 1952). There appeared to be little doubt that cephalosporin N was responsible for the antibacterial activity that had first been observed 4 years earlier in Sardinia.

Cephalosporin N proved to be labile as well as hydrophilic, and for some time progress with its purification was slow. In October 1949 the activity of the aqueous solution remaining after extraction of cephalosporin P from the culture filtrate had been found to be inactivated by a crude preparation of penicillinase from *Bacillus subtilis*, but since the preparation contained enzymes other than penicillinase, the significance of this finding was uncertain. The first clear evidence that cephalosporin N was a new type of penicillin was obtained early in 1952, when E. P. Abraham and G. G. F. Newton showed that a partially purified sample of the antibiotic yielded the characteristic amino acid penicillamine (β,β-dimethylcysteine) on acid hydrolysis.

At this stage it was decided to increase the effort to isolate and characterize cephalosporin N. Between February and May 1952, G. G. F. Newton worked at the Antibiotics Research Station, and it was found that the culture medium became deficient in methionine during the fermentation. Addition to the medium of methionine, in particular the D isomer, was then shown to increase the yield of cephalosporin N (Miller et al., 1956), and following the resulting improvement in supply, this antibiotic was finally isolated by Abraham et al. (1954) in a form that was nearly pure.

Cephalosporin N yielded D-α-aminoadipic acid as well as penicillamine on acid hydrolysis (Abraham et al., 1953). Further studies left no doubt that it had the structure (1) with a residue of D-α-aminoadipic acid linked through its δ-carboxyl group to the nucleus of the penicillin molecule (Newton and Abraham, 1954). It was subsequently renamed penicillin N.

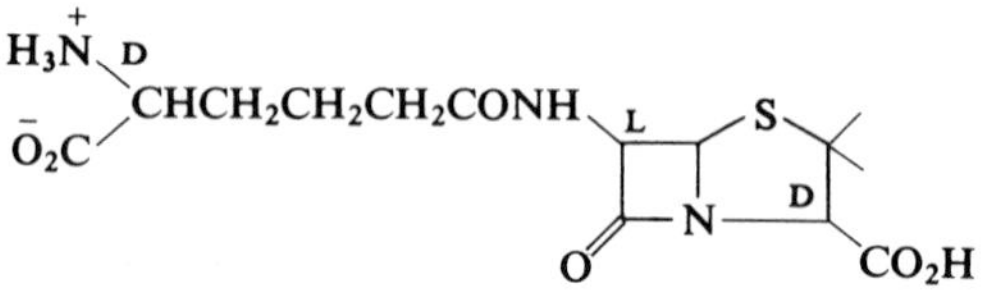

(1)

C. Isolation and Properties of Cephalosporin C

A second hydrophilic antibiotic was discovered by Newton and Abraham among the metabolic products of the Sardinian *Cephalosporium* sp. in September 1953. This substance, cephalosporin C, was first encountered during the chemical study of penicillin N. The penicillin N in a sample of partially purified material was converted to its penillic acid in aqueous solution at pH 2.7 and the resulting product chromatographed on a column of Amberlite IR4B in ammonium acetate buffer. Cephalosporin C was eluted from the column after the penillic acid (Fig. 2) and emerged as a band of ninhydrin-positive material whose ultraviolet absorption spectrum showed λ_{max} at 260 nm. It was readily obtained as a crystalline sodium salt.

At this time research was still concentrated on the isolation and chemistry of penicillin N, and no further study of cephalosporin C was made until 1954. The latter was then found to inhibit the growth of the Oxford strain of *Staphylococcus aureus*, *Salmonella typhi*, and *Escherichia coli* although its specific activity against these organisms was only about 10% of that of penicillin N. However, despite its very low activity, certain other properties of

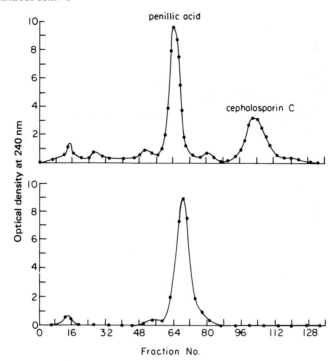

Fig. 2. Separation of cephalosporin C and penicillin N penillic acid by chromatography on Amberlite IR4B. Top curve: crude penillic acid from partly purified penicillin N. Bottom curve: penillic acid from highly purified penicillin N. [From Newton and Abraham, 1956.]

cephalosporin C immediately aroused interest. In some respects it resembled penicillin N but differed from the latter in yielding no penicillamine on hydrolysis and in being much more stable in dilute acid. Moreover, unlike penicillin N and other penicillins known at that time, it was resistant to hydrolysis by penicillinase from *B. subtilis*. This suggested the possibility that cephalosporin C contained a modification of the penicillin ring system with potentially valuable properties (Newton and Abraham, 1955, 1956). Sir Howard Florey, who was informed of these findings while he was on a visit to Australia, expressed the opinion that an effort should be made to prepare cephalosporin C in sufficient quantity for a detailed study of its biological properties to be made.

Early studies showed that cephalosporin C could be separated from impure penicillin N itself and was not formed when the latter was converted to its penillic acid. However, it was present in so small an amount in the culture fluids of the Sardinian *Cephalosporium* sp. C.M.I. 49137 that it could not be detected by antibacterial assay and had only been discovered because it had been concentrated during the purification of penicillin N. The isolation of the new antibiotic in quantity thus appeared at the time to be a formidable undertaking. Nevertheless, relatively small amounts of the antibiotic were gradually accumulated by use of the first stage of the process developed by Abraham *et al.* (1954) for the isolation of penicillin N and the subsequent removal of transformation or degradation products of the acid-labile penicillin N by ion exchange chromatography or by countercurrent distribution in a solvent system consisting of phenol, carbon tetrachloride, and aqueous acetic acid (Abraham and Newton, 1959; Abraham *et al.*, 1966).

By the beginning of 1955 it had been shown that cephalosporin C had a wide range of activity, that it was as effective against a number of penicillin-resistant strains of *Staphylococcus aureus* as against penicillin-sensitive strains, that it was innocuous to mice when given intravenously in very large doses, and that it would protect mice, when given subcutaneously, from streptococcal infections (Florey, 1955). Subsequent experiments showed that it would protect mice from infection with penicillin-resistant staphylococci (Florey, 1956).

Further evidence began to accumulate for the view that the ring system of the cephalosporin C molecule was related to that of the penicillins. Newton and Abraham (1956) reported that crude penicillinase from *Bacillus cereus* 569 contained a minor component which behaved as a cephalosporinase and was absent from the purified penicillinase from the same organism. Abraham and Newton (1956a) showed that cephalosporin C was a competitive inhibitor of the penicillinase from *B. cereus* and Pollock (1957) found that it was a powerful inducer of the enzyme. At this time the prevalence of penicillinase-producing staphylococci in hospitals was causing a serious clinical problem. The need for a substance with the desirable properties of penicillin but without some of the limitations of the latter was therefore clear. Acylation of the amino group in the side chain of penicillin N had been shown to result in a striking change in antibacterial activity (Newton and Abraham, 1954), and it was suggested that further knowledge of cephalosporin C might help to point the way to a structure that would be insensitive to penicillinase but would have much more powerful antibacterial properties than cephalosporin C itself (Abraham, 1957).

D. Chemical Studies

The prospects of obtaining cephalosporin C in relatively large amounts were much improved when a search for higher-yielding mutant strains of the *Cephalosporium* sp., undertaken in 1957 by B. K. Kelly and his colleagues at the Antibiotics Research Station, Clevedon, began to be rewarding. Mutant 8650, which produced much more cephalosporin C than the wild strain, was used in subsequent fermentations. This eventually led to a supply of antibiotic from Clevedon which was sufficient for its chemical structure to be determined.

Progress in studies on the chemical degradation of cephalosporin C enabled a structure to be proposed for this substance at Oxford, in April 1959, which was later confirmed by further chemical work (Abraham and Newton, 1961) and by an X-ray crystallographic analysis (Hodgkin and Maslen, 1961). Attention was then turned by Newton and Abraham, with Bronwen Loder, to the possibility of obtaining the nucleus of the cephalosporin C molecule, stimulated by a report in January 1959, by Batchelor et al. (1959), of the characterization and isolation in quantity of the penicillin nucleus, 6-aminopenicillanic acid, a substance which had previously been stated to exist by workers in Japan (Kato, 1953; Sakaguchi and Murao, 1950) and had also been obtained by total synthesis (Sheehan, 1958). Since cephalosporin C had the same D-α-aminoadipyl side chain as the penicillinase-sensitive penicillin N, it appeared that its resistance to staphylococcal penicillinase depended on its ring system, and a comparison of the antibacterial activities of penicillin N and benzylpenicillin suggested that appropriate changes in the side chain of cephalosporin C would lead to compounds with much higher activities, at least against gram-positive bacteria. The relative stability of the cephalosporin C ring system enabled the. latter to be obtained in 1959, though in very low yield, by mild acid hydrolysis of cephalosporin C itself. By July 1959 small amounts of this substance, 7-aminocephalosporanic acid, had been isolated in a relatively pure state and its N-phenylacetyl derivative had been shown to be much more active than cephalosporin C against a penicillinase-producing strain of S.aureus (Loder et al., 1961). However, the problem of producing 7-aminocephalosporanic acid in quantity remained to be solved.

E. Work in Pharmaceutical Companies

Early in the work on active products of the Sardinian Cephalosporium sp. it seemed possible that one or more of these antibiotics might be of medical interest. In accordance with the policy of the Medical Research Council, applications for patents were made from time to time by those working at Oxford University and the Antibiotics Research Station and assigned to the National Research Development Corporation (N.R.D.C.). This Corporation had been set up in Britain in 1949 under an Act of Parliament—the Development of Inventions Act, 1948—with the function of protecting, developing, and exploiting inventions in the public interest.

Several pharmaceutical companies expressed interest in the cephalosporins at a relatively early stage. The Distillers Company (Biochemicals) Ltd. made contact with the Oxford workers through Sir Howard Florey in 1954 and considered the possibility of providing a supply of penicillin N. In 1955 Imperial

Chemical (Pharmaceuticals) Ltd. initiated a personal connection with the object of becoming acquainted with the current research on penicillin N and cephalosporin C. In the same year an informal suggestion came to Oxford from Eli Lilly and Company that a liaison might be arranged for the purpose of producing cephalosporin C. But when N.R.D.C. asked all British pharmaceutical companies with fermentation facilities to assist in the production of cephalosporin C for further work in Oxford, only Glaxo showed serious interest.

In 1956 N.R.D.C. began to organize meetings between members of Glaxo's staff and research workers at Oxford and Clevedon. The difficulty of producing cephalosporin C in any quantity from the low-yielding *Cephalosporium* sp. then available slowed the pace of further development. However, after the higher-yielding mutant 8650 had become available in 1957, 100 gm of cephalosporin C was ultimately produced in the Glaxo Laboratories and some of this material was used in the last experiments made to confirm the chemical structure which had already been proposed.

In 1958 A. M. Van Arendonk, director of the Eli Lilly patent division, approached the National Research Development Corporation and discussed with B. J. A. Bard and J. C. Cain a proposal for a program aimed at the production of substances related to cephalosporin C, including the nucleus of the molecule, by fermentation. This idea stemmed from work by E. H. Flynn and his colleagues, which was then under way, on the isolation of the penicillin nucleus, 6-aminopenicillanic acid. Eli Lilly signed an agreement with the Corporation in January 1959. Although the project concerned was not successful, they entered into a general option agreement early in 1960 under which they received mutant 8650 of the *Cephalosporium* sp. and access to technical information. From then on they were to make increasingly important contributions to the cephalosporin field.

Other pharmaceutical companies were now showing interest in the cephalosporins. A general option for a licence had been obtained from N.R.D.C. by E. R. Squibb and Company in 1959. In addition to Eli Lilly, three U.S. companies, Merck and Company, Chas. Pfizer and Company, and Smith Kline and French, entered into option agreements in the following year, as did CIBA in Switzerland and Farmitalia in Italy. In 1961 a similar agreement was made with the Fujisawa Pharmaceutical Company in Japan. Until this time it had appeared possible that cephalosporin C itself might find some clinical use for treatment of penicillin-resistant staphylococcal infections, even though its very low specific activity would presumably have required it to be given by intravenous infusion. But this appeared unlikely after the production of 2,6-dimethoxyphenylpenicillin (methicillin) from 6-aminopenicillanic acid and the demonstration of its chemotherapeutic properties (Rolinson *et al.*, 1960; Douthwaite and Trafford, 1960). Thus, a great deal depended on the discovery of a method for the production of 7-aminocephalosporanic acid on a large scale.

Extensive searches in several laboratories for an enzyme which would remove the D-α-aminoadipyl side chain from cephalosporin C had no significant success. But before the end of 1960 an ingenious chemical procedure had been discovered in the Lilly Research Laboratories which enabled the side chain to be removed and 7-aminocephalosporanic acid to be obtained in very much higher yield than was possible by simple hydrolysis (Morin *et al.*, 1962). Details of an improved version of the original process were reported to the N.R.D.C. By this time work at Eli Lilly and at Glaxo had opened the way to the production of cephalosporin C in large amount by fermentation. Thus, 7-aminocephalosporanic acid became available in quantity and an intensive study of the properties of derivatives of this compound soon led to the introduction of two cephalosporins, namely cephalothin and cephaloridine, into medicine.

In comparison with that of many other antibiotics the first stages of the history of the cephalosporins were unusual and prolonged. Eight years elapsed between the isolation of the *Cephalosporium* sp. in Sardinia and the discovery of cephalosporin C in Oxford, largely because the activity of this substance in culture fluids was too low for it to have been detected as an antibiotic in a conventional assay. A further 7 years passed before the isolation of high-yielding mutant strains of the organism and the discovery of a novel method for obtaining the nucleus of the molecule allowed the potentialities of the new ring system of the latter to be adequately explored. During this latter period the difficulties to be overcome appeared at times to be so formidable that it would not have been surprising if the project had been abandoned. Its final success must be attributed to a combination of scientific ability, technical expertise, and willingness to take calculated risks in the pharmaceutical companies that were mainly involved.

III. Chemical Determination of Structure

The molecular formula proposed for cephalosporin C $(C_{16}H_{21}O_8N_3S)$ contained two carbon atoms and two oxygen atoms more than the formula of penicillin N (*1*) (Newton and Abraham, 1956). Like penicillin N, cephalosporin C behaved as a monoaminodicarboxylic acid. It contained a residue of D-α-aminoadipic acid which appeared to be linked to the rest of the molecule through its δ-carboxyl group, since cephalosporin C showed a positive ninhydrin reaction, formed a 2,4-dinitrophenyl derivative which gave dinitrophenyl-α-aminoadipic acid on hydrolysis, and had an ionizable group with pK_a 9.8. A considerably lower pK_a value would have been expected if the

α-carboxyl group of the α-aminoadipic acid had been involved in peptide linkage. The infrared absorption spectrum of the sodium salt of cephalosporin C showed a strong band at 5.61 μ, characteristic of the infrared absorption spectra of the penicillins in which it is associated with the stretching vibration of the C=O moiety of the β-lactam ring. Cephalosporin C yielded D-α-amino-adipic acid and carbon dioxide on hydrolysis with hot acid, and D-α-amino-adipic acid, L-alanine, valine, and glycine when the hydrolysis was preceded by vigorous hydrogenolysis with Raney nickel.

Despite these similarities, cephalosporin C showed some marked differences from penicillin N. On hydrolysis it did not produce penicillamine but yielded sulfur-containing fragments which contained no nitrogen. Under conditions in which 1 mole of ammonia was liberated from penicillin N or benzylpenicillin, it produced 2 moles of ammonia. The valine obtained from cephalosporin C after treatment with Raney nickel was racemic, whereas the valine-containing fragment of penicillin N had the D configuration.

It was first considered possible that a residue of α-hydroxypenicillamine (or its O-acetyl derivative) was present in the molecule (Abraham and Newton, 1956b). However, the hypothesis that cephalosporin C contained a modified β-lactam-thiazolidine ring system threw no light on the nature of the chromophore responsible for the absorption maximum at 260 nm ($\epsilon = 9600$) and further degradation studies led to the abandoning of this hypothesis.

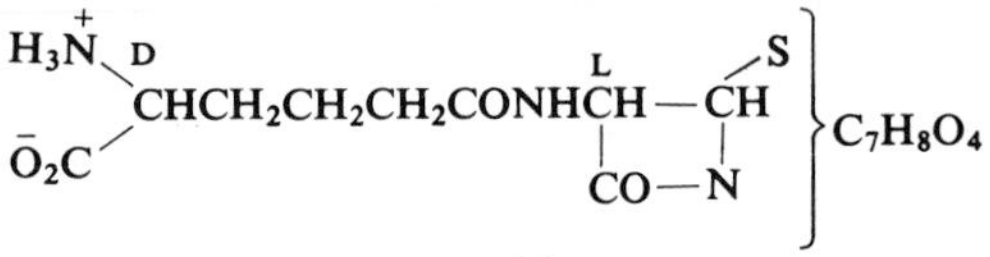

(2)

Consideration of a number of degradation products of cephalosporin C indicated that it contained the partial structure (2). Jeffery et al. (1960) reported that 2-(D-4-amino-4-carboxybutyl)thiazole-4-carboxylic acid (3) was formed when cephalosporin C was kept in neutral aqueous solution at 37°C. The formation of this thiazole from (2) could be accounted for by opening of the β-lactam ring, fission of the bond between the sulfur atom and the remainder of the molecule, and a nucleophilic attack of the sulfur on the amide carbon of the side chain.

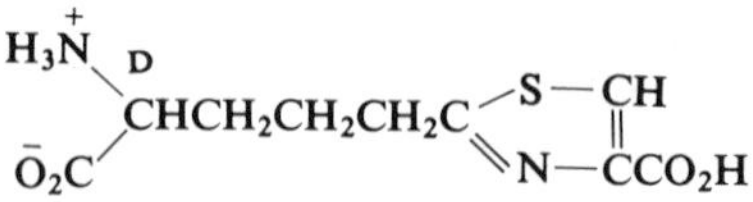

(3)

A further compound, δ-amino-δ-carboxyvalerylglycine (4), which had previously been isolated as a degradation product of penicillin N, was formed in low yield when cephalosporin C was hydrolyzed with acid and the neutral fraction of the resulting material oxidized with silver oxide. Later, a dipeptide of D-α-aminoadipic acid and α,β-diaminopropionic acid (5) was obtained by treatment of cephalosporin C with Raney nickel at room temperature and partial hydrolysis of the product with acid (Abraham and Newton, 1961). Products (4) and (5), like (3), could be formed from (2) by acceptable processes.

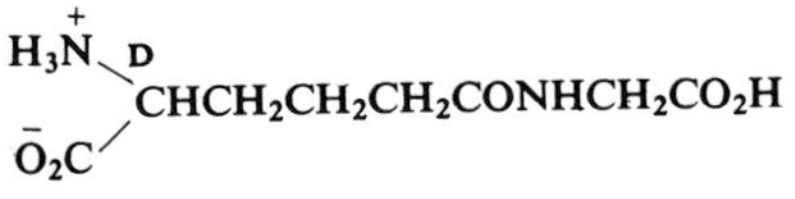

$$\overset{+}{H_3N} \diagdown \underset{\overset{-}{O_2C} \diagup}{} CHCH_2CH_2CH_2CONHCH_2CO_2H$$

(4)

$$\overset{+}{H_3N} \diagdown \underset{\overset{-}{O_2C} \diagup}{} CHCH_2CH_2CH_2CONH\underset{\overset{|}{CO_2H}}{CH}CH_2NH_2$$

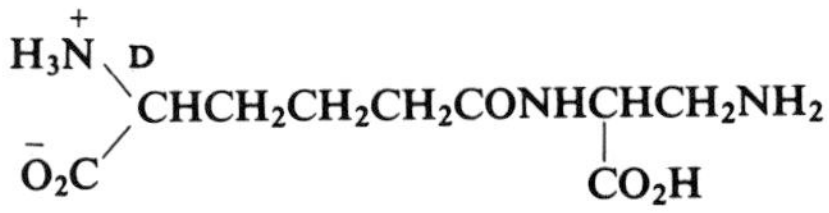

(5)

Of the seven unplaced carbon atoms of the partial structure (2), five formed the carbon skeleton of valine, since DL-valine and some α-ketoisovaleric acid were among the products obtained when the antibiotic was subjected to hydrogenolysis with Raney nickel followed by hydrolysis with hot acid. The finding that 1 mole of acetic acid was liberated from cephalosporin C by mild acid or alkaline hydrolysis established the nature of the remaining C_2 fragment. The presence of a band at 5.77 μ in the infrared spectrum of the antibiotic suggested that the acetic acid was derived from an acetoxyl group.

The next important advance was made when a nuclear magnetic resonance spectrum of cephalosporin C, determined by R. E. Richards and T. Higham, showed that no gem-dimethyl group was present in the molecule. The presence of a single C-methyl group, which had been revealed by a Kuhn–Roth determination, was accounted for by the acetoxyl group. At this stage the structure (6), which contained a fused β-lactam-dihydrothiazine ring system in place of the β-lactam-thiazolidine ring system of the penicillins, was suggested for cephalosporin C as a working hypothesis (Abraham and Newton, 1961). This structure accounted for the failure of cephalosporin C to yield penicillamine

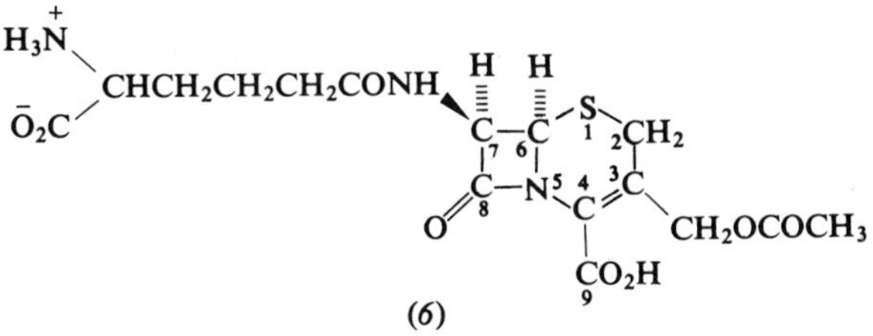

(6)

and for the formation of DL-valine and α-ketoisovaleric acid when hydrolysis was preceded by treatment with Raney nickel. It also accounted for the formation of a neutral compound, known as cephalosporin C$_c$, when cephalosporin C was kept in 0.1 N hydrochloric acid at room temperature. This compound, which showed no net charge when subjected to electrophoresis either at pH 5 or pH 7 and whose infrared absorption spectrum showed bands at 5.62 and 5.69 μ, was clearly the lactone of deacetylcephalosporin C (7) (Jeffery et al., 1961).

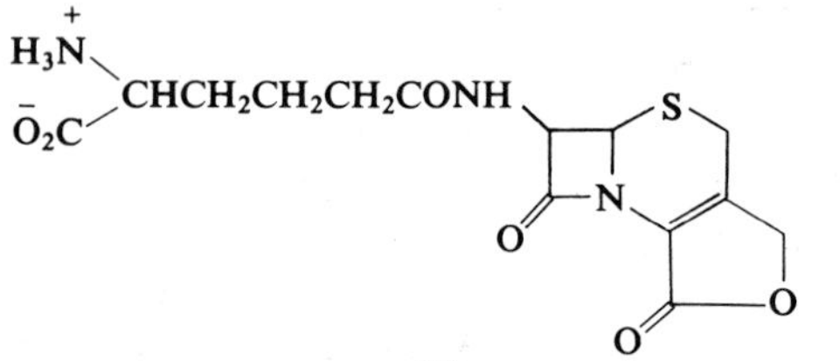

(7)

Soon after structure (6) had been suggested, Dorothy Hodgkin and E. N. Maslen, who had been making an X-ray crystallographic study of the sodium salt of cephalosporin C, were able to discern the presence of a six-membered sulfur-containing ring in the molecule. New degradation products were then isolated which gave further support to structure (6). Among them were γ-hydroxyvaline (8) and α-hydroxy-β-methylbutenolide (9), which were obtained after hydrogenolysis with Raney nickel of cephalosporin C and cephalosporin C$_c$, respectively, and treatment of the products with hot dilute acid. Treatment of cephalosporin C$_c$ with Raney nickel at room temperature yielded a compound which was assigned the structure (10) and which could be regarded as a precursor of (9) (Abraham and Newton, 1961).

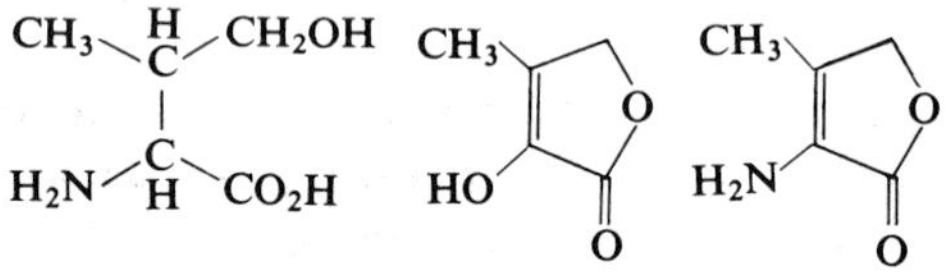

(8)   (9)   (10)

Two degradation products of cephalosporin C, known as compounds 1 and 2, had been obtained earlier by acid hydrolysis of cephalosporin C. The properties of these compounds indicated that they were enolic sulfur-containing lactones formed by condensation of the five-carbon fragments of two molecules of cephalosporin C, and they were assigned structures (11) and (12) respectively. Compound 1 has an α-tetronic acid structure and compound 2 is the corresponding thiolactone.

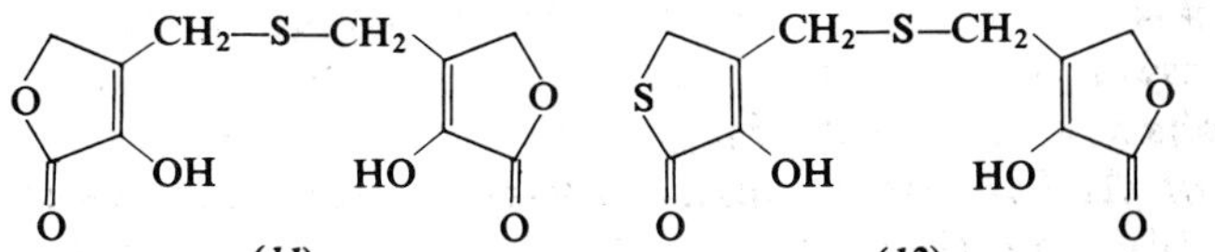

                                (11)   (12)

The isolation of the 2,4-dinitrophenylosazone of hydroxyacetone after ozonolysis of cephalosporin C and treatment of the product with Raney nickel was consistent with the position assigned to the double bond in structure (6). No satisfactory alternative to (6) could be formulated although it would scarcely have been predicted that a compound with this structure would have an ultraviolet absorption spectrum with a maximum at 260 nm. The expected conformation, with *cis* hydrogen atoms attached to C6 and C7, was confirmed by X-ray crystallographic analysis (Hodgkin and Maslen, 1961).

IV. Degradation Products of Cephalosporin C

A. D-δ-Amino-δ-carboxyvalerylglycine

This was synthesized by a process in which the δ azide of *N*-benzyloxy-carbonyl-D-α-aminoadipic acid was coupled with glycine ethyl ester and the protective group removed by hydrogenolysis. The synthetic substance appeared identical with the dipeptide (4) obtained as a degradation product of cephalosporin C. After acid hydrolysis it yielded α-aminoadipic acid and glycine, but when heated in water alone it yielded glycine and 6-oxopiperidine-2-carboxylic acid (Abraham and Newton, 1954).

B. 2-(D-4-Amino-4-carboxybutyl)thiazole-4-carboxylic Acid

The optically active thiazole (3), formed when cephalosporin C was kept in neutral aqueous solution at 37°C, was isolated by chromatography on an anion exchange resin. Although readily soluble in water at pH 7, it separated in crystalline form when the solution was adjusted to pH 3.8. It was unchanged by treatment with hot 6 N hydrochloric acid.

The assignment of structure (3) to this compound by Jeffery *et al.* (1960) was based partly on the following observations. Elementary analysis indicated that the probable molecular formula was $C_9H_{12}O_4N_2S$, and electrometric titration established the presence of a basic group (pK_a 9.9) and two acidic groups (pK_a's 2.6 and 4.0). The ultraviolet absorption spectrum of the substance in water, which showed a maximum at 237 nm, was similar to that recorded by Brookes *et al.* (1957) for 2-(1-amino-2-methylpropyl)thiazole-4-carboxylic acid hydrochloride. A change in λ_{max} from 237 nm in water to 233 nm in 1.0 N hydrochloric acid could be attributed to protonation of the heterocyclic nitrogen atom.

Hydrogenolysis under two different conditions, followed by hydrolysis, provided further support for structure (*3*). Among the products formed with an excess of Adams catalyst were lysine (*13*) and alanine (*14*). Treatment with Raney nickel produced alanine (*14*) and pipecolic acid (*15*).

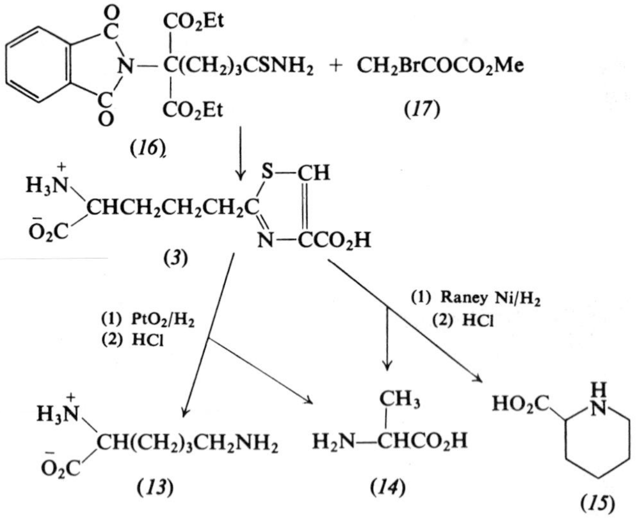

2-(DL-4-Amino-4-carboxybutyl)thiazole-4-carboxylic acid was synthesized by condensation of the thioamide (*16*) with methyl bromopyruvate (*17*) and treatment of the product with 6 N hydrochloric acid at 110°C. The thioamide (*16*) was prepared from the corresponding phthalimidonitrile by heating the latter with liquid hydrogen sulfide at 70°C and was obtained in crystalline form after countercurrent distribution in benzene–methanol–water. The synthetic thiazole was identical with the compound obtained by racemization of the thiazole from cephalosporin C with acetic anhydride (Jeffery *et al.*, 1960).

C. Compounds 1 and 2

When cephalosporin C was heated in 1.25 N hydrochloric acid for 1 hour at 100°C, carbon dioxide was evolved and the ultraviolet absorption maximum shifted from 260 to 237 nm. The products, compounds 1 and 2 (*11* and *12*), were separated on a preparative scale by countercurrent distribution. They could both be detected on paper by their absorption of ultraviolet light and by the fact that they gave an immediate brown color when sprayed with aqueous silver nitrate. The ultraviolet spectrum of compound 1 showed a maximum at 235 nm in water and at 280 nm in 0.05 M sodium hydroxide. That of compound 2 showed a maximum at 243 nm in water and a broad band between 240 and 330 nm in 0.05 M sodium hydroxide.

Analytical data suggested that the molecular formula for compound 1 was $C_{10}H_{10}O_6S$ and the formula for compound 2 was $C_{10}H_{10}O_5S_2$. Both compounds contained two weakly acidic groups, and their infrared spectra showed bands at 3.08 and 5.78 μ which could be attributed to the presence of an OH group and an ester or lactone, respectively. Compound 2 was partly converted into compound 1 by treatment with 1.0 N hydrochloric acid, and both yielded α-hydroxy-β-methylbutenolide (9) after treatment with Raney nickel.

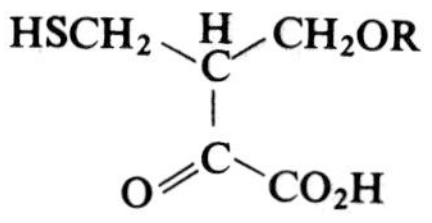

(18)

Since neither showed any C-methyl in a Kuhn–Roth determination but both yielded α-hydroxy-β-methylbutenolide (9) on hydrogenolysis, both compounds could be assigned a structure in which the CH_3 of (9) was replaced by a $-S-CH_2-$ grouping. It was suggested by Abraham and Newton (1961) that these compounds might be formed from the hypothetical intermediate (18) (R = H or $CH_3 \cdot CO$) which is readily derived from cephalosporin C (6). The carboxyl group of (18) could lactonize with either the thiol group or the potential hydroxyl group to give (19) or (20). Condensation of (19) with (20), as shown, would give compound 2 (12). Compound 1 (11) could then be formed by β,γ-elimination of sulfur from the ketone form of the thiolactone ring of (12), followed by elimination of hydrogen sulfide and relactonization.

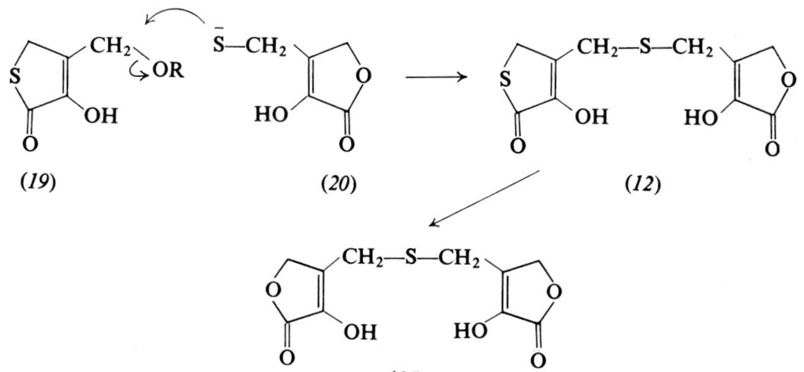

(19)   (20)   (12)

(11)

Synthetic routes to compound 1 start from the Mannich base, β-dimethyl-aminomethyl-α-tetronic acid hydrochloride, first synthesized by Mannich and Bauroth (1924). The free base (*21*) reacted with a sulfhydryl anion in dimethylformamide to yield compound 1 (*11*). The reaction is thought to involve rapid equilibration of the initially formed enolate salt (*22*) with the S anion (*23*) followed by a nucleophilic attack of the latter on the former (Galantay *et al.*, 1964; Long and Turner, 1963).

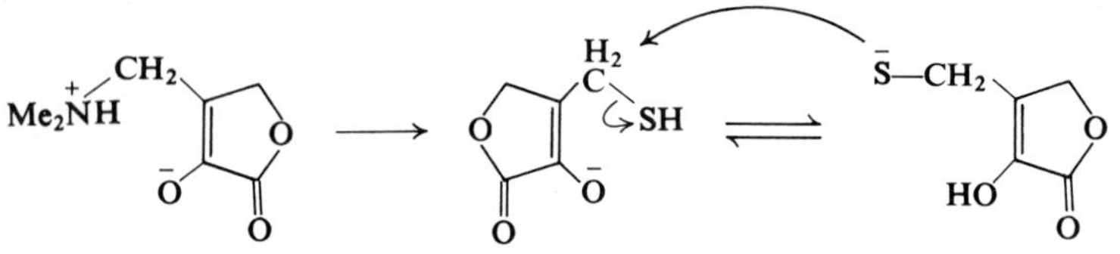

(*21*)   (*22*)   (*23*)

D. α-Amino-β-methylbutenolide

Treatment of cephalosporin C_c (*7*) with Raney nickel produced a substance which was identified as α-amino-β-methylbutènolide (*10*). It migrated as a base when subjected to paper electrophoresis at pH 1.8, gave a weak ninhydrin color and appeared to contain a group which was protonated in the pH range 1–3. Its ultraviolet absorption spectrum, which showed a maximum at 250 nm in water, changed irreversibly to that of α-hydroxy-β-methylbutenolide (*9*) on keeping in 1.0 N hydrochloric acid at 100° for 30 minutes. Hydrogenation with Adams catalyst after the treatment with Raney nickel led to the formation of γ-hydroxyvaline lactone (*24*) (Abraham and Newton, 1961).

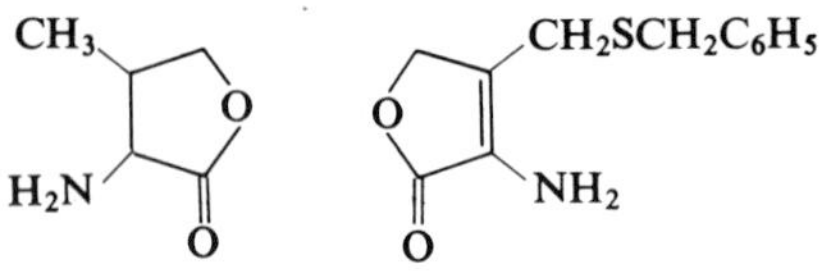

(*24*)   (*25*)

The synthetic route to (*10*) also starts from the Mannich base (*21*) which reacts with toluene-ω-thiol to give β-benzylthiolmethyl-α-tetronic acid. Fusion of the latter with ammonium acetate produced the enamine (*25*), which on treatment with Raney nickel gave α-amino-β-methylbutenolide (*10*) (Barrett *et al.*, 1964).

E. Cephalosporidine

In boiling aqueous solution cephalosporin C yielded a degradation product which was also formed from penicillin N and was given the trivial name cephalosporidine. This optically active product ($C_8H_{10}N_2O_2$) had two ionizable groups with pK_a values of <2.2 and 8.1 and gave no color with ninhydrin. It survived unchanged after heating with hot dilute acid or alkali.

Oxidation with bromine water yielded α-aminoadipic acid and δ-(α-aminoadipyl)glycine (4), showing that the carbon–nitrogen skeleton of α-aminoadipic acid was linked through a second nitrogen to a C_2 fragment. Consideration of these properties, together with its ultraviolet spectrum which showed a maximum of 211 nm in water, suggested that the structure of cephalosporidine (26) consisted of a fused imidazole piperidine-2-carboxylic acid ring system (Abraham and Trown, 1963). Subsequently, it was shown that the nuclear magnetic resonance spectrum of cephalosporidine could be interpreted satisfactorily in terms of (26) (Bishop and Richards, 1963).

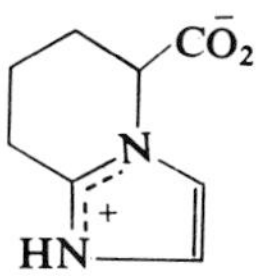

(26)

Structure (26) indicated that cephalosporidine was formed from the δ-(D-α-aminoadipyl)aminoacetaldehyde fragment of cephalosporin C and penicillin N by intramolecular condensation. The DL form of the compound was synthesized by heating DL-δ-(α-aminoadipyl)aminoacetaldehyde diethylacetal at 100° in aqueous acetic acid. The product was found to be identical with the compound formed by racemization of cephalosporidine at 190° (Abraham and Trown, 1963).

V. Derivatives of Cephalosporin C

A. Cephalosporin C_A Compounds

Displacement of the acetoxy group of cephalosporin C by nucleophiles occurs with surprising facility. During the purification of cephalosporin C in pyridine acetate buffer a second substance was encountered which showed antibacterial activity and had no net charge at pH 7. This compound proved to be a pyridinium betaine [(27) $R = C_5H_5\overset{+}{N}$] and was given the trivial name cephalosporin C_A (pyridine) (Hale et al., 1961). Cephalosporin C reacted in a similar fashion with a variety of heterocyclic weak bases and the resulting family of compounds was named the cephalosporin C_A family. Evidence for the quaternary nature of these compounds was provided by their electrophoretic mobility and by the characteristic change in the ultraviolet absorption spectrum of the nicotinamide derivative, resulting in the appearance of a band with λ_{max} 356 nm, when this derivative was reduced with sodium dithionite.

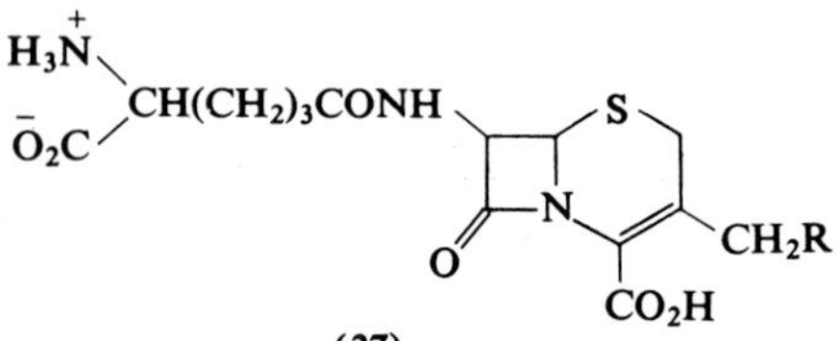

(27)

The antibacterial activity of members of the cephalosporin C_A family varies with the base from which they are formed. Cephalosporin C_A (pyridine) is at least 12 times as active as cephalosporin C against *S. aureus* but somewhat less than twice as active against *Salmonella typhi*.

With sodium thiosulphate cephalosporin C yielded a Bunte salt [(27) $R = S_2O_3Na$] (Demain, 1963).

B. Deacetylcephalosporin C and Its Lactone

Treatment of cephalosporin C with an acetyl esterase prepared from orange peel resulted in hydrolysis of the *O*-acetyl group (Jeffery *et al.*, 1961). The resulting deacetylcephalosporin C (27, R = OH), which was isolated as a crystalline sodium salt with λ_{max} 257 nm, showed a lower R_f value than cephalosporin C on paper in butan-1-ol:acetic acid:water and in propan-1-ol:water. It showed about 20% of the activity of cephalosporin C against *Staphylococcus aureus* and *Salmonella typhi*. Deacetylcephalosporin C lactone (cephalosporin C_c) was formed rapidly from deacetylcephalosporin C at pH values lower than ·1.0. The lactone (7) crystallized with 1 mole of acetic acid and showed λ_{max} 257 nm (Abraham and Newton, 1961).

C. Deacetoxycephalosporin C

Abraham and Newton (1956b) found that hydrogenation of cephalosporin C, with palladium–charcoal as catalyst, resulted in the uptake of almost 1 mole of hydrogen. The product, which still showed the absorption maximum at 260 nm associated with the β-lactam-dihydrothiazine ring system but had only 10% of the antibacterial activity of the parent compound, was not characterized. Later, it was shown that hydrogenation of cephalosporin C in the presence of a large amount of palladium catalyst leads to the formation of deacetoxycephalosporin C [(27) R = H] as a result of hydrogenolysis of the allylic acetoxy group (Morin *et al.*, 1963; Stedman *et al.*, 1964).

D. S-Oxide of Cephalosporin C

Oxidation of cephalosporin C with performic acid at $-6°C$ yielded a product with λ_{max} 258 nm which appeared to be the corresponding sulfoxide (Abraham and Newton, 1961). This compound showed an activity against *Staphylococcus aureus* which was about 10% of that of cephalosporin C.

E. N-Benzoyl and 2,4-Dinitrophenyl Derivatives of Cephalosporin C

The *N*-benzoyl derivative of cephalosporin C was prepared by a Schotten–Baumann reaction with benzoyl chloride in aqueous sodium bicarbonate. The dinitrophenyl derivative was prepared by treatment of cephalosporin C with 1-fluoro-2,4-dinitrobenzene in a solution of sodium bicarbonate in aqueous ethanol (Abraham and Newton, 1956b). Both derivatives are more active against *S. aureus* and considerably less active against *Salmonella typhi* than cephalosporin C itself.

VI. Other Metabolic Products of *Cephalosporium* sp.

A. Penicillin N (Cephalosporin N)

1. PRODUCTION AND ISOLATION

The production of penicillin N by *Cephalosporium* C.M.I. 49,137 was carried out in deep culture with high aeration in a medium containing sucrose, corn-steep liquor, and ammonium acetate (Florey *et al.*, 1956). In studies with *E. salmosynnematum* a production medium containing maize and soya bean meal, ammonium sulphate, and calcium carbonate was used (Olson *et al.*, 1954), and also chemically defined media (Bhuyan and Johnson, 1958; Harvey and Olson, 1958). With both organisms the yield of penicillin N was increased by addition to the medium of methionine, particularly the D isomer (Miller *et al.*, 1956; Kavanagh *et al.*, 1958). However, it was reported that methionine did not enhance penicillin N production by two other species of *Emericellopsis*.

One process of purification of penicillin N involved adsorption of the antibiotic on charcoal at pH 6 and elution with 80% aqueous acetone, followed by adsorption on a column of acid-washed alumina in 80% acetone and elution with 20% acetone. After subsequent countercurrent distribution at pH 6 in a mixture of carbon tetrachloride, phenol, and water containing collidine sulfate as a buffer and carrier, the antibiotic was obtained as a barium salt which was about 80% pure (Abraham et al., 1954). Other processes involved adsorption on and elution from charcoal (Olson et al., 1954) and ion-exchange chromatography (Clark et al., 1956–57).

Later, chromatography in 70% isopropanol on cellulose powder yielded a product whose N-acetyl derivative was isolated as a crystalline N,N-dibenzylethylenediamine salt (Fusari and Machamer, 1957–58).

2. Chemical Structure

Elemental analysis of a purified barium salt of penicillin N indicated that it could have the molecular formula $C_{14}H_{21}O_6N_3S$ (Newton and Abraham, 1954), and this was later confirmed by analysis of the crystalline dibenzylethylenediamine salt of its N-acetyl derivative (Fusari and Machamer, 1957–58). The formation of D-α-aminoadipic acid, penicillamine (D-$\beta\beta$-dimethylcysteine), and CO_2 on acid hydrolysis suggested that the substance was a penicillin with a D-α-aminoadipyl side chain. The fact that the substance titrated as a monoaminodicarboxylic acid with an ionizable group of pK_a 9.8 and that δ-(D-α-aminoadipyl)glycine (4) was obtained on oxidation of the neutral fraction of an acid hydrolyzate with silver oxide showed that the α-aminoadipyl side chain was linked to the nucleus through its δ-carboxyl group. These findings indicated that penicillin N had the structure (1) (Newton and Abraham, 1954).

This structure was confirmed by the isomerization of penicillin N to a penillic acid (28), with λ_{max} 240 nm, in aqueous solution at pH 3.0 and the conversion of the latter by treatment with mercuric chloride to a penillamine (29) which was isolated as a crystalline S-benzyl derivative (Newton and Abraham, 1954). When heated in aqueous solution penicillin N, like cephalosporin C, yielded cephalosporidine (26) from its potential δ-(α-aminoadipyl)aminoacetaldehyde fragment.

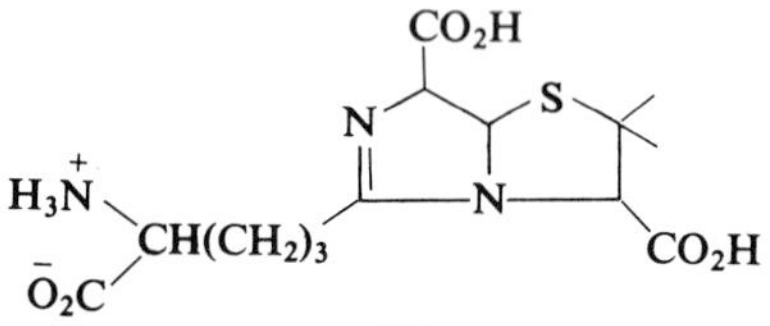

(28) 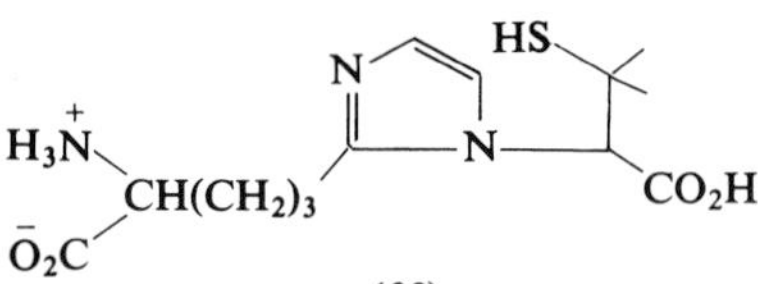   (29)

3. Derivatives

Reaction of penicillin N with 1,2,4-fluorodinitrobenzene, benzoyl chloride, benzyloxycarbonyl chloride, phenylisocyanate, and acetic anhydride, respectively, yielded derivatives which no longer contained the free amino group of the α-aminoadipyl side chain of the parent compound. In contrast to penicillin

N itself, which showed similar activity against *Staphylococcus aureus* and *Salmonella typhi*, the 2,4-dinitrophenyl derivative showed an activity against the latter organism which was only 0.1 % of that against the former. Changes in relative antibacterial activity which were qualitatively similar were found in the other cases although they became progressively smaller with the *N*-benzoyl, *N*-benzyloxycarbonyl, phenylthiocarbamyl, and *N*-acetyl derivatives respectively (Newton and Abraham, 1954).

B. Cephalosporin P

1. PRODUCTION AND ISOLATION

Cephalosporin P was obtained from deep aerated cultures of *Cephalosporium* sp. C.M.I. 49,137 in a medium containing corn steep liquor and glucose (Crawford *et al.*, 1952). It was extracted from the culture filtrate, at pH 6.5, with butyl acetate and purified by countercurrent distribution between solvents and by chromatography (Burton and Abraham, 1951). The active material was found to consist of one major component (P_1) and at least four minor components (P_2 to P_5). Although cephalosporins P_1, P_2, and P_4 were isolated in crystalline form, only P_1 was obtained in amounts sufficient for further study.

2. CHEMICAL STRUCTURE

Burton *et al.* (1956) obtained evidence that cephalosporin P_1 was a monocarboxylic acid containing two acetoxyl groups, two hydroxyl groups, one easily reducible double bond, and one double bond conjugated with the carboxyl group. They suggested that the substance was tetracyclic and related to the steroid group. Further work by Baird *et al.* (1961), who used nuclear magnetic resonance spectra and optical rotatory dispersion measurements in the study of degradation products, led to the proposal of a structure containing the steroid skeleton. This structure needed modification when a mass spectrum showed that the molecular formula was $C_{33}H_{50}O_8$ and not $C_{32}H_{48}O_8$ as had previously been supposed (Lynch *et al.*, 1963). The additional methyl group was shown by an NMR spectrum to be tertiary (Melera, 1963). Further studies indicated that cephalosporin P_1 has the structure (*30*) (Halsall *et al.*, 1966; Oxley, 1966; Chou *et al.*, 1969).

Cephalosporin P_1 is structurally related to helvolic acid, produced by *Aspergillus fumigatus* (Chain *et al.*, 1943; Burton and Abraham, 1951), and to fusidic acid, produced by *Fusidium coccineum* (Godtfredsen *et al.*, 1965) and also by certain strains of *Cephalosporium* and by *Mucor ramannianus* (Vanderhaeghe *et al.*, 1965). All three antibiotics belong to a new group of tetracyclic triterpenes (Okuda *et al.*, 1964; Godtfredsen, 1967).

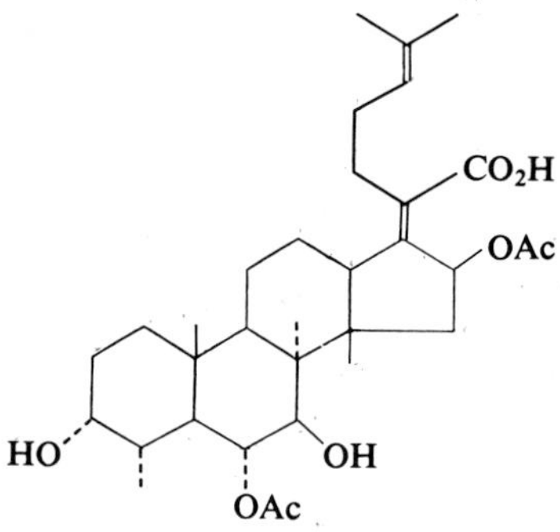

(30)

3. ANTIMICROBIAL PROPERTIES

Cephalosporin P_1 inhibits the growth of staphylococci, corynebacteria, and certain clostridia in high dilutions (Ritchie *et al.*, 1951; Godtfredsen, 1967) but differs from penicillin N and cephalosporin C in showing a relatively low activity against streptococci and no significant activity against gram-negative bacilli.

References

Abraham, E. P. (1957). "Biochemistry of Some Peptide and Steroid Antibiotics," p. 61. Wiley, New York.
Abraham, E. P. (1962). *Pharmacol. Rev.* **14**, 473.
Abraham, E. P., and Newton, G. G. F. (1954). *Biochem. J.* **58**, 266.
Abraham, E. P., and Newton, G. G. F. (1956a). *Biochem. J.* **63**, 628.
Abraham, E. P., and Newton, G. G. F. (1956b). *Biochem. J.* **62**, 658.
Abraham, E. P., and Newton, G. G. F. (1959). Brit. Patent 810196.
Abraham, E. P., and Newton, G. G. F. (1961). *Biochem. J.* **79**, 377.
Abraham, E. P., and Trown, P. W. (1963). *Biochem. J.* **86**, 271.
Abraham, E. P., Newton, G. G. F., Crawford, K., Burton, H. S., and Hale, C. W. (1953). *Nature* **171**, 343.
Abraham, E. P., Newton, G. G. F., and Hale, C. W. (1954). *Biochem. J.* **58**, 94.
Abraham, E. P., Newton, G. G. F., Schenck, J. R., Hargie, M. P., Olson, B. H., Schuurmans, D. M., Fisher, M. W., and Fusari, S. A. (1955). *Nature* **176**, 551.
Abraham, E. P., Newton, G. G. F., and Trown, P. W. (1966). Brit. Patent 1,036,125.
Baird, B. M., Halsall, T. G., Jones, E. R. H., and Lowe, G. (1961). *Proc. Chem. Soc.* 257.
Barrett, G. C., Eggers, S. H., Emerson, T. R., and Lowe, G. (1964). *J. Chem. Soc.* 788.
Batchelor, F. R., Doyle, F. P., Nayler, J. H. C., and Rolinson, G. N. (1959). *Nature* **183**, 257.
Bhuyan, B. K., and Johnson, M. J. (1958). *J. Bacteriol.* **76**, 376.
Bishop, E. O., and Richards, R. E. (1963). *Biochem. J.* **86**, 277.
Brookes, P., Fuller, A. T., and Walker, J. (1957). *J. Chem. Soc.* 689.
Brotzu, G. (1948). Lavori dell'istituto D'Igiene di Cagliari.
Burton, H. S., and Abraham, E. P. (1951). *Biochem. J.* **50**, 168.
Burton, H. S., Abraham, E. P., and Cardwell, H. M. E. (1956). *Biochem. J.* **62**, 171.

Chain, E., Florey, H. W., Jennings, M. A., and Williams, T. I. (1943). *Brit. J. Exp. Pathol.* **24**, 108.

Chou, T. S., Eisenbraun, E. J., and Rapala, R. T. (1969). *Tetrahedron* **25**, 3341.

Clark, R. K., Jr., Fricke, H. H., and Lanius, B. (1956–57). *In* "Antibiotics Annual" (H. Welch and F. Marti-Ibanez, eds.), p. 749. Medical Encyclopedia, New York.

Crawford, K., Heatley, N. G., Boyd, P. F., Hale, C. W., Kelly, B. K., Miller, G. A., and Smith, N. (1952). *J. Gen. Microbiol.* **6**, 47.

Demain, A. L. (1963). *Trans. N.Y. Acad. Sci.* **25**, 731.

Douthwaite, A. H., and Trafford, J. A. P. (1960). *Brit. Med. J.* 687.

Elander, R. P., Stauffer, J. F., and Backus, M. P. (1960). *In* "Antimicrobial Agents Annual" (P. Gray, B. Tabenkin, and S. G. Bradley, eds.), p. 91. Plenum Press, New York.

Florey, H. W. (1955). *Ann. Int. Med.* **43**, 480.

Florey, H. W. (1956). *Giorn. Microbiol.* **2**, 361.

Florey, H. W., Abraham, E. P., Newton, G. G. F., Burton, H. S., Kelly, B. K., Hale, C. W., and Miller, G. A. (1956). Brit. Patent 745208.

Fusari, S. A., and Machamer, H. E. (1957–58). *In* "Antibiotics Annual" (H. Welch and F. Marti-Ibanez, eds.), p. 529. Medical Encyclopedia, New York.

Galantay, E., Engel, H., Szabo, A., and Fried, J. (1964). *J. Org. Chem.* **29**, 3560.

Gams, W. (1971). "Cephalosporium-artige Schimmelpilze-Hyphomycetes." Gustav Fischer Verlag, Stuttgart.

Godtfredsen, W. O. (1967). "Fusidic Acid and Some Related Antibiotics." Doctoral dissertation, University of Copenhagen.

Godtfredsen, W. O., von Daehne, W., Vangedal, S., Arigoni, D., Marquet, A., and Melera, A. (1965). *Tetrahedron* **21**, 3505.

Gottshall, R. Y., Roberts, J. M., Portwood, L. M., and Jennings, J. C. (1951). *Proc. Soc. Exp. Biol. Med.* **76**, 307.

Grosklags, J. H., and Swift, M. E. (1957). *Mycologia* **49**, 305.

Hale, C. W., Newton, G. G. F., and Abraham, E. P. (1961). *Biochem. J.* **79**, 403.

Halsall, T. G., Jones, E. R. H., Lowe, G., and Newall, C. E. (1966). *Chem. Commun.* 685.

Harvey, C. L., and Olson, B. H. (1958). *Appl. Microbiol.* **6**, 276.

Hodgkin, D. C., and Maslen, E. N. (1961). *Biochem. J.* **79**, 393.

Jeffery, J. D'A., Abraham, E. P., and Newton, G. G. F. (1960). *Biochem. J.* **75**, 216.

Jeffery, J. D'A., Abraham, E. P., and Newton, G. G. F. (1961). *Biochem. J.* **81**, 591.

Kato, K. (1953). *J. Antibiot.* **A6**, 130, 184.

Kavanagh, F., Tunin, D., and Wild, G. (1958). *Mycologia* **50**, 370.

Loder, P. B., Newton, G. G. F., and Abraham, E. P. (1961). *Biochem. J.* **79**, 408.

Long, A. G., and Turner, A. F. (1963). *Tetrahedron Lett.* 421.

Lynch, J. F., Wilson, J. M., Budzikiewicz, H., and Djerassi, C. (1963). *Experientia* **19**, 213.

Mangallam, S., Menon, M. R., Sukapure, R. S., and Gopalkrishnan, K. S. (1968). *Hindustan Antibiot. Bull.* **10**, 194.

Mannich, C., and Bauroth, M. (1924). *Chem. Ber.* **24**, 1108.

Melera, A. (1963). *Experientia* **19**, 565.

Miller, G. A., Kelly, B. K., and Newton, G. G. F. (1956). Brit. Patent 759624.

Miller, G. A., Stapley, E. O., and Chaiet, L. (1962). *Bacteriol. Proc.* **49**, 32.

Morin, R. B., Jackson, B. G., Flynn, E. H., and Roeske, R. W. (1962). *J. Amer. Chem. Soc.* **84**, 3400.

Morin, R. B., Jackson, B. G., Mueller, R. A., Lavagnino, E. R., Scanlon, W. B., and Andrews, S. L. (1963). *J. Amer. Chem. Soc.* **85**, 1896.

Newton, G. G. F., and Abraham, E. P. (1954). *Biochem. J.* **58**, 103.

Newton, G. G. F., and Abraham, E. P. (1955). *Nature* **175**, 548.

Newton, G. G. F., and Abraham, E. P. (1956). *Biochem. J.* **62**, 651.

Okuda, S., Iwasaki, S., Tsuda, K., Sano, Y., Hata, T., Udagawa, S., Nakayama, Y., and Yamaguchi, H. (1964). *Chem. Pharm. Bull.* **12**, 121.

Olson, B. H., Jennings, J. C., and Junek, A. J. (1953). *Science* **117**, 76.

Olson, B. H., Jennings, J. C., Pisano, M., and Junek, A. J. (1954). *Antibiot. Chemother.* **4**, 1.

Oxley, P. (1966). *Chem. Commun.* 729.

Pisano, M. A. (1970). *Antonie van Leeuwenhoek J. Microbiol. Serol.* **36**, 445.

Pisano, M. A., Fleischman, A. I., Littman, M. L., Dutcher, J. D., and Pansy, F. E. (1960). *In* "Antimicrobial Agents Annual" (P. Gray, B. Tabenkin, and S. G. Bradley, eds.), p.41. Plenum Press, New York.

Pollock, M. R. (1957). *Biochem. J.* **66**, 419.

Ritchie, A. C., Smith, N., and Florey, H. W. (1951). *Brit. J. Pharmacol.* **6**, 430.

Roberts, J. M. (1952). *Mycologia* **44**, 292.

Rolinson, G. N., Stevens, S., Batchelor, F. R., Cameron-Wood, J., and Chain, E. B. (1960). *Lancet* **ii**, 564.

Sakaguchi, K., and Murao, S. (1950). *J. Agr. Chem. Soc. Japan* **23**, 411.

Sheehan, J. C. (1958). *In* "Amino Acids and Peptides with Antimetabolic Activity" (G. E. W. Wolstenholme and C. M. O'Connor, eds.), Ciba Foundation Symposium, p. 258. Churchill, London.

Stedman, R. J., Swered, K., and Hoover, J. R. E. (1964). *J. Med. Chem.* **7**, 117.

Sukapure, R. S., Deshmukh, P. V., Bringi, N. V., and Thirumalachar, M. J. (1965). *Hindustan Antibiot. Bull.* **8**, 15.

Vanderhaeghe, H., Van Dijck, P., and De Somer, P. (1965). *Nature* **205**, 710.

Waksman, S. A., and Horning, E. S. (1943). *Mycologia* **35**, 47.

Chapter 2

PREPARATIVE METHODS FOR

7-AMINOCEPHALOSPORANIC ACID

AND 6-AMINOPENICILLANIC ACID

FLOYD M. HUBER, ROBERT R. CHAUVETTE,
and BILL G. JACKSON

General Remarks

Prior to determination of the structure of cephalosporin C, studies of structure–activity relationships (Behrens *et al.*, 1948) among the penicillins had shown that biological effectiveness depended to a good extent upon the nature of the acyl moiety attached to the C-6 amino function. Penicillin N (also known as cephalosporin N and synnematin B) was shown (Newton and Abraham, 1954) to have structure (*1*). Knowing the structure of penicillin N

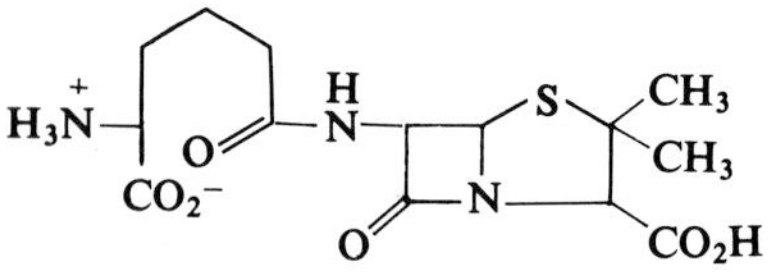

(*1*)

and comparing with the structure of cephalosporin C (Abraham and Newton, 1961; Hodgkin and Maslen, 1961) indicated the potential importance of alteration of the acyl substituent on the C-7 amino group in the cephalosporin case. Loder *et al.* (1961) obtained evidence that this was important in terms of affecting antibacterial activity. The history of these events together with appropriate references are given in Chapter 1. Detailed comments on relative activities of the compounds involved may be found in Chapter 12, together with observations on other differences between the penicillin and cephalosporin compounds. Chapter 10 also contains information substantiating the need for methods of altering the acyl substituent.

Two properties of cephalosporin C made structural modification of the antibiotic especially attractive. These were its acid stability (compared to penicillin) and its resistance to penicillinase, an enzyme produced by certain strains of microorganisms, which destroys the antibiotic activity of penicillins.

Among the first structural modifications investigated was replacement of the aminoadipyl side chain by other acyl radicals. As a prerequisite for acyl modification, methods of removing the amidoadipyl radical were investigated. This chapter summarizes the microbiological and chemical methods which have been attempted or employed to selectively cleave the side chain amide from cephalosporin C (*2*) and other cephalosporanic acids, giving rise to 7-aminocephalosporanic acid (7-ACA) (*3*) and derivatives. Also, the cleavage of penicillins to 6-aminopenicillanic acid is summarized since penicillins have been converted to cephalosporins.

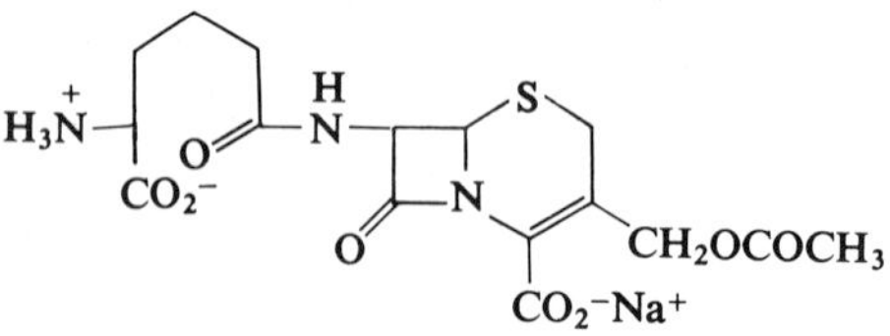

(*2*) 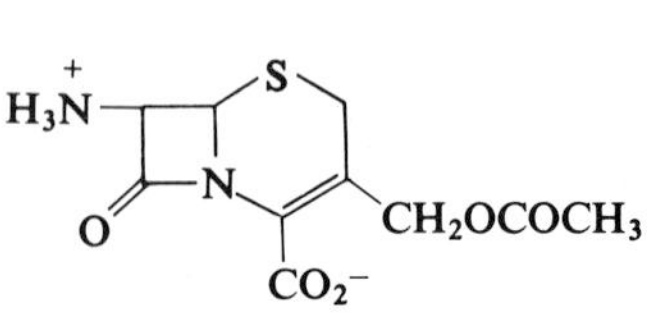   (*3*)

I. Biological Methods*

A. Introduction

Two decades have passed since Sakaguchi and Murao (1950) reported the microbial conversion of benzylpenicillin to phenylacetic acid and a substance described as "Penicin." The characteristics of the latter compound were reported 5 years later by Murao (1955). During the 1950's numerous investigators attempted to reproduce the work reported by Sakaguchi and Murao, but all were unsuccessful. In 1959, Batchelor et al. (1959) reported that a substance, 6-aminopenicillanic acid (6-APA), was produced in *Penicillium chrysogenum* fermentations devoid of side chain precursor. This finding identified the end product of the reaction described by Sakaguchi and Murao as 6-APA, and in 1961 their original observations were confirmed (Murao and Kishida, 1961; Erickson and Bennett, 1961).

Since the original reaction was discovered, its utility has been demonstrated by the many semisynthetic penicillins with excellent therapeutic value. Had it not been that 6-APA was readily available, many of these compounds would not have been synthesized. Doyle and Nayler (1965) have reviewed the uses of the penicillin nucleus. The reaction and its measurement have been reviewed by Hamilton-Miller et al. (1963) and Hamilton-Miller (1966).

The object of this report is to summarize the knowledge of the enzymatic cleavage of both the penicillins and cephalosporins. This summary should aid other investigators in preparing the ring systems of these two important families of antibiotics. Because the nomenclature associated with the catalyst for this reaction has been clouded by its multiple functionality (Spencer and Maung, 1970), the enzyme will be termed acylase for the reasons described in Chapter 9. Because the reversibility of this reaction and its biosynthetic implications will be covered in Chapter 9, little reference will be made to this property in this section.

B. Isolation and Distribution of Microorganisms which Produce Acylase Activity

Although acylase-producing microorganisms may be isolated by conventional techniques, Kameda et al. (1961) reported a medium for selecting microorganisms with acylase activity. This medium contained benzylpenicillin as a sole carbon source and inorganic salts. The exact cultural conditions have been reported to be important in determining if an organism possesses acylase

* Section by Floyd M. Huber, Antibiotic Development Department.

activity. Cole and Sutherland (1966) cultured 148 strains of bacteria at 37°C and observed only one with acylase activity. Subsequently, the strains were cultured at 26°C in another medium containing phenylacetic acid, and 10 were observed with acylase activity. In attempting to detect acylase activity in microorganisms, Batchelor et al. (1961) used a mixture of natural penicillins as a substrate. These investigators found that of the 160 fungi, 30 yeasts, and 25 actinomycetes they examined, 24, 3, and 11, respectively, were observed with acylase activity. Of the 310 strains of Escherichia coli that Holt and Stewart (1964a) tested, 125 were found with acylase activity. English et al. (1960) have reported acylase activity for Aerobacter aerogenes, Proteus vulgaris, Pseudomonas aeruginosa, and P. phaseolicola. Although Holt and Stewart (1964a) reported no activity in numerous gram-positive organisms, Claridge et al. (1960) and Chiang and Bennett (1967) have observed acylase activity in this general class of microorganisms. Acylase activity has been reported by Cole (1966) to be present also in fungi of the genera Aspergillus, Cephalosporium, Epidermophyton, Penicillium, and Trichophyton. Acylase activity is not restricted to microorganisms since Cole (1964) reported that pig kidney acylase I hydrolyzed phenoxymethylpenicillin.

C. Production of Acylase Activity

Because organisms require specific nutrients and unique environmental conditions for enzyme production, only a few selected cases will be discussed. Vigorous aeration and a pH range 6.5–8.5 were required for good acylase activity when E. coli was grown in an inorganic salts medium plus either yeast extract and amino acids or peptides (Kaufmann and Bauer, 1964a). Acylase activity was found to be greatest when the cells were grown at 24°C, and very little activity was observed at 37°C. The addition of phenylacetic acid to the growth medium increased acylase titers. Similarly, Szentirmai (1964) reported that E. coli acylase production was increased when either phenoxyacetic acid, 2,4-dimethoxyphenylacetic acid, or p-methoxyphenylacetic acid was added to the growth medium. The same author reported that readily metabolizable substances such as glucose, fructose, and glycerol repressed acylase activity and that this repression decreased with decreased temperatures of incubation. Similarly, the acylase activity of fungal cultures has been reported to be stimulated by the side chain precursors of the penicillins they hydrolyze. In this respect, Cole (1966) and Uri et al. (1964) demonstrated that the addition of phenoxyacetic acid to fungal cultures increased acylase titers. However, the addition of benzylpenicillin, phenoxymethylpenicillin, or their degradation products had no effect on the production of acylase (Uri et al., 1964).

The production of acylase during the growth of E. coli has been examined by Nyiri (1967). When benzylpenicillin was used as the substrate, only slight activity was observed in the lag phase of growth. The greatest activity was observed during the log phase, and this decreased to almost zero in the decline phase. A direct correlation was also observed between the deacylation of benzylpenicillin and phenylacetylglycine during the growth of the acylase-producing organism.

D. Location of Acylase in Culture Fluids

Prior to the isolation of an enzymatic activity, it is essential to describe its intra- or extracellular location. The acylase activity of *Nocardia* FD4997 and *Proteus rettgeri* (Huang *et al.*, 1963) and *Alcaligenes faecalis* (Claridge *et al.*, 1960) has been reported to be associated with the cellular materials of the culture. In contrast, Batchelor *et al.* (1961) and Chiang and Bennett (1967) reported that the enzyme was mainly found in culture broths of *Streptomyces lavendulae* and *Bacillus megaterium*.

E. Preparation and Properties of Acylase Activity

The most complex preparation to understand is the whole cell system. As representatives of this system, mycelial mats of *Penicillium chrysogenum* and *Aspergillus flavus* have been reported to convert benzylpenicillin to 6-APA and phenylacetic acid (Shimi and Imam, 1966). Singh *et al.* (1969) demonstrated the conversion of phenoxymethylpenicillin to 6-APA by spores of *Fusarium moniliforme*. After the reaction was terminated, the spores were removed from the reaction mixture by centrifugation and could be reused three or four times without significant loss of activity. Similarly, Claridge *et al.* (1960) demonstrated that the cells of *Alcaligenes faecalis*, used for the conversion of benzylpenicillin to 6-APA, could be reused five times. The separation of bacteria from the reaction mixture has been reported to be facilitated by the addition of a quaternary ammonium halide (U.S. Patent 3,278,391). A modification of the whole-cell system includes the use of freeze-dried cells. Such cells of *Nocardia* FD46973, when suspended in phosphate buffer, pH 7.5, and incubated for 16 hours at 28°C converted benzylpenicillin to 6-APA in 80% of theoretical yield.

Procedures have been reported for the hydrolysis of penicillins by simple enzyme preparations. Vanderhaeghe *et al.* (1968) reported that acylase activity of *P. chrysogenum* could be extracted by shaking mycelium in 0.2 *M* sodium chloride. The same authors reported that the acylase activity of *F. avenaceum* could be extracted from freeze-dried cells by 0.2 *M* sodium citrate. The exo-enzyme of *S. lavendulae* has been prepared by ammonium sulfate precipitation, dialysis, and lyophilization (Batchelor *et al.*, 1961). A similar approach was used by Holt and Stewart (1964b) in that the acylase of *E. coli* was purified by cellulose acetate filtration, lyophilization, dialysis, and lyophilization. This preparation was reported to contain 53% protein, 3.7% lipid, and 9.4% ash. The acylase was reported not to be inhibited by *p*-chloromercuriphenylsulfonic acid, a compound known to interact with sulfhydryl groups. A United States patent (U.S. Patent 3,297,546) reported the precipitation of the acylase in *E. coli* broth by the addition of a metal compound (i.e., calcium nitrate) and a quaternary ammonium salt. The acylase from several microbial cultures has also been reported to be prepared by more elegant techniques. Spencer and Maung (1970) reported that the acylase of *P. chrysogenum* could be purified 130-fold by disrupting the cells with a French press and precipitating the activity with ammonium sulfate. The precipitate was then chromatographed on Sephadex G100 and DEAE cellulose. Waldschmidt-Leitz and Bretzel (1964) reported a 300-fold purification of the *F. semitectum* acylase. This degree of purity was accomplished by separations with DEAE cellulose, Sephadex G25, acetone precipitation, Amberlite IRC 50, and Sephadex G25 in sequence. The enzyme had a molecular weight of 65,000 and contained 16.7% nitrogen and two molecules of zinc per molecule of acylase. Chiang and Bennett (1967) obtained a 96-fold purification of the enzyme of *B. megaterium* by sequential chromatography on celite, carboxymethylcellulose, and celite. The resulting material appeared as single component in an ultracentrifugal field and had a molecular weight of 120,000. The cleavage of benzylpenicillin by this enzyme was inhibited by the end products of the reaction (6-APA and phenylacetic acid). The activity was not inhibited by *p*-chloromercuribenzoate, *o*-iodobenzoate, and iodoacetate.

Various investigators have adsorbed or bound acylases to insoluble substances. Adsorption of the acylase of various microorganisms on bentonite and slurries of this substance with penicillin solutions gave 6-APA (U.S. Patent 3,446,705). Self *et al.* (1969) prepared the chloro-*s*-triazine derivative of DEAE cellulose and bound a purified acylase to it. These authors placed this preparation in a column, and when penicillins were percolated through it, 6-APA plus side chain were obtained in the eluate. No loss in the activity of this reactor was observed during an 11-week period.

F. Specificity of Acylase Preparations

Of the many penicillins that have been cleaved, some controversy surrounds the report by Walton (1964a) on the hydrolysis of penicillin N. This investigator claimed that the cleavage was accomplished with an *Achromobacter* species designated MB-1375. A report by Sjöberg *et al.* (1967) indicated that *E. coli* cleaved penicillin N to 6-APA and that the rate of the reaction was approximately 4 % of the rate observed when benzylpenicillin was the substrate. However, these authors noted that low-purity penicillin N was used in their experimentation and that the observed activity might have been associated with an impurity. Other investigators such as Huang et al. (1963), Cole and Rolinson (1961), and Claridge et al. (1963) have tested other bacterial and fungal systems and found none to cleave penicillin N to 6-APA. In addition to reporting the inability of several fungal systems to cleave penicillin N, Vanderhaeghe et al. (1968) reported that isopenicillin N was also not hydrolyzed.

The cleavage of various penicillins by different enzyme sources is summarized in Tables I–III. As will be further discussed in Chapter 9, the enzymes of bacterial origin hydrolyze benzylpenicillin to 6-APA much more rapidly than phenoxymethylpenicillin. The converse is true for enzymes of fungal origin. With respect to the former case, Huang et al. (1963) reported that any deviation from the benzyl side chain decreased the rates of hydrolysis of penicillins by Nocardia and Proteus rettgeri. These two organisms hydrolyzed the following compounds in decreasing order: benzylpenicillin, p-nitrobenzylpenicillin, p-hydroxybenzylpenicillin, o,p-dihydroxybenzylpenicillin, α,α-dimethylbenzylpenicillin, phenoxymethylpenicillin, and phenylmercaptomethylpenicillin. Only weak activity was observed when aliphatic side chain penicillins were tested as substrates. In a similar study, Cole (1969a) reported that the cleavage of penicillins by E. coli occurred in the decreasing order of p-hydroxybenzylpenicillin, benzylpenicillin, 2-furylmethylpenicillin, DL-α-hydroxybenzylpenicillin, D-α-aminobenzylpenicillin, n-propoxymethylpenicillin, isobutoxymethylpenicillin, phenoxymethylpenicillin, α-phenoxyethylpenicillin, phenylpenicillin, and heptylpenicillin. The same preparation was reported to cleave many amides and esters of benzylpenicillin.

Brandl (1965) compared the acylases isolated from E. coli and F. semitectum. The enzyme from the latter organism was active on phenoxymethylpenicillin, much less active on phenylmercaptomethylpenicillin, and not active on benzylpenicillin. The reverse order of activity was found to be true for the enzyme of E. coli. Claridge et al. (1963) reported that acylases of bacterial origin would not hydrolyze synthetic penicillins containing a carboxyl group on the side chain, but a strain of Penicillium chrysogenum was able to hydrolyze some of the substances. Other examples of the preference of fungal systems for side chains other than phenylacetic acid have been reported by Erickson and Bennett (1965) and Uri et al. (1963).

In general, the Michaelis constant (K_m) for the cleavage of either benzylpenicillin or phenoxymethylpenicillin ranges between 1.5 and 10.0 mM (Tables I and II). An exception to this generalization is the K_m of approximately 30 mM reported for E. coli (Cole, 1969a). Usually the temperature optimum for the acylase reaction ranges between 35° and 50°C, but Cole

Table I

ENZYMATIC HYDROLYSIS OF BENZYLPENICILLIN

Enzyme source	Conditions and comments		References
Aerobacter cloacae	—		Claridge *et al.* (1960)
Alcaligenes faecalis	—		Claridge *et al.* (1960)
Bacillus megaterium enzyme	45°C (opt.), pH 8–9 (opt.)	$K_m = 4.5$ mM	Chiang and Bennett (1967)
Bacillus subtilis var. *niger*	—		Claridge *et al.* (1960)
Emericellopsis minima I.M.I. 69015	—		Cole and Rolinson (1961)
Escherichia coli	35°C (opt.), pH 7 (opt.)	$K_m = 1.5$ mM	Brandl (1965)
Escherichia coli	40°C (opt.), pH 7.5–8.5 (opt.)		Rolinson *et al.* (1960b)
Escherichia coli	37°C, pH 9 (opt.)		Sjoberg *et al.* (1967)
Escherichia coli	40°C (opt.), pH 5.5 (opt.)	$K_m = 4.0$ mM	Holt and Stewart (1964b)
Escherichia coli	55°C (opt.)	$K_m = 30.4$ mM	Cole (1969a)
Escherichia coli (enzyme bound to cellulose)	37°C	$K_m = 7.7$ mM	Self *et al.* (1969)
Micrococcus lysodeikticus	—		Claridge *et al.* (1960)
Micrococcus roseus	35°C (opt.), pH 7 (opt.)		Pruess and Johnson (1965)
Mycobacterium phlei	—		Claridge *et al.* (1960)
Nocardia FD4697	pH 8 (opt.)		Huang *et al.* (1963)
Penicillium chrysogenum	pH 8.5 (opt.)		Erickson and Bennett (1965)
Proteus rettgeri	pH 8 (opt.)		Huang *et al.* (1963)
Streptomyces lavendulae	50°C (opt.), pH 9 (opt.)		Batchelor *et al.* (1961)

Table II

ENZYMATIC HYDROLYSIS OF PHENOXYMETHYLPENICILLIN

Enzyme source	Conditions and comments	References
Achromobacter sp. B.R.L. 1755	—	Cole (1964)
Actinoplanes utahensis	34°C, pH 7.5	U.S. Pat. 3,150,059
Aspergillus ochraceous B.R.L. 731	—	Cole (1966)
Cephalosporium sp. CMI 49137	—	Cole (1966)
Emericellopsis minima	—	Cole and Rolinson (1961)
Epidermophyton floccosum B.R.L. 772	—	Cole (1966)
Epidermophyton interdigitale	37°C (opt.), pH 7.5 (opt.)	Uri *et al.* (1963)
Fusarium avenaceum	28°C, pH 6–8	Vanderhaeghe *et al.* (1968)
Fusarium moniliforme spores	$K_m = 2.7$ mM	Singh *et al.* (1969)
Fusarium semitectum	≈ 50°C (opt.), pH 8 (opt.)	Brandl (1965)
Fusarium semitectum purified enzyme	pH 7.5 (opt.)	Waldschmidt-Leitz and Bretzel (1964)
Nocardia FD46973	28°C, pH 7.5	Huang *et al.* (1960)
Penicillium chrysogenum B.R.L. 781, 803	—	Cole (1966)
Penicillium chrysogenum Wis. 49–408	pH 8.5 (opt.)	Erickson and Bennett (1965)
Penicillium sp. B.R.L. 733, 736, 737	—	Cole (1966)
Pig Kidney acylase I	—	Cole (1964)
Streptomyces lavendulae	50°C (opt.), pH 9 (opt.), $K_m = 10$ mM	Batchelor *et al.* (1961); Rolinson *et al.* (1960b)
Trichophyton gypseum	—	Uri *et al.* (1963)
Trichophyton interdigitale	—	Uri *et al.* (1963)
Trichophyton mentagrophytes	—	Uri *et al.* (1963)

Table III

REPORTS OF PENICILLINS THAT HAVE BEEN ENZYMATICALLY
HYDROLYZED OTHER THAN BENZYLPENICILLIN AND
PHENOXYMETHYLPENICILLIN

Reference	Penicillin
Claridge *et al.* (1963)	Ampicillin
	2-Carboxy,3-decenylpenicillin
	3-Carboxypropylpenicillin
	Methicillin
Cole (1964)	*n*-Heptylpenicillin
	n-Pentylpenicillin
Cole (1969a)	D-α-Aminobenzylpenicillin
	DL-α-Hydroxybenzylpenicillin
	Isobutoxymethylpenicillin
	Phenylpenicillin
	α-Phenoxyethylpenicillin
	n-Propoxymethylpenicillin
	2-Thienylmethylpenicillin
Huang *et al.* (1960)	Allylmercaptomethylpenicillin
Huang *et al.* (1963)	*o,p*-Dihydroxybenzylpenicillin
	α,α-Dimethylbenzylpenicillin
	p-Hydroxybenzylpenicillin
	p-Nitrobenzylpenicillin
	Phenylmercaptomethylpenicillin
U.S. Patent 3,150,059	*p*-Tolyloxymethylpenicillin
Rolinson *et al.* (1960b)	*n*-Amylpenicillin
	n-Heptylpenicillin
Vanderhaeghe *et al.* (1968)	*n*-Nonylpenicillin
	n-Propylpenicillin
	n-Undecylpenicillin

(1969a) reported temperature optima for the cleavage of benzylpenicillin and 2-furylmethylpenicillin by *E. coli* of 55° and 60°C, respectively.

Although most enzyme sources have different pH optima for conversions of penicillins to 6-APA, these range between neutrality and 9.0. The importance of this range was demonstrated by several studies in which the reverse reaction was investigated. The hydrolysis of phenoxymethylpenicillin by preparations of *S. lavendulae* was reported to be best at an alkaline pH and the reverse reaction by the same preparation had an optimum pH of 5.0 (Batchelor *et al.*, 1961). Similar pH optima for the reversibility of the reaction have been recorded by other investigators (Cole, 1969c; Kaufmann *et al.*, 1961). In further studying the reversible reaction, Cole (1969c) reported that numerous acids and amides would substitute for the conventional penicillin precursors.

In 1964, Cole reported that benzylpenicillin was not the best substrate for the acylase reaction of *E. coli* since phenylacetylglycine was hydrolyzed at a much more rapid rate. Later, the same author (1969b) found that the enzyme system was specific for L-α-amino acids. Kaufmann and Bauer (1964b) have also described an enzyme system that cleaved acyl and α-aminoacyl compounds and concluded that it was not 6-APA that was important for the substrate specificity of the enzyme.

G. Cleavage of the Cephalosporins

Of the many investigators that have attempted to enzymatically cleave cephalosporin C to 7-aminocephalosporanic acid (7-ACA), only Walton (1964a) has reported success. This investigator reported that species of *Achromobacter*, *Brevibacterium*, and *Flavobacterium* hydrolyzed cephalosporin C to a substance which appeared to be 7-ACA. *Achromobacter* MB-1375 was reported by the same author to rapidly convert cephalosporin C to deacetyl-cephalosporin C and then slowly hydrolyze the latter compound to deacetyl 7-aminocephalosporanic acid. This reaction took place in phosphate buffer at pH 7.5.

In contrast to the foregoing, Demain *et al.* (1963) examined approximately 200 marine microorganisms, 273 known bacterial species, and 99 actinomycete cultures and found none to cleave cephalosporin C to 7-ACA. In a similar study Nuesch *et al.* (1967) tested many actinomycetes, bacteria, and fungi but could not demonstrate the ability of any culture to hydrolyze cephalosporin C. Other investigators such as Huang *et al.* (1963), Claridge *et al.* (1963), Erickson and Bennett (1965), and Sjöberg *et al.* (1967) have tested many different microbial systems and found all inactive with respect to the cleavage of cephalosporin C. It should be noted that Walton (1964b) also reported that he examined 42 bacterial cultures in the presence or absence of a β-lactamase inhibitor (6-APA) and found no evidence for the cleavage of cephalosporin C. Since others have been unable to repeat the work of Walton (1964a), it must be assumed that either this conversion requires a very special set of circumstances or that his test system produced artifacts which were not resolved. The exact reason for the inability of microbiological systems to cleave cephalosporin C to 7-ACA has yet to be described. It seems significant to suggest that further studies be undertaken to elucidate the mechanisms which form the basis for this inadequacy.

Although cephalosporin C appears not to be cleaved, some derivatives of 7-ACA have been enzymatically hydrolyzed (Table IV). In general, the rates of hydrolysis of 7-ACA derivatives are much slower than their corresponding 6-APA analogs. The matter is further complicated since most assay systems

Table IV

ENZYMATIC HYDROLYSIS OF CEPHALOSPORINS

Substrate	Enzyme source	Conditions and comments	Reference
Benzylcephalosporin	Alcaligenes faecalis MB10	Deacetyl 7-ACA also a product	Walton (1964a)
	Escherichia coli B.R.L. 351	37°C, rate = 70% of hydrolysis of benzylpenicillin	Sjöberg et al. (1967)
N-phenoxyacetyl-7-amino-cephalosporanic acid	Nocardia FD4697 (freeze-dried)	pH 8.0	Huang et al. (1963)
	Proteus rettgeri (freeze-dried)	pH 8.0	Huang et al. (1963)
N-phenylmercapto-7-amino-cephalosporanic acid	Nocardia FD4697 (freeze-dried)	pH 8.0	Huang et al. (1963)
	Proteus rettgeri (freeze-dried)	pH 8.0	Huang et al. (1963)
2-thienylmethylcephalosporin (cephalothin)	Escherichia coli N.C.I.B. 8743A	37°C, pH 8.0, reaction rapid and complete	Cole (1969a)
	Escherichia coli B.R.L. 351	37°C, rate = 58% of hydrolysis of benzylpenicillin	Sjöberg et al. (1967)
2-thienylmethylcephalosporin pyridine (cephaloridine)	Escherichia coli N.C.I.B. 8743A	37°C, pH 7.5, reaction fairly rapid and complete	Cole (1969a)
	Escherichia coli B.R.L. 351	37°C, pH 9.0 (opt.), rate = 87% of hydrolysis of benzylpenicillin	Sjöberg et al. (1967)

employ microbiological measurements and most enzyme preparations contain significant esterase activity. This contaminant leads to erroneous results since the deacetyl substances have less biological activity.

The utility of the enzymatic cleavage of cephalosporins other than cephalosporin C is doubtful since these compounds are all synthesized from 7-ACA derived by a chemical cleavage of the antibiotic. Thus, it would not seem logical to cleave a substance to obtain 7-ACA, when 7-ACA was already available.

II. Chemical Methods*

A. Side Chain Cleavage of Cephalosporin C

Direct acid hydrolysis of cephalosporin C to give 7-ACA should, *a priori*, not be an efficient preparative method since other sites on the molecule would be expected to be sensitive to the relatively nonspecific aqueous acid conditions. The first reported conversion (Loder *et al.*, 1961) of cephalosporin C (*2*) to 7-ACA (*3*) was, nonetheless, effected by mild acid hydrolysis. An aqueous solution of cephalosporin C sodium salt was acidified with Dowex 50 × 8 and then further acidified with dilute hydrochloric acid. After 3 days at 20°, the reaction mixture was subjected to ion-exchange chromatography, from which crude 7-ACA was isolated in a yield of 0.6%. Further examination of the hydrolysis mixtures by electrophoresis and bioautography indicated the presence of cephalosporin C_c (*4*) and 7-ACA lactone (*5*).

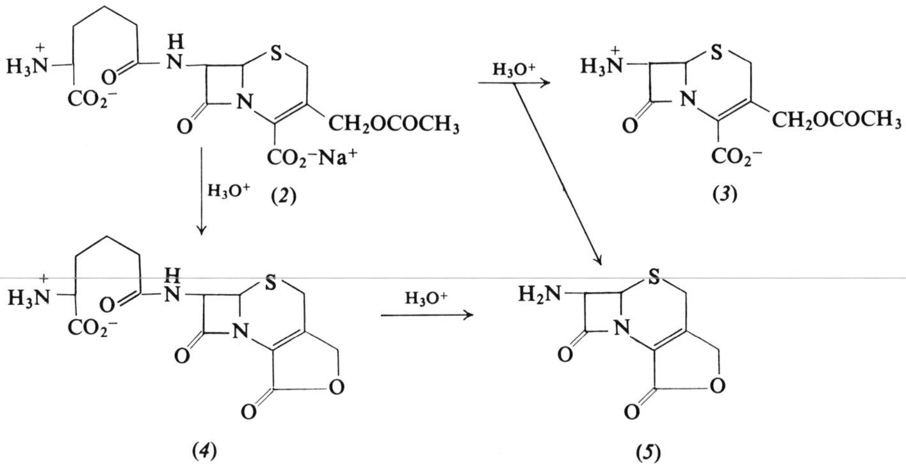

* Section by Robert R. Chauvette, Chemical Research Division, and Bill G. Jackson, Process Research Division, Eli Lilly and Company.

Cephalosporin C_c and cephalosporin C_A (pyridine) (6) were treated with dilute acid. No products were isolated from these hydrolyses; but the electrophoretic behavior of the compounds of the reaction mixtures indicated formation of the respective deacylated products (5) and (7).

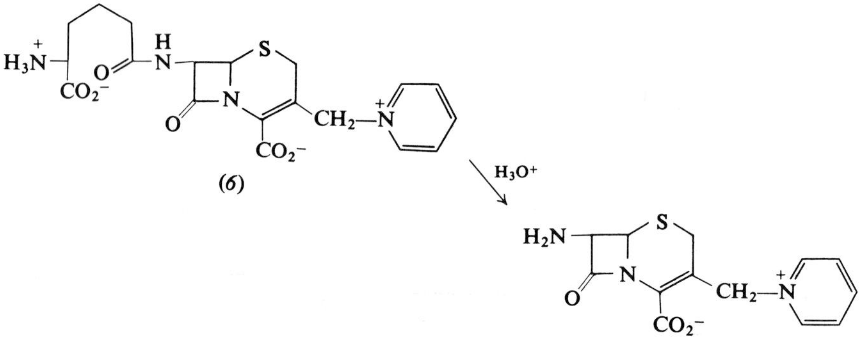

(6)

(7)

The importance of practical methods for the preparation of products discussed in this section will be apparent to many since use in therapy demands efficient and economical recovery of key compounds. The yields reported are those obtained in laboratory processes and probably do not represent optimum results.

The requirement for substantial quantities of 7-ACA to be used in preparing new acylated cephalosporins necessitated a more efficient method of cleaving cephalosporin C to 7-ACA. The first practical selective deacylation method was reported by Morin and co-workers (1962) from the Lilly Research Laboratories. This process evolved from the observation that cephalosporin C furnished 2 moles of nitrogen when treated with aqueous nitrous acid. Since cephalosporin C contains only one diazotizable amine function, the second mole of nitrogen must arise from an additional amino group being liberated as a consequence of the diazotization. The liberation of a second amino nitrogen was rationalized by involving an intramolecularly assisted scission of the C-7 amide bond (8 and 9). Apparently, 7-ACA was an intermediate in the diazotization sequence.

Attempts to isolate the cephalosporin nucleus from aqueous nitrosation mixtures were unsuccessful, nitrosation of 7-ACA ostensibly taking place as fast as hydrolysis of the imino ether (9). Replacement of water by acetic acid for the reaction solvent and use of a volatile nitrosating agent, nitrosyl chloride, made possible the removal of the nitrosating agent prior to contact with water. Rapid diazotization of the amino group following hydrolysis of the imino ether was minimized and isolation of 7-ACA was realized. Formic acid was found to

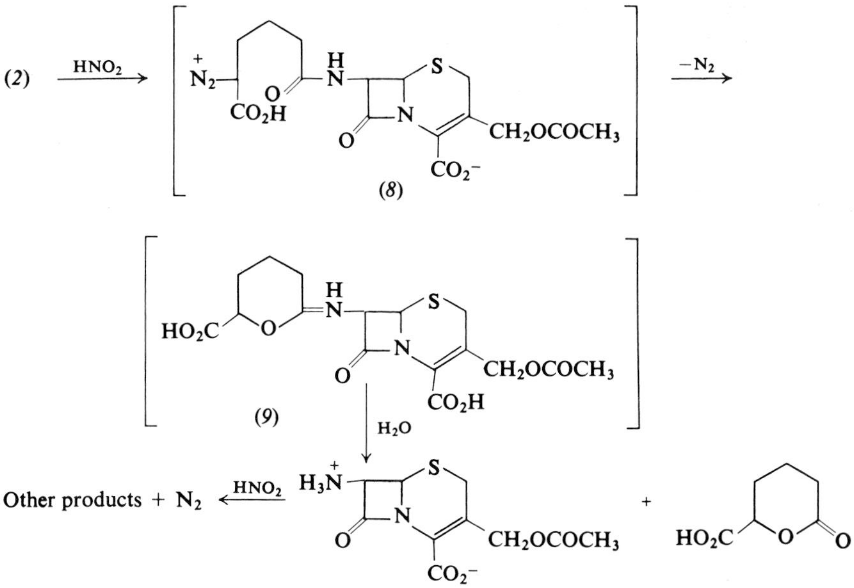

(2) $\xrightarrow{\text{HNO}_2}$ [structure (8)] $\xrightarrow{-\text{N}_2}$

(8)

[structure (9)] $\downarrow$ H$_2$O

(9)

Other products + N$_2$ $\xleftarrow{\text{HNO}_2}$ [7-ACA structure] + [lactone structure]

possess greater solubility for cephalosporin C and, therefore, became the solvent of choice. In addition, yields of 7-ACA were higher ($\approx 40\%$) than when acetic acid was used (7%).

A solution of cephalosporin C (20% w/v) in formic acid was chilled and a cold solution of nitrosyl chloride (2 molar equivalents) in formic acid was added in one portion. After a reaction period of 5 minutes the solvent was removed under reduced pressure and the residue dissolved in water. Addition of mineral base to pH 3.5 precipitated the 7-ACA. Later experiments showed that acetonitrile or nitroparaffins (U.S. Patent 3,367,933) as cosolvents gave improved yields ($\approx 50\%$). Quenching the reaction mixture in large volumes of methanol was effective in destroying the excess nitrosyl chloride (U.S. Patent 3,367,933), eliminating the evaporation under reduced pressure. Yields of 7-ACA can be improved further if 2,2-dimethoxypropane or methyl formate is added to the reaction mixture at the completion of the reaction (U.S. Patent 3,507,862). The total crude product from the reaction of cephalosporin C with nitrosyl chloride was examined carefully to ascertain the fate of cephalosporin C which was not converted to 7-ACA (Morin et al., 1969). The filtrate obtained after separating 7-ACA from the reaction mixture was examined by paper chromatography and was found to contain at least five biologically active components. Extraction of the filtrate at pH 2 with ethyl acetate removed three of the components. The remaining two were identified as cephalosporin C and 7-ACA. Since the antibiotic activity of 7-ACA is negligible compared to cephalosporin C, direct biological assay of the extracted filtrate gave a measure of the amount of unreacted cephalosporin C contained therein. This quantity was found to be 3–5 % of the starting cephalosporin C. Analysis of the whole crude reaction mixture necessitated a different isolation procedure. The residue, obtained after removing excess nitrosyl chloride and formic acid, was separated into acetone-soluble and acetone-insoluble fractions. The acetone-insoluble fraction was found to contain cephalosporin C, 7-ACA, 7-ACA hydrochloride, and inorganic materials. The acetone-soluble portion was treated with diazomethane to convert the mixture of acids into methyl esters, thus facilitating their chromatographic separation.

Column chromatography of the mixture of methyl esters was carried out using 1:1 silica gel and Hyflo Super Cel. Six identifiable compounds were separated.

Two of the substances represented the cleaved aminoadipyl side chain. Dimethyl α-hydroxyadipate (10) was identified by comparison with an independently synthesized sample. The second compound, a $C_7H_{10}O_4$ lactone, was assigned the structure (11) based on its IR and NMR spectra. The side chain residue products amounted to 25–38 % of the starting cephalosporin C, and their yields coincided well with the yield (30 %) of 7-ACA from these runs.

H₃CO₂C ... CO₂CH₃ OH (10)   (11)   (12)

Another component, a noncrystallizable oil, analyzed for $C_{11}H_{12}ClNO_5S$. Its NMR spectrum indicated that it was a cephalosporin. The magnitude of the coupling constant between the C-6 and C-7 hydrogens (Green et al., 1965) indicated that the two hydrogens were *trans* rather than *cis* as in cephalosporin C. All data for this substance were consistent with its being 7-α-chlorocephalosporanic acid methyl ester (12). The chloro derivative was postulated to arise from 7-ACA interacting with nitrosyl chloride; and, in fact, it was prepared independently from 7-ACA and nitrosyl chloride followed by esterification with diazomethane. Although α-chloro carbonyl compounds are well known to possess a reactive chlorine, the chloroester (12) was found to be unreactive toward a variety of nucleophilic reagents.

The three remaining by-products were shown to be adipamido cephalosporanates. All possessed typical cephalosporin UV absorption ($\lambda_{max} \approx 260$ mμ, $\epsilon = 8000$), and their IR spectra indicated presence of a β-lactam ($\nu = 1800$ cm⁻¹). Their NMR spectra were most instructive and confirmed the presence of a cephalosporin nucleus as well as the 7-adipamido function.

Elemental analysis of the least polar of these compounds revealed the presence of a chlorine atom. This fact, coupled with NMR data, allowed assignment of the chloro substituent at C-5′ on the adipyl side chain compound (*13*).

The infrared spectrum of the second adipamido compound possessed a strong band at 1160 cm^{-1}, characteristic of formate esters (Bellamy, 1958). Additionally, the NMR spectrum showed a one proton singlet at $\delta 8.04$. Accordingly, the substance was the C-5′ formate (*14*). The most polar of the three compounds was shown to be the C-5′ hydroxy derivative (*15*) based on IR absorption at 3350 cm^{-1} and an NMR peak at $\delta 3.03$, the proton responsible being exchanged readily with D$_2$O. The products which result from treatment of cephalosporin C with nitrosyl chloride may be interpreted as arising by

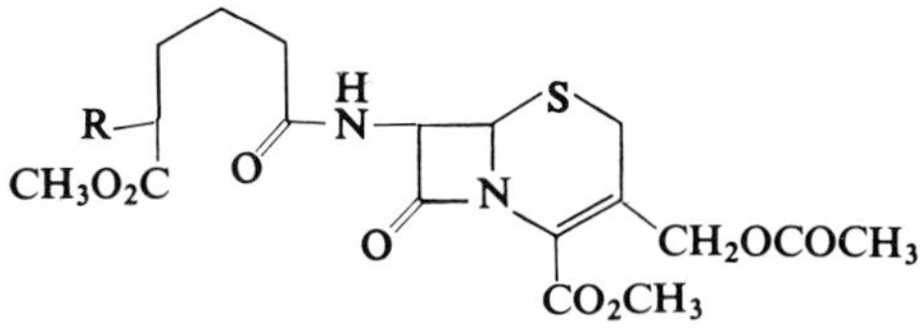

(*13*) R = Cl

(*14*) R = OCHO

(*15*) R = OH

either an intermolecular or intramolecular reaction from a common diazonium ion intermediate (*8*). The intramolecular path, leading to 7-ACA, has been portrayed earlier. Alternately, the ion may undergo displacement by chloride ion, formic acid, or water to produce (*13*)–(*15*). The two modes of reaction are summarized below. The combined yield of esters arising from the intermolecular reaction represents about 40% of the starting cephalosporin C and is approximately the same as the yield of 7-ACA. The chloroester (*12*) was isolated in 7% yield.

Another type of intramolecularly assisted side chain cleavage from cephalosporin C was reported by Fechtig and associates (1968) at CIBA Limited. Cephalosporin C was converted to its *t*-BOC derivative (*16*) using *t*-butyloxycarbonyl azide. Subsequent esterification with phenyldiazomethane afforded the dibenzyl ester (*17*). Removal of the *t*-BOC function with trifluoroacetic acid produced cephalosporin C dibenzyl ester (*18*). When the diester was treated with pyridine and acetic acid in methylene chloride at room temperature, it underwent intramolecular aminolysis, giving a 50% yield of 7-ACA benzyl ester (*19*) and the lactam (*20*).

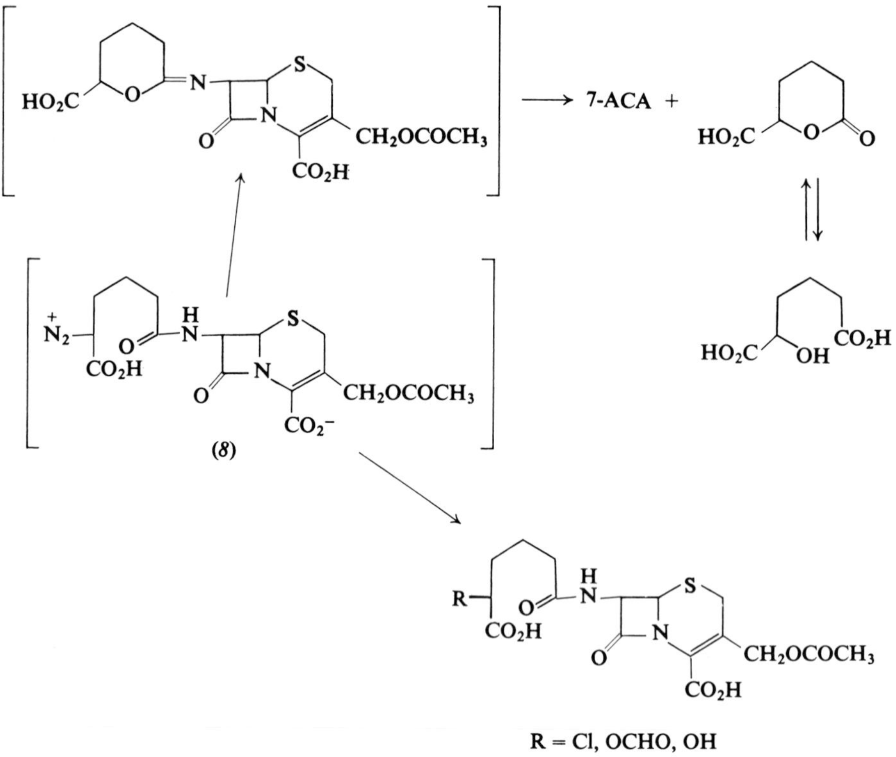

R = Cl, OCHO, OH

Because of the difficulties attendant with removal of the benzyl grouping from 7-ACA benzyl ester (*19*), the aminolysis reaction was investigated using the benzhydryl group as a carboxyl blocking function. Cephalosporin C was converted to its hydrochloride which in turn was treated with diphenyldiazomethane to yield cephalosporin C dibenzhydryl ester (*21*). The dibenzhydryl ester was found to undergo intramolecular aminolysis analogous to the dibenzyl ester (*18*); however, the reaction was further complicated by double-bond isomerization (*22* ⇌ *23*). Deblocking of the mixture of 7-ACA esters obtained by aminolysis gave a 15% yield of 7-ACA. In a sense, the intramolecular aminolysis represents the "reverse" of the intramolecular scission observed with nitrosyl chloride. In the case of the aminoesters the mode of attack is that of a nucleophilic amine upon a weakly *electrophilic* amide carbonyl. With nitrosyl chloride the weakly *nucleophilic* carbonyl attacks the strongly electrophilic C-5′ carbon in the adipic side chain.

The foregoing discussion makes evident the fact that the more successful methods for removing the 7-acyl side chain derive from chemical reactions

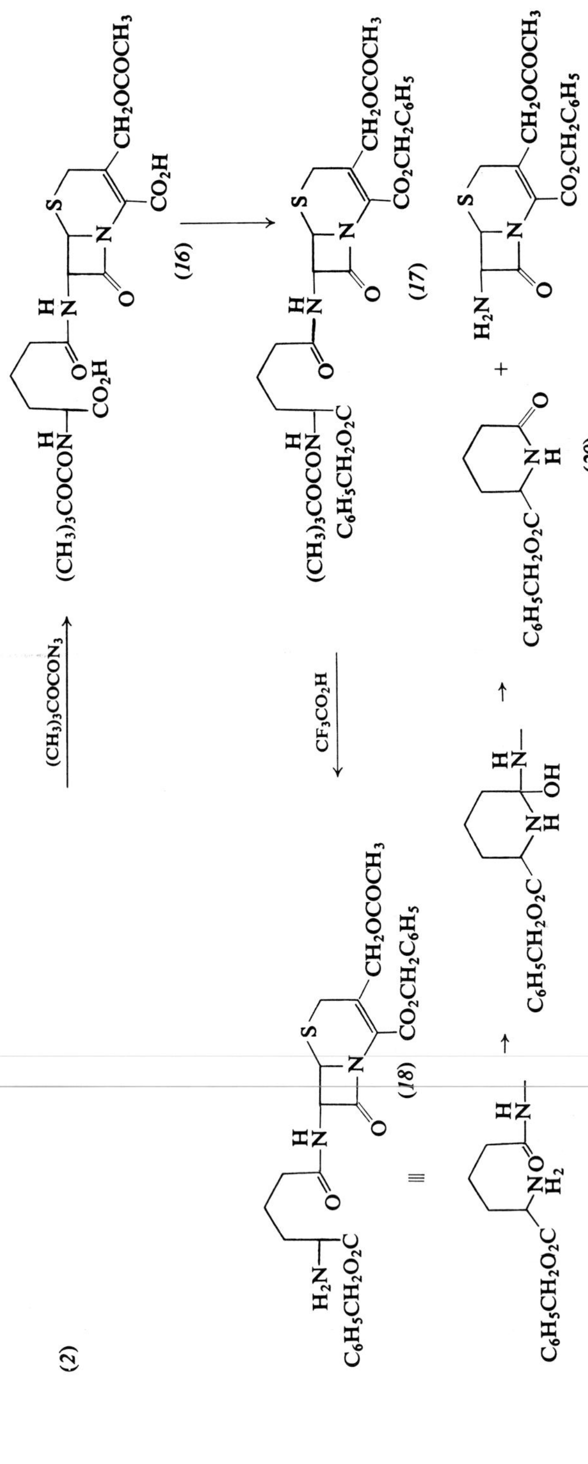

(2)
(CH3)3COCON3
(16)
CF3CO2H
(17)
(18)
(19)
(20)

involving the formation of a 7-imino intermediate, easily hydrolyzed under mild conditions (as in the NOCl cleavage), as opposed to a direct hydrolysis of the 7-amide bond, requiring more rigorous treatment.

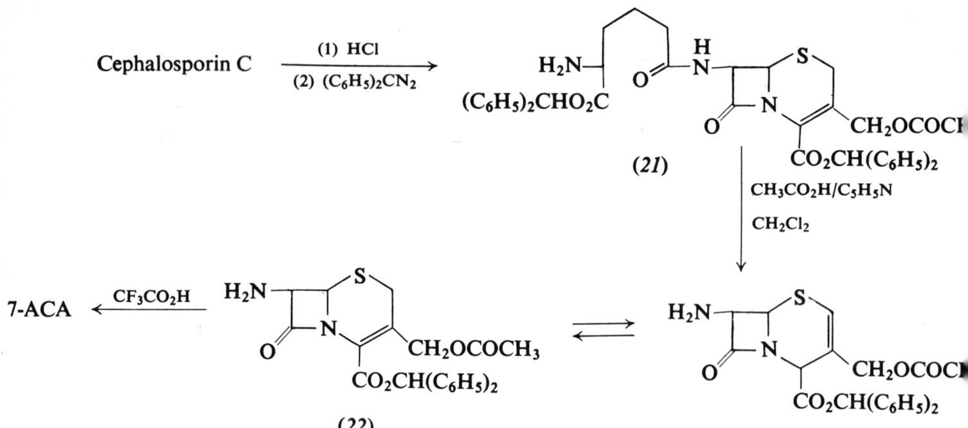

Two early attempts at side chain cleavage of cephalosporin C indeed produced small quantities of the same 7-imino ether that was to figure later as a key intermediate in a very successful reaction to produce 7-ACA. In the first of these, cephalosporin C, with its amino function protected by a 2,4-dinitrophenyl group (24), was reacted at room temperature with Meerwein's reagent (triethyloxonium fluoroborate) in dioxane–ethylene chloride solution to produce an ethyl imino ether in modest yield (Belg. Patent 628,493; U.S. Patent 3,234,223). Subsequent hydrolysis of this imino ether led to some 7-ACA. As it stands, however, the method seems to be impractical and no published evidence of a concentrated effort at improving it is available. In the second attempt, an ethyl imino ether was presumed to be formed during a reaction of cephalosporin C with ethyl orthoformate and boron trifluoride etherate in absolute alcohol (Fr. Patent 1,376,905). The mixture was examined by electrophoresis and reported to contain 7-ACA.

Then, in an ingenious series of reactions, CIBA scientists developed a practical side chain cleavage of cephalosporin C which proceeds through an imino chloride to an imino ether at the C-7 amide linkage. A selective hydrolysis of the latter intermediate leads to isolation of a 7-aminocephalosporanate ester; an exhaustive hydrolysis affords 7-ACA directly. Initial disclosures of the method (Gr. Brit. Patent 1,041,985) described side chain cleavage reactions of a cephalosporin C derivative whose amino and carboxyl functions were blocked in preceding, separate steps. The side chain elimination was best achieved in methylene chloride (CH_2Cl_2) or in chloroform ($CHCl_3$) solvents in which these fully protected derivatives of cephalosporin C are most soluble. The reaction scheme for converting these derivatives to 7-ACA is represented in a general way in the equations below.

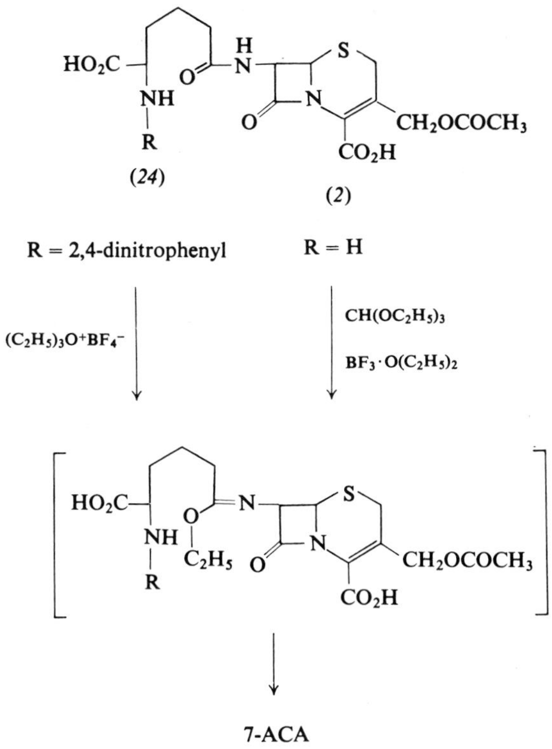

In early reports of this cleavage method, the use of phosphorus oxychloride to form the imino chloride intermediate required several days at room temperature and produced only moderate yields of 7-ACA esters. In time, phosphorus pentachloride was recognized to be a more effective chlorinating agent. In the presence of excess pyridine, phosphorus pentachloride gave a nearly complete conversion of the 7-amide function to imino chloride in a few hours at room temperature, or even in the cold, and afforded higher yields of 7-ACA esters. On treatment with an alcohol, the imino chloride was converted to an imino ether which hydrolyzed with ease to an ester of 7-ACA and, presumably, an N-acylaminoadipic acid diester. A separate and more rigorous hydrolysis, dependent upon the nature of the ester-protecting group, afforded 7-ACA. The 7-ACA was isolated as a crystalline precipitate from aqueous solution at a pH near 3.5, its isoelectric point.

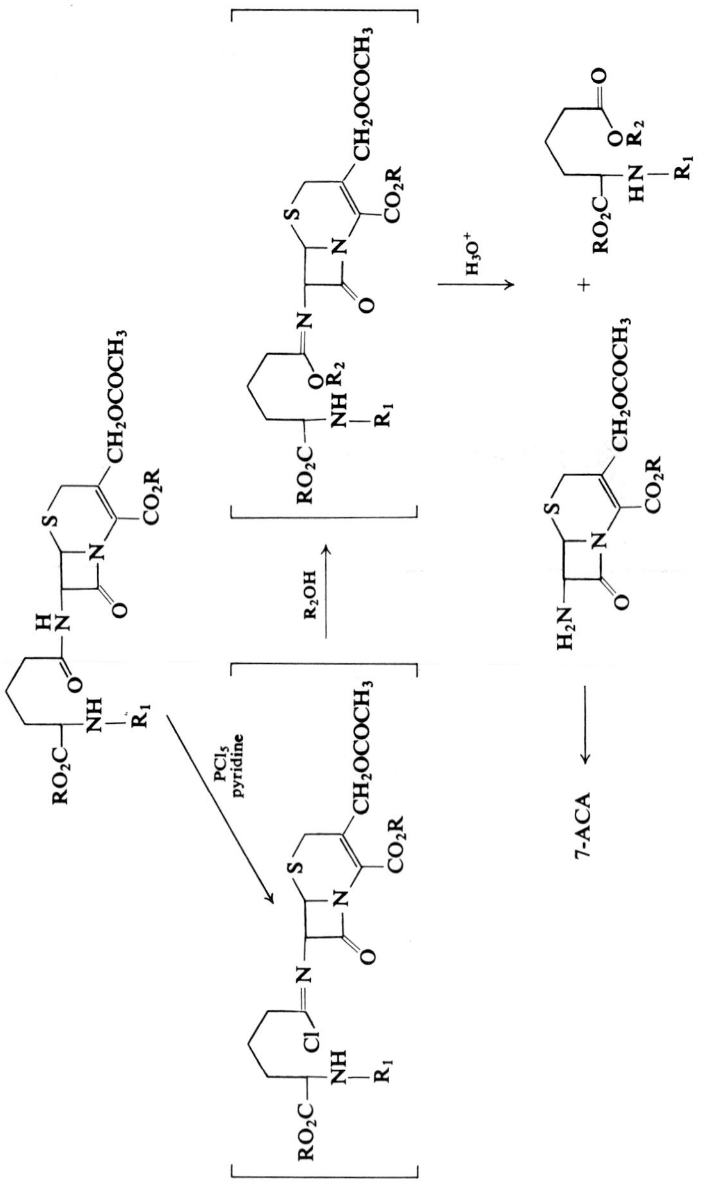
PCl5
pyridine
R2OH
H3O+
7-ACA

A list of fully protected cephalosporin C derivatives which were tested as starting material in this cleavage procedure is extensive. Notable ones are mentioned here. Methods of preparation for a number of these compounds can be found in patents describing attempts to remove the side chain through acid hydrolysis (Aust. Patent 19,908) and through intramolecular aminolysis (Belg. Patent 645,157) as described earlier in this chapter. Methods for the preparation of others appear, together with cleavage procedures, using phosphorus oxychloride or pentachloride (Gr. Brit. Patent 1,041,985). Both *N*-phenylacetyl (*25a*) and *N*-carbobenzoxy (*25b*) cephalosporin C dibenzyl esters gave benzyl 7-aminocephalosporanate (*26a*).

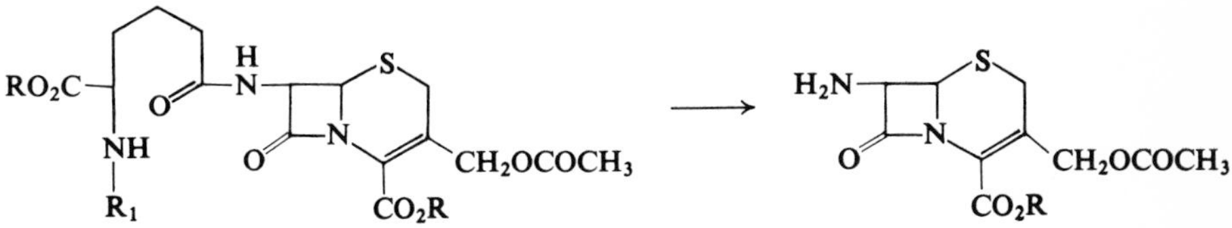

(*25*)   (*26*)

(*25a*) R = CH$_2$C$_6$H$_5$; R$_1$ = COCH$_2$C$_6$H$_5$

(*25b*) R = CH$_2$C$_6$H$_5$; R$_1$ = CO$_2$CH$_2$C$_6$H$_5$

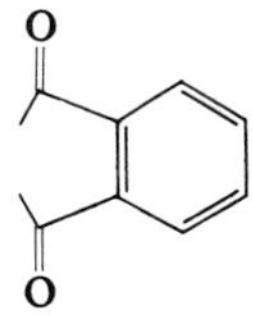

(*26a*) R = CH$_2$C$_6$H$_5$

(*26b*) R = CH$_2$— —OCH$_3$

(*25c*) R = CH$_2$C$_6$H$_5$; R$_1$ = —NO$_2$

(*26c*) R = CH(C$_6$H$_5$)$_2$

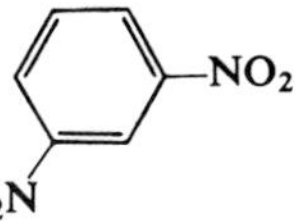

(*25d*) R = CH$_2$C$_6$H$_5$; R$_1$ =

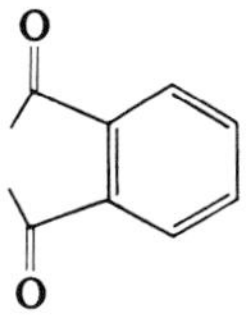

(*25e*) R = .CH$_2$C$_6$H$_5$; R$_1$ = COC$_6$H$_5$

(*25f*) R = CH$_2$— —OCH$_3$; R$_1$ =

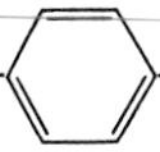

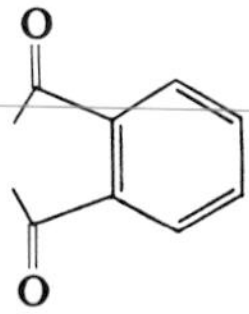

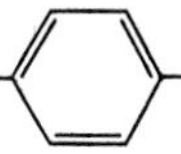

(*25g*) R = CH(C$_6$H$_5$)$_2$; R =

The same amino ester (*26a*) was obtained from N(2,4-dinitrophenyl)-cephalosporin C dibenzyl ester (*25c*) in 58% yield, from N,N-phthaloyl cephalosporin C dibenzyl ester (*25d*) in 45% yield, and from N-benzoyl cephalosporin C dibenzyl ester (*25e*) in 32% yield. N,N-Phthaloylcephalosporin C p-methoxybenzyl ester (*25f*) gave p-methoxybenzyl 7-aminocephalosporanate (*26b*) in 48% yield.

A favored substrate was the N,N-phthaloyl cephalosporin C dibenzhydryl ester (*25g*) (Gr. Brit. Patent 1,041,985; Fechtig et al., 1968). It was prepared in excellent yield from an acylation of cephalosporin C in aqueous acetone solution buffered at pH 9, using a slight excess of N-carbethoxyphthalimide. The reaction proceeded at room temperature. N,N-Phthaloyl cephalosporin C (*27*) was isolated by ethyl acetate extraction of the reaction mixture acidified to pH 2. The esterification was done in dioxane–methanol solution at room temperature, using slightly over 2 moles of diphenyldiazomethane. The product crystallized when triturated with petroleum ether and was recrystallized from methylene chloride–ethyl acetate. Removal of the side chain from N,N-phthaloyl cephalosporin C dibenzhydryl ester (*25g*) was effected in methylene chloride, using excess dry pyridine and phosphorus oxychloride. The reaction

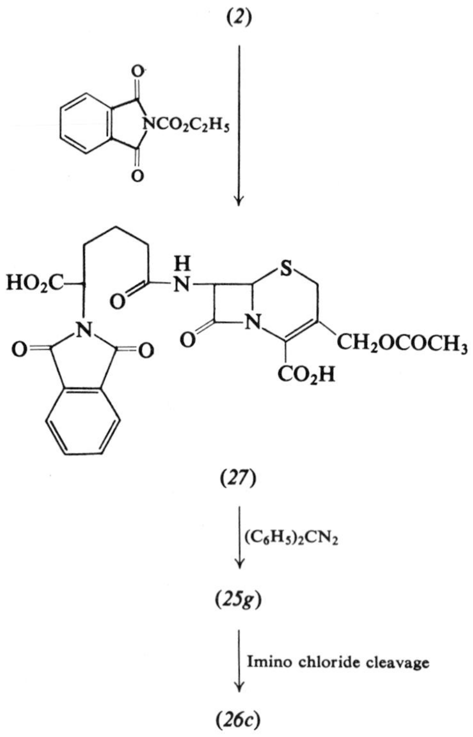

(*2*)

(*27*)

(*25g*)

(*26c*)

required 10 days at 22°. Treatment with methanol at room temperature for 8.5 hours, then with aqueous phosphoric acid in dioxane gave benzhydryl 7-aminocephalosporanate (*26c*). It was separated from the aqueous phase by ethyl acetate extraction at neutral pH. The yield was 66%.

In a separate step, the benzhydryl ester (*26c*) was hydrolyzed at room temperature, using anhydrous trifluoroacetic acid with anisole. The trifluoroacetic acid was replaced by water–ethyl acetate and 7-ACA precipitated from the aqueous phase at pH 3.5 in 91% yield.

The same workers described another cleavage of *N,N*-phthaloyl cephalosporin C dibenzhydryl ester (*25g*). A 10% solution of phosphorus pentachloride in methylene chloride was used in place of phosphorus oxychloride. After a half-hour at 20°, methanol was added. After another 6 hours at room temperature, the reaction solution was poured into aqueous phosphoric acid and dioxane to effect hydrolysis. The amino ester (*26c*) was isolated and immediately hydrolyzed as before, to give 7-ACA in 75% overall yield.

Eventual refinements in the cleavage of *N,N*-phthaloyl cephalosporin C dibenzhydryl ester (*25g*) contributed to even higher yields of 7-ACA, in significantly improved purity (Gr. Brit. Patent 1,119,806). These included a lower temperature (−20° to −10°) and a shorter reaction time (30–40 minutes) to minimize side reactions in the imino chloride step. In the alcoholysis step, methanol (preferred over ethanol) was used in a ratio of 100 moles per mole of imino chloride to assure a quick and quantitative conversion to imino ether. As this reaction is exothermic, the alcohol was precooled and allowed to react at −10° for 30 minutes and then at room temperature for 1 hour. Addition of dilute acid with vigorous stirring of the two-phase mixture for about 45 minutes was judged adequate for hydrolysis. The benzhydryl ester (*26c*) was separated in the methylene chloride layer after the mixture was made basic with aqueous alkali. Following further hydrolysis, using trifluoroacetic acid with anisole, cold water was added and the aqueous layer was titrated to pH 3.5. 7-ACA crystallized in over 80% yield. That three of the foregoing reactions were done in the same vessel and carried out on a kilogram of the starting material attested to the feasibility of this synthetic scheme as a large-scale process for making 7-ACA.

Subsequent patents issued to Nederlandsche Gistern Spiritus Fabriek (N.G.S.F.) (Belg. Patent 718,824), Glaxo Labs. (Belg. Patent 719,712), and CIBA Limited (Neth. Patent 68,12413) described a successful phosphorus pentachloride cleavage of cephalosporin C using silylating agents to simultaneously protect the amino and carboxylic acid groupings. Silylation was, in fact, a logical sequel to N.G.S.F.'s earlier experience in applying the imino chloride cleavage procedure to a penicillin silyl ester. The latter represented the first published report of 6-APA derived by a chemical degradation of commercially available penicillins (Neth. Patent 66,06872). This latest innovation, silylation as a means of protecting the carboxyl groups in N-acyl cephalosporin C derivatives or both type functional groups in cephalosporin C itself during side chain cleavage, represented a distinct improvement in the overall chemical scheme. Particularly, simultaneous blocking of both the amino and carboxyl groups eliminated the isolation and purification of two intermediates. As fully silylated cephalosporin C derivatives are soluble in chlorinated hydrocarbons, the cleavage reactions could follow silylation using the same solvent without interruption of a work-up. With silyl esters being especially sensitive to hydroxylic solvents, their hydrolysis entailed no separate step; the addition of water as a final operation merely expedited the isolation of 7-ACA. Doing away with a separate, rigorous hydrolysis of an ester minimized deacetylation at the C-3 methyl, a serious side reaction with the former procedure.

Available data indicated that best results with the imino chloride cleavage, using silyl protection, are obtained with anhydrous forms of cephalosporin C. Anhydrous cephalosporin C sodium salt was silylated using dimethyldichlorosilane and dimethylaniline in methylene chloride at room temperature, then cleaved using phosphorus pentachloride at $-55°$ for 2.5 hours, n-butanol for 2.5 hours, and a cold mixture of methanol–water for hydrolysis. The yield of isolated 7-ACA was 92.5% (Belg. Patent 718,824). In like manner, but using trimethylchlorosilane and anhydrous cephalosporin C free acid, a 91% yield was achieved. With N,N-phthaloyl cephalosporin C as substrate, the reaction gave an 85% yield of 7-ACA (Fechtig et al., 1968).

The six-step chemical sequence described earlier in this chapter was thus reduced to four reactions that could be carried out in one reaction vessel in a relatively short time. In terms of simplicity, yield, and purity of product, the imino chloride cleavage, in the form last described, represents the most important side chain removal method for cephalosporin C since the development of the nitrosyl chloride method. The chemistry appears to be reasonably workable as an economical process for manufacturing 7-ACA.

Scientists at the Lilly Research Laboratories have investigated the feasibility of applying the imino chloride cleavage process to an N-acylated form of cephalosporin C with an alternate possibility of protecting the carboxyl groups as mixed anhydrides (Chauvette et al., in press). The blocking step was envisioned as a preliminary treatment of the N-acyl derivative, before cleavage, in a common reaction vessel. The mixed anhydride of benzylpenicillin with acetic acid has long been known and was a relatively stable and useful intermediate in penicillin chemistry (Cooper and Binkley, 1948). This alternate route to 7-ACA was made feasible by success in the utilization of chloroacetyl chloride or chloroacetic acid anhydride in the isolation of cephalosporin C from production fermentation broth (Belg. Patent 759,064). By this procedure, cephalosporin C was isolated as a N-chloroacetyl derivative and crystallized as a quinoline salt (28). The method was simpler and more efficient than the traditional crystallization of the sodium salt dihydrate. As this N-chloroacetyl derivative was not amenable to the nitrosyl chloride reaction which requires a free amino group, the more general imino chloride cleavage was logically applied. Through silylation with dimethyldichlorosilane, equivalent yields of 7-ACA were obtained in phosphorus pentachloride cleavage of the N-chloroacetyl derivative as with cephalosporin C sodium salt.

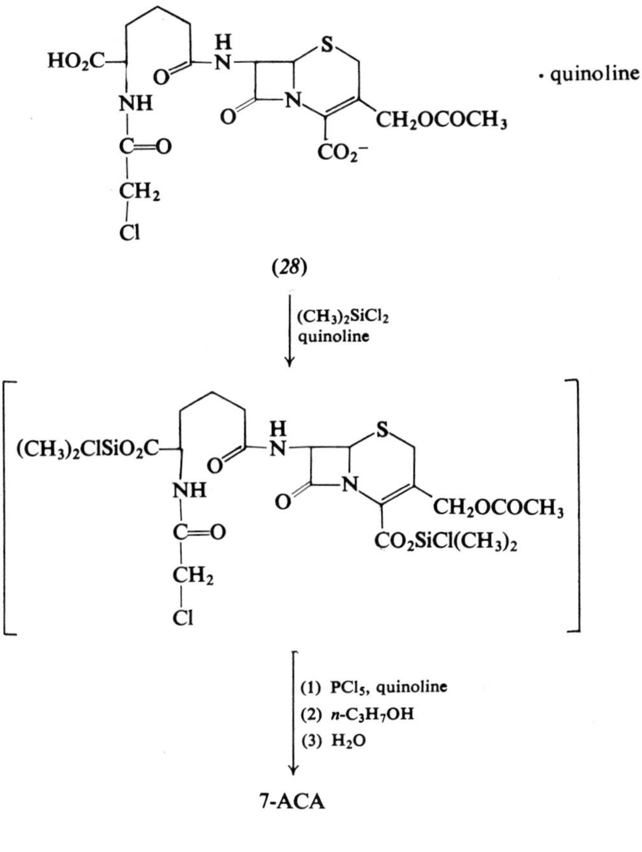

(28)

|
| (CH₃)₂SiCl₂
| quinoline
↓

|
| (1) PCl₅, quinoline
| (2) n-C₃H₇OH
| (3) H₂O
↓

7-ACA

A previous experience with the esterification of cephalosporins, which resulted in double-bond isomerization to Δ^2 or isocephalosporins (Chauvette and Flynn, 1966), was no assurance that mixed anhydride formation at the C-4 carboxyl in cephalosporin C would give isomeric products.

When N-chloroacetyl cephalosporin C quinoline salt was suspended in methylene chloride at room temperature and treated with the required molar amounts of acetyl chloride, an organic base and a catalytic amount of dimethylformamide, the N-acylated derivative went into solution, usually within 30 minutes. The mixture underwent imino chloride cleavage at −20° in the normal way, giving 7-ACA in yield and purity comparable to that obtained through silylation (Belg. Patent 758,800).

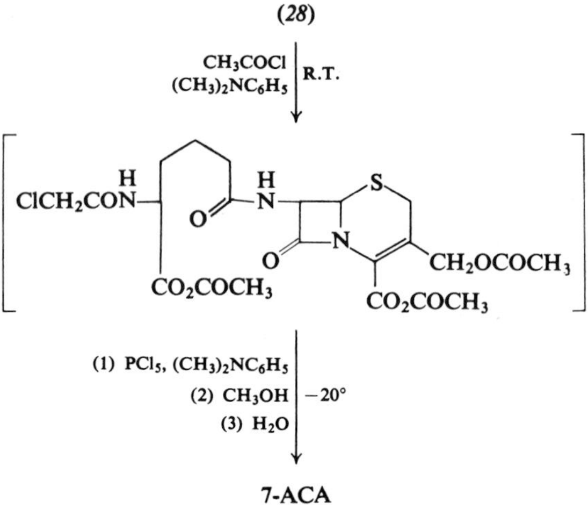

(28)

Double-bond migration resulting in the Δ^2 form of 7-ACA was evident only when all the organic base necessary to accommodate both the mixed anhydride and the imino chloride formation was introduced initially in the reaction mixture. This complication was circumvented when the acid chloride and the base were employed in equal molar ratios in the mixed anhydride formation step at room temperature; the remainder of the base was then added only after cooling to −20° for the phosphorus pentachloride reaction. The nature of the base was also critical. Either pyridine or quinoline afforded lower yields of 7-ACA than did dimethyl- or diethylaniline. The hydrolysis step in this cleavage procedure was notably simple. Addition of cold water, with vigorous stirring of the two-phase reaction mixture for about 12–15 minutes at the existing pH, was adequate for complete decomposition of the imino ether and the mixed anhydride linkages if they were still intact at this stage of the reaction. It is quite conceivable that the mixed anhydrides had already decomposed during prolonged contact with excess alcohol in the imino ether formation.

The same workers devised an alternate method for preparation of the mixed anhydride, which involved treatment of the free acid of cephalosporin C with excess ketene in chloroform solution. Presumably, N-acylation occurred simultaneously with the formation of mixed anhydrides. This reaction solution was subjected to imino chloride cleavage in the usual way and gave 7-ACA in 57% yield.

In the evaluation of the various side chain cleavage reactions of cephalo-sporin C reported to date, serious consideration must be given to the availability of the form of cephalosporin C subjected to the reaction. The yield and

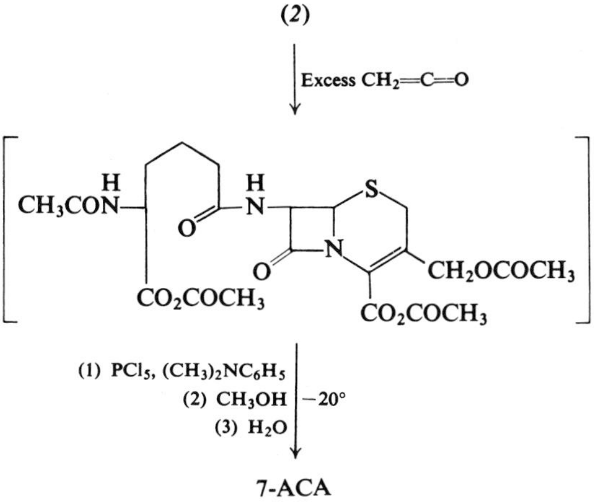

(2)

Excess $CH_2\!=\!C\!=\!O$

$$\left[CH_3CON-\overset{H}{} \quad \underset{O}{\parallel} \quad \overset{H}{\underset{\underset{\displaystyle CO_2COCH_3}{O}}{N}} \quad \underset{\underset{\displaystyle CO_2COCH_3}{N}}{S} \quad CH_2OCOCH_3 \right]$$

(1) PCl_5, $(CH_3)_2NC_6H_5$
(2) CH_3OH $-20°$
(3) H_2O

7-ACA

purity of the 7-ACA forthcoming in a cleavage reaction is of necessity, impor-tant. But the method of isolation of cephalosporin C itself, which historically has been a cumbersome task and a low yielding operation, must be considered together with the cleavage reaction to which it is coupled. Therefore, any derivative of cephalosporin C which will form in good yield and allow a ready separation of the antibiotic from its complex broth, in a form already adapt-able to an efficient side chain cleavage, would predictably net an economically feasible process for the production of 7-ACA. The foregoing amide cleavage of N-chloroacetyl cephalosporin C with phosphorus pentachloride, either through silyl or mixed anhydride protection fulfills such requirements. All yields reported here are those obtained in laboratory preparations.

Recent patents awarded to CIBA Limited (Ger. Patent 1,928,142; Belg. Patent 720,185, 734,565) claim yet another variant of the imino chloride cleavage sequence, wherein cephalosporin C was precipitated as a zinc (or copper) complex by simple addition of these cations to relatively crude extracts. This isolation appears to be remarkably selective. The zinc complex is crystalline, reasonably pure, and was reported to give 7-ACA in good yield via direct silylation and imino chloride cleavage. As a method of isolation, the precipitation of a zinc complex of cephalosporin C appears more attractive (from an economic standpoint) than does the N-picryl derivative which CIBA workers developed earlier for this express purpose (Neth. Patent 67,16487).

B. Side Chain Cleavage of Miscellaneous Cephalosporins

In connection with a synthesis of cephalexin (29) from penicillin, the imino chloride cleavage was modified (Belg. Patent 717,741) and an acid catalyzed N-deacylation was developed (Belg. Patent 746,860) to efficiently remove the arylacetyl side chain from a variety of deacetoxycephalosporanate esters. In this synthesis (Chauvette et al., 1971) either phenoxymethyl penicillin (30a) or benzyl penicillin (30b) was esterified and oxidized to the sulfoxide in preparation for a thermal, acid catalyzed rearrangement to the corresponding deacetoxycephalosporin (32a–c) (see Chapter 5). Penicillin sulfoxide esters evaluated in this synthetic scheme were the trichloroethyl (31a), p-methoxybenzyl (31b), and p-nitrobenzyl (31c) esters.

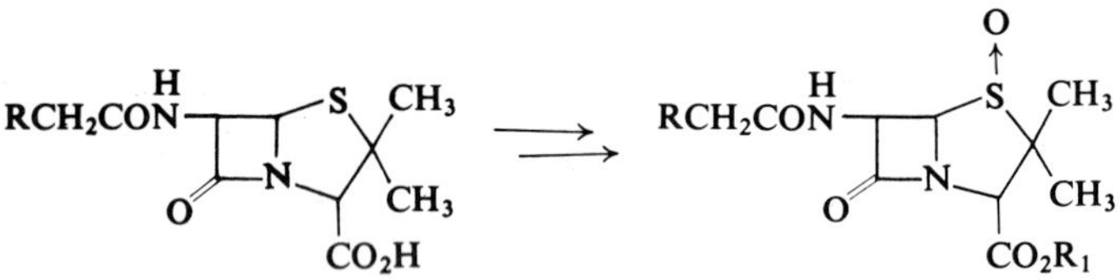

(30)

(30a) R = C_6H_5O

(30b) R = C_6H_5

(31)

(31a) R_1 = CH_2CCl_3

(31b) R_1 = CH_2—⟨benzene⟩—OCH_3

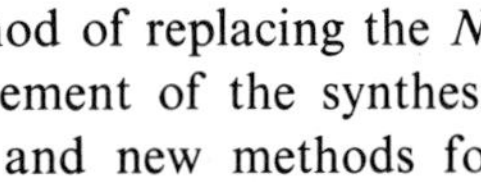

(31c) R_1 = CH_2—⟨benzene⟩—NO_2

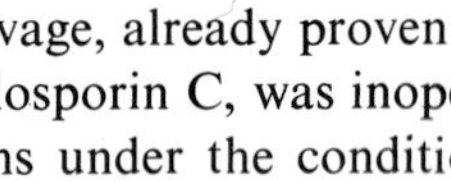

Following the ring expansion reaction, a method of replacing the N-acyl function of the original penicillin was a requirement of the synthesis. A number of known cleavages were reexamined and new methods for N-deacylation were sought. The imino chloride cleavage, already proven useful in removing the aminoadipyl side chain in cephalosporin C, was inoperative with these arylacetamido deacetoxycephalosporins under the conditions as originally published and available at the time. It was found, however, that phenoxy- and phenylacetamidodeacetoxycephalosporanate esters required elevated reaction temperatures with phosphorus pentachloride and pyridine in an anhydrous, nonpolar solvent to form 7-imino chlorides in good yield. Benzene was the most satisfactory solvent. Dioxane and chlorinated hydro-carbons were markedly inferior. A slight excess of phosphorus pentachloride and dry pyridine (in equimolar ratio) over the amount of amide, gave an opti-mum yield of 7-aminodeacetoxycephalosporanate ester (33). Phosphorus

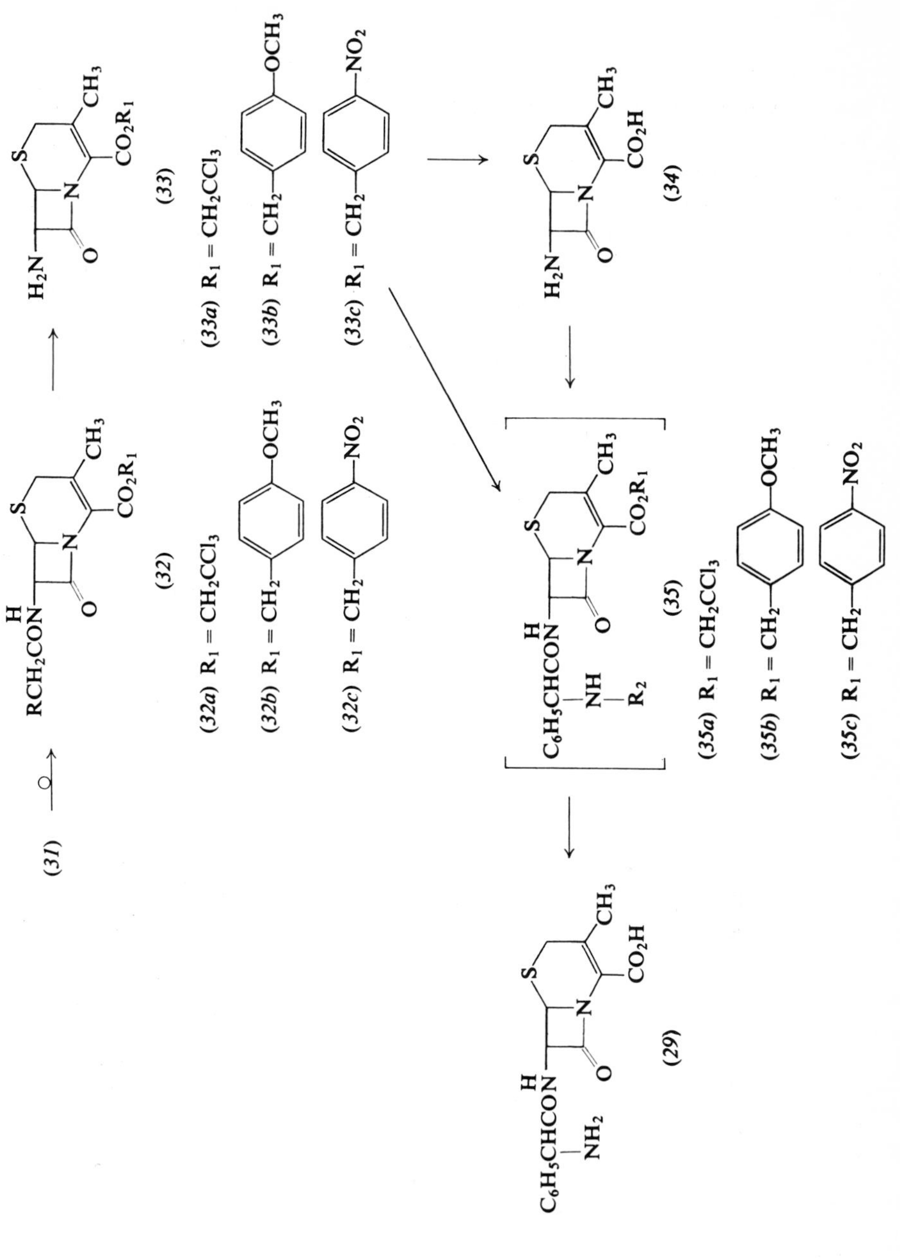

(31)

(32)

(32a) $R_1 = CH_2CCl_3$

(32b) $R_1 = CH_2$—⟨⟩—OCH_3

(32c) $R_1 = CH_2$—⟨⟩—NO_2

(33)

(33a) $R_1 = CH_2CCl_3$

(33b) $R_1 = CH_2$—⟨⟩—OCH_3

(33c) $R_1 = CH_2$—⟨⟩—NO_2

(34)

(35)

(35a) $R_1 = CH_2CCl_3$

(35b) $R_1 = CH_2$—⟨⟩—OCH_3

(35c) $R_1 = CH_2$—⟨⟩—NO_2

(29)

oxychloride and thionyl chloride were virtually unreactive. Alcohols reacted as anticipated, converting the imino chlorides completely to imino ethers at room temperature in just a few hours. On contact with water, the imino ethers hydrolyzed readily at the existing pH (≈ 2) in about 20 minutes. By design, the ester was isolated in lieu of 7-amino-3-methyl-3-cephem-4-carboxylic acid (7-ADCA) (34) to facilitate reacylation with an N-protected D-α-phenylglycine in a mixed anhydride coupling reaction. The intermediate cephalexin derivative (35) was thus formed in nearly quantitative yield. The equivalent acylation of 7-ADCA (34) in its zwitterionic form goes less smoothly (Ryan et al., 1969). As a convenient means of separating the product in pure form from so complex a reaction mixture, sulfonic acids were employed to precipitate the 7-ADCA esters as stable, highly crystalline salts from ethyl acetate extracts. The yield of 2',2',2'-trichloroethyl 7-amino-3-methyl-3-cephem-4-carboxylate (33a), isolated as a tosylate salt, was consistently 80%; of p-methoxybenzyl 7-amino-3-methyl-3-cephem-4-carboxylate (33b), tosylate salt, was 47%; and of p-nitrobenzyl 7-amino-3-methyl-3-cephem-4-carboxylate (33c), tosylate salt, was 75%.* A Belgian patent (Belg. Patent 719,712) likewise reports the obtention of both 2',2',2'-trichloroethyl 7-amino-3-methyl-3-cephem-4-carboxylate (33a), tosylate salt in 24% yield, and benzylhydryl 7-amino-3-methyl-3-cephem-4-carboxylate, tosylate salt in 66% yield, from imino chloride cleavages of 7-phenylacetamidodeacetoxycephalosporanate esters.

In general, the deacetoxycephalosporins should be a more attractive substrate for direct acid hydrolysis than cephalosporanic acids since one route of decomposition, namely, lactone formation, is no longer possible. In addition, the β-lactam in deacetoxy cephalosporins is apparently more stable, for nucleophilic cleavage of the β-lactam is accompanied by expulsion of the substituent at C-3'.

The first reported synthesis of 7-ADCA (34) was accomplished by acid hydrolysis of deacetoxy cephalosporin C (U.S. Patent 3,124,576). No yields were reported for that process, however. Studies by B. G. Jackson (Belg. Patent 746,860) of the Lilly Research Laboratories have shown that direct acid hydrolysis of deacetoxycephalosporanic acids and esters to 7-ADCA and 7-ADCA esters is practical. Successful direct acid hydrolysis was effected by heating the deacetoxycephalosporin with aqueous acid for a relatively short period of time. Sulfonic acids were the acids of choice, and an organic co-solvent was employed.

Optimum conditions for both the acids and esters were essentially the same. The amide was dissolved in ≈ 3.5 volumes of tetrahydrofuran; 0.7–1 volume of water was introduced and sufficient p-toluenesulfonic acid was added to give an acid concentration of 1 M. The mixture was heated under reflux for

---

* L. R. Peters, personal communication.

2.5–3 hours. Unreacted starting material was recovered by extraction at low pH, and the amino acid or ester was separated after raising the pH.

The rate of hydrolysis was dependent upon the concentration of p-toluene sulfonic acid. Maximum efficiency was attained when the acid concentration was about 1 M. Longer reaction times caused more hydrolysis, but the efficiency diminished ($\approx 60\%$ after 7 hours).

Only a small amount of β-lactam cleavage was found to occur under these conditions. Approximately 80–90% of β-lactam-containing materials could be recovered from the reaction mixtures. Careful examination of the reaction mixtures resulted in isolation of the thiolactone (36).

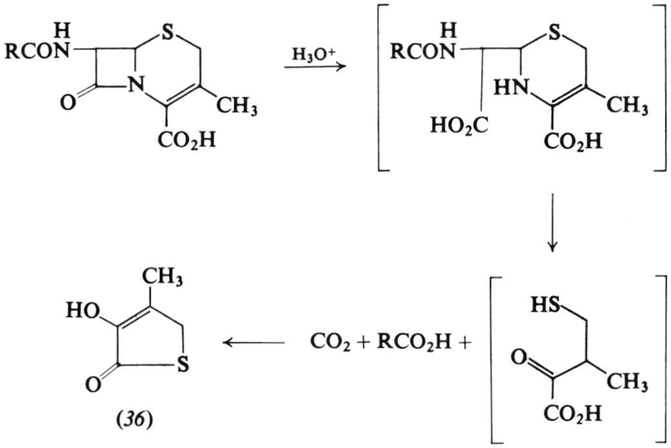

This substance was presumed to be the end product resulting from β-lactam hydrolysis. The isolated yield of (36) corresponded well with the loss of β-lactam noted previously. Further, the acid (RCO$_2$H above) recovered was roughly equal to the combined yields of 7-ADCA and thiolactone. When 7-phenoxyacetamido-3-methyl-3-cephem-4-carboxylic acid (37) was hydrolyzed under the conditions described above, a 41% yield of 7-ADCA resulted. The starting acid was recovered in 43% yield and a 12% yield of thiolactone was obtained. Phenoxyacetic acid was isolated to the extent of 55%.

Two esters of deacetoxycephalosporanic acids were subjected to direct acid hydrolysis. The trichloroethyl ester (38) was hydrolyzed and the aminoester product isolated as the tosylate salt (39) in a yield of 40%. Unreacted ester was recovered to the extent of 47%. The p-nitrobenzyl ester (40) was an especially attractive substrate for acid hydrolysis since unreacted ester could be recovered by simply diluting the reaction mixture with water. The purity of the recovered ester was quite high, and its separation from the product was nearly quantitative. Typically, the recovered ester amounted to 50–52% of the starting quantity. Correspondingly, the aminoester [isolated as a tosylate monohydrate (41)] was obtained in a 35–37% yield upon vacuum evaporation of the filtrate from the recovered ester. Taking into account the recovery of starting ester gives this process an efficiency of 73–75%, which is comparable to yields obtained when the same ester is cleaved with phosphorus pentachloride.

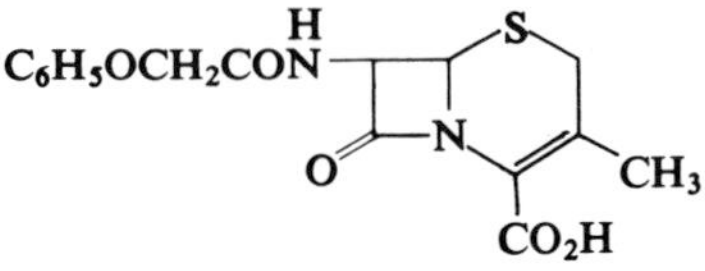

(37)

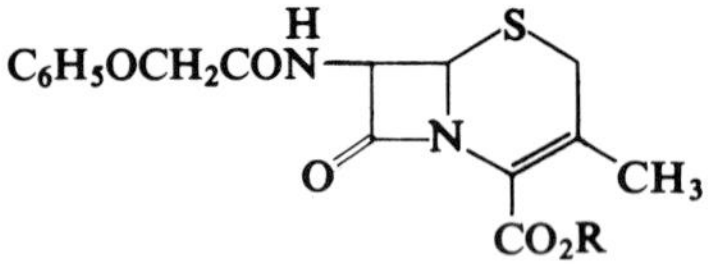

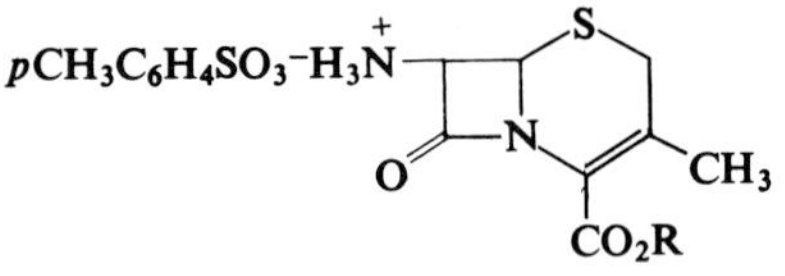

(38) R = CH$_2$CCl$_3$

(39) R = CH$_2$CCl$_3$

(40) R = CH$_2$—⟨benzene⟩—NO$_2$

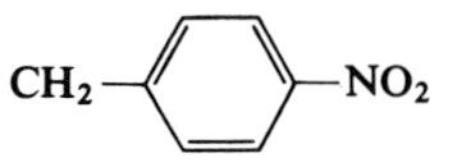

(41) R = CH$_2$—⟨benzene⟩—NO$_2$

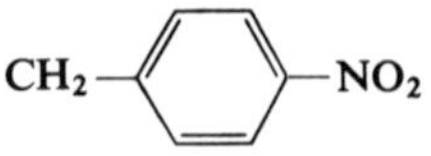

The filtrate from the aminoester (41) was found to contain p-nitrobenzyl alcohol and the thiolactone (36), both present to the extent of 5% of the starting ester. Phenoxyacetic acid was also present and could be isolated in a 37% yield.

The amide cleavage of analogous Δ^2 isomers was also investigated. Hydrolysis of 7-phenoxyacetamido-3-methyl-2-cephem-4-carboxylic acid (42) gave a 43% yield of the Δ^2-7-ADCA (43). Unreacted starting material amounted to 40% and about 2% was converted to the thiolactone (36). From the corresponding Δ^2-p-nitrobenzyl ester (44), neither the starting ester nor anticipated aminoester (45) was isolated. Instead, crude Δ^2 acid (42) was recovered to the extent of 20%. Since it was known that esters of Δ^2-cephalosporins are much more susceptible to hydrolysis than their corresponding Δ^3 isomers, the results were rationalized by assuming that hydrolysis of the ester had occurred. Isolation of p-nitrobenzyl alcohol in 95% yield supported this hypothesis.

Less rewarding than the preceding reactions was an investigation* into the generation of a 7-thioamide intermediate and its alkylation for the cleavage of

* R. R. Chauvette and P. A. Pennington, unpublished results.

deacetoxycephalosporanate esters. Trichloroethyl 7-phenoxyacetamidode-acetoxycephalosporanate (32a) was made to react with phosphorus penta-sulfide in dry benzene at reflux temperature, to give the 7-thioamide

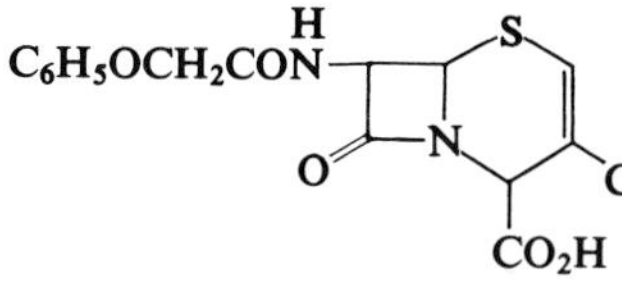

(42)

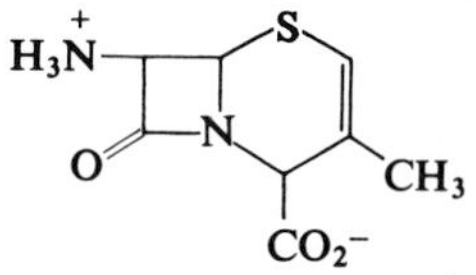

(43)

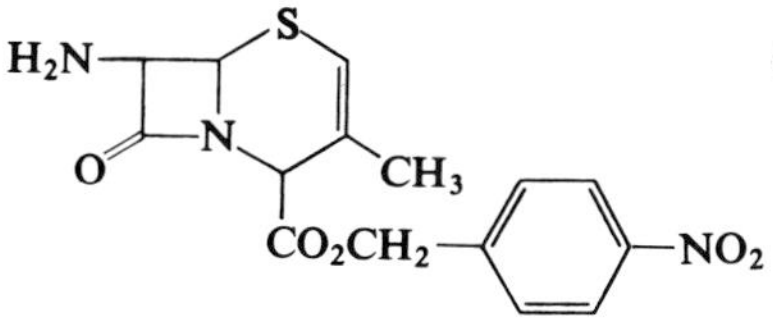

(45)

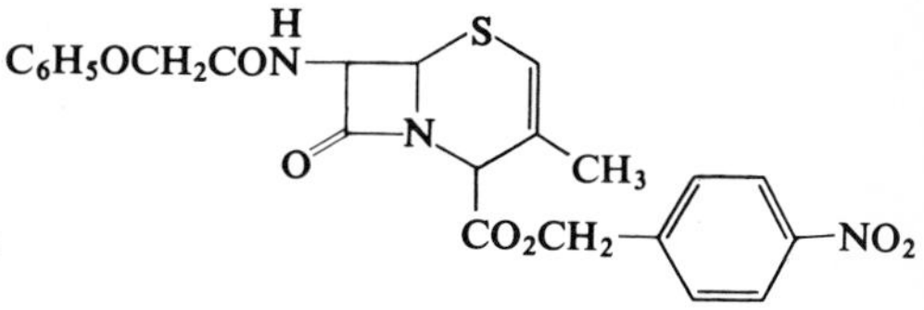

(44)

exclusively. Examination of the filtered and water-washed reaction mixture with silica gel thin layer chromatography (using 7:3 benzene and ethyl acetate for eluent) showed the reaction to be complete in a few hours. In this solvent system, the thioamide moved slightly ahead of starting material and showed a characteristic bright yellow color when visualized in an iodine chamber. Trichloroethyl 7-phenoxythioacetamidodeacetoxycephalosporanate (46) was isolated in 60% yield by crystallization from ethanol.

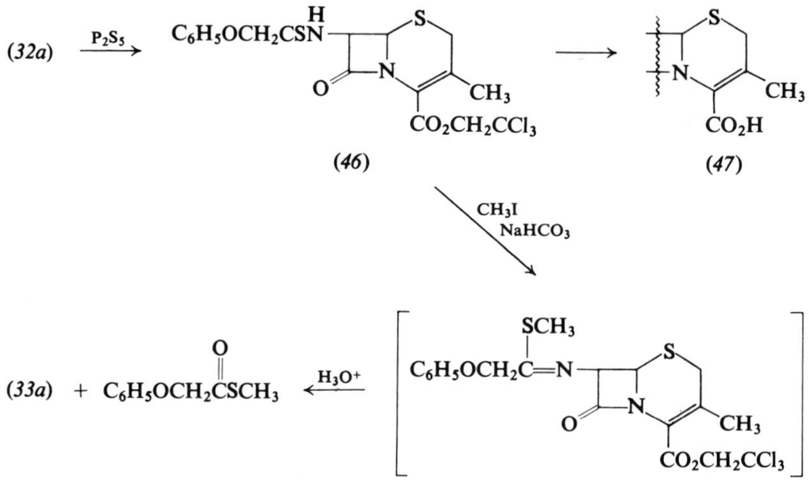

(32a)

(46)

(47)

(33a)

The free acid (47) was obtained following reductive removal of the ester with zinc in acetic acid. An acetone solution of the thioamide ester (46) was heated under reflux overnight with large excesses of methyl iodide and sodium bicarbonate in suspension. An S-methyl imino thioether intermediate was presumed. Its hydrolysis in the usual manner gave trichloroethyl 7-amino-deacetoxycephalosporanate (33a). Routinely, the product was best isolated as a tosylate salt in 90% yield. A serious disadvantage was the need for isolating the thioamide in pure, crystalline form for alkylation. Other activated alkyl halides could not be substituted for methyl iodide to give the same yield. The thioamide reactions did not transfer well to cephalosporin C, penicillins, and other cephalosporins.

In connection with the preparation of new cephalosporins for biological evaluation, the side chain cleavage of a wide variety of cephalosporins using the general imino chloride cleavage method may be found in the literature.

The 7-acyl side chain of a substituted 2-methylene-deacetoxycephalospora-nate ester (Kaiser et al., 1971) was removed under those same imino chloride cleavage conditions previously described: 2',2',2'-Trichloroethyl-2-(4-bromo-phenyl)thiomethylene-3-methyl-7-phenoxyacetamido-3-cephem-4-carboxyl-ate (48) gave a 66% yield of 2',2',2'-trichloroethyl 7-amino-2-(4-bromophenyl)-thiomethylene-3-methyl-3-cephem-4-carboxylate (49) tosylate salt.

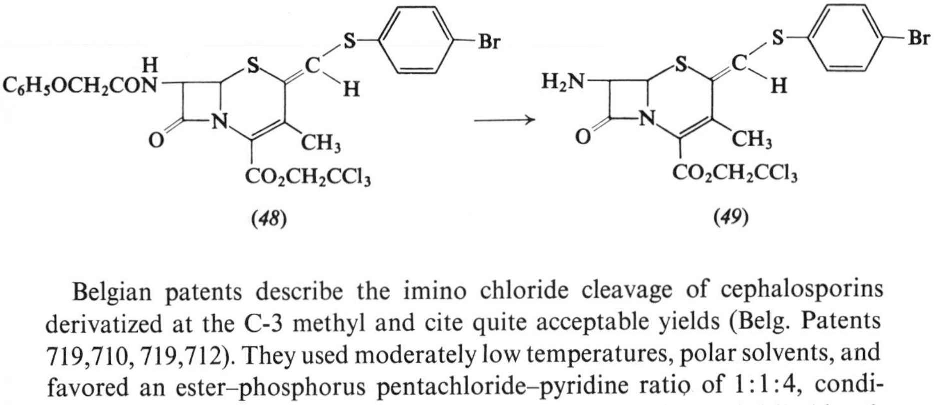

(48)   (49)

Belgian patents describe the imino chloride cleavage of cephalosporins derivatized at the C-3 methyl and cite quite acceptable yields (Belg. Patents 719,710, 719,712). They used moderately low temperatures, polar solvents, and favored an ester–phosphorus pentachloride–pyridine ratio of 1:1:4, condi-tions akin to those used with cephalosporin C. Diphenylmethyl 7-(2-thienyl-acetamido)3-methoxymethyl-3-cephem-4-carboxylate (50a) gave diphenyl-methyl 7-amino-3-methoxymethyl-3-cephem-4-carboxylate (51a) tosylate salt in 67% yield.

The corresponding 3-ethoxymethyl derivative (50b) gave diphenylmethyl 7-amino-3-ethoxymethyl-3-cephem-4-carboxylate (51b), tosylate salt.

The 3-n-propoxymethyl derivative (50c) gave diphenylmethyl 7-amino-3-n-propoxymethyl-3-cephem-4-carboxylate (51c), tosylate salt.

The 3-isopropoxymethyl derivative (*50d*) gave diphenylmethyl 7-amino-3-isopropoxymethyl-3-cephem-4-carboxylate (*51d*) tosylate salt.

The 3-(2-ketocyclohexyl)methyl derivative (*50e*) gave diphenylmethyl 7-amino-3-(2-ketocyclohexyl)methyl-3-cephem-4-carboxylate (*51e*) tosylate salt in 33% yield.

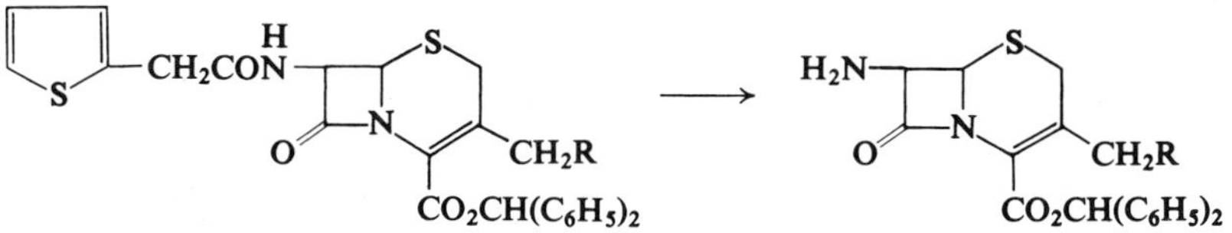

(*50*)

(*51*)

(*50a*) R = OCH$_3$ (*51a*) R = OCH$_3$

(*50b*) R = OC$_2$H$_5$ (*51b*) R = OC$_2$H$_5$

(*50c*) R = OC$_3$H$_7$ (*51c*) R = OC$_3$H$_7$

(*50d*) R = OCH(CH$_3$)$_2$ (*51d*) R = OCH(CH$_3$)$_2$

(*50e*) R = 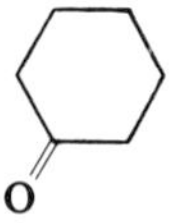   (*51e*) R =

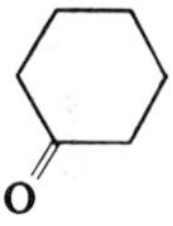

(*50f*) R = OCOC$_6$H$_5$ (*51f*) R = OCOC$_6$H$_5$

The 3-benzoyloxymethyl derivative (*50f*) gave diphenylmethyl 7-amino-3-benzoyloxymethyl-3-cephem-4-carboxylate (*51f*) tosylate salt in 83% yield.

In addition, a patent (Belg. Patent 719,712) reported the imino chloride cleavage of close analogs of cephalosporin C. Diphenylmethyl 7-valeramido-cephalosporanate (*52a*) gave diphenylmethyl 7-amino-3-acetoxymethyl-3-cephem-4-carboxylate as an oil. Without further purification, the amino ester

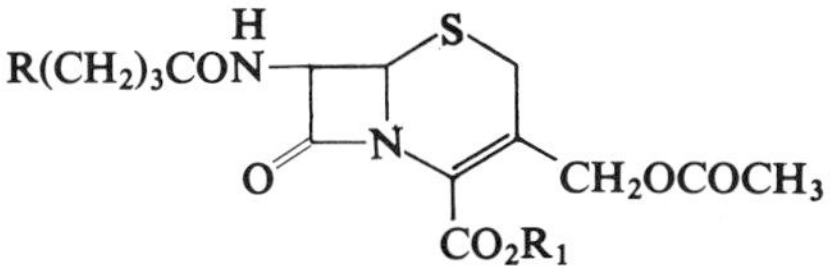

(*52*)

7-ACA

(*52a*) R = CH$_3$; R$_1$ = CH(C$_6$H$_5$)$_2$

(*52b*) R = CH$_3$; R$_1$ = H

(*52c*) R = CO$_2$H; R$_1$ = H

was hydrolyzed using trifluoroacetic acid with anisole to give 7-ACA in 75%
overall yield. The same cephalosporin, without the benzhydryl protecting
group (52b), was silylated using trimethylchlorosilane and subjected to the
same cleavage conditions to give 7-ACA in 72% yield. 7-(4-Carboxybutyr-
amido)cephalosporanic acid (52c) was silylated and cleaved to give 7-ACA in
a 20% yield.

The same workers (Cocker et al., 1965) showed that 7-ACA was spon-
taneously produced from ω-chloroalkanamido cephalosporins by an intramolecular cyclization onto the 7-amide position. 7-(4-Chlorobutanamido)
and 7-(5-chloropentanamido)cephalosporanic acids were examples cited in this
side chain cleavage.

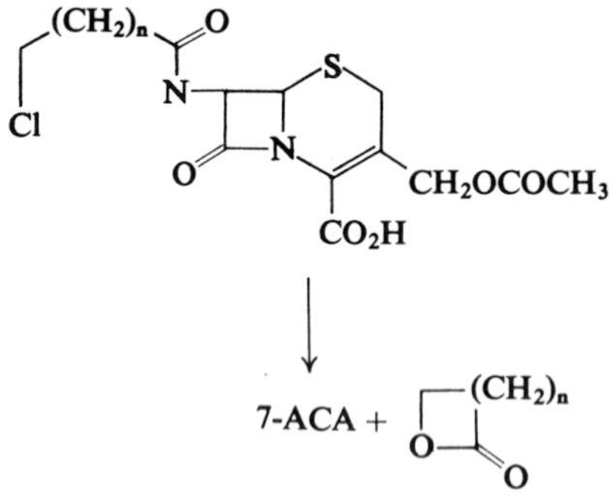

C. Side Chain Cleavage of Penicillins

Direct fermentation of precursor-free penicillin broths (Batchelor et al.,
1959) and enzymatic hydrolysis of the side chain of natural penicillin
(Rolinson et al., 1960a; Claridge et al., 1960; Huang et al., 1960; Kaufmann
and Bauer, 1960) were for many years the only available sources of 6-amino-
penicillanic acid (6-APA) (53). The penicillin nucleus was totally synthesized
(Sheehan and Henery-Logan, 1959, 1962) but in too complex a fashion for
useful application. Therefore, 6-APA obtained by microbiological methods
was the starting material in an extensive research effort made by numerous
laboratories in search of new penicillins during the early 1960's.

In late 1967, the announcement of a practical route to 6-APA, alluded to
earlier in this chapter (Neth. Patent 66,06872; U.S. Patent 3,499,909), represented an important achievement. The introduction of silyl esters as a means
of protecting the C-3 carboxyl in penicillin during imino chloride cleavage
went beyond a laboratory preparation of 6-APA. We have already seen its
corresponding use in cephalosporin chemistry where it brought about significant improvements of handling, yield, and quality in the process of making
7-ACA.

(30) $\longrightarrow$

(30a) R = C$_6$H$_5$O

(30b) R = C$_6$H$_5$

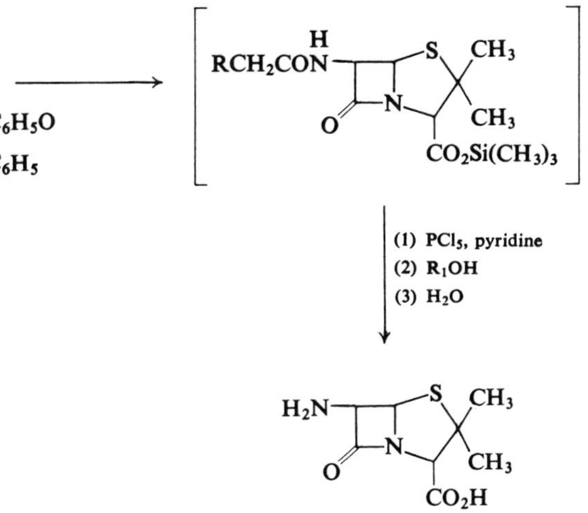

(1) PCl$_5$, pyridine
(2) R$_1$OH
(3) H$_2$O

(53)

The silylation of both phenoxymethylpenicillin free acid (30a) and benzyl-penicillin potassium salt 30b was described using either trimethylchlorosilane or dimethyldichlorosilane in methylene chloride or chloroform at room temperature in the presence of pyridine, triethylamine, or quinoline. The esterification was generally complete within 30–40 minutes. The cleavage step which followed began with cooling the reaction mixture to as low as −50° for addition of phosphorus pentachloride as a solid or in solution in the same solvent. After 3 hours in the cold, a large excess of an alcohol was added at 10°–20° lower than the temperature used in the preceding reaction. The alcoholysis was allowed to proceed for a few hours. Water was then added and immediately the pH was adjusted to near 4 with ammonium bicarbonate. The precipitated 6-APA was separated by filtration and washed with cold 50% aqueous acetone. In this way, 6-APA was obtained in 85–95% yields. Its purity was reported to be as high as 95%.

While penicillins in other ester forms (notably benzyl and benzhydryl) were reportedly subjected to the same cleavage by workers at N.G.S.F., their use necessitated an added hydrogenolysis or hydrolysis step, which was a definite disadvantage. A case in point is the side chain removal from phenoxymethyl-penicillin (54a) and benzylpenicillin (54b) trichloroethyl esters.* These compounds were converted to trichloroethyl 6-aminopenicillanate (55) in dry benzene with phosphorus pentachloride and pyridine. No difference in yield of amino ester (55) was observed with reaction temperatures of −10° or 25°.

* R. R. Chauvette and P. A. Pennington, unpublished results.

The imino chloride reacted with methanol in the usual manner and the hydrolysis was best effected with a pH 4.5 phosphate buffer in an ice bath. The product was isolated as a tosylate salt that crystallized readily from ethyl acetate. Trichloroethyl 6-benzylpenicillanate (*54b*) gave a 60% yield of trichloroethyl 6-aminopenicillanate (*55*), tosylate salt.

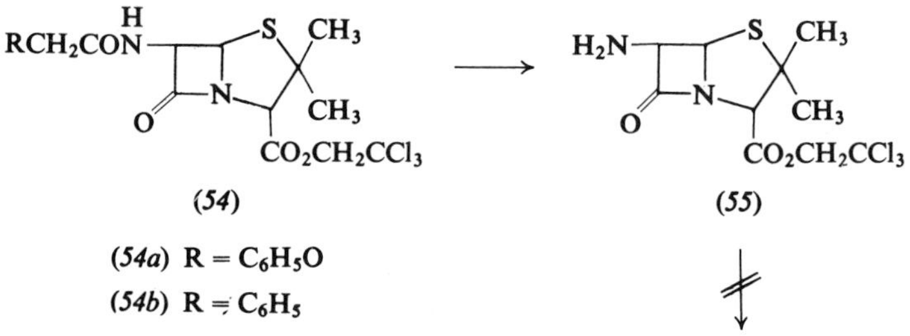

(*54*)

(*54a*) R = C_6H_5O
(*54b*) R = C_6H_5

(*55*)

6-APA

Trichloroethyl 6-phenoxymethylpenicillanate (*54a*) gave a 40% yield of the same aminoester (*55*), tosylate salt. Trichloroethyl 6-phenoxymethylpenicillanate-1-oxide gave only a 10% yield of trichloroethyl 6-aminopenicillanate-1-oxide, tosylate salt.

An unfortunate setback awaited the final deblocking reaction for generating 6-APA. It was not possible to remove the trichloroethyl ester without extensive β-lactam ring opening, using zinc in 90% aqueous acetic acid and with conditions that satisfactorily reduced the trichloroethyl ester of many penicillins and cephalosporins.

A recent patent issued to Beecham Group Limited (Ger. Patent 1,937,962) discloses the preparation of several esters of 6-APA via imino chloride cleavage of benzylpenicillanate esters. The cleavage reactions were reportedly done at −25°, using carbon tetrachloride as solvent and N-methylmorpholine as proton acceptor. The aminoesters were isolated as both benzenesulfonate and p-toluenesulfonate salts. No mention is made of their conversion to 6-APA. Trichloroethyl (*55*) and p-chlorophenylmercapto (*56a*) 6-aminopenicallanates were obtained in 80% yields. Benzylidineaminooxy (*56b*) and furfurylidineaminooxy (*56c*) 6-aminopenicillinates were obtained in somewhat lower yields.

Daehne *et al.* (1970) published on acyloxymethyl esters of penicillins that were N-deacylated using the imino chloride cleavage procedure. Pivaloyloxymethyl benzylpenicillanate (*57*) gave pivaloyloxymethyl 6-aminopenicillanate (*58*), hydrochloride salt, in about 90% yield. These esters are known to impart an improved oral absorption to penicillins (Jansen and Russell, 1965) and cephalosporins (U.S. Patent 3,488,729). They undergo hydrolysis in serum and

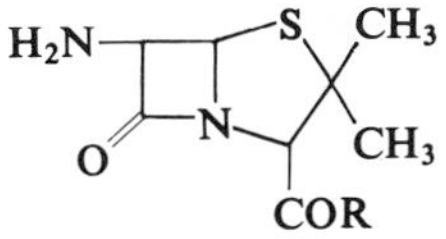

(56)

(56a) R = S—⟨benzene⟩—Cl

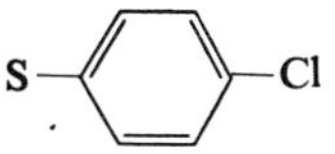

(56b) R = O—N=CHC$_6$H$_5$

(56c) R = O—N=CH—⟨furan⟩

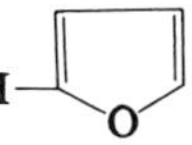

tissue by nonspecific esterases to regenerate the biologically active free acid. The preparation of these penicillin esters was clearly intended to improve the oral efficacy of β-lactam antibiotics. The motive behind their side chain cleavage was that of replacing the phenylacetyl moiety of benzylpenicillin by the phenylglycyl grouping in the ampicillin derivative (59) and not for generating 6-APA. It is conceivable, however, that the aminoester (58) would easily convert to 6-APA.

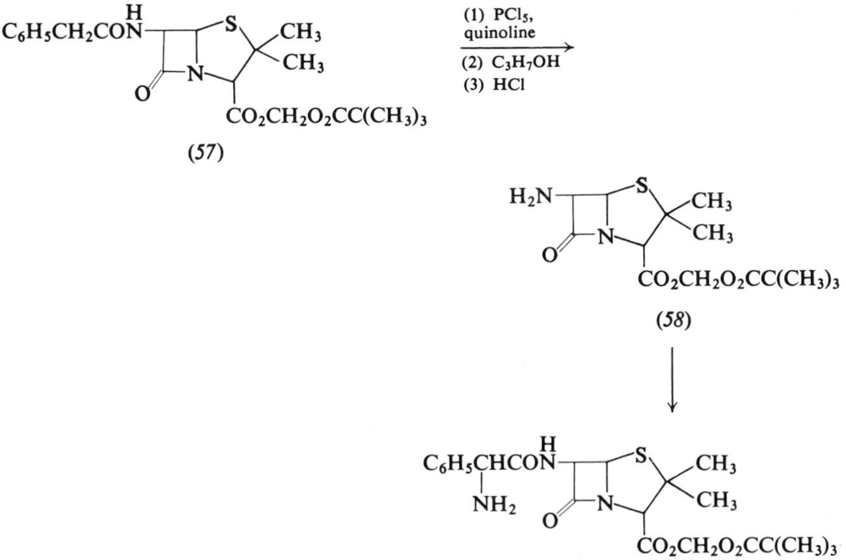

(57)

(1) PCl$_5$, quinoline
(2) C$_3$H$_7$OH
(3) HCl

(58)

(59)

Penicillin side chains have been removed in the imino chloride cleavage, using acetic mixed anhydride protection (Chauvette *et al.*, 1972) in a manner analogous to cephalosporin C. Both benzyl penicillin, sodium salt, and phenoxymethyl penicillin free acid were converted to mixed anhydrides by reaction with acetyl chloride and diethylaniline in methylene chloride at room temperature. In each case, the mixture was chilled to −60° for addition of more diethylaniline and phosphorus pentachloride in methylene chloride solution. After 1.5 hours, cold methanol was added. After another 30 minutes, the mixture was poured into water and stirred for 5 minutes. The aqueous layer was separated and immediately adjusted to pH 3.4. The crystalline product was filtered, washed successively with cold 50% aqueous methanol, cold acetone, and vacuum dried. Yields of 6-APA approached 60%.

An interesting nonenzymatic conversion of a penicillin to 6-APA has been reported (Johnson *et al.*, 1966; U.S. Patent 3,271,409). The reduction of *o*-nitrophenoxymethylpenicillin (*60*) was accompanied by a ring closure of the

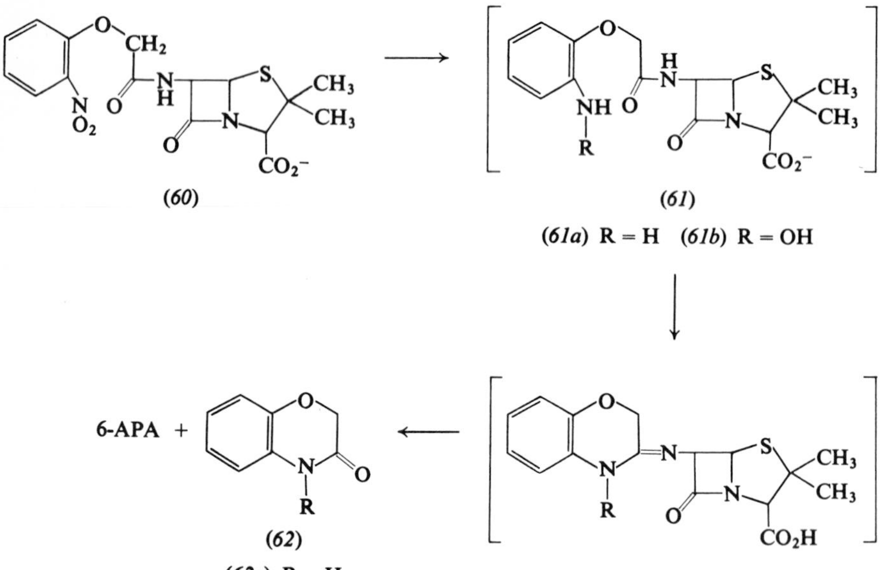

(*60*)　　　　　　　　　　(*61*)

(*61a*) R = H　(*61b*) R = OH

6-APA +

(*62*)

(*62a*) R = H
(*62b*) R = OH

newly formed amino group onto the 6-amide linkage, resulting in a spontaneous cleavage of the side chain. A variety of *o*-nitrophenyl substituted penicillins were reduced in cold, aqueous solutions to their corresonding 2-amino (*61a*) intermediates using hydrogen and palladium catalysts or to 2-hydroxylamino (*61b*) intermediates with sodium borohydride, in the presence of a catalytic amount of 5 % palladium on carbon. The anilino intermediates were unstable at room temperature and degraded to 6-APA and benzoxazine (*62a*) or *N*-hydroxybenzoxazine (*62b*). The 6-aminopenicillanic acid was conveniently isolated in 46 % yield by a direct crystallization from solvent extracts containing the weakly basic amines from the filtered reduction mixtures, when acidified to pH 2. While the substrates for this study were prepared in the laboratory by appropriate acylations of 6-APA, *o*-nitrophenoxymethylpenicillin (*60*) could presumably be made by direct fermentation with *o*-nitrophenoxyacetic acid-precursed penicillin broth (U.S. Patents 2,479,295; 2,479,296; 2,502,410; 2,623,876).

Still another potentially workable nonenzymatic side chain cleavage of penicillin has been indicated by work in the cephalosporins. In the mid-1960's, Cocker *et al.* (1965) observed a spontaneous deacylation of 7-chloroacetamidocephalosporanic acid (*63*) by thiourea, during attempts to displace the acetoxyl radical at the C-3 methyl by sulfur nucleophiles. Using conditions which normally displaced the acetoxyl group of 7-phenylacetamidocephalosporanic acid to give a 3-amidinothiomethyl-3-cephem derivative as an inner salt, the 7-chloroacetamido compound was suspended in water, dissolved by adjusting to pH 7, then heated at 31° for 65 hours with excess thiourea. 7-ACA precipitated during the course of the reaction.

The aqueous filtrate was shown to contain both iminothiazolidone (*64*) and thiourea.

Chloromethylpenicillin from biosynthesis or from acylation of 6-APA (U.S. Patent 2,941,995) would be expected to undergo a like intramolecular displacement of the acyl grouping with thiourea to generate 6-APA. This reaction has not been reported previously. It must be assumed that the idea, as applied to penicillin, was completely overlooked or was not successfully exploited. The generality of the action of thiourea in the removal of the *N*-chloroacetyl block has now been recognized (Masaki *et al.*, 1968).

It should be pointed out that the amide cleavage reactions just described for *o*-nitrophenoxymethylpenicillin (*60*) and prophesized for 6-chloromethylpenicillin do not have the same merit in the corresponding cephalosporins, as a source of 7-ACA. Unlike penicillins, cephalosporins cannot be precursed by addition of a chosen substituted acetic acid to their fermentation. Neither *o*-nitrophenoxyacetamido- nor chloroacetamidocephalosporanic acid is attainable by direct fermentation. As an added consideration, however, were these penicillins economically produced biosynthetically, they could conceivably become the starting materials for making 7-ADCA (*34*) via the penicillin sulfoxide ester rearrangement route.

Beyond the scope of this chapter are a substantial number of *N*-deacylation reactions of both penicillin and cephalosporin derivatives that do not constitute side chain degradations to 6-APA or 7-ACA in a preparative sense. The catalytic hydrogenolysis of N-carbobenzoxy-6-aminopenicillanic acid (Gr. Brit. Patent 894,368; U.S. Patent 3,107,250) and the acid hydrolysis of N-formyl 7-aminocephalosporanic acid (Neth. Patent 69,16634) are examples of

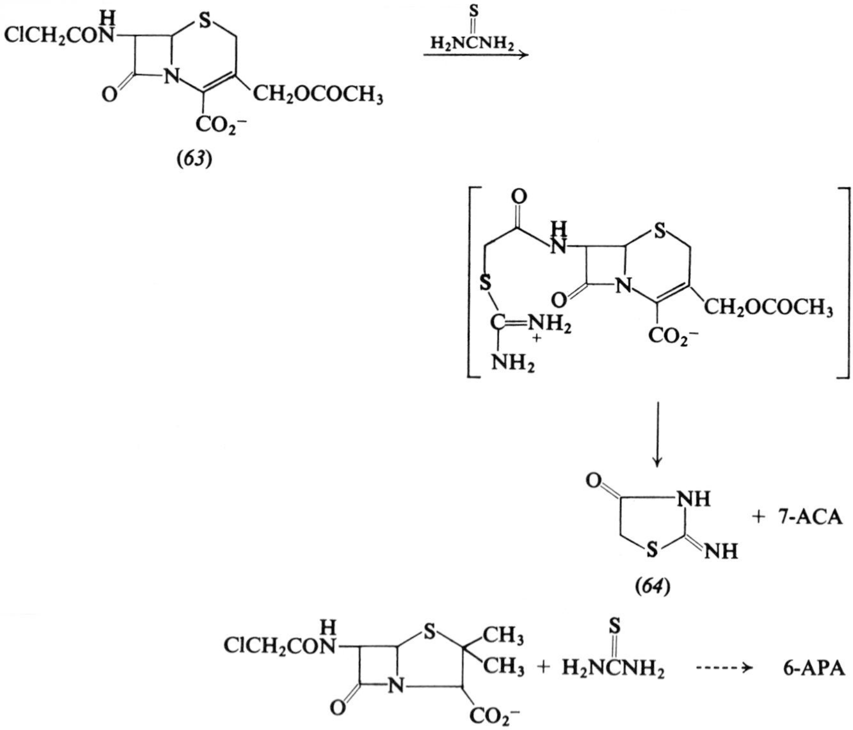

(63)

(64)

+ 7-ACA

(65)

N-deblocking procedures applied to β-lactam molecules but well recognized in synthetic organic chemistry. Regenerations of 6-APA and 7-ACA of this type have not been reviewed here.

References

Abraham, E. P., and Newton, G. G. F. (1961). *Biochem. J.* **79**, 373.
Australia Patent 19,908.
Batchelor, F. R., Doyle, F. P., Nayler, J. H. C., and Rolinson, G. N. (1959). *Nature* **183**, 257.
Batchelor, F. R., Chain, E. B., Richards, M., and Rolinson, G. N. (1961). *Proc. Roy. Soc.* (*London*) *Ser. B.* **154**, 522.
Behrens, O. K., Corse, J., Edwards, J. P., Garrison, L., Jones, R. G., Soper, Q. F., Van Abeele, F. R., and Whitehead, C. W. (1948). *J. Biol. Chem.* **175**, 793.
Belgium Patent 628,493.
Belgium Patent 645,157.

Belgium Patent 717,741.
Belgium Patent 718,824.
Belgium Patent 719,710.
Belgium Patent 719,712.
Belgium Patent 720,185.
Belgium Patent 734,565.
Belgium Patent 746,860.
Belgium Patent 758,800.
Belgium Patent 759,064.
Bellamy, L. J. (1958). "The Infrared Spectra of Complex Molecules," 2nd ed., p. 189. Methuen, London.
Brandl, E. (1965). *Z. Physiol. Chem.* **342**, 86.
Chauvette, R. R., and Flynn, E. H. (1966). *J. Med. Chem.* **9**, 741.
Chauvette, R. R., Pennington, P. A., Ryan, C. W., Cooper, R. D. G., Jose, F. L., Wright, I. G., Van Heyningen, E. M., and Huffman, G. W. (1971). *J. Org. Chem.* **36**, 1259.
Chauvette, R. R., Hayes, H. B., Huff, G. L., and Pennington, P. A. (1972). *J. Antibiotics* in press.
Chiang, C., and Bennett, R. E. (1967). *J. Bacteriol.* **93**, 302.
Claridge, C. A., Gourevitch, A., and Lein, S. (1960). *Nature* **187**, 237.
Claridge, C. A., Luttinger, J. R., and Lein, S. (1963). *Proc. Soc. Exp. Biol. Med.* **113**, 1008.
Cocker, J. D., Cowley, B. R., Cox, J. S. G., Eardley, S., Gregory, G. I., Lazenby, J. K., Long, A. G., Sly, J. C. P., and Somerfield, G. A. (1965). *J. Chem. Soc.* 5015.
Cole, M. (1964). *Nature* **203**, 519.
Cole, M. (1966). *Appl. Microbiol.* **14**, 98.
Cole, M. (1969a). *Biochem. J.* **115**, 733.
Cole, M. (1969b). *Biochem. J.* **115**, 741.
Cole, M. (1969c). *Biochem. J.* **115**, 747.
Cole, M., and Rolinson, G. N. (1961). *Proc. Roy. Soc. (London) Ser. B.* **154**, 490.
Cole, M., and Sutherland, R. (1966). *J. Gen. Microbiol.* **42**, 345.
Cooper, D. E., and Binkley, S. B. (1948). *J. Amer. Chem. Soc.* **70**, 3966.
Daehne, W. v., Frederiksen, E., Gundersen, E., Lund, F., Mørch, P., Petersen, H. J., Roholt, K., Tybring, L., and Godtfredsen, W. O. (1970). *J. Med. Chem.* **13**, 607.
Demain, A. L., Walton, R. B., Newkirk, J. F., and Miller, I. M. (1963). *Nature* **199**, 909.
Doyle, F. P., and Nayler, J. H. C. (1965). *In* "Advances in Drug Research" (N. J. Harper and A. B. Simmonds, eds.), Vol. I, pp. 1–69. Academic Press, London and New York.
English, A. R., Huang, H. T., and Sobin, B. A. (1960). *Proc. Soc. Exp. Biol. Med.* **104**, 405.
Erickson, R. C., and Bennett, R. E. (1961). *Bacteriol. Proc.* 65.
Erickson, R. C., and Bennett, R. E. (1965). *Appl. Microbiol.* **13**, 738.
Fechtig, B., Peter, H., Bickel, H., and Vischer, E. (1968). *Helv. Chim. Acta* **51**, 1108.
France Patent 1,376,905.
Germany Patent 1,928,142.
Germany Patent 1,937,962.
Great Britain Patent 894,368.
Great Britain Patent 1,041,985.
Great Britain Patent 1,119,806.
Green, G. F. H., Page, J. E., and Staniforth, S. E. (1965). *J. Chem. Soc.* 1595.
Hamilton-Miller, J. M. T. (1966). *Bacteriol. Rev.* **30**, 761.
Hamilton-Miller, J. M. T., Smith, J. T., and Knox, R. (1963). *J. Pharm. Pharmacol.* **15**, 81.
Hodgkin, D. C., and Maslen, E. N. (1961). *Biochem. J.* **79**, 393.
Holt, R. J., and Stewart, G. T. (1964a). *J. Gen. Microbiol.* **36**, 203.

Holt, R. J., and Stewart, G. T. (1964b). *Nature* **201**, 824.
Huang, H. T., English, A. R., Seto, T. A., Shull, G. M., and Sobin, B. A. (1960). *J. Amer. Chem. Soc.* **82**, 3790.
Huang, H. T., Seto, T. A., and Shull, G. M. (1963). *Appl. Microbiol.* **11**, 1.
Jansen, A. B. A., and Russell, T. R. (1965). *J. Chem. Soc.* 2127.
Johnson, D. A., Panetta, C. A., and Smith, R. R. (1966). *J. Org. Chem.* **31**, 2560.
Kaiser, G. V., Ashbrook, C. W., Goodson, T., Wright, I. G., and Van Heyningen, E. M. (1971). *J. Med. Chem.* **14**.
Kameda, Y., Kimura, Y., Toyoura, E., and Omori, T. (1961). *Nature* **191**, 1122.
Kaufmann, W., and Bauer, K. (1960). *Naturweissenschaften* **47**, 474.
Kaufmann, W., and Bauer, K. (1964a). *J. Gen. Microbiol.* **35**, iv.
Kaufmann, W., and Bauer, K. (1964b). *Nature* **203**, 520.
Kaufmann, W., Bauer, K., and Offee, H. A. (1961). *Antimicrob. Ag. Ann.* **1960**, 1.
Loder, B., Newton, G. G. F., and Abraham, E. P. (1961). *Biochem. J.* **79**, 408.
Masaki, M., Kitahara, T., Juriba, H., and Ohta, M. (1968). *J. Amer. Chem. Soc.* **90**, 4508.
Morin, R. B., Jackson, B. G., Flynn, E. H., and Roeske, R. W. (1962). *J. Amer. Chem. Soc.* **84**, 3400.
Morin, R. B., Jackson, B. G., Flynn, E. H., and Roeske, R. W. (1969). *J. Amer. Chem. Soc.* **91**, 1396.
Murao, S. (1955). *J. Agr. Chem. Soc. Japan* **29**, 404.
Murao, S., and Kishida, Y. (1961). *J. Agr. Chem. Soc. Japan* **35**, 607.
Netherlands Patent 66,06872.
Netherlands Patent 67,16487.
Netherlands Patent 68,12413.
Netherlands Patent 69,16634.
Newton, G. G. F., and Abraham, E. P. (1954). *Biochem. J.* **58**, 103.
Nuesch, J., Gruner, J., Knuesel, F., and Treichler, H. J. (1967). *Pathol. Microbiol.* **30**, 880.
Nyiri, L. (1967). *Nature* **214**, 1348.
Pruess, D. L., and Johnson, M. J. (1965). *J. Bacteriol.* **90**, 380.
Rolinson, G. N., Batchelor, F. R., Butterworth, D., Cameron-Wood, J., Cole, M., Eustace, G. C., Hart, M. V., Richards, M., and Chain, E. B. (1960a). *Nature* **187**, 236.
Rolinson, G. N., Batchelor, F. R., Butterworth, D., Cameron-Wood, J., Cole, M., Eustace, G. C., Hart, M. V., Richards, M., and Chain, E. B. (1960b). *Nature* **187**, 4733.
Ryan, C. W., Simon, R. L., and Van Heyningen, E. M. (1969). *J. Med. Chem.* **12**, 310.
Sakaguchi, K., and Murao, S. (1950). *J. Agr. Chem. Soc. Japan* **23**, 411.
Self, D. A., Kay, G., Lilly, M. D., and Dunnill, P. (1969). *Biotech. Bioeng.* **11**, 337.
Sheehan, J. C., and Henery-Logan, K. R. (1959). *J. Amer. Chem. Soc.* **81**, 5838.
Sheehan, J. C., and Henery-Logan, K. R. (1962). *J. Amer. Chem. Soc.* **84**, 2983.
Shimi, I. R., and Imam, G. M. (1966). *Biochem. J.* **101**, 831.
Singh, K., Schgal, S. N., and Vezina, C. (1969). *Appl. Microbiol.* **17**, 643.
Sjöberg, B., Nathorst-Westfelt, L., and Ortengren, B. (1967). *Acta Chem. Scand.* **21**, 547.
Spencer, B., and Maung, C. (1970). *Biochem. J.* **118**, 29P.
Szentirmai, A. (1964). *Appl. Microbiol.* **12**, 185.
United States Patent 2,479,295.
United States Patent 2,479,296.
United States Patent 2,502,410.
United States Patent 2,623,876.
United States Patent 2,941,995.
United States Patent 3,107,250.
United States Patent 3,124,576.

United States Patent 3,150,059.
United States Patent 3,234,223.
United States Patent 3,271,409.
United States Patent 3,278,391.
United States Patent 3,297,546.
United States Patent 3,367,933.
United States Patent 3,446,705.
United States Patent 3,488,729.
United States Patent 3,499,909.
United States Patent 3,507,862.
Uri, J., Valu, G., and Bekesi, I. (1963). *Nature* **200**, 896.
Uri, J., Valu, G., and Bekesi, I. (1964). *Naturweissenschaften* **51**, 298.
Vanderhaeghe, H., Claesen, M., Vlietinck, A., and Parmentier, G. (1968). *Appl. Microbiol.* **16**, 1557.
Waldschmidt-Leitz, E., and Bretzel, G. (1964). *Z. Physiol. Chem.* **337**, 222.
Walton, R. B. (1964a). *Develop. Ind. Microbiol.* **5**, 349.
Walton, R. B. (1964b). *Science* **143**, 1438.

Chapter 3

MODIFICATIONS OF THE β-LACTAM SYSTEM

GARY V. KAISER and STJEPAN KUKOLJA

I. Reactions of the Side Chain Amino Group

A. Introduction

In the early stages of research on penicillin antibiotics, the significance of different N-acyl side chains was recognized. All of the several hundred natural penicillins contain the bicyclic ring system, 6-aminopenicillanic acid (6-APA) as a common feature, but they differ in the side chain amide group. The side chains were incorporated into the compounds biochemically by adding various N-acyl precursors, mostly derivatives of acetic acid, to fermentation media. The structures of some representative naturally occurring and precursed penicillins are shown in Table I.

Table I

SIDE CHAINS IN NATURAL PENICILLINS

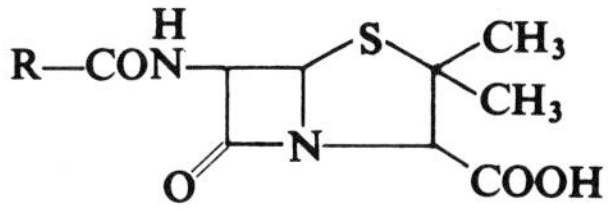

R	Name	Penicillin
$CH_3CH_2CH{=}CHCH_2-$	2-Pentenyl	F
$CH_3(CH_2)_3CH_2-$	n-Amyl	Dihydro F
$CH_3(CH_2)_5CH_2-$	n-Heptyl	K
$CH_2{=}CHCH_2SCH_2-$	Allylthiomethyl	O
$CH_3{-}C{=}CHCH_2SCH_2-$ $\quad\vert$ $\quad Cl$	3-Chloro-2-butenyl-thiomethyl	S
$CH_3(CH_2)_3SCH_2-$	Butylthiomethyl	BT
$NH_2C(CH_2)_2CH_2-$ $\quad\vert$ $\quad CO_2H$	Aminoadipyl	N
$C_6H_5{-}CH_2-$	Benzyl	G
$C_6H_5{-}OCH_2-$	Phenoxymethyl	V
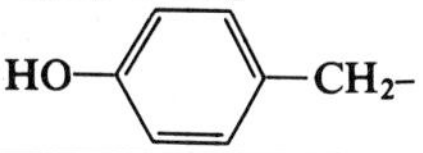 $HO-\bigcirc-CH_2-$	p-Hydroxybenzyl	X

Many of these antibiotics display antibacterial potency comparable to that of penicillin G, and the structural formulas show that a wide variation of the side chain is possible without loss of activity. Although the available penicillins were considered to be outstanding antibiotics, extensive application in chemotherapy revealed serious limitations, two of which were the susceptibility to inactivation by the enzyme penicillinase and low activity against gram-negative bacteria. When 6-APA became available on a large scale by fermentation, more significant modifications of the 6-amino substituents were possible. Limitations previously encountered were the result of selective incorporation of N-acyl precursors by the *Penicillium* fungus.

The discovery of cephalosporin C and its successful cleavage to 7-aminocephalosporanic acid (7-ACA) stimulated further interest in the investigation of β-lactam antibiotics—specifically the preparation of semisynthetic cephalosporins. Within the last few years several excellent reviews covering chemistry (Sheehan, 1964, 1967; Doyle and Nayler, 1964; Van Heyningen, 1967; Manhas and Bose, 1969), stucture activity relationships (Abraham,

1968; Price, 1969), pharmacology (Lynn, 1966; Busch and Lane, 1967; Smith et al., 1969), and clinical aspects (Herrell, 1968) of semisynthetic β-lactam antibiotics have been published. The problems concerning the methods of introducing various N-acyl groups into 6-APA and 7-ACA will be discussed in the next section.

B. Acylation of the Amino Group

1. Acylation of 6-Aminopenicillanic Acid

The procedures used for introduction of N-acyl groups into 6-APA and 7-ACA depend upon the particular properties of the acylating group, as well as on the sensitivity of the β-lactam function. In general, many of the techniques employed in peptide chemistry are applicable to the preparation of semisynthetic penicillins and cephalosporins.

Batchelor and co-workers (1959) disclosed the first isolation of 6-aminopenicillanic acid (6-APA) (1). Soon after, this compound was available in quantity, which resulted in the synthesis of numerous new semisynthetic penicillins.

Perron and associates (1960) reported the acylation of 6-APA with a variety of DL, L, and D α-aryloxyalkanoic acids (2) through the acid chloride or the mixed anhydride method. The acid chlorides were reacted with 6-APA in aqueous acetone in the presence of sodium bicarbonate. The reactions with mixed anhydrides were performed in nonaqueous solvents in the presence of triethylamine. The new penicillins (3) were obtained in good yield and isolated as potassium salts. Potassium 2-ethylhexanoate was frequently used to prepare the salts. Some α-substituted phenoxypenicillins (3) prepared according to the above procedure have increased acid stability.

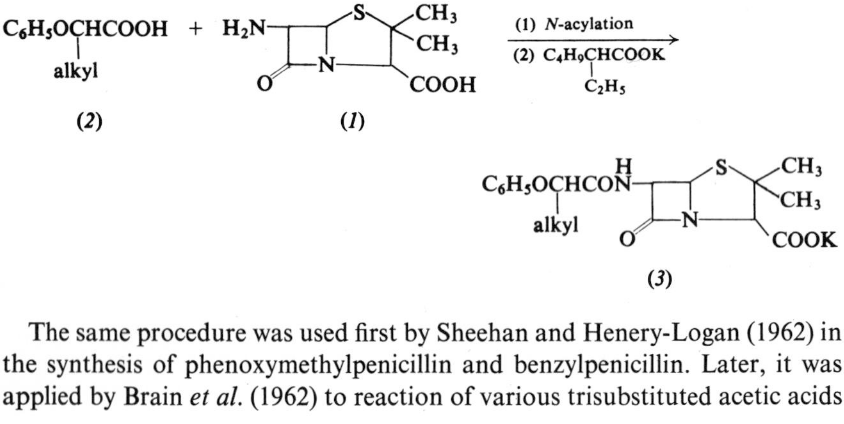

The same procedure was used first by Sheehan and Henery-Logan (1962) in the synthesis of phenoxymethylpenicillin and benzylpenicillin. Later, it was applied by Brain et al. (1962) to reaction of various trisubstituted acetic acids with 6-APA, by Doyle *et al.* (1962b) in preparation of a series of 2,6-dialkoxy-phenylpenicillins and by Pala *et al.* (1970) in the synthesis of terpenyl penicillins.

Perron *et al.* (1961) found that 6-APA reacts readily with isocyanates and isothiocyanates (*4*) in dimethylformamide or methylene chloride in the presence of an excess of triethylamine to give triethylammonium 6-(substituted ureido)- and 6-(substituted thioureido)penicillanates (*5*). Yields varied from 28 to 91%. The same investigators treated 6-APA in dimethylformamide in the presence of triethylamine with a variety of cyclic anhydrides and isolated crystalline monotriethylammonium salts (*6*) of the corresponding carboxy penicillins.

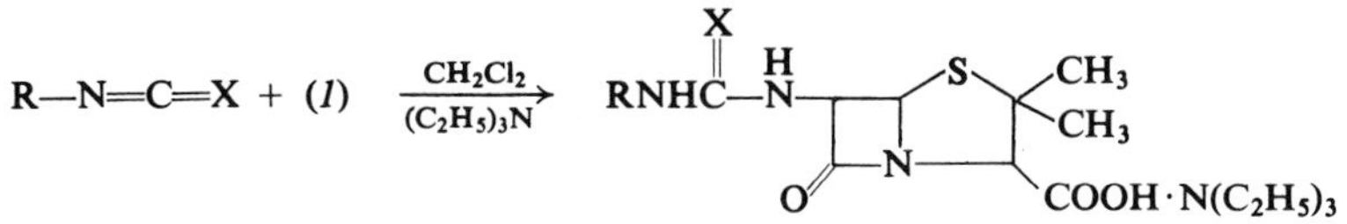

R = alkyl or aryl
X = O or S

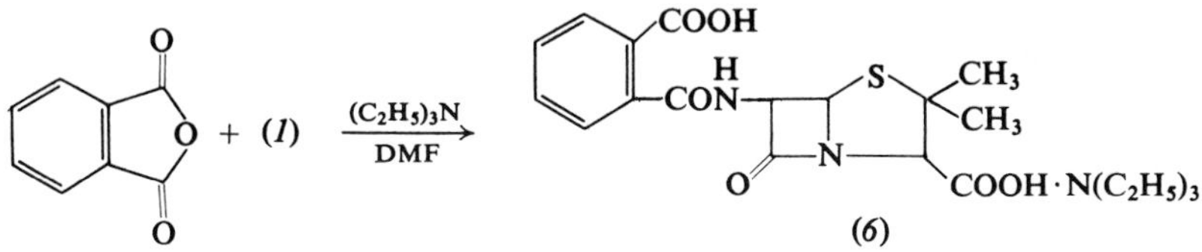

The same group of workers have described a number of 6-(*N*-substituted *N'*-phthalamido)penicillanic acids (*8*), isolated as sodium or potassium salts (Perron *et al.*, 1962). They prepared these penicillins by condensing N-substituted phthalamic acids (*7*) with 6-APA via the mixed anhydride method using either ethyl or isobutyl chloroformate. Treatment of 6-APA with phthalamic

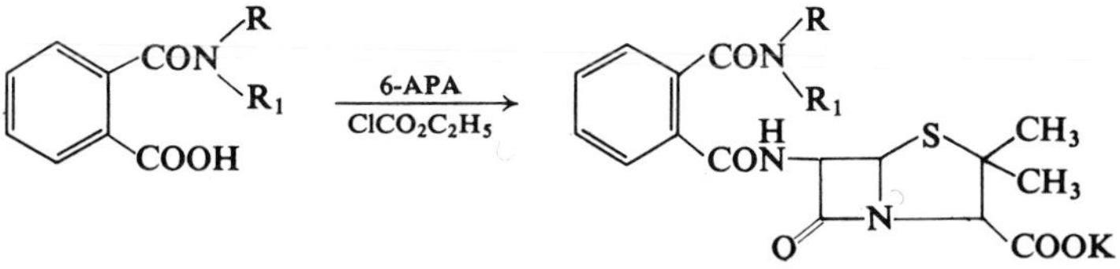

acid (*9*) did not result in the desired product. Application of the mixed anhydride procedure to this acid gave *o*-cyanobenzoic acid (*10*) as a major product and a minute quantity of 6-(*o*-cyanobenzamido)penicillanic acid (*11*). The mixed anhydride method when applied to *N*-carbethoxyphthalamic acid

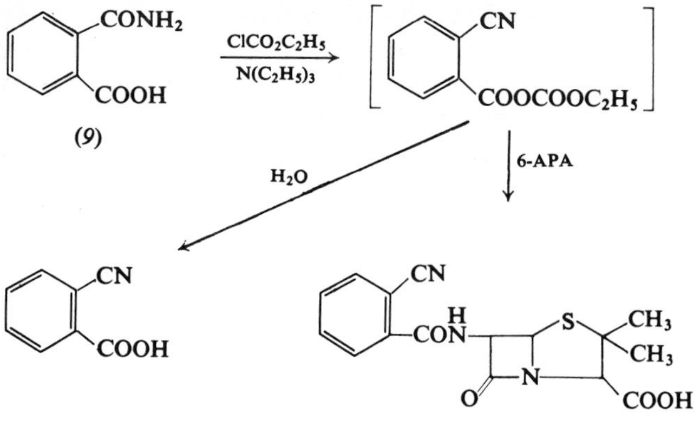

(12) afforded 6-phthalimidopenicillanic acid (13), also obtained from 6-APA and N-carbethoxyphthalimide (14) previously by Nefkens et al. (1960) and by Sheehan and Henery-Logan (1962).

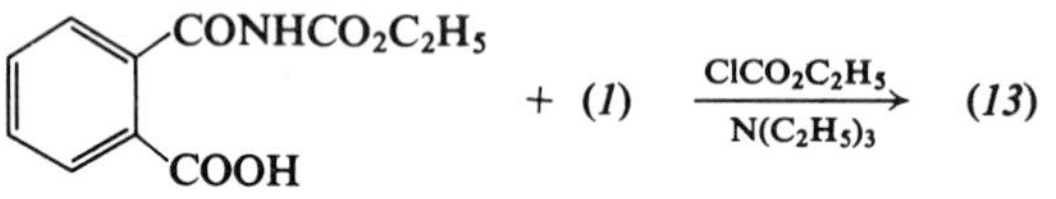

Doyle and co-workers (1962a) have described the synthesis of α-amino-benzylpenicillins. They prepared N-benzyloxycarbonyl-α-aminopenicillins (16) by condensation of the corresponding N-benzyloxycarbonylamino acids (15) and 6-APA via the mixed anhydride coupling. The mixed anhydride was prepared using ethyl chloroformate and triethylamine and, without isolation, was reacted with 6-APA in cold sodium bicarbonate solution. The N-protecting group was removed by catalytic hydrogenation with palladium catalyst to give the α-amino-substituted penicillin (17).

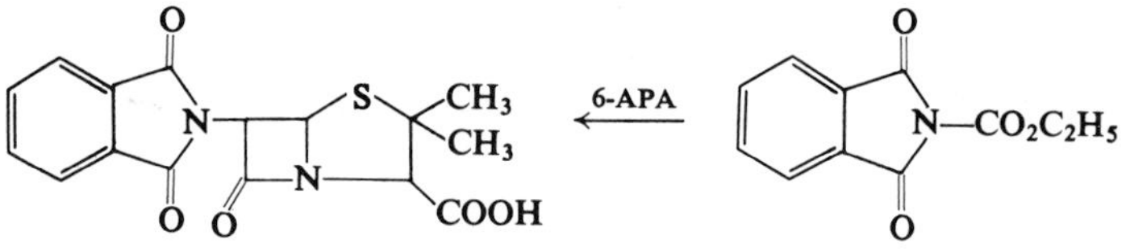

The preceding reference describes only L(+)- and D-α-aminobenzylpenicil-lins. Other derivatives are described in detail in a patent (Gr. Brit. Patent 873,049).

Ekstrom *et al.* (1965) discussed the problems encountered in the selection of protecting groups for the synthesis of amino acid derivatives of penicillin. They used α-azido acid intermediates (*18*) for the acylation of 6-APA since the

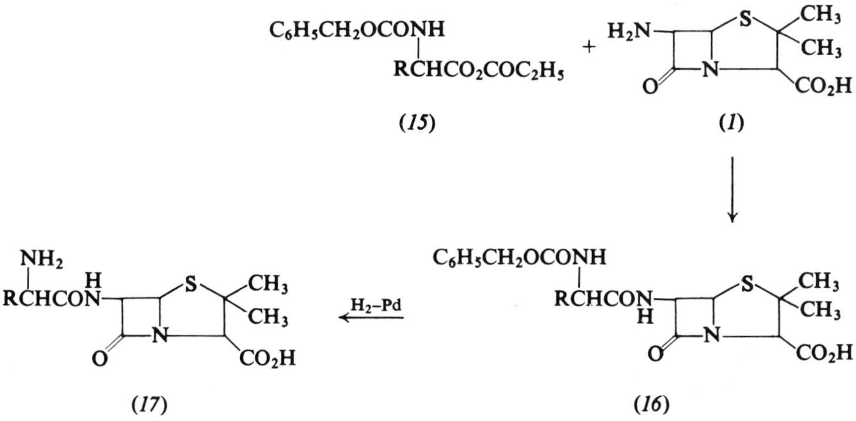

(*15*) (*1*)

(*17*) (*16*)

azido function could later be hydrogenated to the amino group. The α-azido acid chlorides [(*18*) Y = Cl] were usually employed. They were synthesized by treating the appropriate acid with an excess of thionyl chloride in dry ether. In some cases they used the mixed anhydrides or the acid azides [(*18*), Y = N$_3$] for the coupling reaction. For the acylation of 6-APA, a solution of acid chloride in acetone was added to a suspension of 6-APA in aqueous acetone, and neutral pH was maintained by the addition of sodium bicarbonate. Condensation with the acid azide was performed in a mixture of ether and water.

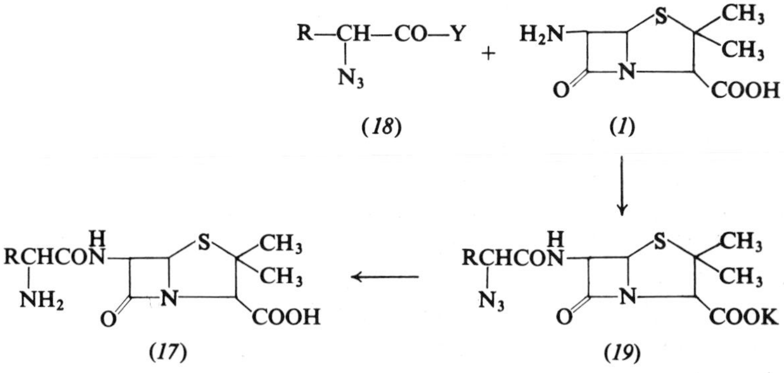

(*18*) (*1*)

(*17*) (*19*)

Mixed anhydride condensations were carried out in aqueous dimethylformamide, using triethylamine as base. Hydrogenations of the azido group in (*19*) were carried out in water using prehydrogenated palladium on calcium carbonate or a Raney nickel catalyst. The amino-substituted penicillins (17) were isolated in 60–90% yield.

Dane and Dockner (1965) described an improved method for the synthesis of α-amino substituted penicillins (17). They demonstrated the usefulness of the β-dicarbonyl-blocking group for the protection of the amino function in amino acids. By the interaction of D-phenylglycine (20) and ethyl acetoacetate (21) in warm methanol in the presence of potassium hydroxide, the corresponding potassium salt of the N-protected phenylglycine (22) was obtained in 81% yield.

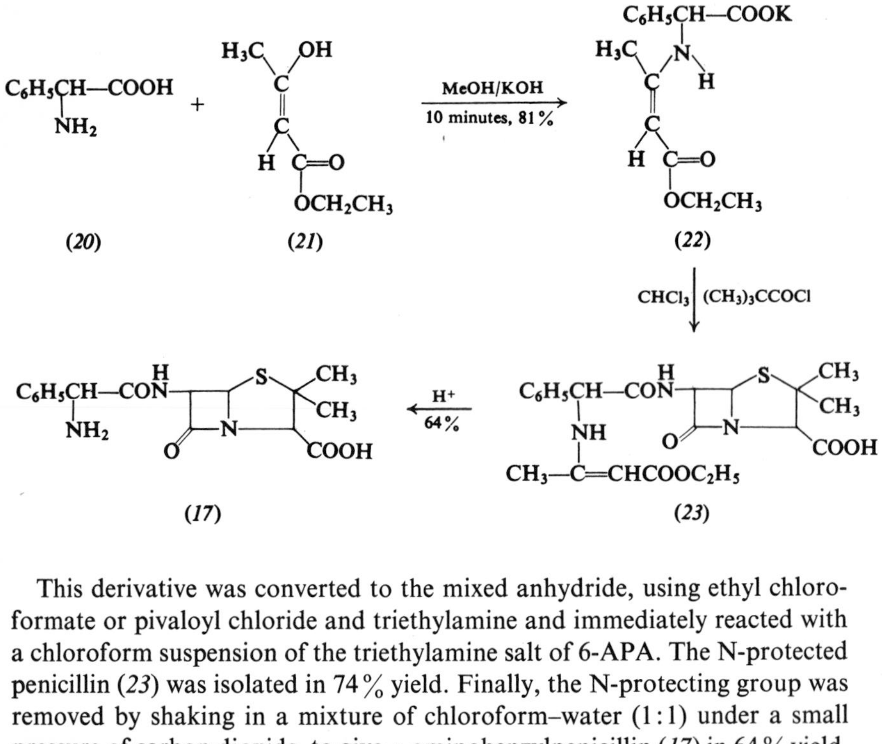

This derivative was converted to the mixed anhydride, using ethyl chloroformate or pivaloyl chloride and triethylamine and immediately reacted with a chloroform suspension of the triethylamine salt of 6-APA. The N-protected penicillin (23) was isolated in 74% yield. Finally, the N-protecting group was removed by shaking in a mixture of chloroform–water (1:1) under a small pressure of carbon dioxide, to give α-aminobenzylpenicillin (17) in 64% yield.

Daehne et al. (1970) discovered a similar pathway for the preparation of ampicillin (17) by acylating pivaloyloxymethyl 6-aminopenicillanate via the acid chloride or mixed anhydride method.

When 6-APA was reacted with the unprotected D-phenylglycyl moiety (24) in aqueous acetone, an interesting imidazolidinone penicillin (25) (hetacillin) was obtained in 50% yield (Hardcastle et al., 1966). The same product was prepared by the reaction of (17) with acetone and the structure was determined by X-ray diffraction analysis.

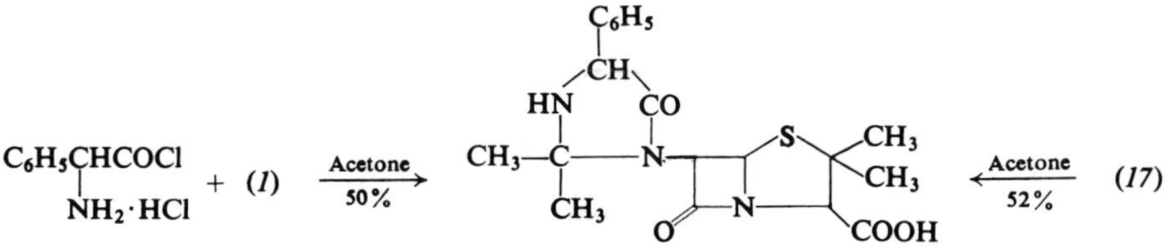

$$\begin{array}{c} C_6H_5 \\ CH \\ HN \quad CO \\ CH_3-C-N \\ CH_3 \end{array} \quad S \quad CH_3$$

$$C_6H_5CHCOCl \quad + \quad (1) \quad \xrightarrow[\text{50%}]{\text{Acetone}} \quad \text{(25)} \quad \xleftarrow[\text{52%}]{\text{Acetone}} \quad (17)$$

$$\underset{NH_2 \cdot HCl}{|}$$

(24)   (25)

The acylation of 6-aminopenicillanate esters having an easily removable carboxyl protecting group and, therefore, soluble in organic solvents has been reported. Glombitza (1964) discovered that 6-APA trialkylsilyl esters (26) could be readily obtained by reacting 6-APA with hexamethyldisilazane in chloroform; the ester (26) was successfully acylated with acid chlorides or by the mixed anhydride method. The advantage of this sequence is that the silyl group in (27) was removed merely by treatment with water during the workup procedure. The penicillins (28) were synthesized in high yields (65–98%).

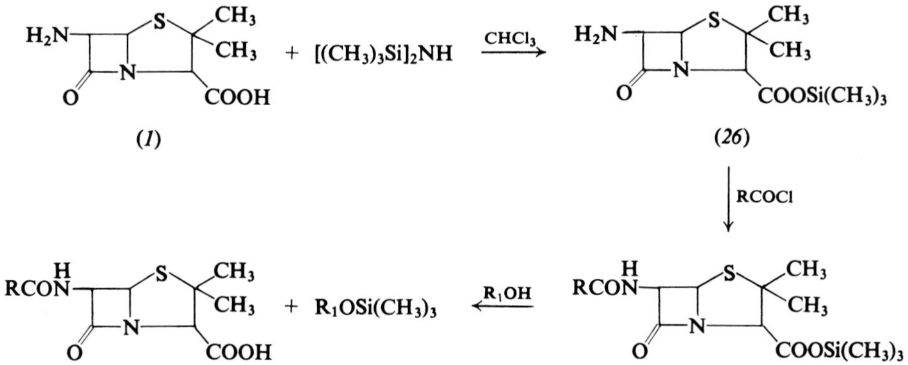

$$H_2N \quad S \quad CH_3 \qquad + \quad [(CH_3)_3Si]_2NH \quad \xrightarrow{CHCl_3} \quad H_2N \quad S \quad CH_3$$
$$\qquad N \quad CH_3 \qquad\qquad\qquad\qquad\qquad\qquad\qquad N \quad CH_3$$
$$O \qquad COOH \qquad\qquad\qquad\qquad\qquad\qquad O \qquad COOSi(CH_3)_3$$

(1)   (26)

$$\Big\downarrow RCOCl$$

$$RCON \overset{H}{\quad} S \quad CH_3 \qquad + \quad R_1OSi(CH_3)_3 \quad \xleftarrow{R_1OH} \quad RCON \overset{H}{\quad} S \quad CH_3$$
$$\qquad N \quad CH_3 \qquad\qquad\qquad\qquad\qquad\qquad\qquad N \quad CH_3$$
$$O \qquad COOH \qquad\qquad\qquad\qquad\qquad\qquad O \qquad COOSi(CH_3)_3$$

(28)   (27)

$R = C_6H_5CH_2-; \quad C_6H_5OCH_2-; \quad C_6H_5OCH-; \quad C_6H_5OCH- \quad ; \quad C_6H_5OCH-;$
$\qquad\qquad\qquad\qquad\qquad\qquad\qquad CH_3 \qquad\quad CH_2CH_3 \qquad\quad C_6H_5$

$$C_6H_5OC- \; ; \qquad \underset{OCH_3}{\overset{OCH_3}{\bigodot}} \quad ; \qquad \bigodot - \underset{\underset{O \quad CH_3}{N \quad C}}{C-C-}$$
$$\underset{CH_3}{\overset{CH_3}{|}}$$

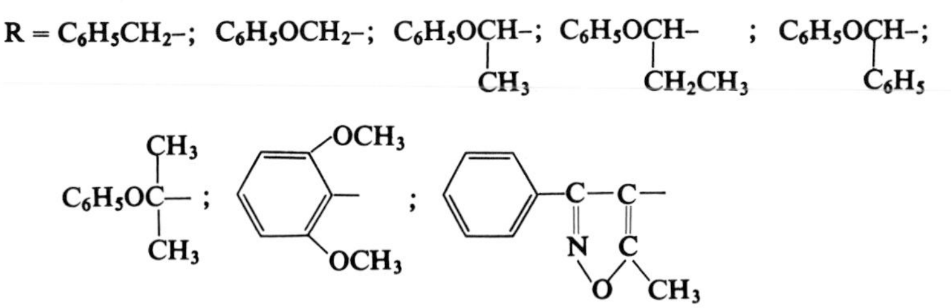

Similarly, the reaction of silyl ester (26) with δ-butyrolactone-α-carboxylic acids followed by mild acid hydrolysis afforded 6-(δ-butyrolactone-α-carb-amido)penicillanic acid or its α-butyl derivative (Rozanova and Strukov, 1969).

Bamberg and associates (1967) demonstrated the use of 6-APA phenacyl esters in the preparation of various pyridylmethyl penicillins. They found that good yields were obtained by coupling of the pyridylacetic acids and 6-APA phenylacyl ester (29) in dimethylformamide with dicyclohexylcarbodiimide. Following the procedure of Sheehan and Daves (1964), the carboxyl protecting group in (30) was removed with potassium thiophenoxide in dimethylformamide, giving the potassium salt of the penicillins (31). Crystalline salts could be isolated in as much as 64% yield.

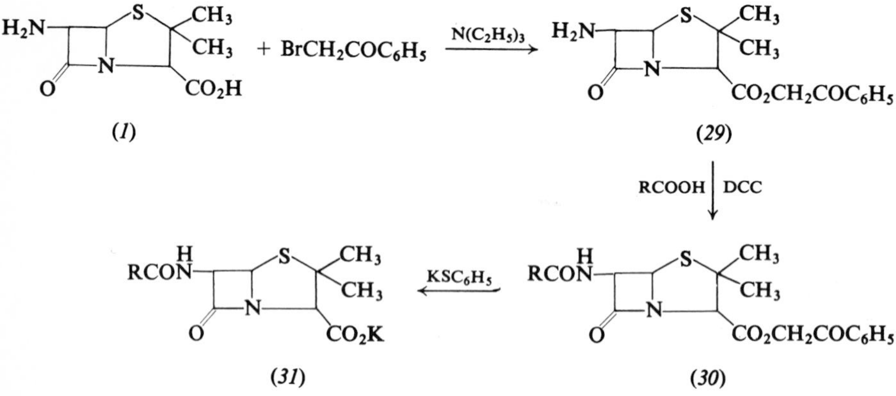

R = pyridylmethyl

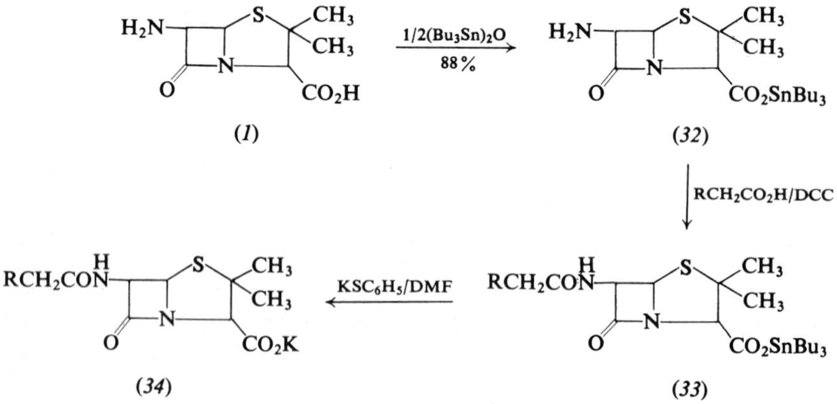

Bamberg et al. (1968) also reported the use of tributyltin 6-aminopenicillanate in penicillin synthesis. 6-APA tributyltin ester (32) was prepared in 88% yield by treatment of 6-APA with tributyltin oxide in benzene with azeotropic removal of the water formed. The resulting ester was acylated with heterocyclic acetic acids in methylene chloride using dicyclohexylcarbodiimide. After acylation, the tributyltin group in (*33*) was hydrolyzed with potassium thio-phenoxide in dimethylformamide and the potassium salts (*34*) were isolated in 40–60 % yield.

Coupling of α-guanidinophenylacetic acid (*35*) with benzyl ester (*36*) in the presence of dicyclohexylcarbodiimide was reported by Leanza *et al.* (1965). After acylation was completed, the benzyl group in (*37*) was removed by cataly-tic hydrogenolysis. The guanidinopenicillins (*38*) were isolated as the zwitterions.

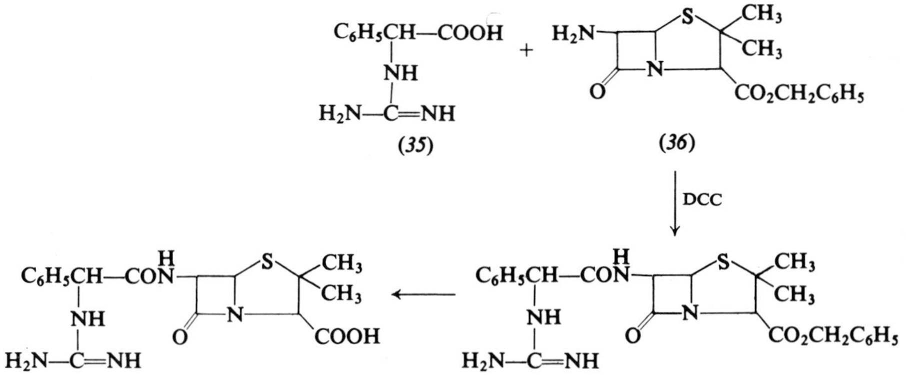

(*35*)   (*36*)

DCC

(*38*)   (*37*)

2. ACYLATION OF 7-AMINOCEPHALOSPORANIC ACID

The first acylation of 7-ACA was reported by Loder and associates (1961). While working on the structure of cephalosporin C they isolated a minute amount of 7-ACA (*39*) and were able to acylate the 7-amino group with phenylacetyl chloride to produce cephaloram (*40*).

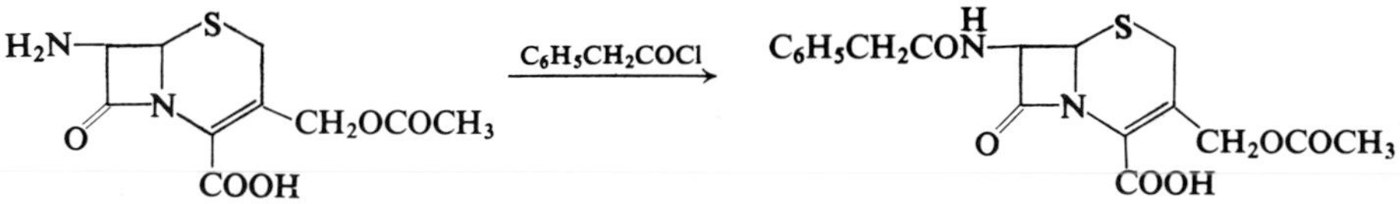

(*39*)   (*40*)

The general procedures used most frequently for the acylation of 6-APA, i.e., (a) acid chloride, (b) mixed anhydride, or (c) dicyclohexylcarbodiimide method were also employed successfully for the acylation of 7-ACA. Reac-tions have been carried out in aqueous or nonaqueous solvents using sodium bicarbonate or an organic base as an acid acceptor. In order to avoid the prob-lem of the insolubility of 7-ACA, esters have frequently been used in the acyla-tion step. Subsequent removal of the ester grouping yields the new cephalo-sporins.

A large number of 7-arylamidocephalosporanic acids have been synthesized, using modified Schotten–Baumann conditions, by the reaction of acid chlorides of substituted arylacetic acids with 7-ACA (Chauvette *et al.*, 1962; Cocker *et al.*, 1965; Kurita *et al.*, 1966; Kariyone *et al.*, 1970). For example, cephalothin (*42*), a widely used broad spectrum antibiotic, was prepared by treating 7-ACA with 2-thienylacetyl chloride (*41*) in aqueous acetone and sodium bicarbonate. The resulting product was isolated as the potassium or sodium salt in good yield (U.S. Patent 3,218,318).

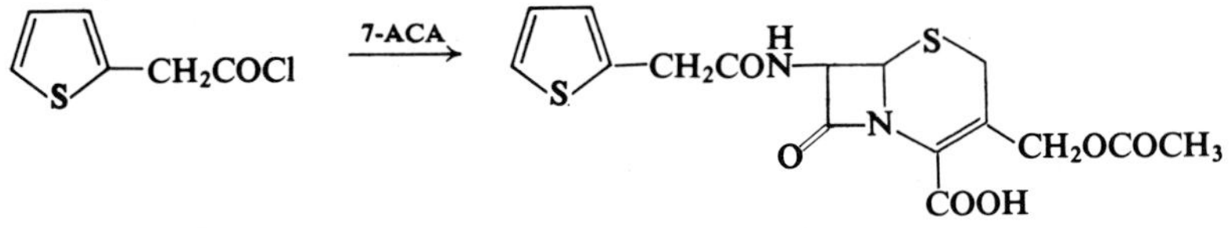

(*41*)   (*42*)

Kariyone *et al.* (1970) published a synthesis of 7-[1-(1H)-tetrazolylacetamido]cephalosporanic acid (*45*) carried out by a sequence of *N*-acylation followed by nucleophilic displacement of the acetoxy group. First the sodium salt of 7-ACA was acylated with 1-(1H)-tetrazolylacetyl chloride (*43*) in aqueous acetone and then the acetoxy substituent in (*44*) was displaced by 2-mercapto-5-methyl-1,3,4-thiadiazole in phosphate buffer (pH 6.4) to give (*45*) in good yield. This cephalosporin is known as cefazolin.

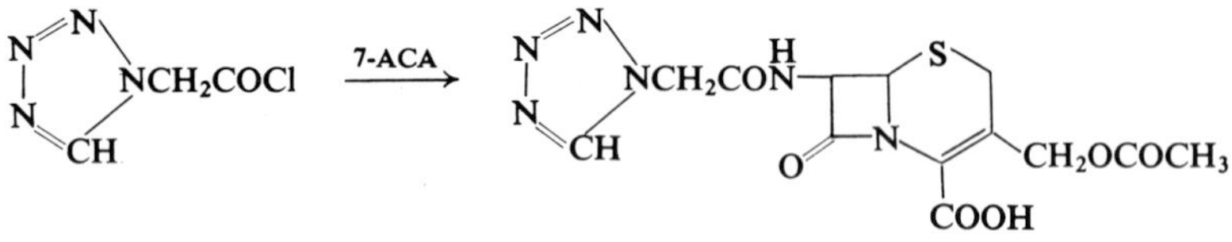

(*43*)   (*44*)

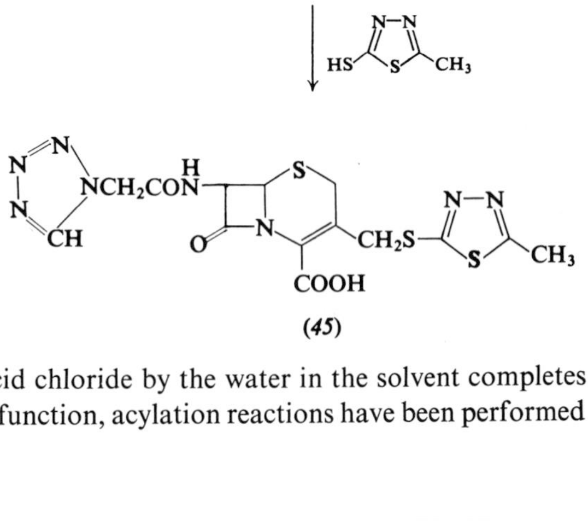

(*45*)

When hydrolysis of an acid chloride by the water in the solvent completes with acylation of the amino function, acylation reactions have been performed in dry organic solvents such as chloroform or methylene chloride in the presence of triethylamine. This technique was used to acylate 6-APA and 7-ACA with pyridineacetyl chlorides by Stedman *et al.* (1967) and with 3- and 4-substituted sydnoneacetyl chlorides by Naito *et al.* (1968a, b). It was also used in the preparation of 7-(4-pyridylthio)acetamidocephalosporanic acid (*47*), an antibacterial agent known as cephapirin (U.S. Patent 3,503,967). Freshly prepared 4-pyridylmercaptoacetyl chloride (*46*) was added to a solution of 7-ACA in methylene chloride and triethylamine, and the resulting cephalosporin (*47*) was isolated in 75% yield.

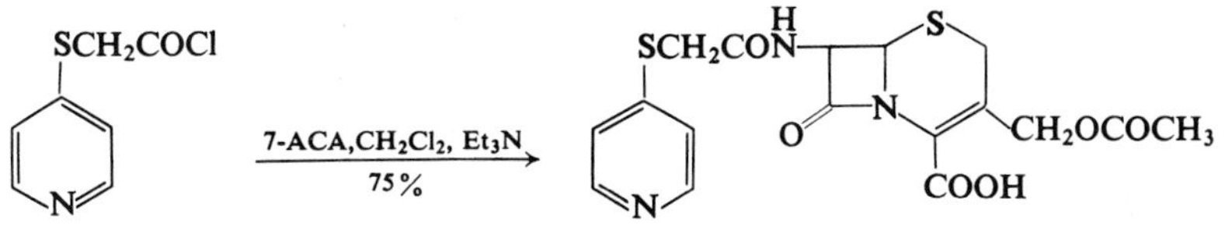

This cephalosporin derivative was also obtained by the interaction of 7-(α-bromoacetamido)cephalosporanic acid (*49*) and 4-mercaptopyridine (*48*) in sodium bicarbonate.

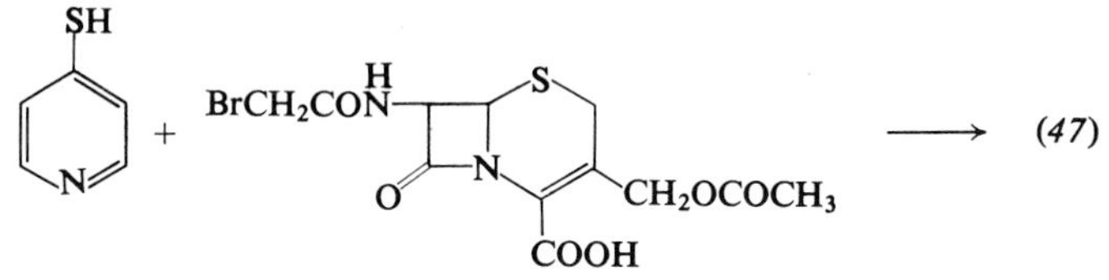

Application of the mixed anhydride technique for the acylation of 7-ACA was demonstrated in the preparation of cephacetrile (*51*), another promising cephalosporin antibiotic (Neth. Patent 6,600,586). The interaction of cyanoacetic acid [(*50*) X = OH] and trichloroacetyl chloride or pivaloyl chloride in tetrahydrofuran in the presence of triethylamine afforded the reactive anhydride which was immediately coupled with 7-ACA in tetrahydrofuran to give 7-cyanoacetamidocephalosporanic acid (*51*) in almost quantitative yield. An alternative preparation of cephacetrile (*51*) was also achieved in high yield by condensing cyanoacetyl chloride [(*50*) X = Cl] with 7-ACA in methylene-chloride in the presence of tributylamine.

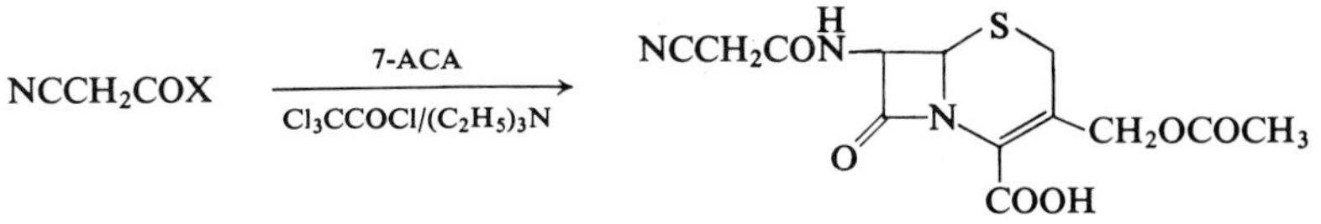

Kurita *et al.* (1966) and Spencer *et al.* (1966) carried out the acylation of 7-ACA with DL, L, and D amino acids. These reactions presented a problem frequently encountered in peptide chemistry, namely, the selection of a convenient amino protective group removable under conditions in which the bicyclic ring system remains intact. Spencer and associates discovered that the *t*-butoxycarbonyl protective group could be removed successfully under acidic conditions after the preparation of cephalosporin amino acid derivatives while the same conditions, as reported by Ekstrom *et al.* (1965), destroyed the corresponding penicillin derivatives. This result clearly demonstrated a greater acid stability of the cephalosporin nucleus relative to the penicillin nucleus. Both groups of investigators employed the mixed anhydride technique to couple 7-ACA with the N-protected amino acids. For example, the synthesis of cephaloglycin (*54*) is presented below. First, the mixed anhydride was prepared by condensing D-α-*t*-butoxycarboxamidophenylacetic acid (*52*) with isobutyl chloroformate in tetrahydrofuran in the presence of triethylamine. This derivative was added to a cold solution of 7-ACA triethylammonium salt in 50% aqueous tetrahydrofuran. The resulting product (*53*) was isolated in 74% yield. The *N-t*-butoxycarbonyl protecting group in (*53*) was removed with 50% aqueous formic acid, and cephaloglycin (*54*) was isolated in 32% yield. When the cleavage of (*53*) was performed with trifluoroacetic acid, the corresponding trifluoroacetate salt of cephaloglycin was obtained and subsequently converted to cephaloglycin by treatment with Amberlite LA-1. Similar reactions were also run using *p*-nitrobenzyl, benzyloxycarbonyl, and

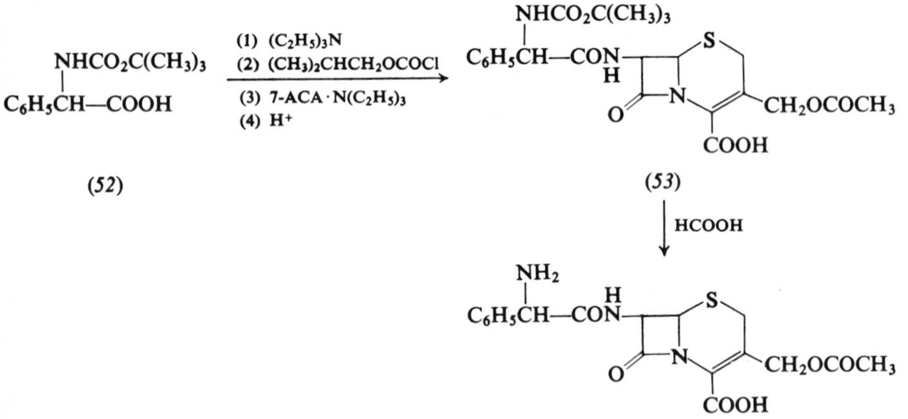

β-dicarbonyl protecting groups. Since the problem of racemization during formation of the amide linkage was constantly present, Spencer and associates monitored the purity of optical isomers using a Moore–Stein amino acid analyzer. This analytical technique was especially useful when the D isomers proved to be more potent than the corresponding L isomers against most microorganisms.

Kurita *et al.* (1966) described an alternative synthesis of cephaloglycin. α-Azidophenylacetyl chloride (*55*) was reacted with 7-ACA in aqueous acetone in the presence of sodium bicarbonate. The resulting α-azidophenylacetamidocephalosporanic acid (*56*) was then reduced with Raney nickel catalyst in aqueous solution at a pressure of 3 atm for 45 minutes. The desired product (*54*) was isolated in low yield.

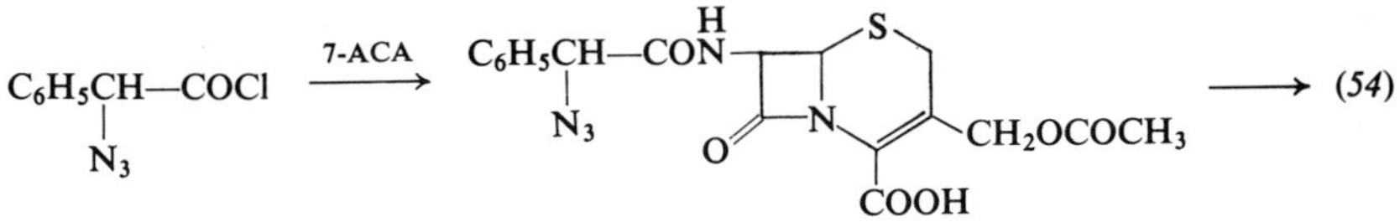

The availability of 7-aminodeacetoxycephalosporanic acid (7-ADCA) (*57*) enabled Ryan and co-workers (1969) to prepare many amino acid derivatives of 7-ADCA on a laboratory scale. They used a method similar to that employed in the synthesis of cephaloglycin. *N-t*-Butoxycarbonyl-D-phenylglycine (*58*) was condensed with 7-ADCA (*57*) by the mixed anhydride method. The *t*-butoxycarbonyl protecting group in (*59*) was removed with trifluoroacetic acid and the desired D-phenylglycine derivative of 7-ADCA (*60*), known as cephalexin, was isolated by treatment with Amberlite LA-1 exchange resin. The same product (*60*) was also obtained by reductive cleavage of the acetoxyl group from cephaloglycin.

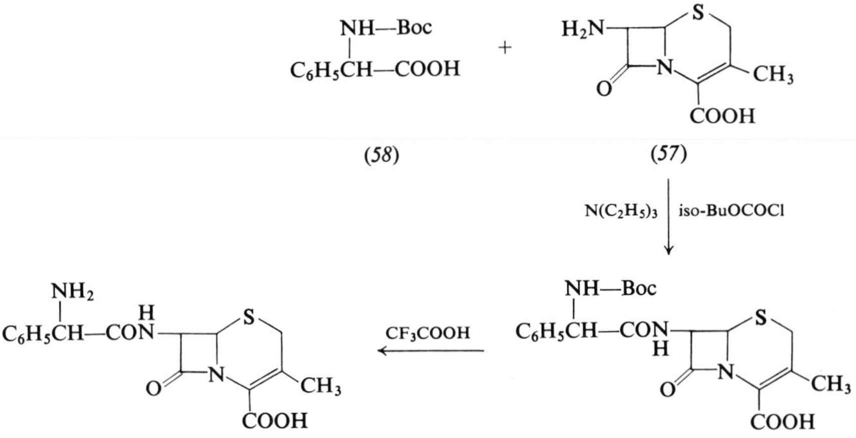

Chauvette and associates (1971) reported an improved synthesis of cephalexin. The *N*-*t*-butoxycarbonyl-D-α-phenylglycine (*61b*) or *N*-trichloroethyloxycarbonyl-D-α-phenylglycine (*61a*) was condensed with 7-ADCA trichloroethyl ester (*62*) in a mixed anhydride coupling reaction in a wide variety of solvents, using methyl chloroformate to form the mixed anhydride. The doubly protected derivatives (*63a, b*) were isolated in nearly quantitative yields. Both trichloroethyl groups in (*63a*) were removed using zinc dust in 90% aqueous formic acid and the desired cephalexin (*60*) was isolated in approximately 60% yield. In the case of the *N*-*t*-butoxycarbonyl derivative [(*63b*) $R_1 = CH_2CCl_3$], the protective groups were removed by a stepwise procedure. First the trichloroethyl ester group was removed with zinc dust and acetic or formic acid in dimethylformamide to give *N*-*t*-butoxycarbonyl cephalexin [(*63b*) $R_1 = H$] in approximately 90% yield. Then the second protective group in (*63b*) was easily removed with *p*-toluenesulfonic acid in acetonitrile, and the resulting cephalexin (*60*) was isolated in 70% yield as the zwitterion.

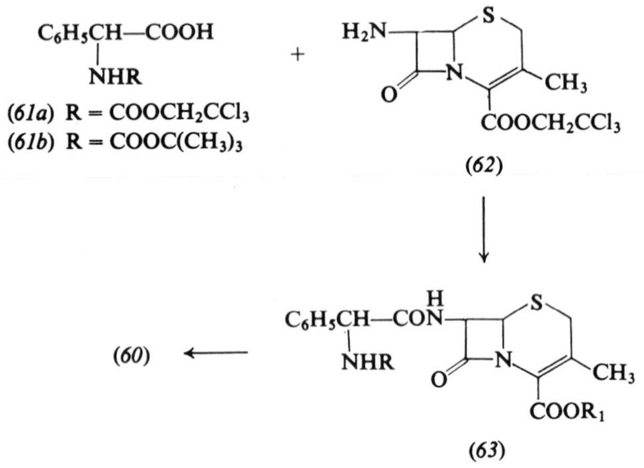

C_6H_5CH—COOH
NHR
(*61a*) R = $COOCH_2CCl_3$
(*61b*) R = $COOC(CH_3)_3$
+
H_2N
S
N
O
CH_3
$COOCH_2CCl_3$
(*62*)
(*60*)
H
C_6H_5CH—CON
NHR
S
N
O
CH_3
$COOR_1$
(*63*)

The dicyclohexylcarbodiimide method has been used less often than the other two methods for *N*-acylation of 7-ACA. Nevertheless, several heterocyclic acids have been activated with dicyclohexylcarbodiimide and coupled with 7-ACA in organic solvents (U.S. Patent 3,218,318).

An improved procedure for the preparation of 7-acylamidocephalosporanic acids by acylating the 7-ACA esters which are soluble in organic solvents was also reported. The best results were achieved by using the silyl esters of 7-ACA since the ester group was easily removed by mildly acidic conditions during the workup procedure (Gr. Brit. Patent 1,073,530; Jackson, 1971).

A less usual acylation of 7-ACA and 6-APA was discovered by Gottstein *et al.* (1970). They observed that 7-ACA was thioacylated with *S*-carboxymethyl *N,N*-diethyldithiocarbamate (*64*) in phosphate buffer (pH 7) in the presence of sodium iodide–iodine solution. The sodium salt of 7-(*N,N*-diethylcarbamoylmercaptoacetamido)cephalosporanate (*65*) was isolated in 24% yield. The same product was also obtained by direct acylation of 7-ACA

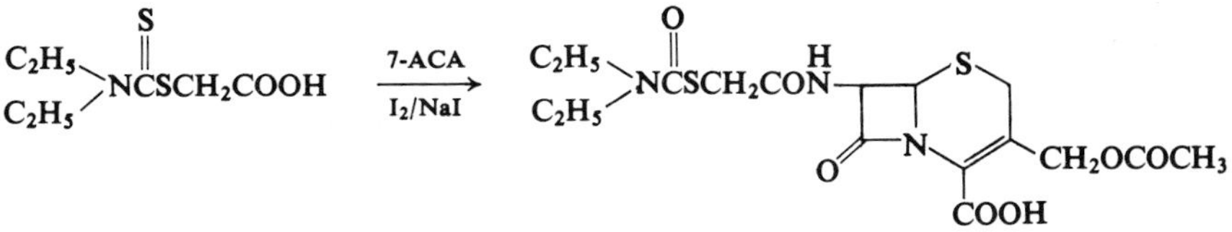

(*64*)   (*65*)

with *S*-carboxymethyl *N,N*-diethyldithiocarbamate mixed anhydride in tetrahydrofuran. It was suggested that this reaction proceeded through the cyclic intermediate (*66*) and nucleophilic attack of the amino function of 7-ACA.

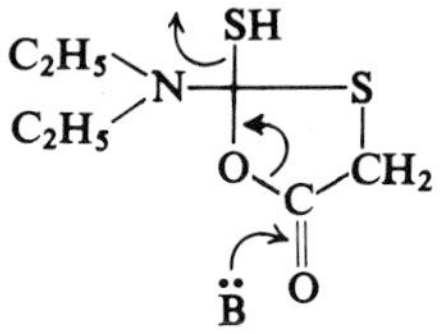

(*66*)

Cocker *et al.* (1965) described phenacetylation of a modified 7-ACA nucleus. The acetoxyl group of 7-ACA was displaced with thiourea to form the thiouronium derivative (*67*) as a methanol solvate. Phenacetylation of (*67*) under carefully controlled conditions gave the 7-phenylacetamido thiouronium derivative (*68*).

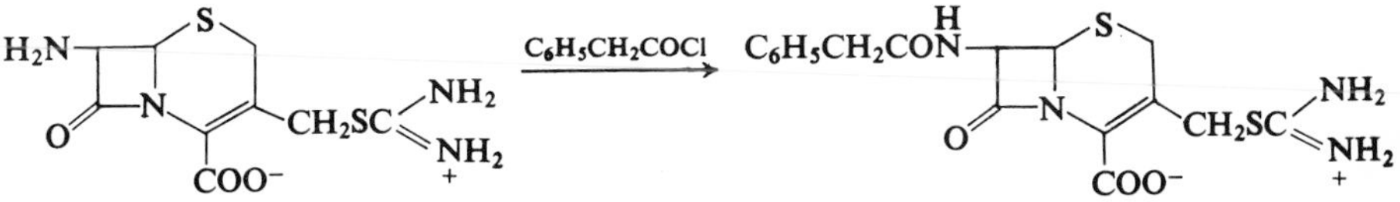

(*67*)   (*68*)

Kaiser and associates (1971b) also reported the synthesis of an amide derivative of a modified 7-ACA. Acylation of the amino ester (*69*) with phenylmercaptoacetyl chloride in acetone containing urea as an acid acceptor gave the trichloroethyl ester in 93% yield. After reductive cleavage of the ester group with zinc and acetic acid in dimethylformamide, the new cephalosporin (*70*) was obtained in 74% yield.

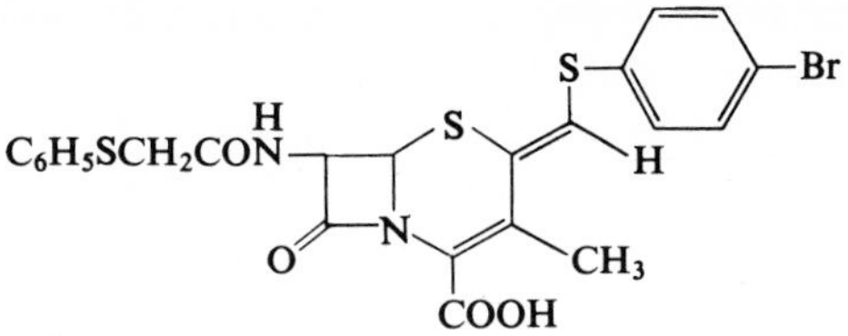

(70)

(1) $C_6H_5SCH_2COCl$
(2) Zn/CH_3COOH

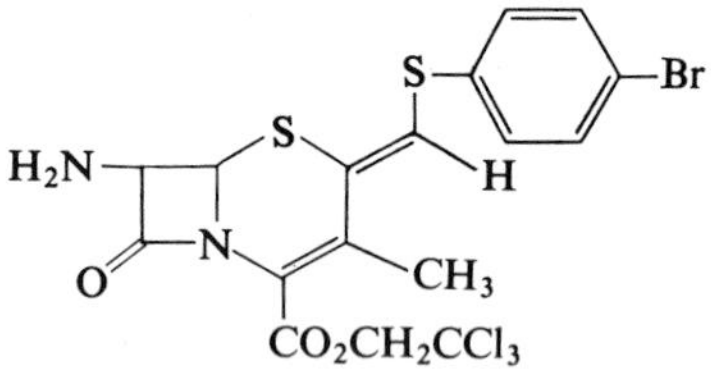

(69)

The 3-alkoxymethyl and 3-alkylthiomethyl-3-cephem derivatives (esters or acids) were acylated by acid chloride or mixed anhydride method. In the case of esters, the protecting group was removed after acylation (Webber *et al.*, 1971; Belg. Patents 734,532, 734,533). For example, 3-alkoxymethyl-7-phenoxy-acetamidocephalosporin acids (72) were prepared by acylation of 7-amino-3-alkoxymethyl-3-cephem-4-carboxylate esters (71) with phenoxyacetyl chloride followed by ester cleavage.

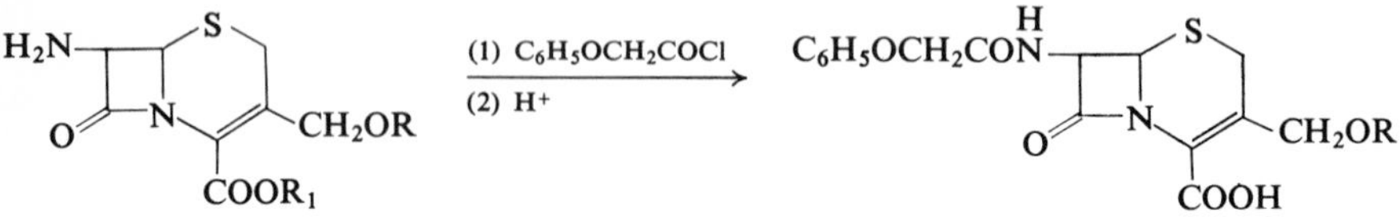

(71)   (72)

Condensation of alkylisocyanates (73) with the triethylammonium salt of 7-ACA in methylene chloride afforded 7-alkylureidocephalosporanic acid (74) (Fr. Patent 1,397,509).

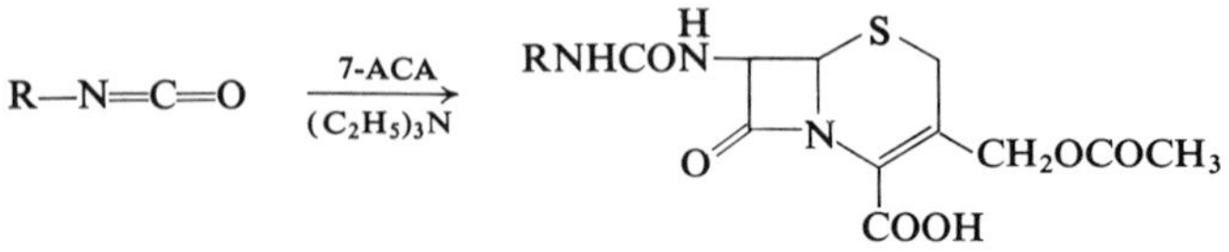

(73)   (74)

Archer and Kitchell (1966) reported that the amino group in 7-ACA (*39*) was converted with sodium bicarbonate to the carbamate (*75*), isolated as the methylcarbamate methyl ester (*76*). The same ester was prepared by acylation of 7-ACA (*39*) with methyl chloroformate and subsequent esterification of the acid (*77*) with diazomethane. Reaction of the methylcarbamate–potassium salt (*78*) with methyl iodide in dimethylformamide also produced (*76*).

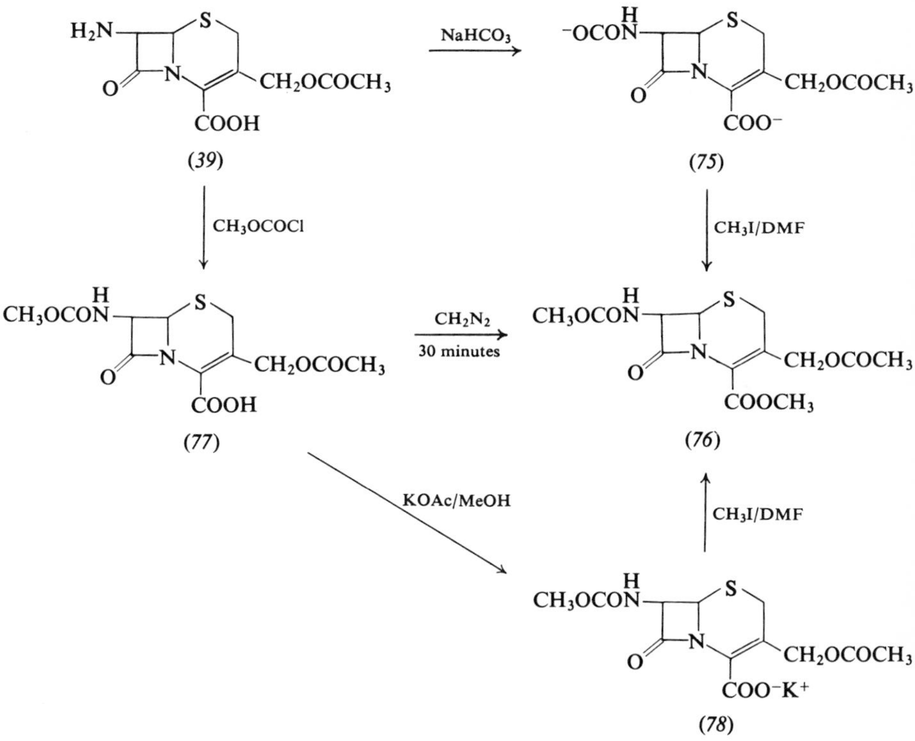

C. Alkylation of the Amino Group

A few reports of N-alkyl derivatives of penicillins have appeared in the literature. The first N-alkylation of 6-APA was reported by Sheehan and Henery-Logan (1962). They treated 6-APA with trityl chloride in aqueous isopropanol containing diethylamine. The resulting 6-tritylaminopenicillanic acid (*79*) was obtained in good yield and characterized as the crystalline diethylamine salt.

The trityl group, which can be easily removed under mildly acidic conditions, was utilized by Koe (1962) to synthesize 6-aminopenicillanamide and methyl 6-aminopenicillanate. The free acid (*79*) was converted to the mixed anhydride with isobutyl chloroformate and triethylamine in dry acetone. Treatment with aqueous dibasic ammonium phosphate gave 6-tritylaminopenicillanamide (*80*) in 87% yield. The latter was hydrolyzed with a solution of *p*-toluenesulfonic acid in acetone. Crystalline 6-aminopenicillanamide *p*-toluenesulfonate (*81*) was collected in 83% yield. Similarly, the free acid (*79*) was converted with diazomethane into methyl 6-aminopenicillanate *p*-toluenesulfonate in 76% yield.

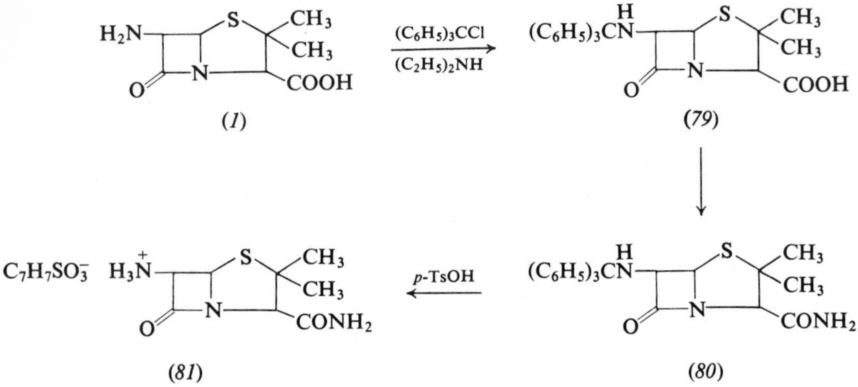

Leigh (1965) reported *N*-alkylation of 6-aminopenicillanic acid by reductive condensation with aldehydes and ketones. Catalytic hydrogenation of a mixture of an aliphatic aldehyde and one equivalent of 6-aminopenicillanic acid in the presence of platinum oxide, gave mixtures of 6-alkylamino- (*83*), 6-dialkylamino- (*82*), and unchanged 6-aminopenicillanic acids (*1*). The crude mixtures from the alkylation reaction were treated with phenoxyacetyl chloride and the resulting mixtures of 6-dialkylamino- (*82*), 6-(*N*-alkyl-*N*-phenoxyacetamido)- (*84*), and 6-phenoxyacetamidopenicillanic acids were then separated. With ketones, only monosubstitution occurred. Reductive alkylations were carried out with formaldehyde, butyraldehyde, isobutyraldehyde, salicylaldehyde, 3,5-dichlorosalicylaldehyde, acetone, and *p*-chlorobenzylmethylketone. Quaternary ammonium salts were prepared from 6-dimethylaminopenicillanic acid and alkyl halides.

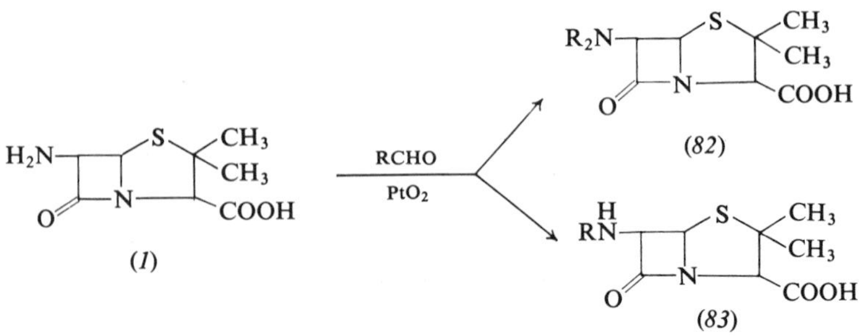

(83) $\xrightarrow{\text{C}_6\text{H}_5\text{OCH}_2\text{COCl}}$ (84)

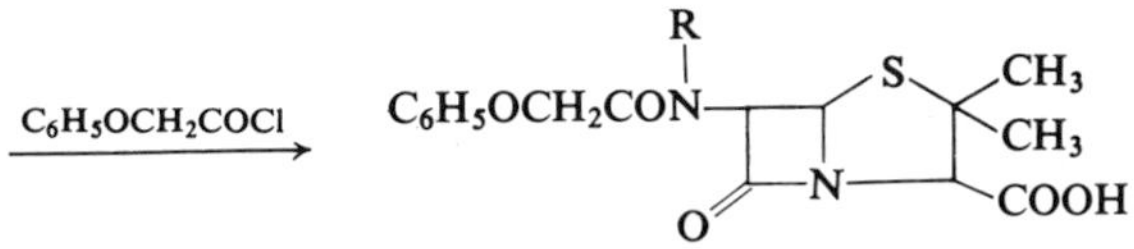

Kaiser and Ashbrook (1970) have used the procedure of Leigh (1965) to prepare the corresponding deacetoxycephalosporin derivative (85).

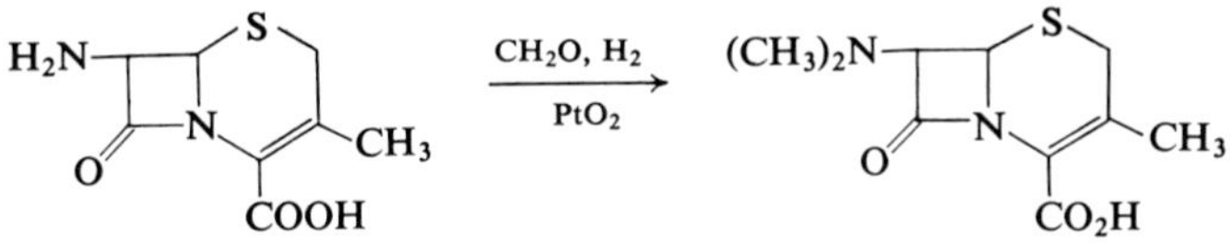

(57) $\xrightarrow[\text{PtO}_2]{\text{CH}_2\text{O, H}_2}$ (85)

Moll and Hannig (1970) described the preparation of the methyl esters of 6-aminopenicillanic acid (87), N-methyl 6-aminopenicillanic acid (86), and N,N-dimethylaminopenicillanic acid (88) by reaction of 6-aminopenicillanic acid (1) with diazomethane. The mixture was separated by chromatography and the esters characterized by the infrared, mass, and NMR spectra.

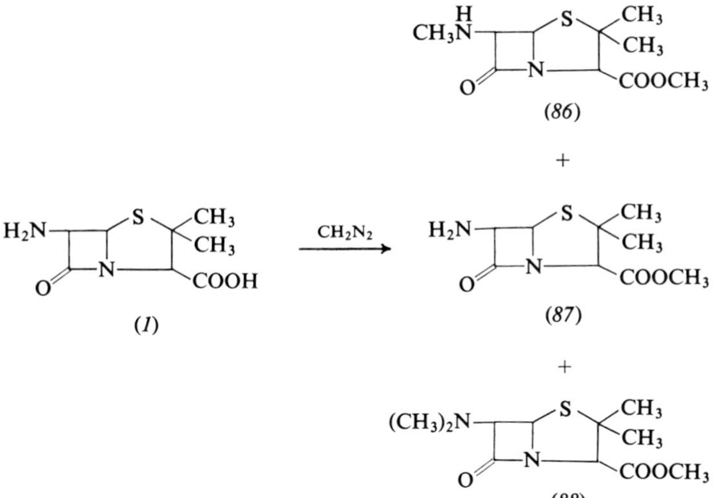

(86)

+

(1) $\xrightarrow{\text{CH}_2\text{N}_2}$ (87)

+

(88)

Jackson and Stoodley (1970) prepared methoxymethyl 6-aminopenicillanate (89) in 62% yield by treatment of the triethylammonium salt of 6-APA with chloromethyl methyl ether. This ester was converted with p-nitrobenzaldehyde to the Schiff base (90) in 66% yield. Compound (90) later rearranged to the corresponding thiazepine derivative (see Section II).

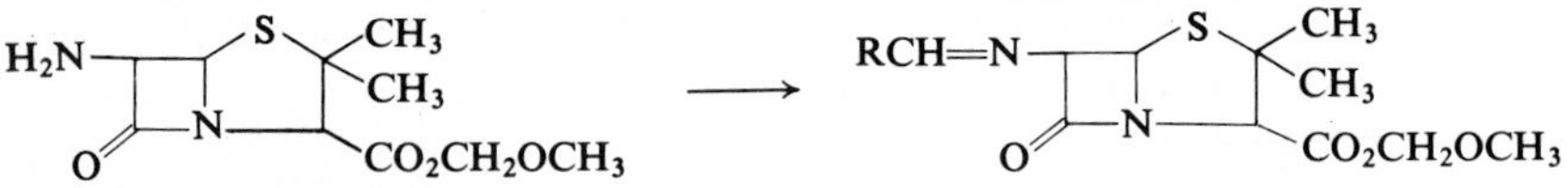

(89)   (90)

$$R = p\text{-}NO_2\cdot C_6H_4$$

In order to activate the C-6 position in the penicillin nucleus for an eventual *C*-alkylation, Reiner and Zeller (1968) studied the reactivity of Schiff base derivatives of 6-APA. The Schiff base (*91*), prepared by treating 6-APA with a 10 *M* excess of salicylaldehyde in aqueous solution, was isolated as a crystalline acid in 78% yield. This acid was converted with an excess of diazomethane in ether to the corresponding methyl ester (*92*) in almost quantitative yield, which upon hydrolysis with hydrochloric acid yielded methyl 6-aminopenicillanate (*93*) as a light yellow oil in 69% yield. Compound (*92*) was reacted with copper acetate and sodium bicarbonate in a mixture of water and chloroform at 0° to give the crystalline copper complex (*94*) in 95% yield (see also, Section II,C).

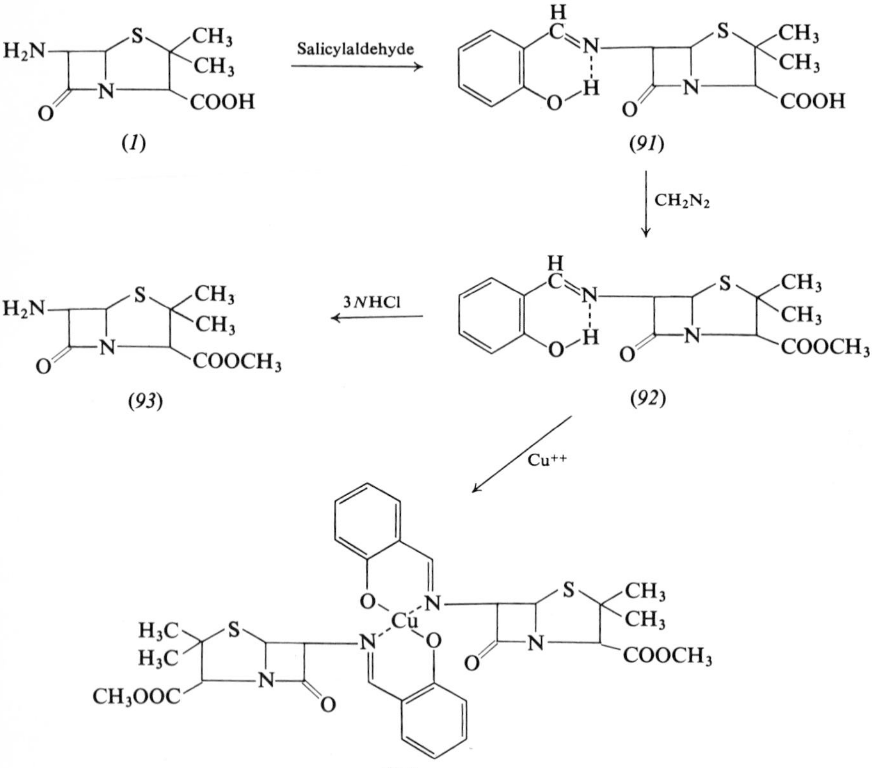

(1)   (91)

(93)   (92)

(94)

The reaction of 6-APA with a 6 M excess of benzaldehyde in ethanol gave the N-benzylidene derivative (*95*) in 90% yield.

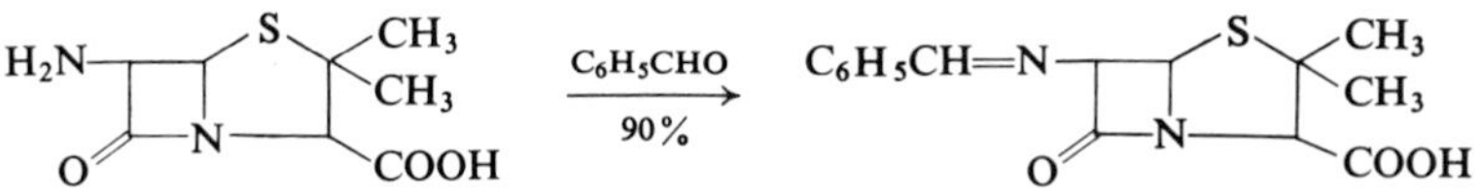

II. Modifications at the β-Lactam Carbons

Since the mechanism of action of penicillins and cephalosporins is thought to involve irreversible acylation of a key enzyme by the strained β-lactam system, modifications directly at the β-lactam should have profound effects upon antimicrobial activity. Structural studies on penicillins and cephalosporins have established that the β-lactam of each is substituted with an acylamino function *cis* to the sulfur in the fused heterocycle (Fig. 1). When considering

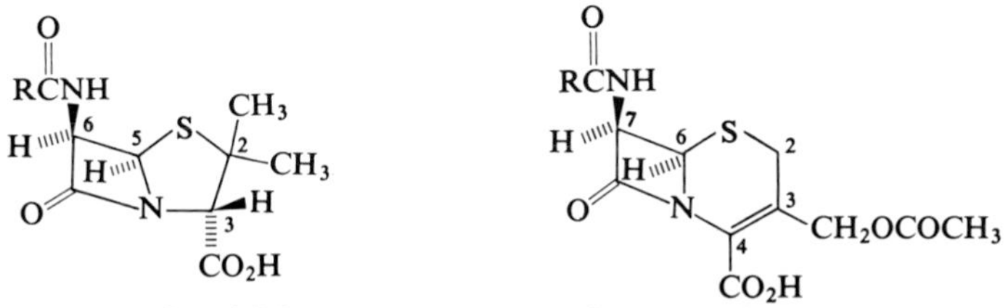

Structure of Penicillin   Structure of Cephalosporin

Fig. 1. β-Lactam ring systems.

reactions involving the β-lactam carbons of these compounds, a fundamental question arises: What substituent and conformational requirements at the β-lactam are necessary for antimicrobial activity? The answer should be forthcoming in the near future because at the time of this writing the knowledge of reactions at the β-lactams of penicillins and cephalosporins is expanding rapidly.

For convenience the reactions in this section are classified as deaminations, epimerizations, and alkylations. To date none of the deaminated, epimerized, or alkylated derivatives have shown substantial antimicrobial activity when compared to their natural precursors, but investigators continue to search for a substitution pattern which will improve on that found in the natural compounds.

A. Deamination

Cignarella and associates (1962) reported the first deamination of 6-amino-penicillanic acid (6-APA) (*1*). When treated with sodium nitrite and hydrochloric acid, 6-APA was converted to 6-chloropenicillanic acid (*96*), isolated as the dibenzylethylenediamine salt. Substitution of hydrobromic acid in the reaction gave the 6-bromo derivative (*97*). Both deaminated products were devoid of microbiological activity against *M. pyogenes aureus* 209P.

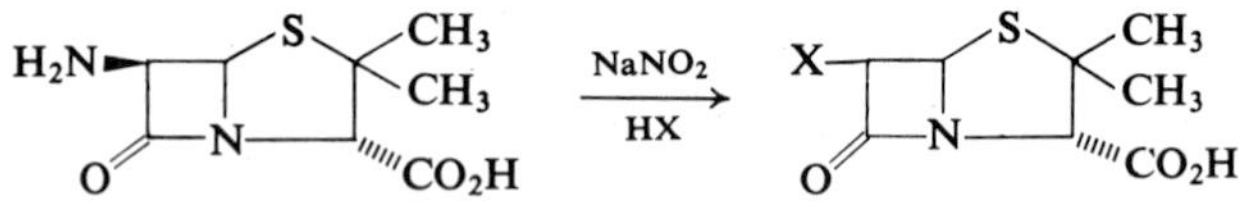

(*1*)

(*96*) X = Cl
(*97*) X = Br

Evrard and co-workers (1964) prepared the methyl esters of (*96*) and (*97*) and showed that (*97*) could be hydrogenated to penicillanic acid (*98*). Their study emphasized the value of gas chromatography in the separation of penicillanates including methyl penicillanate (*99*).

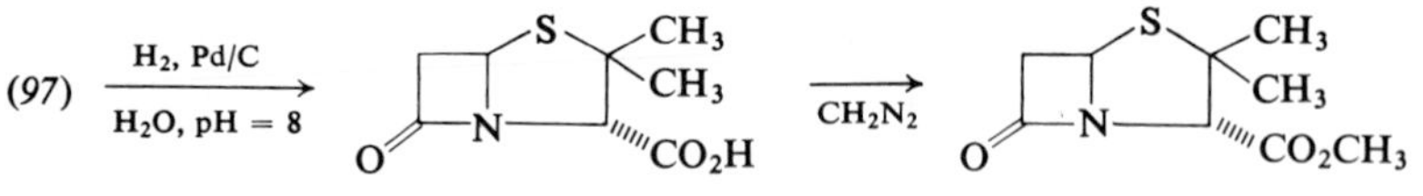

(*98*)   (*99*)

The yield of 6-chloropenicillanic acid from the nitrous acid deamination of 6-APA was improved to 75% by McMillan and Stoodley (1966, 1968) who used ice-cold 70% aqueous methanolic hydrochloric acid. They established that deamination proceeds with inversion at C-6, i.e., the β-lactam protons in (*100*) are *trans*.

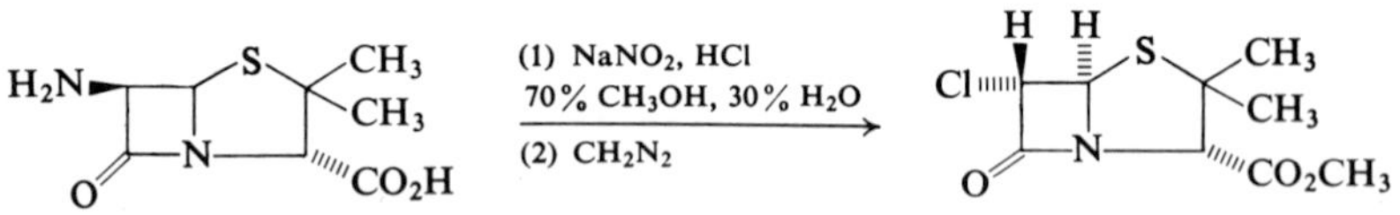

(*1*)   (*100*)

Hauser and Sigg (1967) reached the same conclusion with respect to product stereochemistry in their studies of the deamination of 6-APA. When 90% acetic acid was used, the product was 6-α-acetoxypenicillanic acid (*101*). In water, with perchloric, sulfuric, phosphoric, or *p*-toluenesulfonic acid as the hydrogen ion source, 6-α-hydroxypenicillanic acid (*102*) was formed. Benzyl

6-α-hydroxypenicillanate (*103*) was treated with phenoxyacetyl chloride, *p*-bromophenylsulfonyl chloride, and methanesulfonyl chloride to give new α-substituted penicillanates (*104–106*). None of these 6-α-substituted penicillanate esters or the acid (*107*) had an inhibiting effect against a selection of gram-positive and gram-negative bacteria at concentrations of 1 mg/ml.

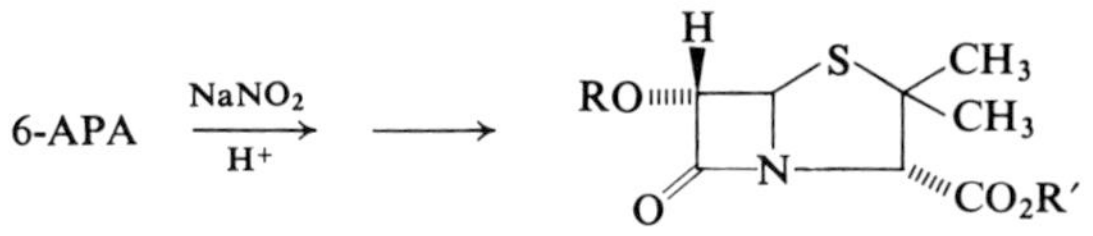

6-APA $\xrightarrow[\text{H}^+]{\text{NaNO}_2}$

(*1*)

(*101*) R = CH$_3$CO; R' = H
(*102*) R = H; R' = H
(*103*) R = H; R' = CH$_2$C$_6$H$_5$
(*104*) R = C$_6$H$_5$OCH$_2$CO; R' = CH$_2$C$_6$H$_5$
(*105*) R = 4-BrC$_6$H$_4$SO$_2$; R' = CH$_2$C$_6$H$_5$
(*106*) R = CH$_3$SO$_2$; R' = CH$_2$C$_6$H$_5$
(*107*) R = C$_6$H$_5$OCH$_2$CO; R' = H

Both McMillan and Stoodley (1966) and Hauser and Sigg (1967) based their stereochemical assignments on the NMR coupling constants of the β-lactam protons (see Chapter 8). The following paragraph discusses the data leading to these assignments.

Kagan and associates (1964) examined a number of pairs of *cis* and *trans* β-lactams. Applying the Karplus equation, which relates the dihedral angles between vicinal protons in cyclohexane to their coupling constants (Karplus, 1959, 1962) to β-lactams, Kagan concluded that J_{cis} should be larger than J_{trans}. Thus, the products with the larger J values ($J = 5.5$–6.0 Hz) were assigned the *cis* proton configuration while β-lactams with the smaller J values ($J = 2.3$–2.5 Hz) were assigned the *trans* proton configuration. A later report by Luche and co-workers (1968) verified these assignments. The structures of two *cis* β-lactams, (*108*) and (*109*), were determined by X-ray crystallography. Both of

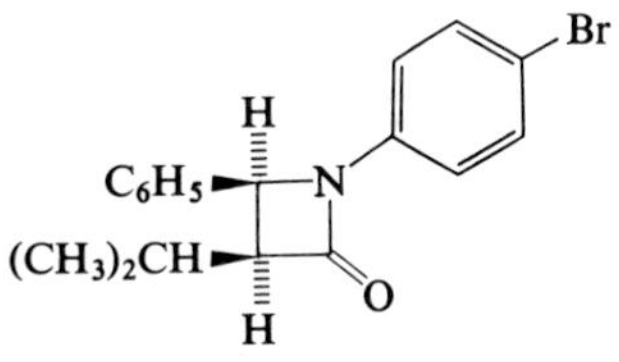

(*108*) 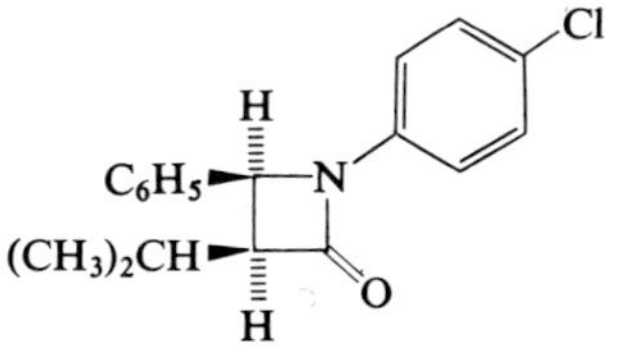   (*109*)

these isomers had $J_{HH} = 6$ Hz. Barrow and Spotswood (1965) reported NMR spectra of 14 monocyclic β-lactams. They, too, concluded that the Karplus equation qualitatively predicted $J_{cis} > J_{trans}$ for the vicinal protons. Experimentally they found J_{cis} to be 4.9–5.9 Hz and J_{trans} to be 2.2–2.8 Hz. Green

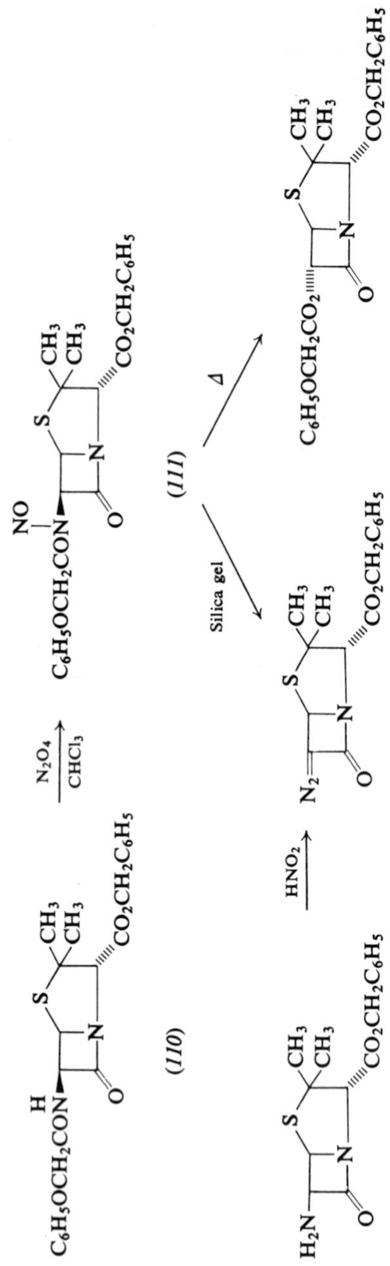

C6H5OCH2CON
H
O
N
S
CH3
CH3
CO2CH2C6H5
(110)
N2O4
CHCl3
NO
(111)
Silica gel
Δ
C6H5OCH2CO2
(104)
H2N
(36)
HNO2
N2
(112)

and co-workers (1965, 1966), who tabulated NMR data for dozens of penicillins and cephalosporins, concluded that cis β-lactam protons have J values of ≈ 4 Hz while trans β-lactam protons have J values of ≈ 2 Hz.

Hauser and Sigg (1967) also prepared benzyl 6-α-phenoxyacetoxypenicillanate (104) via a nitrosoamide rearrangement. Penicillin V benzyl ester (110) was treated with dinitrogen tetroxide in chloroform to give the N-nitrosoamide (111). Heating in warm benzene for 24 hours caused rearrangement of (111) to (104), identical to material obtained from the sodium nitrite route. When (111) was chromatographed over silica gel, benzyl 6-diazopenicillanate (112) formed as a yellow oil. The same compound was formed when benzyl 6 aminopenicillanate (36) was treated with nitrous acid. Both procedures to (104) gave very low yields.

McMillan and Stoodley (1968) postulated that deamination of 6-APA (1) in the presence of sodium nitrite and hydrochloric acid involved an intermediate 6-diazopenicillanic acid (113). When the reaction was run in deuterochloric acid, the 6-α-chloropenicillanic acid produced contained a deuterium atom at C-6. Control experiments demonstrated that both 6-APA and 6-α-chloropenicillanic acid failed to incorporate deuterium under the reaction conditions. Consequently, deuterium must have been incorporated at an intermediate stage. These workers, like Hauser and Sigg, reported that treatment of benzyl 6-aminopenicillanate (36) with nitrous acid gave benzyl 6-diazopenicillanate (112) in low yield. This result, coupled with the deuteration data, strongly suggests that (113) is an intermediate in the deamination of 6-APA.

When the deamination was run in aqueous methanol to achieve higher yields of (96), competing reactions had to be considered. McMillan and Stoodley (1968) using 70% methanol, obtained an optimal yield of 75%. Increasing the concentration of methanol to 90%, Stoodley (1968) obtained (96) in only 15% yield. Use of methanolic hydrogen chloride resulted in no (96) at all. Instead, in the latter two cases a new compound (114), the result of a series of rearrangements, was isolated. Its structure was assigned on the basis of analytical and spectral data and was confirmed by independent synthesis.

Stoodley (1968) concluded that methanolysis of 6-APA had preceded deamination when (114) was produced. To support this conclusion, he showed that (115), when treated with sodium nitrite in methanolic hydrogen chloride, gave (*114*). Furthermore, compound (*116*) was not an intermediate since it was not converted to (*114*) under reaction conditions. This route explains the yield dependence of (*96*) on the concentration of methanol. In methanolic hydrochloric acid and sodium nitrite, (*1*) undergoes methanolysis faster than deamination, whereas the reverse is true in 70% methanolic hydrochloric acid.

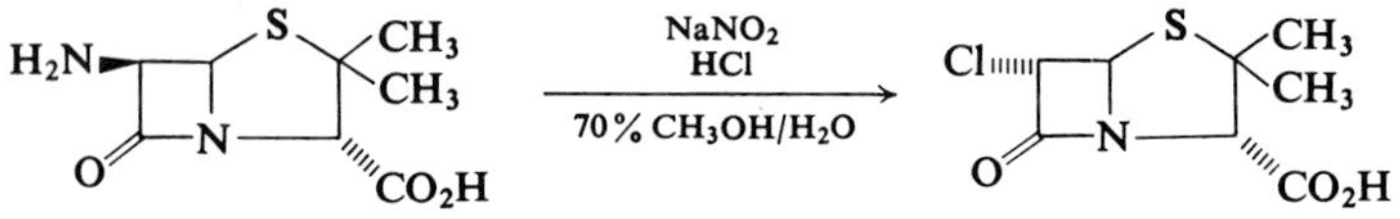

(*1*)   (*96*)

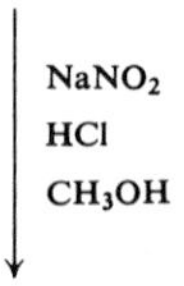

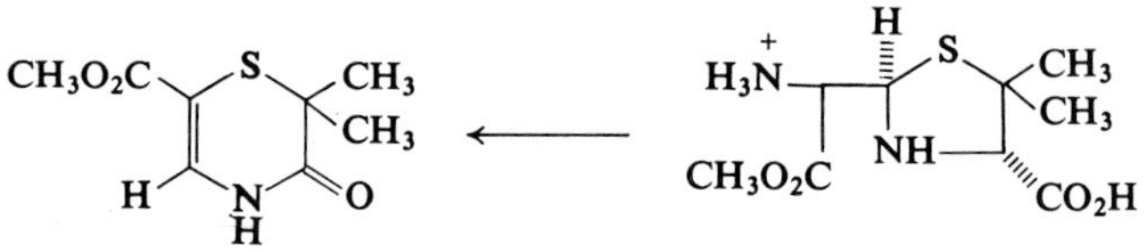

(*114*)   (*115*)

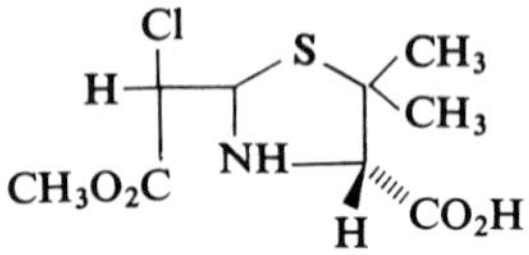

(*116*)

McMillan and Stoodley (1966, 1968) attempted nucleophilic displacement reactions on 6-α-chloropenicillanate derivatives. They reacted 6-α-chloropenicillanic acid (*96*) and its methyl ester (*100*) with sodium azide in dimethylformamide. In each case, β-lactam rupture, ring expansion, and loss of chloride were noted. Spectroscopic considerations suggested the products were the thiazine (*117*) and its methyl ester (*118*). Sodium methoxide in methanol gave analogous ring-opened rearrangement products (*119*) and (*120*). In the latter cases the structural assignments were confirmed by independent synthesis. Reactions of methyl 6-α-chloropenicillanate (*100*) with sodium iodide in methylethylketone, silver cyanide in acetonitrile, or sodium benzoate in dimethylformamide gave unreacted starting material.

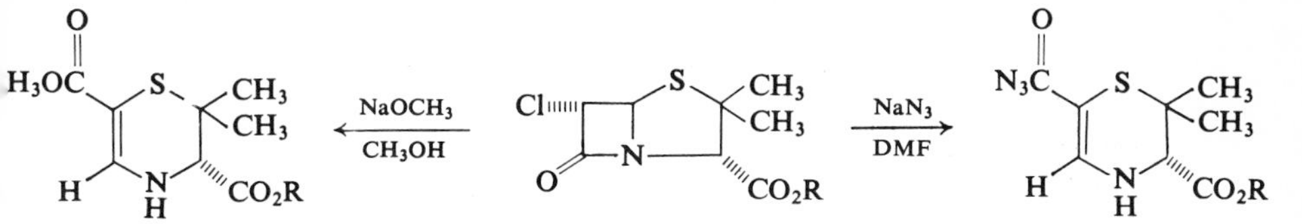

(*119*) R = H (47%)

(*120*) R = CH₃ (85%)

(*96*) R = H

(*100*) R = CH₃

(*117*) R = H (52%)

(*118*) R = CH₃ (12%)

Hauser and Sigg (1967) reported that the 6-α-sulfonate esters (*105*) and (*106*) were unreactive toward a variety of nucleophiles, i.e., sodium iodide, sodium acetate, sodium azide, sodium thioacetate, and sodium thiophenylate. Under mild conditions, with prolonged heating in the presence of these nucleophiles, the β-lactam was cleaved.

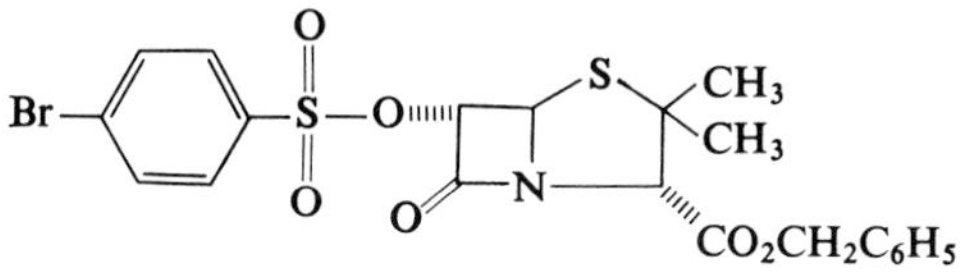

(*105*)

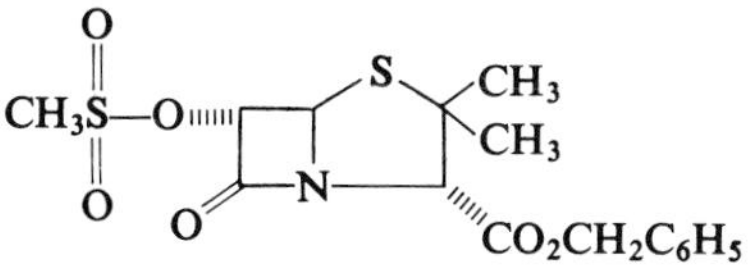

(*106*)

In an effort to provide electrophilic assistance for the ionization of methyl 6-α-chloropenicillanate (*100*), Clayton and associates (1970) used antimony pentachloride in methylene chloride. A ring expansion product (*121*) was obtained. Methyl penicillanate (*99*) and methyl β-phthalimidopenicillanate (*122*) gave analogous reaction products (*123*) and (*124*). The investigators suggested two possible pathways for the conversion: formation of an enethiolate (*125*), which undergoes self condensation of sulfur on the β-lactam carbonyl, or ring expansion of an intermediate such as (*126*) [see related studies by Wolfe and Lee (1968) and Kovacs *et al.* (1969) in Section I,B].

Clayton (1969) reported that diazotization of 6-APA with sodium nitrite and hydrobromic acid in the presence of sodium bromide gave two compounds. They were converted to a mixture of methyl esters and separated by chromatography. The main product (85% of the mixture) was methyl 6-α-bromo-penicillanate (*127*). The second product (15% of the mixture) was identified as

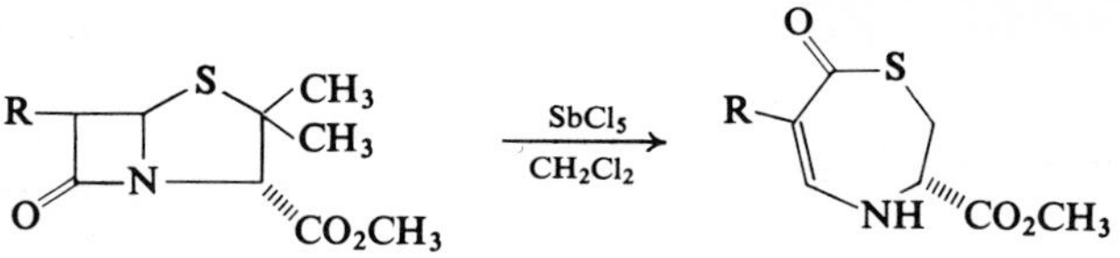

(100) R = α-Cl

(99) R = H

(122) R = β phthalimido

(121) R = Cl (30%)

(123) R = H (48%)

(124) R = phthalimido (32%)

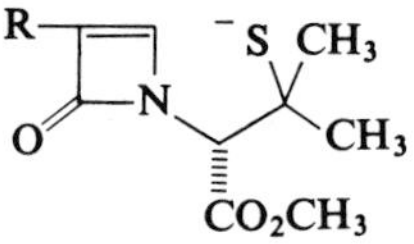

(125)

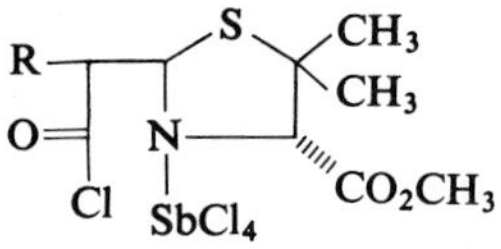

(126)

methyl 6,6-dibromopenicillanate (128). When sodium iodide was substituted for sodium bromide, the crude acid mixture contained 55% 6,6-diiodopenicillanic acid (130) and 45% 6-α-iodopenicillanic acid (129). Clayton reasoned that the reaction involved oxidation of halide ion to halogen, which then reacted with the diazo intermediate. He argued that since iodide ion is more readily oxidized to iodine than bromide ion to bromine, a greater proportion of 6,6-disubstituted acid to 6-monosubstituted acid would be expected in the sodium iodide reaction. When 6-APA, dissolved in 2.5 N sulfuric acid, was

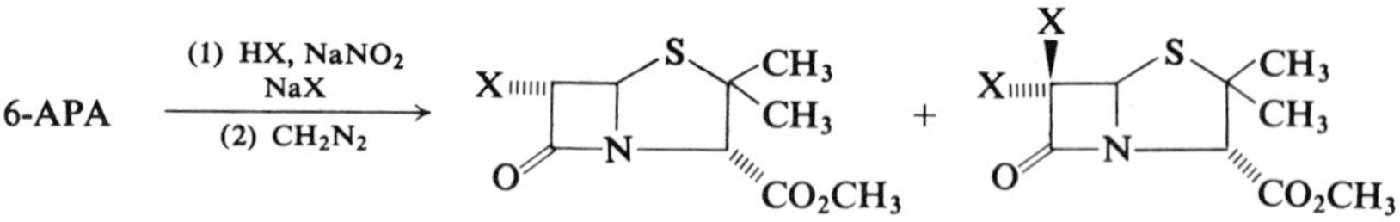

6-APA

(1)

(127) X = Br

(129) X = I

(128) X = Br

(130) X = I

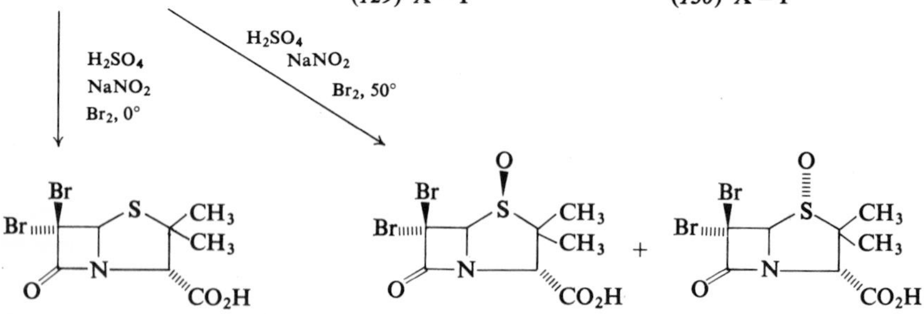

(131)

(132)

(133)

treated with sodium nitrite and bromine at 0°, the dibromo acid (*131*) crystallized in 35% yield.

If the temperature of the bromine reaction was allowed to reach 50°, the corresponding sulfoxide was obtained in 6% yield as a mixture of epimers at the sulfur atom. NMR showed that 73% of the mixture was the 1-β oxide (*132*) while 27% was the 1-α oxide (*133*). The same ratio of sulfoxides was obtained when (*131*) was oxidized with sodium periodate in ethanol.

Attempts to hydrolyze the geminal dibromide function of (*128*) were unsuccessful. With silver acetate in refluxing acetic acid and with silver trifluoroacetate in acetonitrile, (*128*) was recovered unchanged. Like the monohalo compounds, compound (*128*) was unreactive to azide and cyanide ions under mild conditions while more vigorous conditions resulted in cleavage of the β-lactam. When (*128*) was hydrogenated at atmospheric pressure and room temperature in methanol using 5% Pd/CaCO₃, after 40 minutes, the product was methyl 6-α-bromopenicillanate (*127*) in 85% yield. When the reduction was allowed to proceed for 3 hours, both bromine atoms were replaced and methylpenicillanate (*99*) was isolated in 80% yield. Penicillanic acid (*98*) could be prepared in 72% yield by hydrogenating 6,6-dibromopenicillanic acid (*131*) with 5% Pd/CaCO₃ in water at pH 7.5 for 2 hours at room temperature.

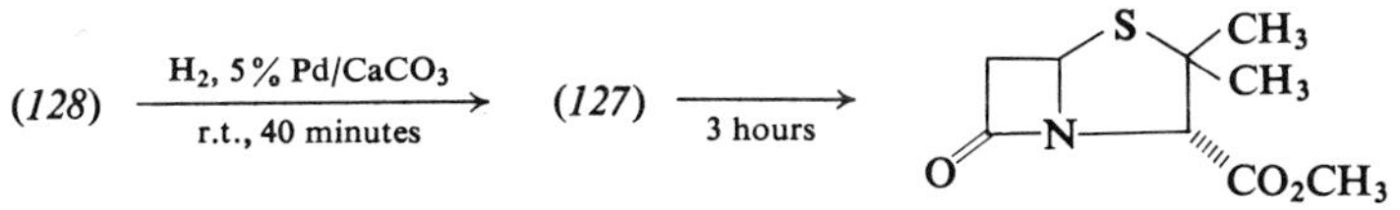

(99)

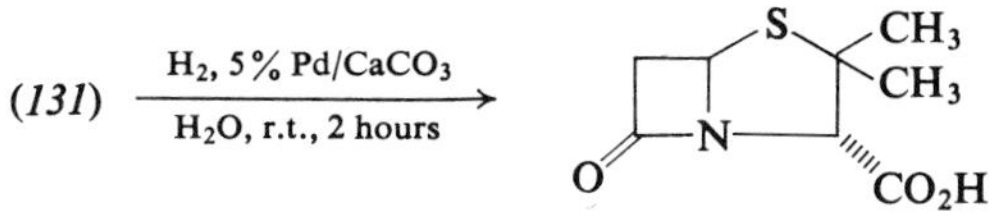

(98)

The dibromo acid (*131*) reacted with ethylchloroformate to give a crystalline mixed anhydride. Upon treatment with triethylamine, the mixed anhydride underwent the anhydropenicillin rearrangement (Wolfe *et al.*, 1963) to give the thiolactone (*134*) along with another compound which was assigned structure (*135*).

Clayton reported that none of the new compounds in his study had significant antibacterial properties.

Morin and co-workers (1969a) obtained 7-chlorocephalosporanic acid (*136*) as a by-product of the nitrosyl chloride cleavage of cephalosporin C (*137*) (see

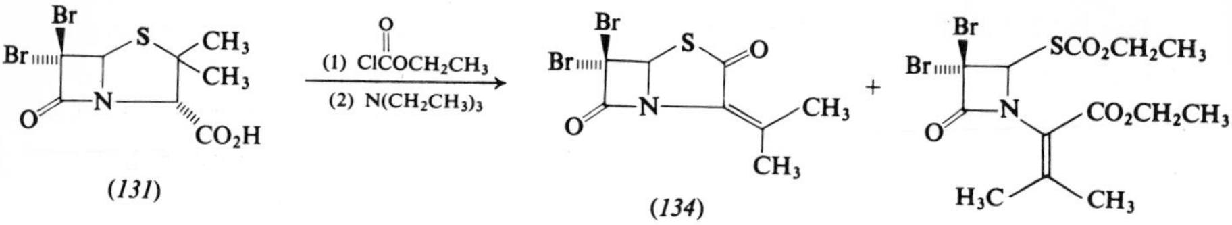

(131)　　　　(1) ClCOCH₂CH₃　(2) N(CH₂CH₃)₃　→　(134)　　+　　(135)

Chapter 2, Section II). They proposed that (*136*) could arise from any 7-amino-cephalosporanic acid (*39*) produced by premature hydrolysis of the intermediate iminolactone (*138*). In a separate experiment 7-ACA (*39*) was treated with nitrosyl chloride in formic acid, and the product was esterified with diazomethane to give a methyl ester (*139*) which was identical to the methyl ester derived from the cephalosporin C reaction.

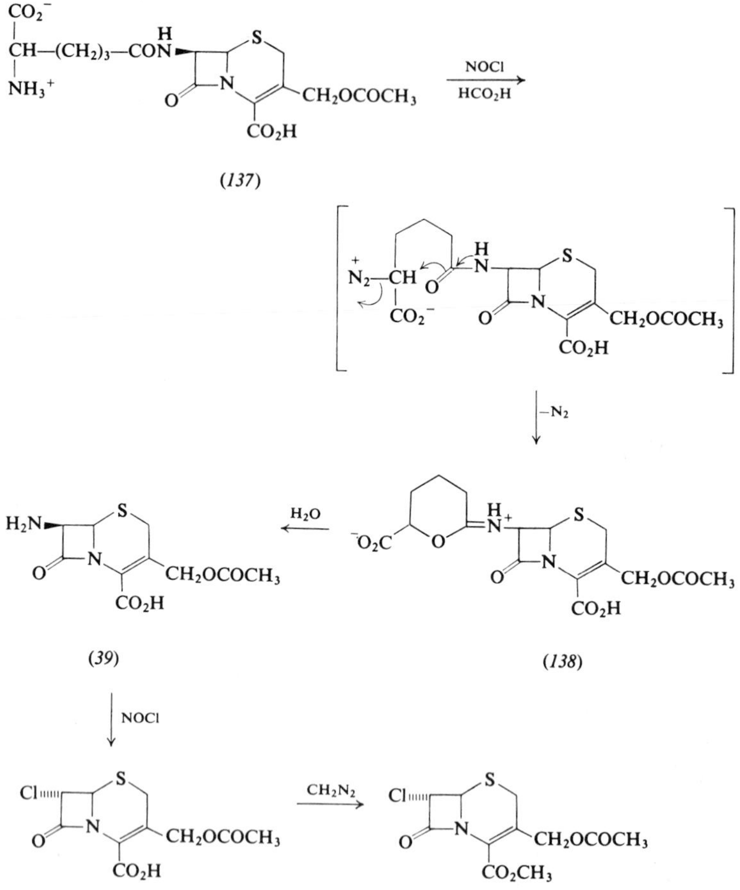

(137)

(39)　　　　　　(138)

(136)　　　　　　(139)

The NMR spectrum of (*139*) showed $J = 1.7$ Hz for the β-lactam protons, suggesting an α orientation for the 7-chloro group. As with methyl 6-α-chloropenicillanate (*100*), compound (*139*) was inert at room temperature to a variety of nucleophiles (methylamine, azide ion, acetate ion, and potassium phthalimide). More vigorous conditions caused rupture of the β-lactam.

Using the optimal conditions developed by McMillan and Stoodley (1968) for the deamination of 6-APA, Kaiser and Ashbrook (1970) converted 7-aminodeacetoxycephalosporanic acid, 7-ADCA (*140*), to its α-chloro derivative (*141*) ($J_{\text{H-6, H-7}} = 1.5$ Hz).

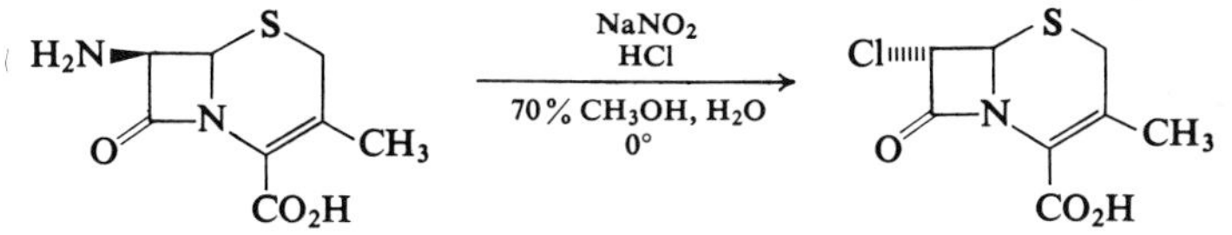

(*140*)   (*141*)

Like the penicillin-derived compounds, the α-chlorocephalosporanic acids (*136*) and (*141*) had negligible antimicrobial activity.

B. *Epimerization*

Johnson and co-workers (1968) reported the first example of epimerization at C-6 of a penicillin. Treatment of hetacillin (*25*) with aqueous sodium hydroxide (pH 11.5) for 30 minutes at room temperature, followed by acidification to pH 2, caused formation of epihetacillin (*142*) in 85% yield. Esterification with diazomethane gave methyl epihetacillinate (*143*) in 91% yield. The epimerization also proceeded in nonaqueous systems. Treatment of methyl hetacillinate (*144*) in dimethyl sulfoxide with triethylamine for 5.5 hours gave (*143*), shown to be identical to the diazomethane esterification product of (*142*).

When (*25*) isomerized to (*142*), a sharp drop in specific rotation from $[\alpha]_D^{23}$ +343° to $[\alpha]_D^{23}$ +232° and loss of biological activity was noted. The infrared spectrum showed that the β-lactam band at 1775 cm^{-1} in (*25*) had shifted to 1800 cm^{-1} in (*142*). The NMR spectrum showed that the protons at C-5 and C-6, which had $J = 4.5$ Hz in (*25*), had $J = 1.5$ Hz in (*142*) and (*143*). This indicated a *trans* proton relationship in the epimerized compounds (see Chapter 8).

Treatment of (*25*) in D_2O with sodium deuteroxide (pH 11.5) followed by acidification with deuterium chloride (pH 2.0) gave deuteroepihetacillin in 79% yield. The NMR spectrum showed that the doublet for the C-6 proton was absent, and that a singlet had replaced the doublet for the C-5 proton in epi-hetacillin.

When Johnson and Mania (1969) attempted a direct epimerization of 6-APA and benzylpenicillin, they were unsuccessful. They did, however, achieve their

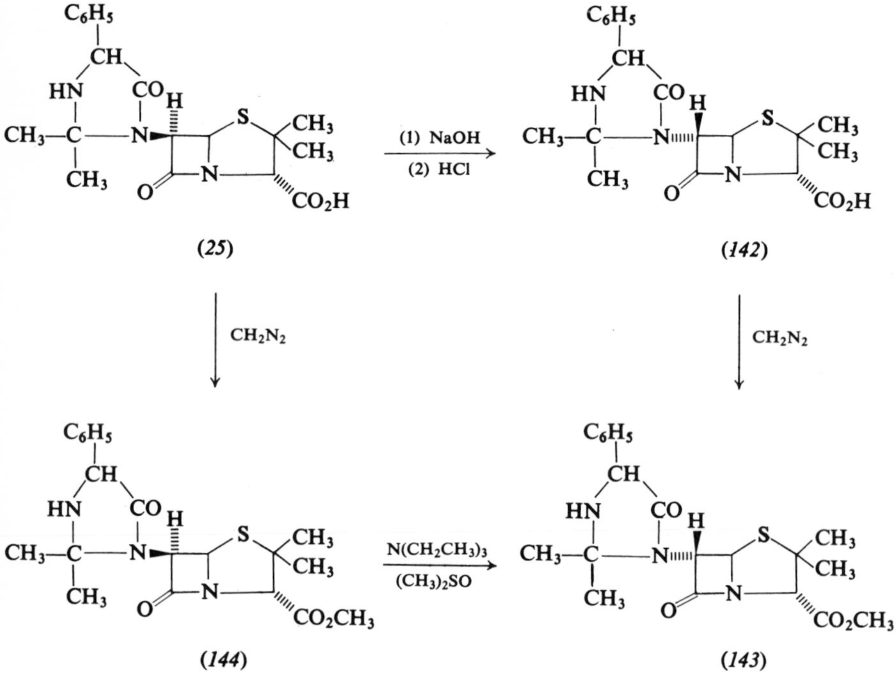

goal by starting with (142). Alkylation of (142) with methyl 4-fluoro-3-nitro-benzoate in aqueous alkaline tetrahydrofuran gave crude (145) in 83% yield. Hydrogenation of (145) in neutral, aqueous solution using 30% palladium on alumina presumably yielded the amine (146), but no attempt at isolation was made. Spontaneous cyclization of (146) in moist, weakly acidic methyl isobutylketone at room temperature gave 6-amino-6-epipenicillanic acid (147) in 15% yield and 13% of the side chain reaction product, (148).

Acylation of (147) with phenylacetylchloride gave benzyl-6-epipenicillin (149) isolated as the potassium salt in 71% yield. Potassium benzylepipenicillin exhibited negligible antimicrobial activity against standard test organisms (see Chapter 12).

Wolfe and Lee (1968) caused epimerization of methyl 6-phthalimidopeni-cillanate (122) in >50% yield using three sets of conditions: (a) sodium hydride

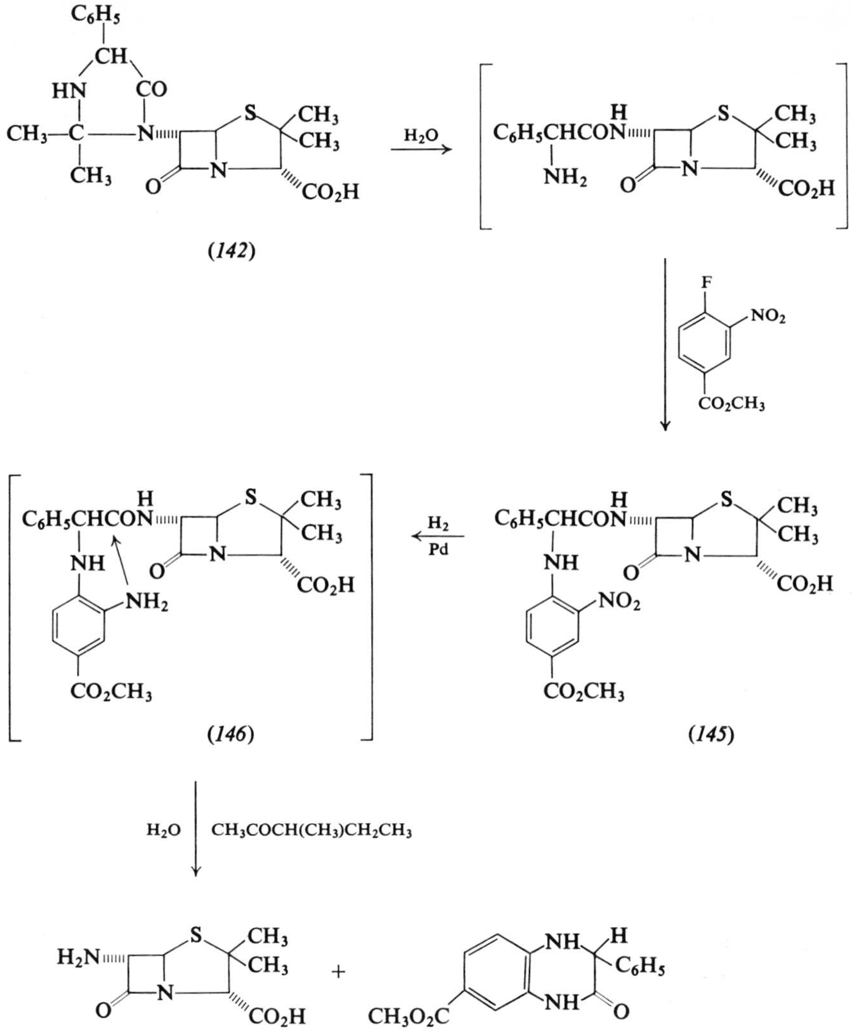

(142) (145) (146) (147) (148)

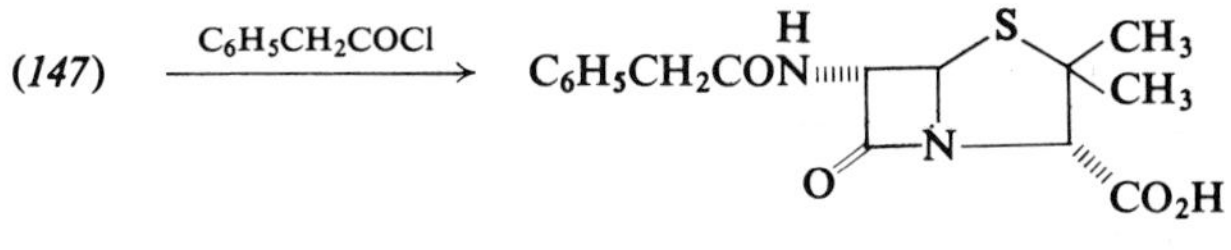

(149)

in tetrahydrofuran, (b) potassium *t*-butoxide in *t*-butanol, and (c) triethylamine in methylene chloride.

Procedure (b) in *t*-BuOD produced (*150*), containing one deuterium at C-6. Recovered (*122*) from procedure (b) in *t*-BuOD, however, contained no deuterium. When undeuterated (*150*) was treated with potassium *t*-butoxide in *t*-BuOD, it was recovered quantitatively with no incorporation of deuterium. These observations indicated that the epimerization was irreversible under reaction conditions (b).

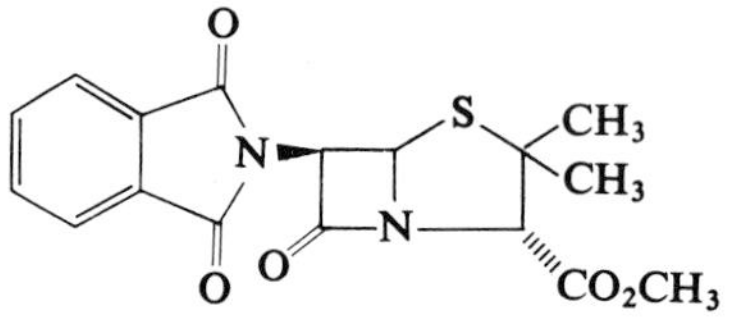

(*122*)

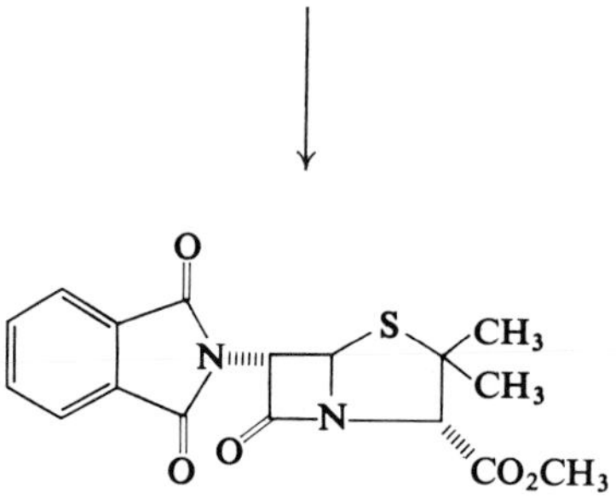

(*150*)

Wolfe and Lee believed that simple deprotonation–reprotonation did not occur. As an alternate pathway, they suggested a β elimination involving intermediate (*151*). They could not trap (*151*) under conditions (a) or (b) in the presence of methyl iodide, benzyl chloride, benzyl bromide, *p*-nitrobenzyl bromide, methyl acrylate, phenoxy-epoxypropane, or acetonitrile. In fact, none of these reagents had any effect on the epimerization of (*122*)–(*150*).

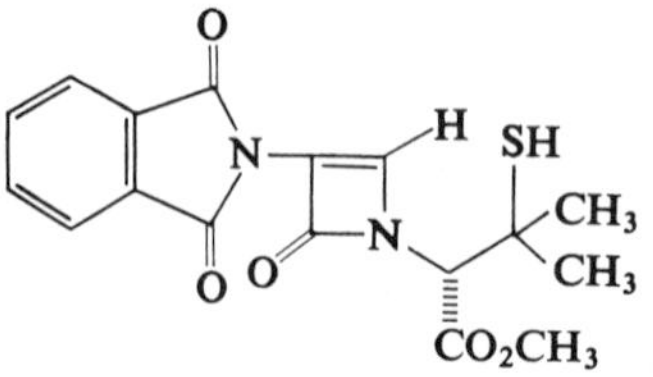

(*151*)

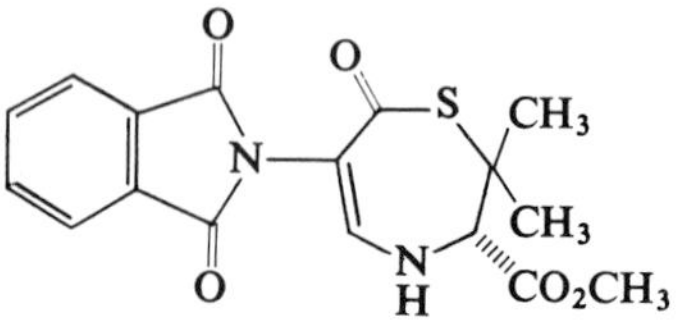

(*124*)

Kovacs and associates (1969) observed that compound (*124*) was produced in 25% yield when methyl 6-phthalimidopenicillanate (*122*) was treated with three equivalents of trimethylamine. This result was compatible with Wolfe's β-elimination intermediate (*151*) undergoing nucleophilic attack of the sulfur on the β-lactam carbonyl group.

Similarly, Jackson and Stoodley (1970) reported that methoxymethyl 6-β-*p*-nitrobenzylideniminopenicillanate (*90*) was rapidly converted to thiazepine (*152*) with one equivalent of triethylamine in chloroform. No C-6 epimerized material was noted. Compound (*152*) was subsequently transformed to thiazine (*153*) in a slower step. These workers suggested that the formation of (*152*) involved cleavage of the S-1–C-5 bond by a β elimination followed by an intramolecular attack of the thiol at the β-lactam carbonyl.

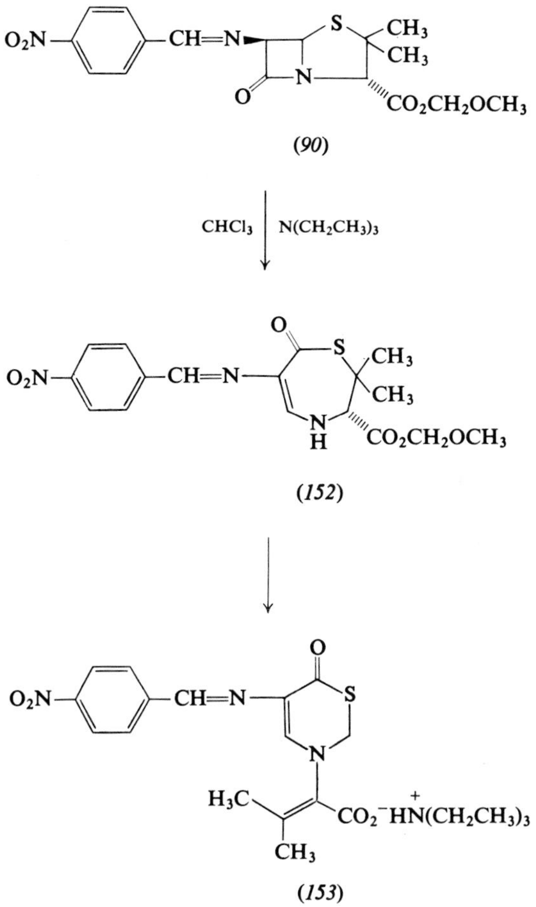

(*90*)

CHCl₃ │ N(CH₂CH₃)₃

(*152*)

(*153*)

Cooper and co-workers (1969) reported the preparation of the 6-α-phthalimidopenicillin sulfoxide esters (154) and (155). Methyl 6-β-phthalimidopenicillanate (122) was epimerized to the 6-α isomer (150) with sodium hydride-tetrahydrofuran as reported by Wolfe and Lee (1968) (see Chapter 5). Oxidation of (150) using m-chloroperbenzoic acid in chloroform gave the two sulfoxides, (154) and (155), in the ratio of 4:1, respectively. Oxidation of (122) under the same conditions gave the β-phthalimido-α-sulfoxide (156) which epimerized to (155) with triethylamine in methylene chloride.

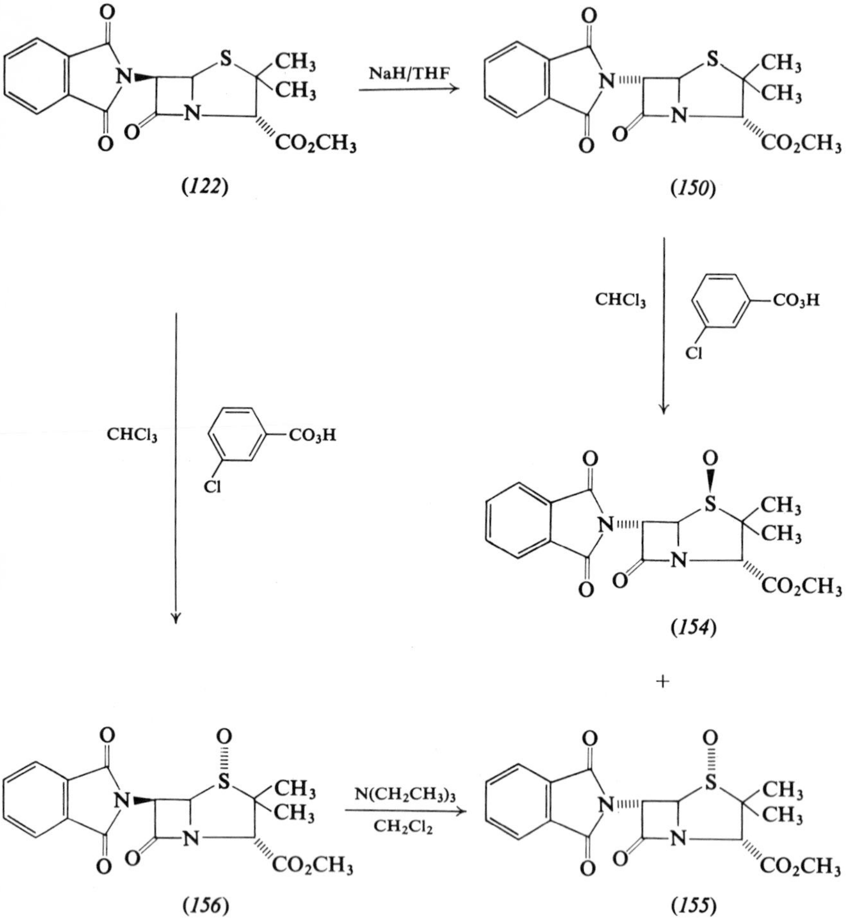

Clayton and associates (1969) examined the general requirements for epimerization at C-6 for various penicillanic acids. Attempting to equilibrate 6-α-bromopenicillanic acid (97) with its 6-β epimer, they dissolved (97) in sodium hydroxide solution at pH 10–11. The solution was acidified after 5 hours, but the recovered acid was unchanged (97). Epimer (97) was similarly treated in NaOD–D$_2$O while the reaction was monitored with NMR spectroscopy. The 6-H doublet at δ4.82 slowly disappeared while the 5-H doublet at δ5.41 sharpened to a singlet. The investigators concluded that the C-6 proton in (97) was sufficiently acidic for ionization but that the anion (157) deuterated exclusively from the β side to give (158). This result corroborated the report of Johnson et al. (1968) of the irreversible conversion of hetacillin to epihetacillin in aqueous alkali.

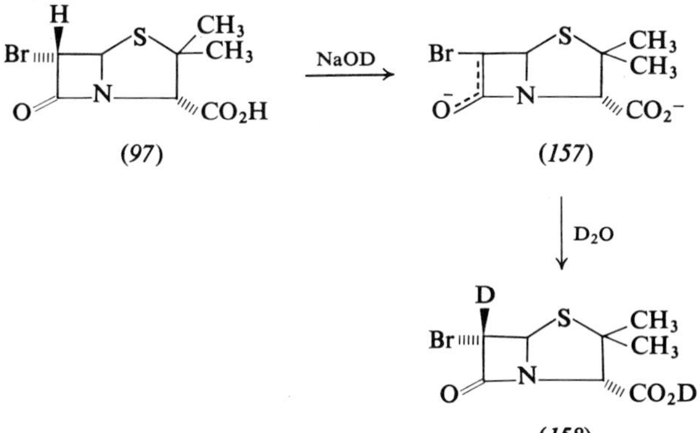

Clayton and associates (1969) noted that 6-β-aminopenicillanic acid (1), 6-β-dimethylaminopenicillanic acid (159), and 6-β-tritylaminopenicillanic acid (79) did not epimerize when treated with NaOH at pH 10–11 for 30 minutes. Similarly, penicillanic acid (98) in deuterated alkali showed no evidence of deuterium incorporation. More vigorous treatment of these compounds cleaved the β-lactam. The investigators concluded that the prime factor determining anion formation was the electronegativity of the C-6 substituent. For the 6-β-acylaminopenicillanic acids which failed to epimerize at pH 11, it was suggested that base first removed the secondary amido proton. The proximity of the resulting negative charge inhibited proton loss from C-6.

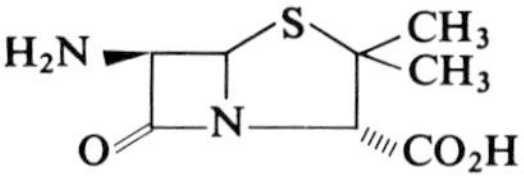

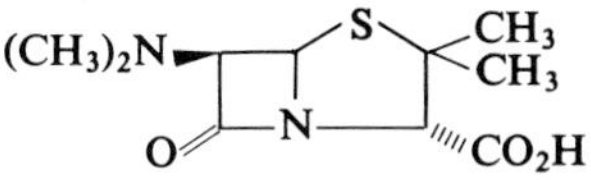

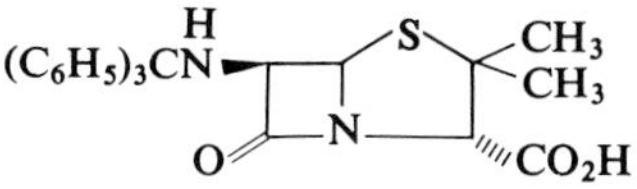

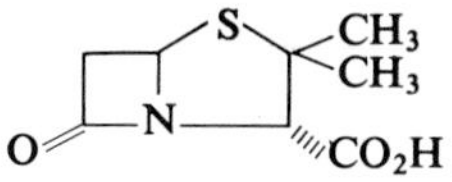

A highly electron withdrawing trimethylammonium substituent at C-6 facilitated proton removal. Merely dissolving the hemihydroiodide (*160*) in water and adjusting the pH to 7 with sodium bicarbonate solution resulted in epimerization. The NMR spectrum of the epibetaine (*161*) in $(CD_3)_2SO$ showed $\delta 6.03$ (d, 5-H) and $\delta 5.23$ (d, 6-H) with $J_{H-5, H-6} = 1.5$ Hz. Addition of D_2O to the $(CD_3)_2SO$ solution or dissolution of (*161*) in D_2O resulted in rapid replacement of the C-6 proton.

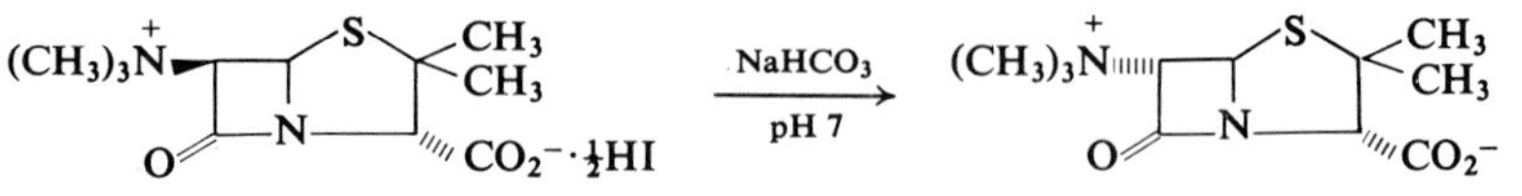

The hemihydroiodides (*160*) and (*162*) were each dissolved in D_2O, buffered at pH 5.9, and monitored with NMR spectroscopy. After 45 minutes, the sample which originally contained (*160*) had lost 86 % of the C-6 proton intensity while only 12 % had been replaced in (*162*). Conversion of (*160*) and (*162*) into deuterated (*161*) was rapid and complete above pH 7 but was not observed at all below pH 4.

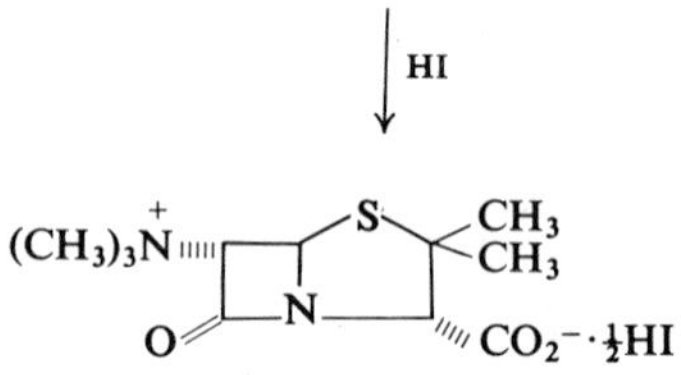

In a further series of experiments, hetacillin (*25*) and epihetacillin (*142*) were each dissolved in D_2O–NaOD at pH 9.5. After 30 minutes, the solutions were acidified with DCl and the precipitated solid (70 %) was collected and examined by NMR spectroscopy. The product from (*25*) contained 60 % of epimer (*142*) which was deuterated at C-6, and 40 % of undeuterated epimer (*25*). The product from (*142*) contained approximately 30 % deuterium at C-6 but no detectable (*25*).

Clayton and associates (1969) concluded that the ionization step was faster in the conversion of β epimer to anion than of α epimer to anion. But they thought that this difference was too small to explain complete conversion to α epimer at equilibrium. They attributed the production of α epimers to greater relative steric compression in going from anion to β epimer than to α epimer.

Commenting on the proposal of a β-elimination mechanism for the non-aqueous epimerization of methylphthalimidopenicillanate (*122*) (Wolfe and

Lee, 1968), Clayton and co-workers (1969) concluded that a simple ionization mechanism was adequate to explain their results.

Wolfe and co-workers (1970) acknowledged that penicillanic acids with strong electron-withdrawing substituents at C-6 underwent epimerization in aqueous hydroxide via carbanionic intermediates. They suggested that β elimination and carbanion formation at C-6 were competing reaction pathways. The latter process was facilitated by an appropriate combination of electron withdrawing C-6 substituent [Br, $\overset{+}{N}(CH_3)_3$, $C_6H_4(CO)_2N$] and strong base [OH^-, NaH, $NaNH_2$, $(CH_3)_3CO^-$]. Beta elimination was favored when the base was triethylamine. Reaction of anhydro-6-β-phthalimidopenicillin (*163*) (see Chapter 5) with sodium hydroxide in tetrahydrofuran ("carbanion conditions") or with triethylamine in methylene chloride ("β-elimination conditions") gave anhydro-6-α-phthalimidopenicillin (*164*) as the sole product. With triethylamine in CH_2Cl_2-$(CH_3)_3COD$, the conversion of (*163*) to (*164*) proceeded without incorporation of deuterium. The change in the NMR spectrum of the β-lactam protons from $\delta 5.60$ and $\delta 5.90$ ($J = 4.2$ Hz) in (*163*) to $\delta 5.58$ and $\delta 5.62$ ($J = 1.8$ Hz) in (*164*) indicated the *cis* to *trans* epimerization.

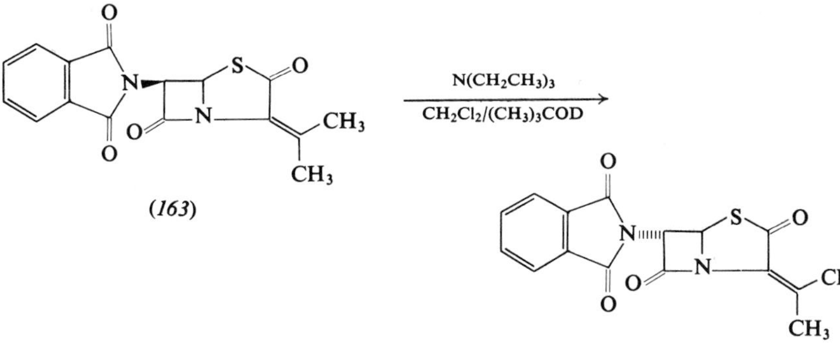

(*163*)

$$\xrightarrow[CH_2Cl_2/(CH_3)_3COD]{N(CH_2CH_3)_3}$$

(*164*)

Wolfe and Hasan (1970) reexamined the Raney nickel desulfurization of penicillins. When the antibiotics (*165*) and (*166*) were desulfurized in deuterium oxide solution, following pretreatment of the Raney nickel by repeated washing with deuterium oxide, the products (*167*) and (*168*) contained one deuterium at C-5. Comparing the NMR coupling constants for the deuterated and nondeuterated products, they showed that replacement of sulfur by deuterium at C-5 had proceeded with retention of configuration.

Sassiver and Shepherd (1969) effected C-7 epimerization in the cephalosporin sulfoxide series. Decarboxylation of cephalothin sulfoxide (*169*) with triethylamine in refluxing chloroform for 16 hours gave two products. The

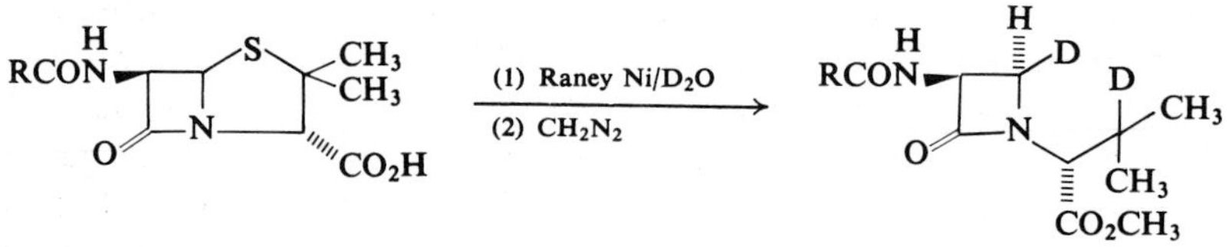

(165) R = C$_6$H$_5$CH$_2$–   (167) R = C$_6$H$_5$CH$_2$–

(166) R = C$_6$H$_5$OCH$_2$–   (168) R = C$_6$H$_5$OCH$_2$–

expected *cis* epimer (170) and the *trans* epimer (171) were present in a 1:4 ratio. Decarboxylation of (169) with one equivalent of *N*-methylmorpholine in refluxing tetrahydrofuran gave pure (170) in 71% yield. One equivalent of triethylamine in dimethyl sulfoxide (48 hours, 50°) completely isomerized (170) to (171). Compound (171) was identical to (170) by thin layer chromatography, IR and UV spectra, and microanalysis. However, the NMR spectrum of (171) showed the coupling constant for the β-lactam protons was $J_{H-6, H-7} = 2.5$ Hz in (171), whereas, $J_{H-6, H-7} = 5$ Hz in (170). When the epimerization of (170) to (171) was carried out with triethylamine in (CD$_3$)$_2$SO–D$_2$O, NMR spectroscopy showed nearly complete exchange at the C-7 position in (171). Also nearly complete exchange at the C-2 methylene and thienylacetyl methylene was noted.

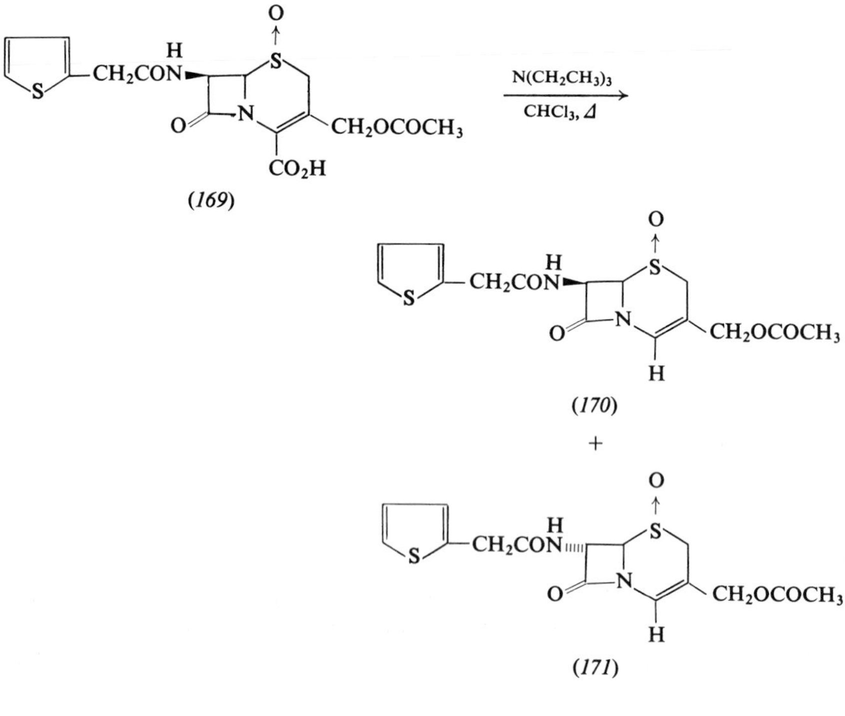

(169)

(170)

+

(171)

Sassiver and Shepherd (1969) carried out the C-7 epimerization without decarboxylation, using a 9-fluorenyl ester (*172*) prepared from cephalothin sulfoxide and diazofluorene. Compound (*173*) had $J_{\text{H-6, H-7}} = 3$ Hz while (*172*) had $J_{\text{H-6, H-7}} = 5$ Hz. These workers noted that cephalothin (*42*) did not epimerize at C-7 under conditions which transformed (*169*) and (*170*) to (*171*). They suggested that the sulfoxide function facilitated epimerization by allowing homoenolic stabilization of the anion at C-7, or simply by acting inductively as an electron-withdrawing group.

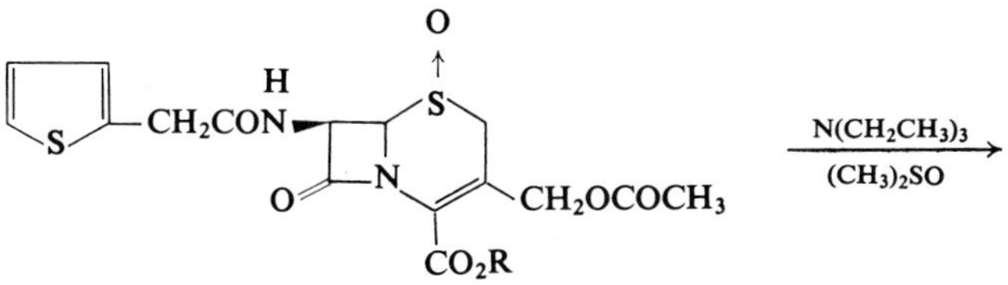

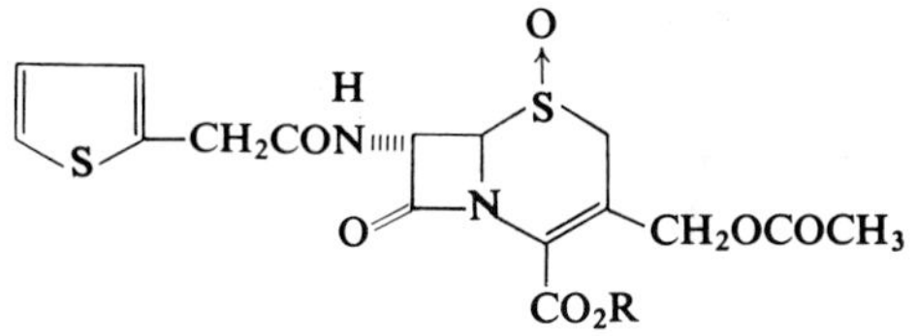

Gutowski (1970) reported a reversible, nonbasic epimerization of penicillin sulfoxide esters. Trichloroethyl ester (*174*), when treated with *N,O-bis*-(trimethylsilyl)acetamide (BSA) for several days at room temperature, reached

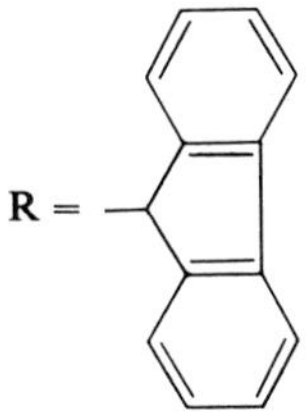

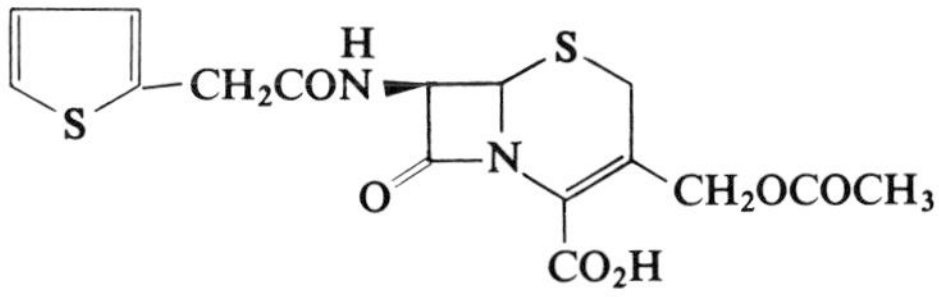

equilibrium with its *trans* epimer (*175*). The ratio of (*175*) to (*174*) at equilibrium was 4:1. Compound (*175*) was easily separated from (*174*) by fractional
crystallization from methanol. The conversion of pure (*175*) to the same
equilibrium mixture with BSA is the first successful transformation of a 6-
epipenicillin derivative to its epimer with the natural configuration at C-6.

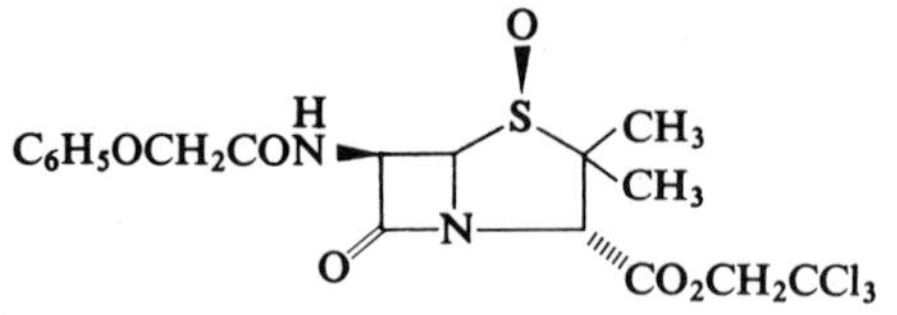

(*174*)

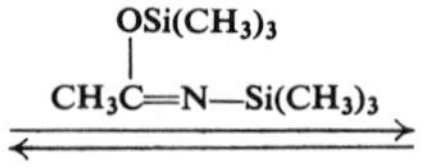

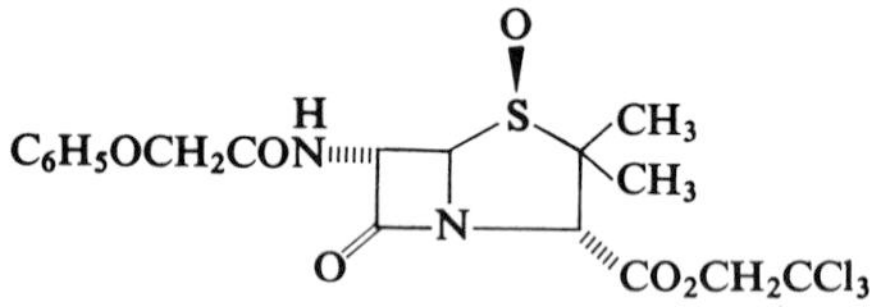

(*175*)

The reaction probably involves formation of a silyl enol ether (*176*) which
reverts to a mixture of epimers by a desilylation–reprotonation process from
either the α or β face. The sulfoxide is necessary for the BSA catalyzed epimerization perhaps because it increases the ease of removal of the C-6 proton.
Cephalosporins and cephalosporin sulfoxides failed to epimerize at C-7 under
these conditions.

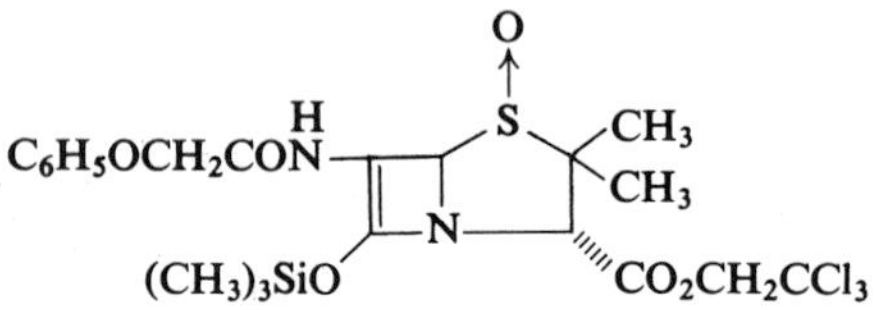

(*176*)

The acid catalyzed ring expansion (Morin *et al.*, 1969b) (see Chapter 5) of
(*175*) gave the 7-epideacetoxycephalosporanate (*177*) in 24% yield. Compound
(*177*) was deesterified with zinc and hydrochloric acid in acetonitrile to give
the deacetoxyepicephalosporanic acid (*178*), which had no significant antimicrobial activity.

Once again, examination of the coupling constants for the β-lactam protons
allowed immediate assignment of configuration. Compound (*175*) had

(175) ⟶ C₆H₅OCH₂CON ⫴⫴

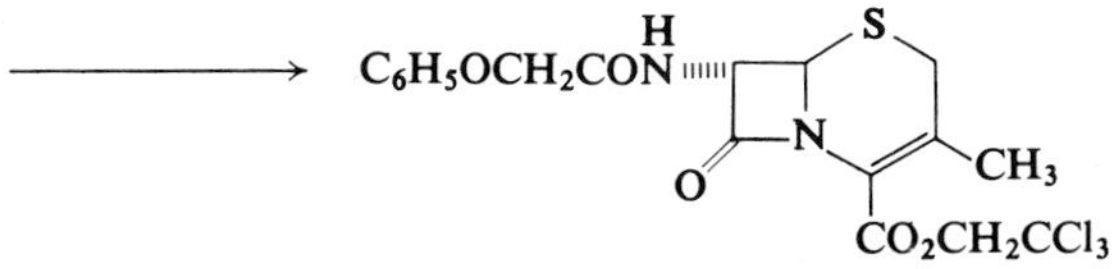

(177)

CH₃CN | Zn/HCl

C₆H₅OCH₂CON ⫴⫴

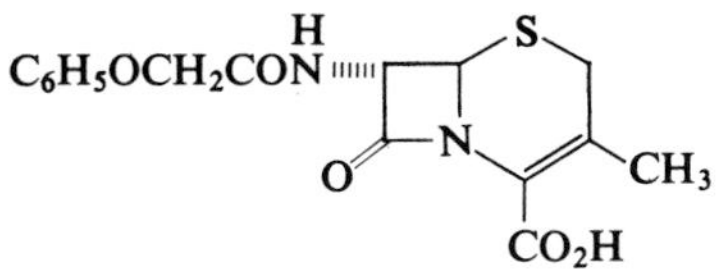

(178)

$J_{H-5,H-6} = 1.5$ Hz compared to $J_{H-5,H-6} = 4$ Hz in (174). In the cephem series, compound (177) had $J_{H-6,H-7} = 1.8$ Hz and compound (178) had $J_{H-6,H-7} = 2.0$ Hz, while deacetoxy 7-β-phenoxyacetamidocephalosporanic acid (179) had $J_{H-6,H-7} = 4.5$ Hz.

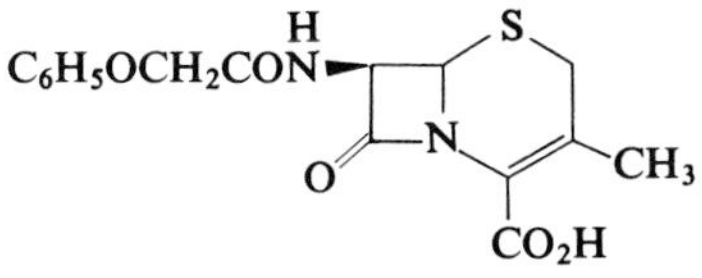

C₆H₅OCH₂CON

(179)

Bose and co-workers (1968) reported the total synthesis of 5,6-*trans*-phenoxymethylpenicillin methyl ester (180). Reaction of methyl-5,5-dimethyl-2-thiazoline-4-carboxylate (181) with azidoacetyl chloride in the presence of triethylamine gave a 5–8% yield of the bicyclic azide (182). The coupling constant between protons at C-5 and C-6 ($J = 1.5$ Hz) indicated a *trans* relationship. Compound (182) was reduced to methyl 6-α-aminopenicillanate (183) in moderate yield, using hydrogen and Adams catalyst in benzene. Impure (183) was acylated directly with phenoxyacetyl chloride and triethylamine to give the 5,6-*trans* amido ester (180) in 17% yield from the azide. Since Gutowski (1970) has shown that phenoxymethylpenicillin sulfoxide esters are equilibrated to a mixture of C-6 epimers with N,O-bis(trimethylsilyl)acetamide, product (180) could probably be converted to the sulfoxide with the natural configuration at C-6.

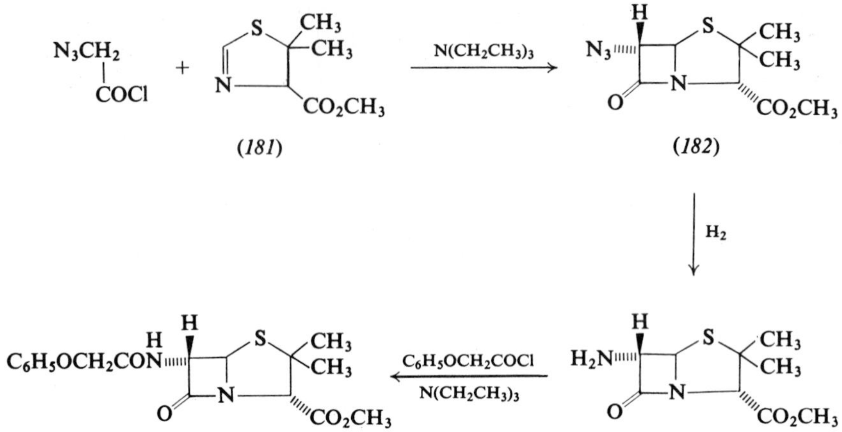

N₃CH₂—COCl + (181) →[N(CH₂CH₃)₃] (182)

(182) →[H₂] (183)

(180) ←[C₆H₅OCH₂COCl / N(CH₂CH₃)₃] (183)

(181) (182)

(180) (183)

In the course of developing a totally synthetic route to cephalothin lactone (*184*) and lactam (*185*), Heymes *et al.* (1966) and Nomine (1970) had occasion to prepare the corresponding 7-epi derivatives (*186*) and (*187*). A key intermediate was compound (*188*), present as both the *threo* and *erythro* diastereomers. Dolfini *et al.* (1969) have worked out a similar approach to cephalosporin

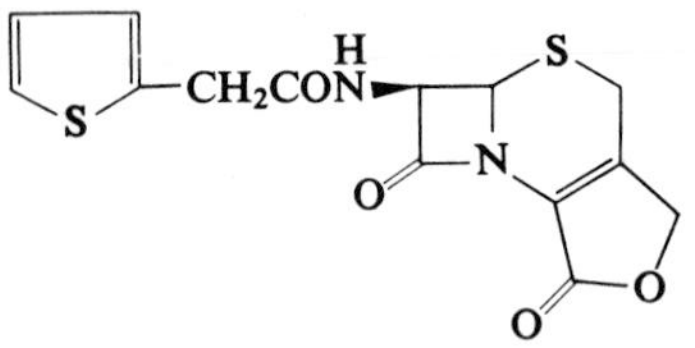

(184)

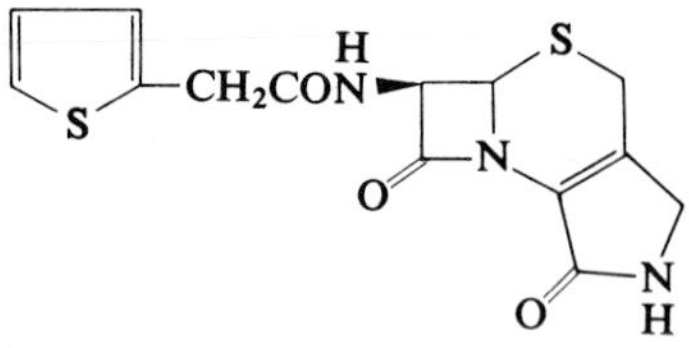

(185)

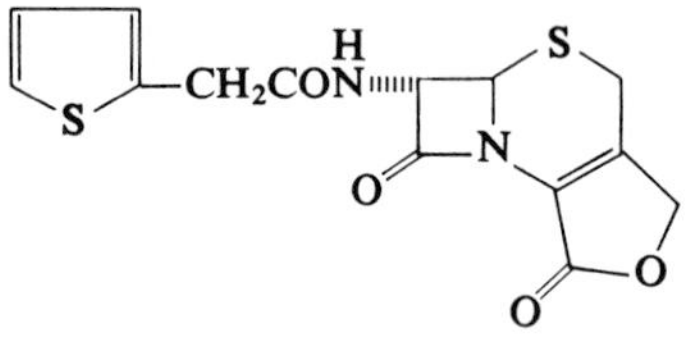

(186)

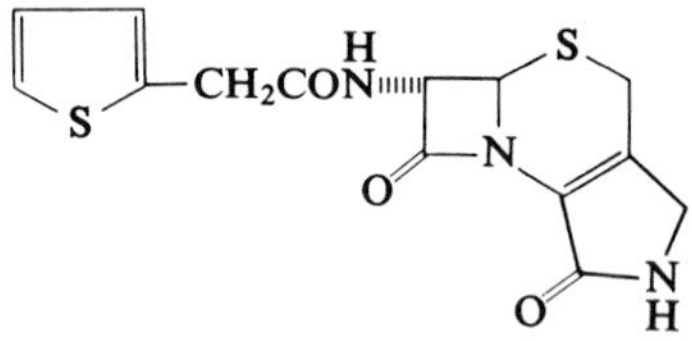

(187)

lactone also using intermediate (*188*). Ring closure of the *threo* trityl derivative (*189*) with dicyclohexylcarbodiimide in nitromethane gave product (*190*) with the natural configuration at C-7, whereas, closing the *erythro* derivative (*191*) led to the C-7 epimer (*192*). Removal of the trityl group from (*190*) with hydrochloric acid in nitromethane yielded the nucleus (*193*), which was acylated with 2-thienylacetyl chloride to give (*184*). The *N*-phthaloyl group was removed from (*192*) with hydrazine, and the resulting 7-epi nucleus (*194*) was converted to (*186*). The same *erythro–threo* relationships hold in the routes to lactams (*185*) and (*187*).

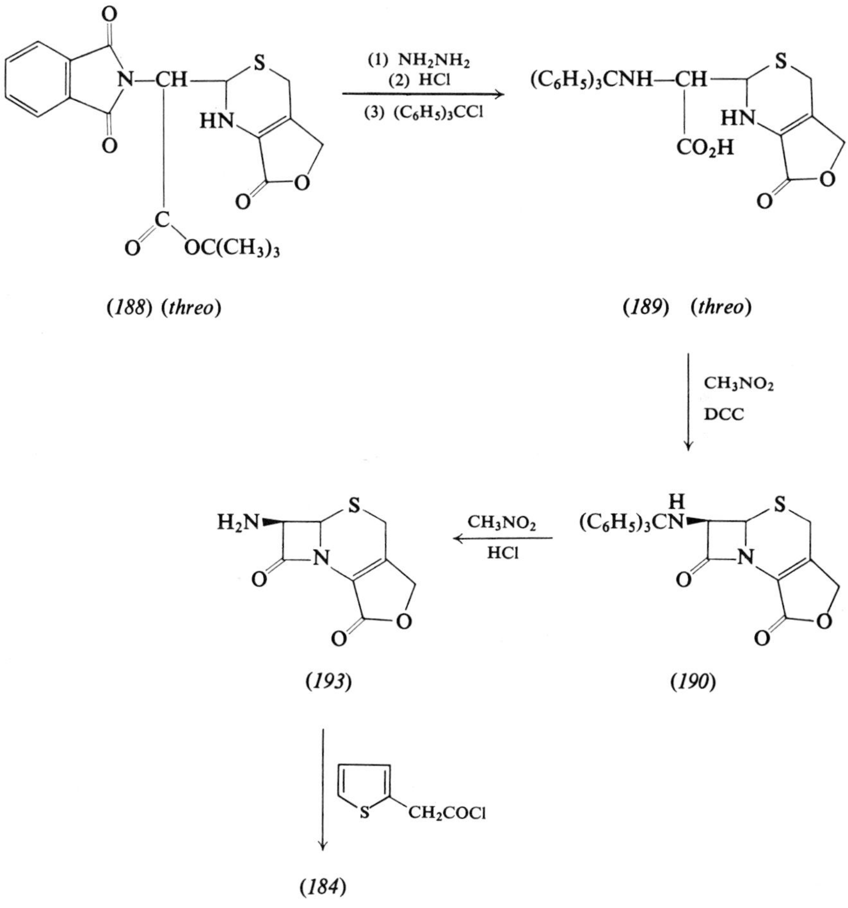

(*188*) (*threo*)   (*189*) (*threo*)

(*193*)   (*190*)

(*184*)

Fortunately, conditions were developed to convert the *erythro* diastereomer to the *threo* diastereomer, thus making the syntheses stereospecific. The synthetic β-lactam derivatives (*184*) and (*185*) from the *threo* series, after resolution, were identical in all respects to the semisynthetic antibiotics which originated from fermentation processes. The products from the *erythro* series (*186*) and (*187*) were devoid of antibiotic activity.

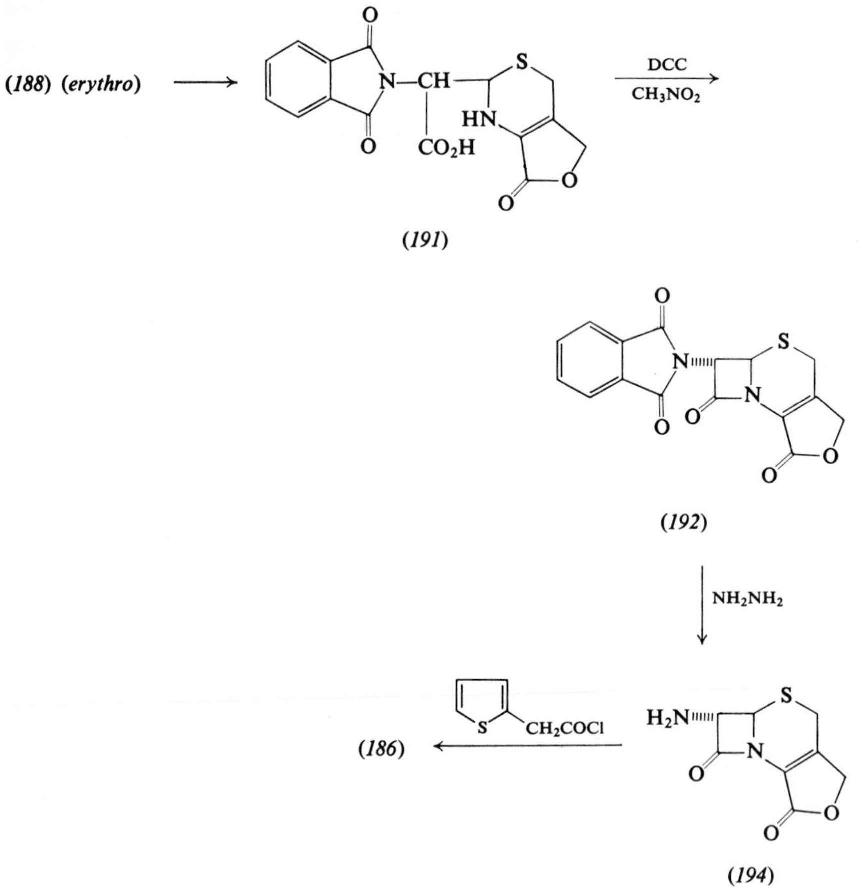

(191)

(192)

NH₂NH₂

(186)   ←   [thienyl]S—CH₂COCl

(194)

C. Alkylation

Reiner and Zeller (1968) studied the C-6 alkylation of the penicillin nucleus—partly because of the suggestion that introducing an α-methyl group at this position could give a penicillin having increased antibiotic activity (Strominger and Tipper, 1965) (see Chapters 7 and 10).

The imine (92) which Reiner and Zeller (1968) prepared from salicylaldehyde and 6-APA, followed by esterification with diazomethane, did not undergo alkylation in the presence of sodium hydride. Instead the β-lactam ring was cleaved. [Similarly, Wolfe and Lee (1968) were unable to alkylate methyl N-phthalimidopenicillanate (122) with sodium hydride and various alkylating agents.]

To protect the phenolic hydroxyl group, which probably interferes in the alkylation, and to further intensify the acidity of the C-6 proton, (*92*) was converted to its crystalline copper complex (*94*) with copper acetate and sodium bicarbonate in chloroform–water at 0°. It was possible to benzylate (*94*) with benzylchloride and sodium hydride in *N*,*N*-dimethylformamide, but the product (*195*) was difficult to purify. The paramagnetic property of copper prevented the use of NMR, and the workers were unable to establish whether one or two benzyl groups had been added.

Compound (*94*) condensed with benzaldehyde and formaldehyde with sodium hydride to give (*196*) and (*197*), but it was not possible to assign stereochemistry at C-6. All attempts to break down the copper complexes to the corresponding C-6 substituted penicillins failed.

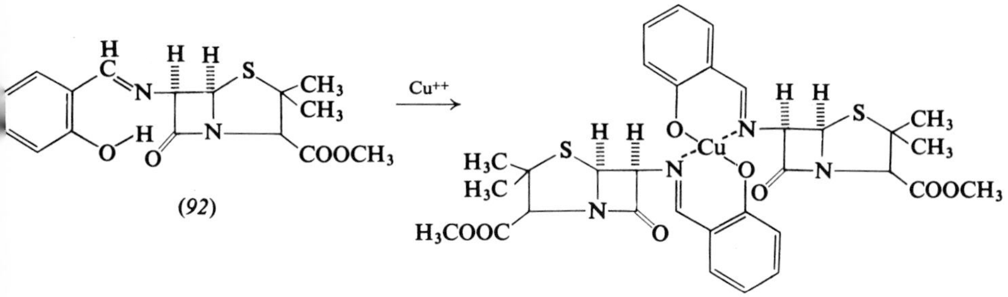

(*92*)

(*94*)

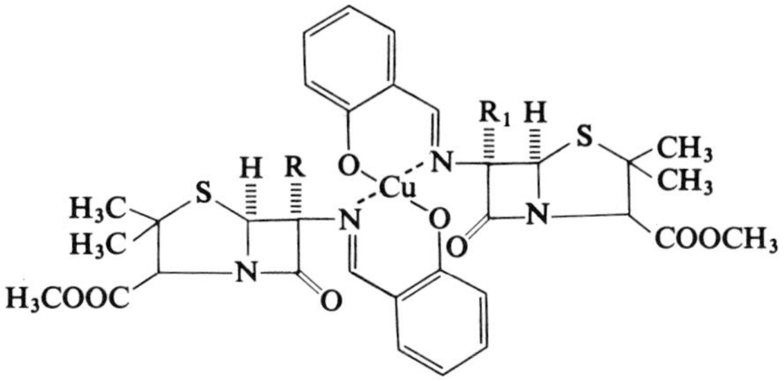

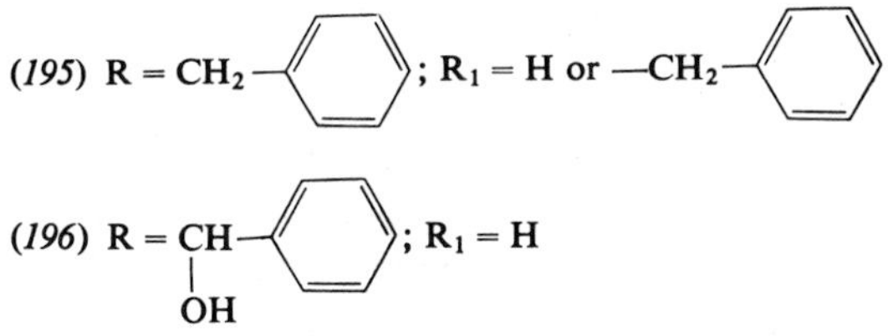

(*195*) R = CH$_2$—〈 〉; R$_1$ = H or —CH$_2$—〈 〉

(*196*) R = CH—〈 〉; R$_1$ = H
        |
       OH

(*197*) R = CH$_2$OH; R$_1$ = CH$_2$OH

Subsequently, Reiner and Zeller (1968) noted that 6-APA itself reacted with benzaldehyde in isopropyl alcohol–water at pH 7.5 to form (*198*) in 76 % yield. Hydrolysis of (*198*) with sulfuric acid in acetone gave 6-amino-6-(α-hydroxybenzyl)penicillanic acid (*199*) in 50 % yield. Product (*199*) was a single compound, not a mixture of C-6 epimers, but the specific configuration was not assigned. Acetylation of (*199*) with phenylacetyl chloride gave the amide (*200*) in 51 % yield. Compound (*200*) had very weak activity—a result which Reiner and Zeller attributed to either the "wrong" configuration of the hydroxybenzyl group or its large space requirement.

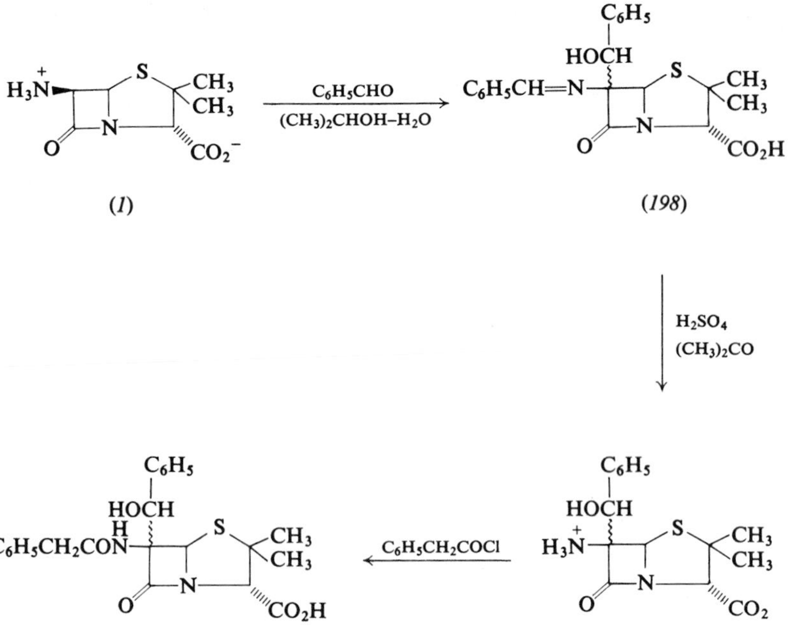

(*1*)   (*198*)

H₂SO₄
(CH₃)₂CO

(*200*)   (*199*)

6-APA condensed with formaldehyde in the presence of salicylaldehyde to form in 24 % yield, an amorphous acid which was assigned structure (*201*). Unfortunately, the desired product (*202*) could not be isolated. Treatment of (*201*) with ethanol–water containing excess dimedon resulted in the crystallization of exactly one equivalent of formaldehyde–dimedon adduct, but after subsequent concentration of the filtrate, only 6-APA was isolated. The investigators believed that (*202*) formed but suffered a retro-aldol reaction.

Kaiser and associates (1971a) carried out a stereospecific C-6 alkylation of a penicillin derivative by employing the rearrangement of a nitrogen ylide. The dimethylamino hydrochloride (*203*) (Leigh, 1965) was reacted with diazomethane in ether to give the amino ester (*204*), which yielded the quaternary salt (*205*) upon treatment with allyl bromide in acetone. Compound (*205*) was

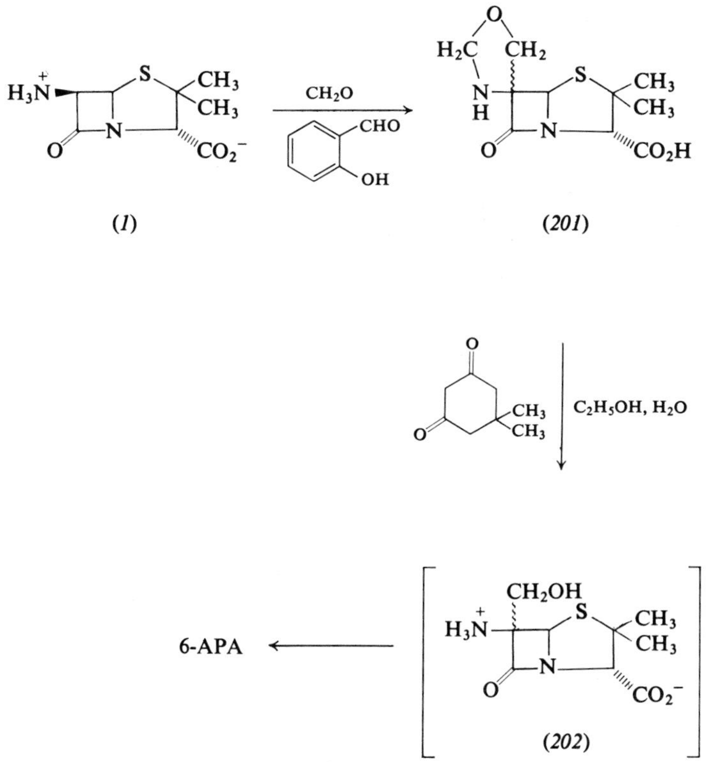

(1)

(201)

(202)

6-APA

rearranged to the amine (*206*) in 75% yield by using 1.5 equivalents of sodium hydride in 5:2 benzene–dimethylformamide at room temperature. The reaction probably involves a cyclization of the nitrogen ylide (*207*). The methiodide derivative (*208*) of the rearrangement product was shown to have the trialkylammonium group in the β (natural) orientation by comparing its NMR properties with those of known pairs of 6-α- and 6-β-trialkylammonium penicillanates.

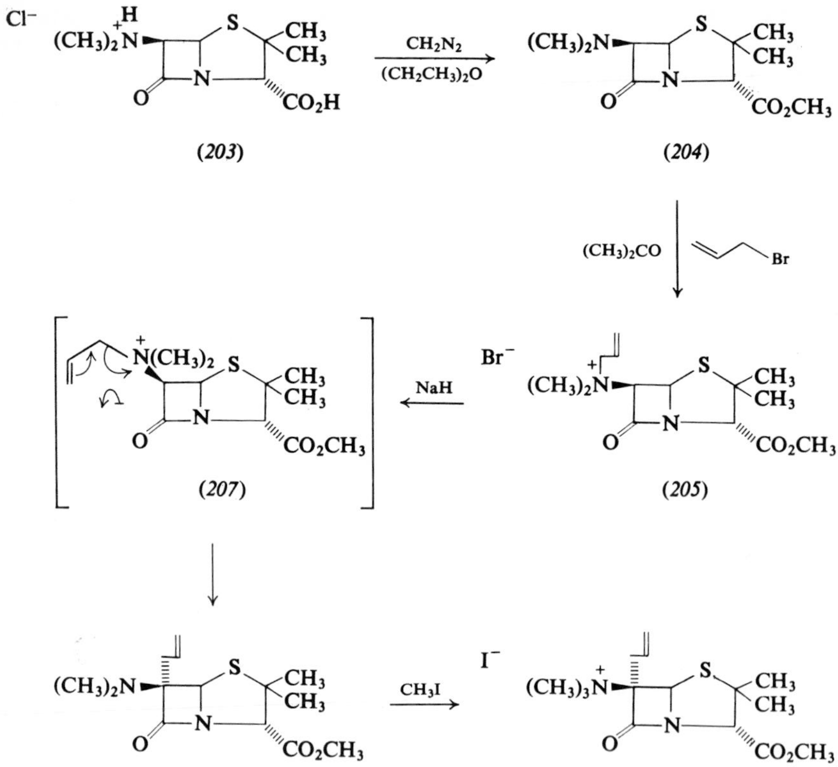

(203)   (204)   (207)   (205)   (206)   (208)

In contrast to the rearrangement of (205) in benzene–dimethylformamide, quantitative epimerization to (209) was observed in aqueous sodium bicarbonate solution.

(205) $\xrightarrow[\text{(2) HBr/H}_2\text{O}]{\text{(1) NaHCO}_3/\text{H}_2\text{O}}$

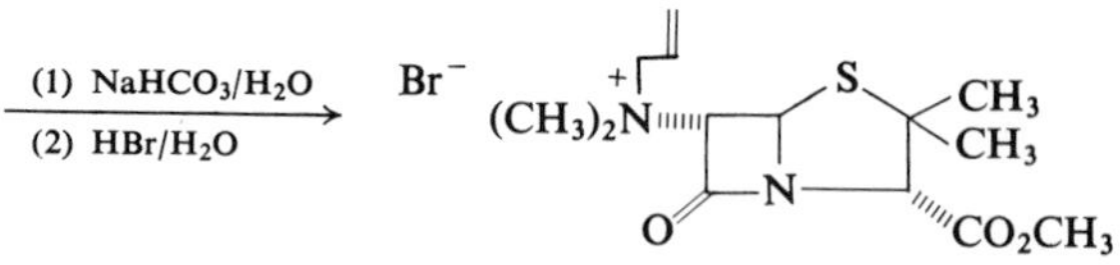

(209)

The deacetoxycephalosporin analog (210), prepared exactly as in the penam case, appeared to follow the same reaction course (Kaiser and Ashbrook, 1970). The product (211) characterized as the hydrochloride (212) is thought to have the β (natural) configuration of the C-7 dimethylamino group by analogy with the result in the penam case.

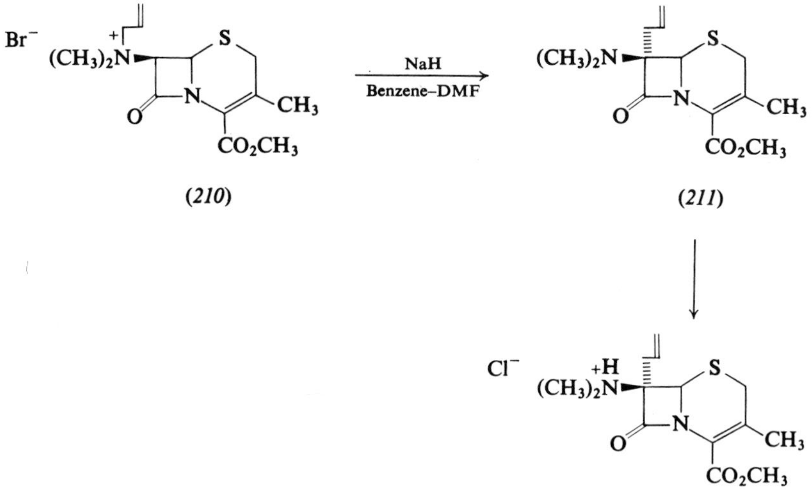

(210)   (211)

(212)

III. Cleavage of the β-Lactam

The strained β-lactam ring, common to the structure of the penicillins and cephalosporins, is susceptible to a wide variety of cleavage reactions. Since the reactivity of the β-lactam in these antibiotics is fundamentally linked to antimicrobial activity and bacterial resistance, further understanding of the reactions discussed in this section could lead to clinically important results.

In spite of the structural similarity between the penicillins and the cephalosporins, there are major differences in the way the compounds undergo β-lactam ring cleavage. Hydrolysis of penicillins (213) by dilute alkali, penicil-

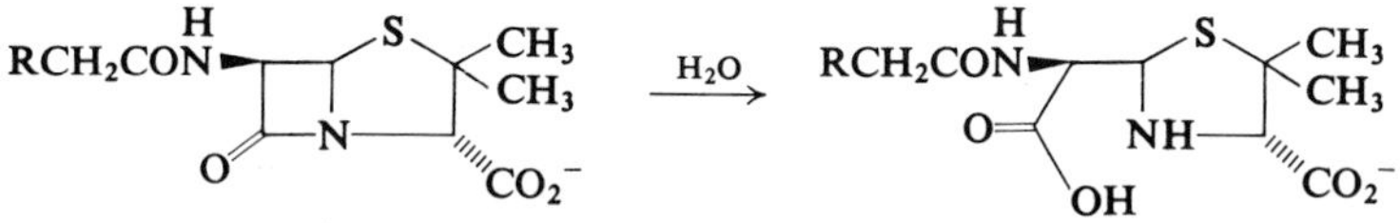

(213)   (214)

linase, or amino groups yield chiefly the corresponding penicilloates (214), which can be isolated and are well characterized (Mozingo and Folkers, 1949).

Nucleophilic ring opening of cephalosporins (*215*) presents a more complicated case because the corresponding "cephalosporoate" (*216*) is unstable. Expulsion of acetate with the assistance of the electron pair on the enamine
nitrogen is likely. In fact, extensive fragmentation along with production of
free acetate is evident when cephalosporin C is subjected to aqueous cleavage
conditions (Newton and co-workers, 1968).

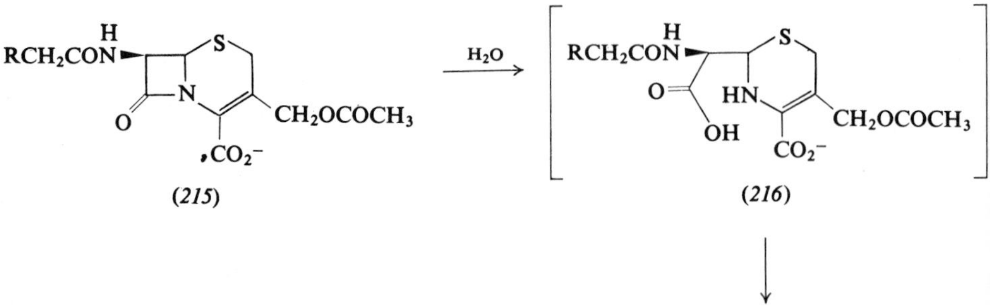

(*215*)   (*216*)

Fragmentation products

The cephalosporoate (*217*) of cephalosporin C γ-lactone (*218*) is unique
because the α,β-unsaturated lactone function stabilizes the β-lactam hydrolysis
product (*217*) (Jeffery *et al.*, 1961).

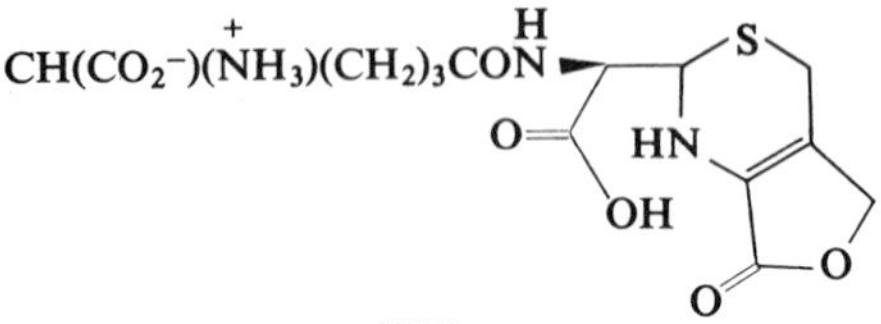

(*217*)

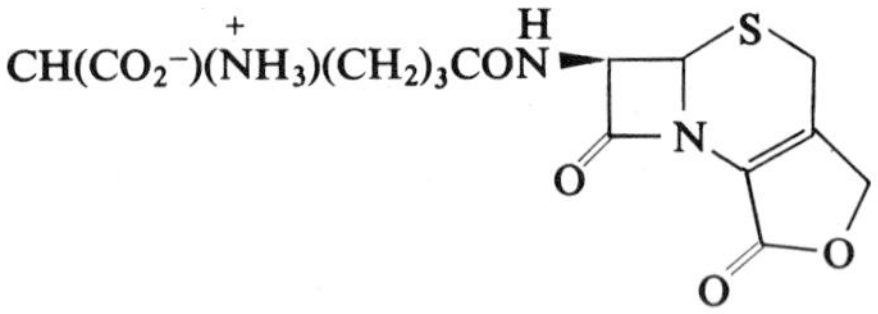

(*218*)

Eggers and associates (1965) studied the reaction of cephaloram (*40*) with
sodium benzyloxide in benzyl alcohol. The product (*219*), which has lost the
acetoxy function, probably arises by the scheme illustrated below. The structure of compound (*219*) was verified by independent synthesis.

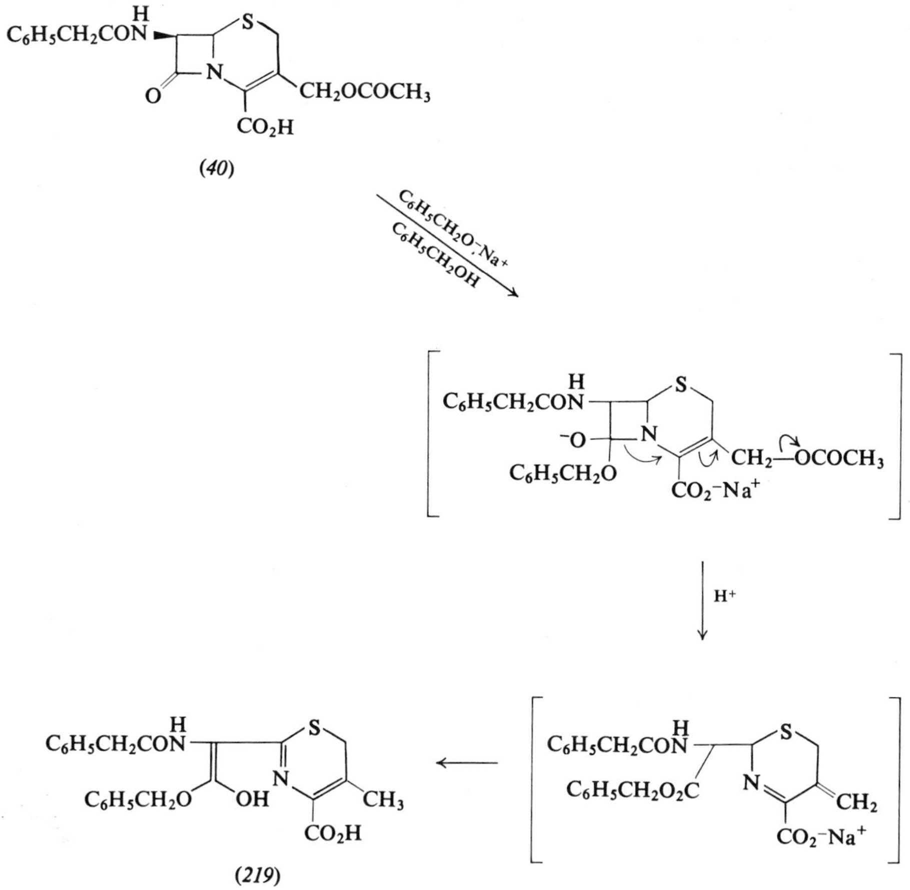

(40)

(219)

Sabath and co-workers (1965) reported that β-lactam cleavage of cephalosporin C (*137*), cephalothin (*42*), and cephaloridine (*220*) with a β-lactamase was accompanied by the appearance of two equivalents of acid per mole of antibiotic. One equivalent was attributed to the β-lactam hydrolysis while the other resulted from the liberation of acetate ion or pyridine. By comparison, deacetoxycephalosporin C (*221*) yielded only one equivalent of acid.

Studies by Hamilton-Miller *et al.* (1970a, b) on the aminolysis and enzymatic hydrolysis of cephalosporins have shed considerable light on the complex breakdown pattern of the cephalosporins. The degradation of 7-*n*-butyramido-cephalosporanic acid (*222*) with ND_3–D_2O was monitored by NMR and UV spectra. Analysis of the data and comparison with model compounds led to the conclusion that the *exo*-methylene compound (223) was formed as a semistable

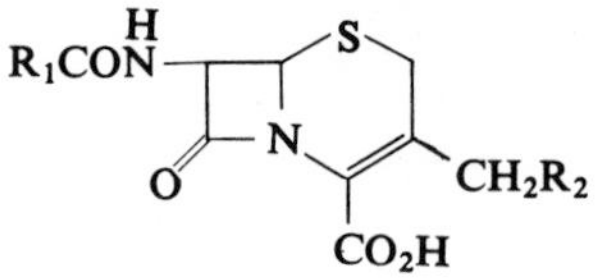

$$R_1CON\overset{H}{-}\left[\begin{array}{c}S\\N\\O\end{array}\right]CH_2R_2$$
$$CO_2H$$

(42) $R_1 = $ ⟨thienyl⟩$CH_2—$; $R_2 = OCOCH_3$

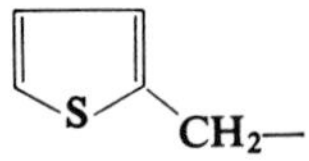

(137) $R_1 = CH(CO_2^-)(\overset{+}{N}H_3)(CH_2)_3—$; $R_2 = OCOCH_3$

(220) $R_1 = $ ⟨thienyl⟩$CH_2—$; $R_2 = \overset{+}{N}$⟨pyridinium⟩

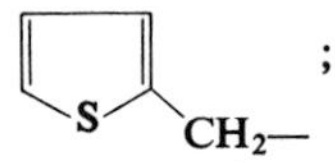

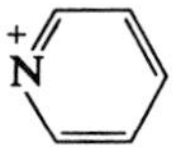

(221) $R_1 = CH(CO_2^-)(\overset{+}{N}H_3)(CH_2)_3—$; $R_2 = H$

(222) $R_1 = CH_3(CH_2)_3—$; $R_2 = OCOCH_3$

intermediate. Compound (223) (λ_{max} 230 mμ) underwent further degradation to a new compound (λ_{max} 270 mμ) which was assigned structure (224). Corresponding results were obtained with cephalosporin C.

(222) $\longrightarrow$

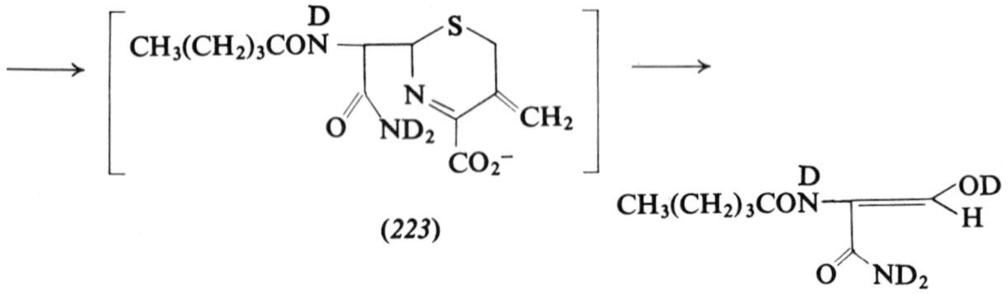

$$\left[CH_3(CH_2)_3CON\overset{D}{-}\left[\begin{array}{c}S\\N\\O\quad ND_2\end{array}\right]CH_2 \right] \longrightarrow$$
$$CO_2^-$$

(223)

$$CH_3(CH_2)_3CON\overset{D}{-}\underset{O\quad ND_2}{\overset{}{\diagup}}\overset{OD}{\underset{H}{\diagdown}}$$

(224)

$$CH_3(CH_2)_3CON\overset{H}{-}\left[\begin{array}{c}S\\N\\O\end{array}\right]CH_2X \qquad \xrightarrow{ND_3-D_2O} \qquad CH_3(CH_2)_2CON\overset{D}{-}\left[\begin{array}{c}S\\HN\\O\quad ND_2\end{array}\right]CH_2X$$
$$CO_2H \qquad\qquad\qquad\qquad\qquad\qquad\qquad\qquad CO_2^-$$

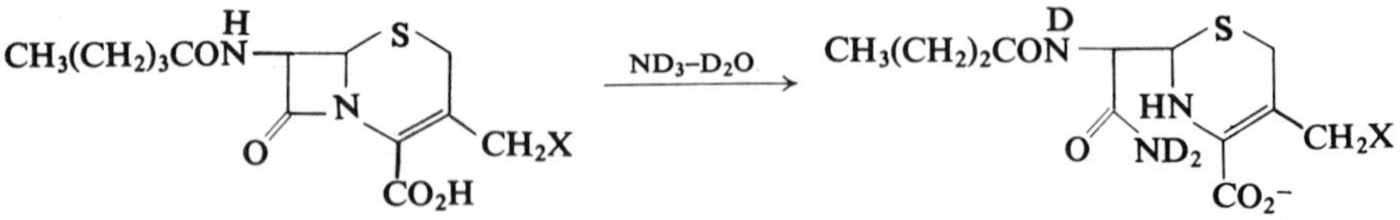

(225) X = H

(226) X = OH

(227) X = H

(228) X = OH

Aqueous aminolysis of 7-*n*-butyramidodeacetoxycephalosporanic acid (*225*) and 7-*n*-butyramidodeacetylcephalosporanic acid (*226*), however, gave inter-mediate deacetoxy and deacetyl cephalosporoates (*227*) and (*228*). Δ^2-Cepha-loram (*229*) upon aqueous aminolysis formed the deacetyl derivative which was subsequently converted to (*230*).

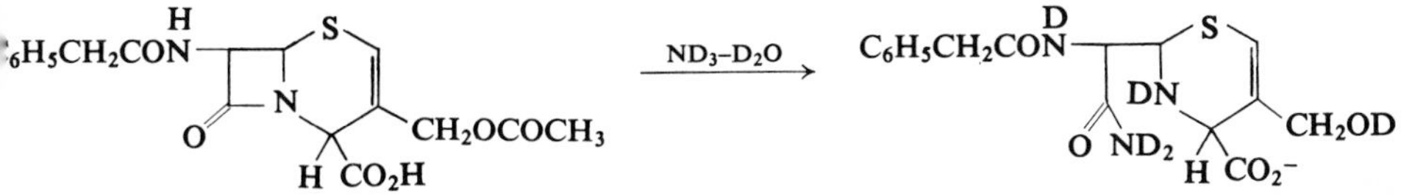

(*229*)   (*230*)

Experiments with β-lactamase on cephalosporin C (*137*) established that the compounds having UV absorption maxima at 230 mμ were also inter-mediates in the enzymatic hydrolyses. β-Lactamase treatment of deacetyl-cephalosporins, however, also gave intermediates with λ_{max} 230 mμ—a dif-ferent result from the aminolysis. The investigators speculated that enzymatic treatment could have converted the hydroxyl groups of the deacetyl com-pounds into better leaving groups resulting in behavior similar to that of cephalosporins.

Conversion of small amounts of penicillins to reactive penicillenates (*231*) has been implicated as a factor in penicillin allergy (Abraham, 1968). The peni-cillenates are thought to react with amino groups of proteins to form haptens of antigens. This subject is discussed in detail in Chapter 10.

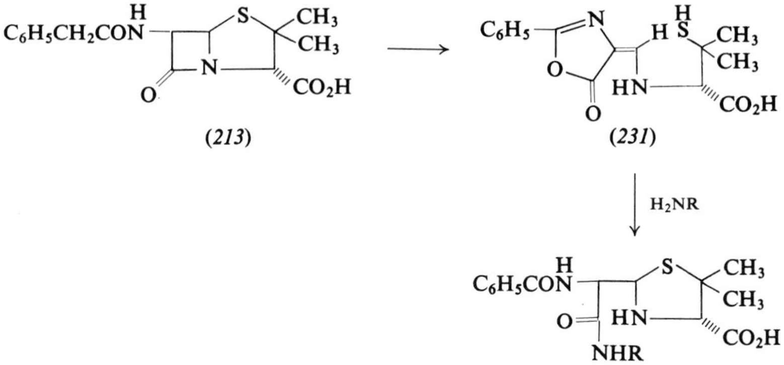

(*213*)   (*231*)

In the case of cephalosporins, stable compounds analogous to those of the penicillenates apparently are not formed. When cephalosporin C (*137*) is kept at 37° in neutral aqueous solution, a small amount of the thiazine (*232*) is obtained (Jeffery and co-workers, 1960). Compound (*232*) results from β-lactam cleavage and nucleophilic attack of sulfur on the acyl side chain.

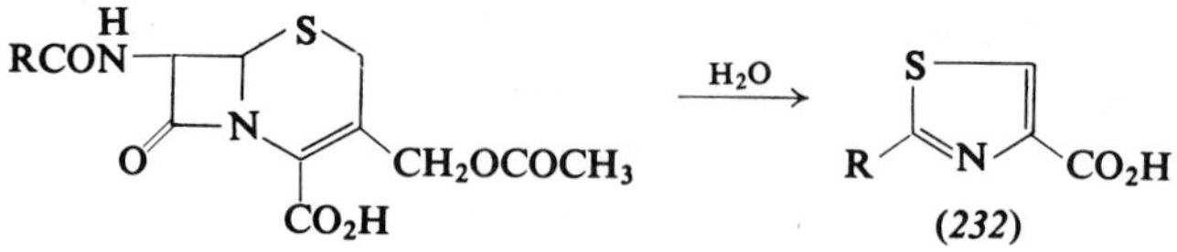

$$R = (CO_2^-)(\overset{+}{N}H_3)CH(CH_2)_3-$$

Another key problem encountered with benzylpenicillin is its instability in dilute acid—a factor which accounts for its destruction in the stomach. The sensitivity of penicillin to acid parallels the ease of formation of oxazoline (*233*), which subsequently is transformed to the penillic acid (*234*).

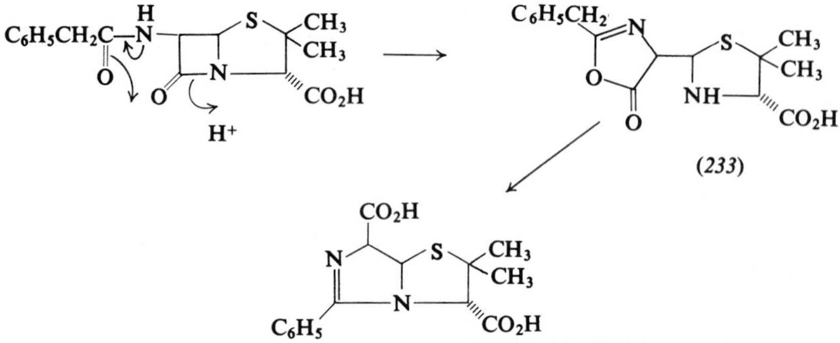

(*233*)

(*234*)

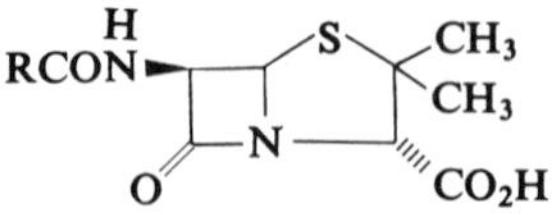

(*17*) R =

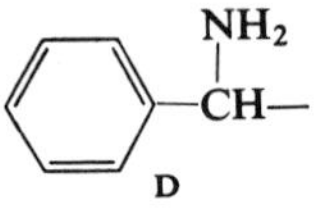

(*235*) R =

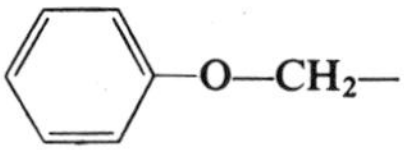

(*236*) R = N=

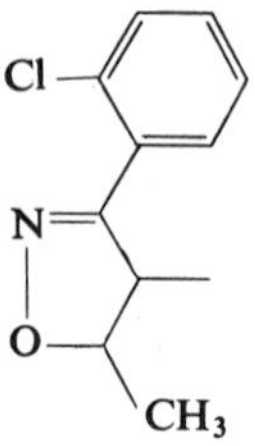

Formation of penillic acid has been minimized by introducing electron withdrawing groups at the N-acyl side chain. For example, phenoxymethyl-penicillin (235), ampicillin (17), and cloxacillin (236) (all important clinically useful compounds) are relatively stable to acid.

Compared to the penicillins, cephalosporins are relatively insensitive to acid regardless of the N-acyl side chain because of the decreased nucleophilicity of the nitrogen in the dihydrothiazine ring (Abraham, 1968).

References

Abraham, E. P. (1968). In "Topics in Pharmaceutical Sciences" (D. Perlman, ed.), Vol. 1, pp. 1–31. Wiley (Interscience), New York.
Archer, R. A., and Kitchell, B. S. (1966). J. Org. Chem. **31**, 3409.
Bamberg, P., Ekstrom, B., and Sjoberg, B. (1967). Acta Chem. Scand. **21**, 2210.
Bamberg, P., Ekstrom B., and Sjoberg, B. (1968). Acta Chem. Scand. **22**, 367.
Barrow, K. D., and Spotswood, T. M. (1965). Tetrahedron Lett. 3325.
Batchelor, F. R., Doyle, F. P., Nayler, J. H. C., and Rolinson, G. N. (1959). Nature **183**, 257.
Belgium Patent 734,532.
Belgium Patent 734,533.
Bose, A. K., Spiegelman, G., and Manhas, M. S. (1968). J. Amer. Chem. Soc. **90**, 4506.
Brain, E. G., Doyle, F. P., Hardy, K., Long, A. A. W., Mehta, M. D., Miller, D., Nayler, J. H. C., Soulal, M. J., Stove, E. R., and Thomas, G. R. (1962). J. Chem. Soc. 1445.
Busch, H., and Lane, M. (1967). In "Chemotherapy," pp. 29–46, 88–91. Year Book Medical Publ., Chicago, Illinois.
Chauvette, R. R., Flynn, E. H., Jackson, B. G., Lavagnino, E. R., Morin, R. B., Mueller, R. A., Pioch, R. P., Roeske, R. W., Ryan, C. W., Spencer, J. L., and Van Heyningen, E. (1962). J. Amer. Chem. Soc. **84**, 3401.
Chauvette, R. R., Pennington, P. A., Ryan, C. W., Cooper, R. D. G., José, F. L., Wright, I. G., Van Heyningen, E. M., and Huffman, G. W. (1971). J. Org. Chem. **36**, 1259.
Cignarella, G., Pifferi, G., and Testa, E. (1962). J. Org. Chem. **27**, 2668.
Clayton, J. P. (1969). J. Chem. Soc. C 2123.
Clayton, J. P., Nayler, J. H. C., Southgate, R., and Stove, E. R. (1969). Chem. Commun. 129.
Clayton, J. P., Southgate, R., Ramsay, B. G., and Stoodley, R. J. (1970). J. Chem. Soc. C 2089.
Cocker, J. D., Cowley, B. R., Cox, J. S. G., Eardley, S., Gregory, G. I., Lazenby, J. K., Long, A. G., Sly, J. C. P., and Somerfield, G. A. (1965). J. Chem. Soc. 5015.
Cooper, R. D. G., Demarco, P. V., and Spry, D. O. (1969). J. Amer. Chem. Soc. **91**, 1528.
Daehne, W. v., Frederiksen, E., Gundersen, E., Lund, F., Morch, P., Petersen, H. J., Roholt, K., Tybring, L., and Godtfredsen, W. O. (1970). J. Med. Chem. **13**, 607.
Dane, E., and Dockner, T. (1965). Chem. Ber. **98**, 789.
Dolfini, J. E., Schwartz, J., and Weisenborn, F. (1969). J. Org. Chem. **34**, 1582.
Doyle, F. P., and Nayler, J. H. C. (1964). In "Advances in Drug Research" (N. J. Harper and A. B. Simmonds, eds.), Vol. 1, pp. 1–69. Academic Press, London and New York.
Doyle, F. P., Fosker, G. R., Nayler, J. H. C., and Smith, H. (1962a). J. Chem. Soc. 1440.
Doyle, F. P., Hardy, K., Nayler, J. H. C., Soulal, M. J., Stove, E. R., and Waddington, H. R. J. (1962b). J. Chem. Soc. 1453.
Eggers, S. H., Kane, V. V., and Lowe, G. (1965). J. Chem. Soc. 1262.
Ekstrom, B., Gomez-Revilla, A., Mollberg, R., Thelin, H., and Sjoberg, B. (1965). Acta Chem. Scand. **19**, 281.

Evrard, E., Claesen, M., and Vanderhaeghe, H. (1964). *Nature* **201**, 1124.

France Patent 1,397,509.

Glombitza, K. W. (1964). *Ann.* **673**, 166.

Gottstein, W. J., Eachus, A. H., and Cheney, L. C. (1970). *J. Org. Chem.* **35**, 1693.

Great Britain Patent 873,049.

Great Britain Patent 1,073,530.

Green, G. F. H., Page, J. E., and Staniforth, S. E. (1965). *J. Chem. Soc.* 1595.

Green, G. F. H., Page, J. E., and Staniforth, S. E. (1966). *Chem. Commun.* 597.

Gutowski, G. E. (1970). *Tetrahedron Lett.* 1779.

Hamilton-Miller, J. M. T., Newton, G. G. F., and Abraham, E. P. (1970a). *Biochem. J.* **116**, 371.

Hamilton-Miller, J. M. T., Richards, E., and Abraham, E. P. (1970b). *Biochem. J.* **116**, 385.

Hardcastle, G. A., Johnson, D. A., Panetta, C. A., Scott, A. I., and Sutherland, S. A. (1966). *J. Org. Chem.* **31**, 897.

Hauser, D., and Sigg, H. P. (1967). *Helv. Chim. Acta* **50**, 1327.

Herrell, W. E. (1968). *Clin. Med.* **75**, 19.

Heymes, R., Amiard, G., and Nomine, G. (1966). *C. R. Acad. Sci. Paris Ser. C* **263**, 170.

Jackson, B. G. (1971). Personal communication.

Jackson, J. R., and Stoodley, R. J. (1970). *Chem. Commun.* 14.

Jeffery, J. D'A., Abraham, E. P., and Newton, G. G. F. (1960). *Biochem. J.* **75**, 216.

Jeffery, J. D'A., Abraham, E. P., and Newton, G. G. F. (1961). *Biochem. J.* **81**, 591.

Johnson, D. A., and Mania, D. (1969). *Tetrahedron Lett.* 267.

Johnson, D. A., Mania, D., Panetta, C. A., and Silvestri, H. H. (1968). *Tetrahedron Lett.* 1903.

Kagan, H. B., Basselier, J. J., and Luche, J. L. (1964). *Tetrahedron Lett.* 941.

Kaiser, G. V., and Ashbrook, C. W. (1970). Unpublished results.

Kaiser, G. V., Ashbrook, C. W., and Baldwin, J. E. (1971a). *J. Amer. Chem. Soc.* **93**, 2342.

Kaiser, G. V., Ashbrook, C. W., Goodson, T., Wright, I. G., and Van Heyningen, E. M. (1971b). *J. Med. Chem.* **14**, 426.

Kariyone, K., Harada, H., Kurita, M., and Takano, T. (1970). *J. Antibiot.* **23**, 131.

Karplus, M. (1959). *J. Chem. Phys.* **30**, 11.

Karplus, M. (1962). *J. Amer. Chem. Soc.* **84**, 2458.

Koe, B. K. (1962). *Nature* **195**, 1200.

Kovacs, O. K. J., Ekstrom, B., and Sjoberg, B. (1969). *Tetrahedron Lett.* 1863.

Kurita, M., Atarashi, S., Hattori, K., and Takano, T. (1966). *J. Antibiot. Ser. A* **19**, 243.

Leanza, W. J., Christensen, B. G., Rogers, E. F., and Patchett, A. A. (1965). *Nature* **207**, 1395.

Leigh, T. (1965). *J. Chem. Soc.* 3616.

Loder, B., Newton, G. G. F., and Abraham, E. P. (1961). *Biochem. J.* **79**, 408.

Luche, J. L., Kagan, H. B., Parthasarathy, R., Tsoucaris, G., deRango, C., and Zelwer, C. (1968). *Tetrahedron* **24**, 1275.

Lynn, B. (1966). *Pharm. J.* **196**, 115.

Manhas, M. S., and Bose, A. K. (1969). *In* "Synthesis of Penicillin, Cephalosporin C and Analogs." Dekker, New York.

McMillan, I., and Stoodley, R. J. (1966). *Tetrahedron Lett.* 1205.

McMillan, I., and Stoodley, R. J. (1968). *J. Chem. Soc. C* 2533.

Moll, F., and Hannig, M. (1970). *Arch. Pharm.* **303**, 321.

Morin, R. B., Jackson, B. G., Flynn, E. H., Roeske, R. W., and Andrews, S. L. (1969a). *J. Amer. Chem. Soc.* **91**, 1396.

Morin, R. B., Jackson, B. G., Mueller, R. A., Lavagnino, E. R., Scanlon, W. B., and Andrews, S. L. (1969b). *J. Amer. Chem. Soc.* **91**, 1401.

Mozingo, R., and Folkers, K. (1949). *In* "The Chemistry of Penicillin" (H. T. Clarke, J. R. Johnson, and R. Robinson, eds.), p. 535. Princeton Univ. Press, Princeton, New Jersey.

Naito, T., Nakagawa, S., Takahashi, K., Fujisawa, K., and Kawaguchi, H. (1968a). *J. Antibiot.* **21**, 300.

Naito, T., Nakagawa, S., Takahashi, K., Masuko, K., Fujisawa, K., and Kawaguchi, H. (1968b). *J. Antibiot.* **21**, 290.

Nefkens, G. H. L., Tesser, G. I., and Nivard, R. J. F. (1960). *Rec. Trav. Chim. Pays-Bas* **79**, 688.

Netherlands Patent 6,600,586.

Newton, G. G. F., Abraham, E. P., and Kuwabara, S. (1968). *Antimicrob. Ag. Chemother.* **1967**, 449.

Nomine, G. (1970). Text of plenary lecture presented at *Eur. Meeting Medicinal Chem., Brussels* September.

Pala, G., Casadio, S., Coppi, G., Crescenzi, E., and Mantegani, A. (1970). *Arzneim. Forsch.* **20**, 62.

Perron, Y. G., Minor, W. F., Holdrege, C. T., Gottstein, W. J., Godfrey, J. C., Crast, L. B., Babel, R. B., and Cheney, L. C. (1960). *J. Amer. Chem. Soc.* **82**, 3934.

Perron, Y. G., Minor, W. F., Crast, L. B., and Cheney, L. C. (1961). *J. Org. Chem.* **26**, 3365.

Perron, Y. G., Minor, W. F., Crast, L. B., Gourevitch, A., Lein, J., and Cheney, L. C. (1962). *J. Med. Chem.* **5**, 1016.

Price, K. E. (1969). *In* "Advances in Applied Microbiology" (D. Perlman, ed.), Vol. 11, pp. 17–75. Academic Press, New York.

Reiner, R., and Zeller, P. (1968). *Helv. Chim. Acta* **51**, 1905.

Rozanova, T. N., and Strukov, I. T. (1969). *Khim.-Farm. Zh.* **3**, 30.

Ryan, C. W., Simon, R. L., and Van Heyningen, E. M. (1969). *J. Med. Chem.* **12**, 310.

Sabath, L. D., Jago, M., and Abraham, E. P. (1965). *Biochem. J.* **96**, 739.

Sassiver, M. L., and Shepherd, R. G. (1969). *Tetrahedron Lett.* 3993.

Sheehan, J. C. (1964). *In* "Molecular Modification in Drug Design," Advances in Chemistry Series, No. 45, pp. 15–24. Amer. Chem. Soc., Washington, D.C.

Sheehan, J. C. (1967). *Ann. N.Y. Acad. Sci.* **145**, 216.

Sheehan, J. C., and Daves, D. G. J., Jr. (1964). *J. Org. Chem.* **29**, 2006.

Sheehan, J. C., and Henery-Logan, K. R. (1962). *J. Amer. Chem. Soc.* **84**, 2983.

Smith, J. T., Hamilton-Miller, J. M. T., and Knox, R. (1969). *J. Pharm. Pharmacol.* **21**, 337.

Spencer, J. L., Flynn, E. H., Roeske, R. W., Siu, F. Y., and Chauvette, R. R. (1966). *J. Med. Chem.* **9**, 746.

Stedman, R. J., Swift, A. C., Miller, L. S., Dolan, M. M., and Hoover, J. R. E. (1967). *J. Med. Chem.* **10**, 363.

Stoodley, R. J. (1968). *J. Chem. Soc. C* 2891.

Strominger, J. L., and Tipper, D. J. (1965). *Amer. J. Med.* **39**, 708.

United States Patent 3,218,318.

United States Patent 3,503,967.

Van Heyningen, E. (1967). *In* "Advances in Drug Research" (N. J. Harper and A. B. Simmonds, eds.), Vol. 4, pp. 1–70. Academic Press, London and New York.

Webber, J. A., Huffman, G. W., Koehler, R. E., Murphy, C. F., Ryan, C. W., Van Heyningen, E. M., and Vasileff, R. T. (1971). *J. Med. Chem.* **14**, 113.

Wolfe, S., and Hasan, S. K. (1970). *Chem. Commun.* 833.

Wolfe, S., and Lee, W. S. (1968). *Chem. Commun.* 242.

Wolfe, S., Godfrey, J. C., Holdrege, C. T., and Perron, Y. G. (1963). *J. Amer. Chem. Soc.* **85**, 643.

Wolfe, S., Lee, W. S., and Misra, R. (1970). *Chem. Commun.* 1067.

Chapter 4

ALTERATION OF THE DIHYDROTHIAZINE

RING MOIETY

CHARLES F. MURPHY and J. ALAN WEBBER

I. Introduction

The dihydrothiazine ring of the cephalosporins is unique in the history of natural products and antibiotics. The functionalities of the dihydrothiazine ring have made the chemistry not only difficult but oftentimes exciting and unexpected. The possibilities of sulfur oxidation or alkylation, substitution at the C-2 position (adjacent both to sulfur and a double bond), double-bond addition reactions, double-bond isomerizations, substitution reactions (on the C-3 methylene group), changes involving α,β-unsaturated esters or carboxylic acids, and reactions of an enamide system where the amide is part of a β-lactam moiety must be considered when reactions on a cephalosporin molecule are performed. It is this array of interrelated functionalities that has made chemical studies of this particular dihydrothiazine moiety complex. Publications now have appeared describing some of the chemistry of cephalosporins and, more particularly, that of the dihydrothiazine ring.

Our discussions of this moiety of the cephalosporins will include frequent references to structure. The atoms are numbered as shown below:

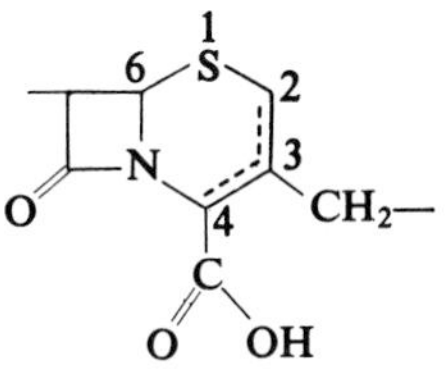

When the double bond is in the C-3–C-4 or C-2–C-3 position, it will be denoted as a 3-cephem (Δ^3) or 2-cephem (Δ^2) cephalosporin, respectively. When the stereochemistries of sulfoxides are described, R configuration will refer to the group being in back of the plane of the paper; S configuration, forward. Similarly, when substitution occurs at C-2, C-3, or C-4, α substitution denotes the group in back of the plane of the paper, and β, forward of the plane. This chapter is arranged according to the numbering of atoms, i.e., S-1, C-2, C-3, C-4, C-3 substituted methyl, and C-4 carboxyl. Discussions of N-5 and C-6 are included in Chapter 3.

II. Reactions at Sulfur (S-1)

Well-known reactions of sulfide sulfur include oxidation, alkylation, and metal abstraction. In cephalosporin chemistry, only oxidation of (and reduction to) the sulfide sulfur has been reported.

Cocker *et al.* (1965) first studied oxidation of cephalosporanic acids (*1*) to their corresponding sulfoxides (*2*). The most effective conversion was obtained with sodium periodate in aqueous solution. Further studies by Cocker *et al.* (1966) showed that 2-cephem acids (*3*) upon periodate oxidation gave 3-cephem sulfoxide acids. The gas evolution noted by these workers was postulated to be the result of a decarboxylative double-bond isomerization reaction to give the 3-cephem compound (4).

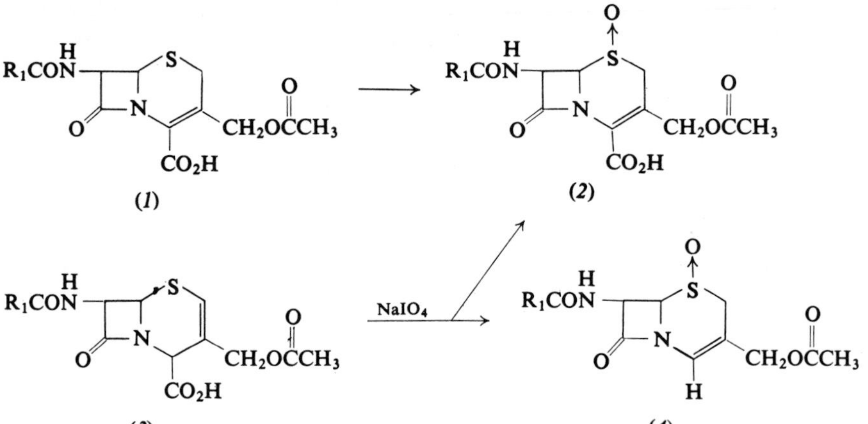

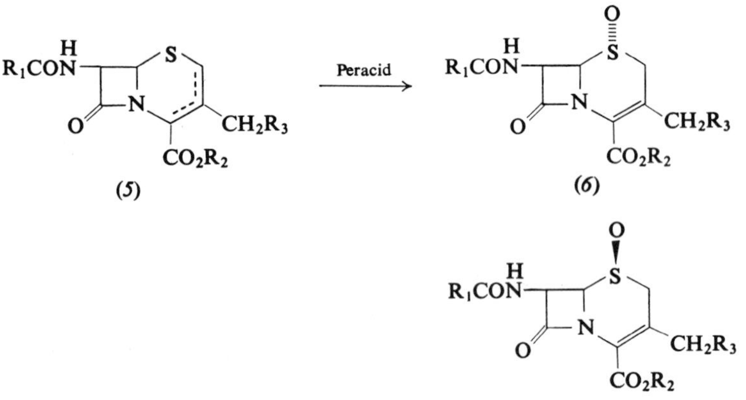

Although Cocker et al. (1966) achieved partial success in oxidizing cephalosporin esters to their corresponding sulfoxides, another study (Kaiser et al., 1970) has shown that either 2-cephem or 3-cephem esters (5) are easily oxidized by strong percarboxylic acids (m-chloroperbenzoic, trifluoroperacetic, performic) in nonaqueous solutions. In many cases the high reactivity of the oxidizing agent requires lower temperatures and dilute solutions to minimize sulfone formation. The peracid oxidations generally produce a mixture of the epimeric R and S sulfoxides (6) and (7). The stereochemistry of the major isomer has been assigned the S configuration in a comprehensive NMR study (Cooper et al., 1970) (see Chapters 5 and 8 for discussion). A downfield shift of the amide NH resonance of the S-sulfoxide isomer relative to the corresponding resonance of the R-sulfoxide isomer indicates hydrogen bonding and implies that the sulfoxide oxygen and 7-amido group are *cis* in the S isomer.

An explanation for the major isomer also being the most sterically hindered has been advanced by Cooper *et al.* (1969) in terms of "reagent approach control." These workers suggest that an initial hydrogen bond between the amide-NH and oxidizing agent forces the oxidation to take place on the β face to give the sulfoxide with the S configuration. Additional discussion may be found in Chapter 5.

Although 3-cephem sulfoxide is generally the product of either 2-cephem or 3-cephem oxidation, it was found that the 2-cephem sulfoxide could be isolated from 2-cephem sulfide (*8*) ($R_1 = C_6H_5OCH_2$) oxidations if no hydroxylic solvent was brought into contact with the product (Cooper *et al.*, 1970). The R and S 2-cephem sulfoxides (*9*) and (*10*) were isolated and NMR studies showed that the S-sulfoxide isomer predominates.

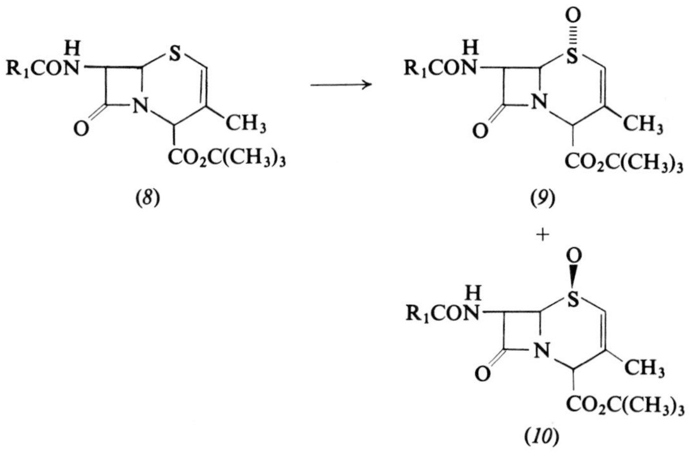

(*8*) $\longrightarrow$ (*9*)

+

(*10*)

Although an early attempt to reduce cephalosporin sulfoxides was unsuccessful (Cocker *et al.*, 1966), it has been found (Kaiser *et al.*, 1970) that activated sulfoxides are reduced with a wide variety of agents. Thus, in the presence of certain acyl halides, cephalosporin sulfoxides (*11*) are readily reduced to their corresponding sulfides (*12*) with reducing agents such as iodide, stannous,

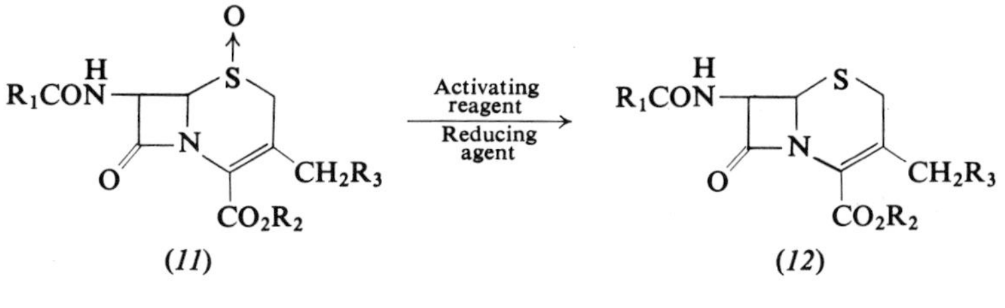

(*11*) Activating reagent / Reducing agent (*12*)

cuprous, thiosulfate, and ferrous ions. The need for activation is attributed to additional stability derived from the hydrogen bond between the sulfoxide and amide proton. Reagents such as imino chlorides, silanes, and phosphorous trihalides served both as activating and reducing agents. The oxidation and reduction of cephem sulfur has been used as a method of controlling the double bond position in cephalosporins. Examples of this technique are discussed in Section IV,B.

Cephem sulfones have been reported only as undesirable over-oxidation products formed during the preparation of sulfoxides.

III. Modifications at C-2

The allylic position at C-2 in the 3-cephem ring might appear to the organic chemist to be a highly reactive position. Only recently, however, have C-2 substituted cephalosporins been reported. There have been no examples of compounds prepared by simple alkylations or acylations. Direct halogenation (N-bromosuccinimide) has led to unstable intermediates and unidentified products (R. D. G. Cooper and I. G. Wright, unpublished).

Lead tetraacetate has been found to react with 2,2,2-trichloroethyl 3-methyl-7-phenoxyacetamido-3-cephem-4-carboxylate-1-oxide (13) to give 2,2,2-trichloroethyl 2-acetoxy-3-methyl-7-phenoxyacetamido-3-cephem-4-carboxylate (14) (Cooper et al., 1970). Although the structure of this compound is well documented, no further chemistry has been reported.

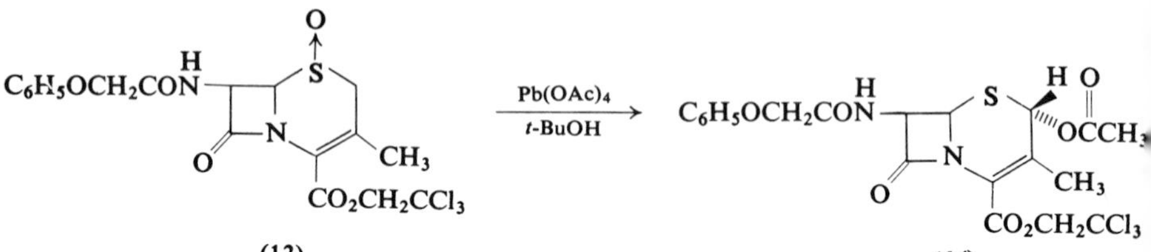

(13)   Pb(OAc)₄ / t-BuOH →   (14)

Another type of substitution at C-2 was discovered (Wright et al., 1971) when a cephalosporin sulfoxide ester (15) was reacted under Mannich reaction conditions (formaldehyde, secondary amine salts) to give a product which did not contain the usual β-substituted amino group of normal Mannich reaction products. The identification of a methylene group substituted at C-2 in compound (16) indicated that the expected amino group had been eliminated under reaction conditions. The reaction was found to be generally applicable to cephalosporin sulfoxides; however, electron-withdrawing ester groups (trichloroethyl) facilitate the reaction. Hydrogenation of the C-2 exomethylene

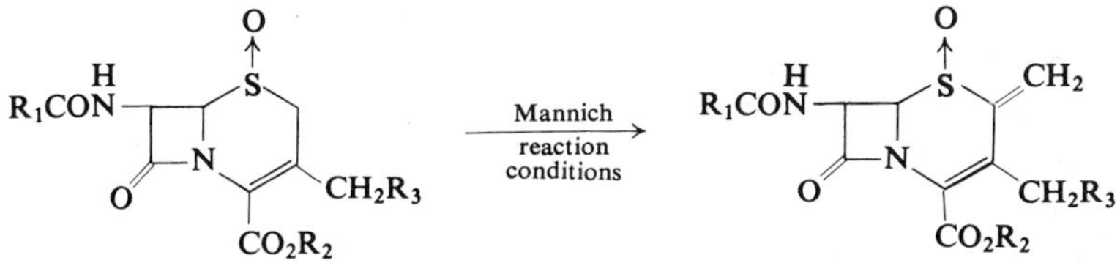

(16a) $R_1 = C_6H_5OCH_2$, $R_2 = CH_2CCl_3$, $R_3 = H$

(16b) $R_1 = C_6H_5OCH_2$, $R_2 = C(CH_3)_3$, $R_3 = H$

(16c) $R_1 =$ 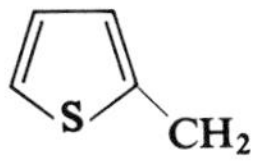 , $R_2 = CH_2CCl_3$, $R_3 = OCCH_3$

(16d) $R_1 =$ 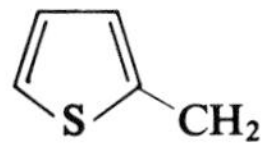 , $R_2 = C(CH_3)_3$, $R_3 = OCCH_3$

compounds gave mixtures of α- and β-2-methyl cephalosporins [(17) and (18) ($R_1 = C_6H_5OCH_2$, $R_2 = CH_2CCl_3$)] (Wright et al., 1971).

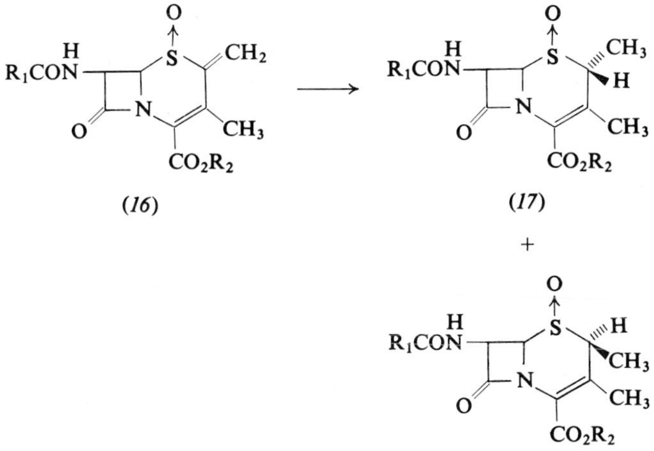

The β configuration was assigned to the major isomer on the basis of NMR studies and on the presumption that the catalyst would attack from the least hindered side. The C-2 methyl derivatives were readily epimerized to a mixture with 83 % α and 17 % β isomers, under the conditions of the Mannich reaction.

Another product isolated after hydrogenation of the C-2 exomethylene derivative was the 2-cephem derivative (19).

$(16) \longrightarrow$ (19)

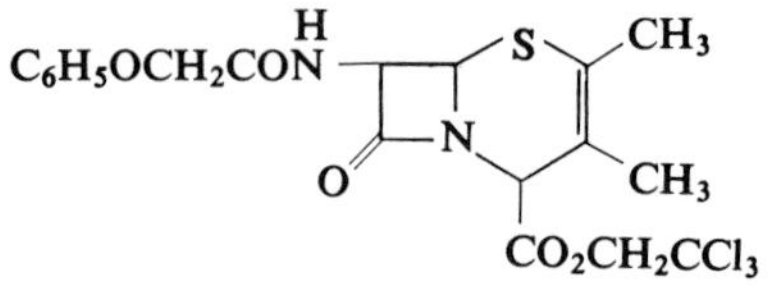

Reduction of the sulfoxide group of (16) with stannous chloride and acetyl chloride at −40° gave the C-2 methylene cephalosporin (20).

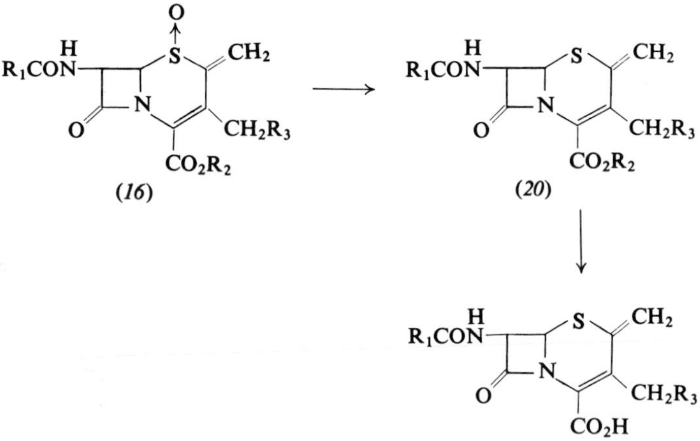

(16)   (20)

(21)

(20a) $R_1 = C_6H_5OCH_2$, $R_2 = CH_2CCl_3$, $R_3 = H$

(20b) $R_1 = C_6H_5OCH_2$, $R_2 = C(CH_3)_3$, $R_3 = H$

(20c) $R_1 = $ 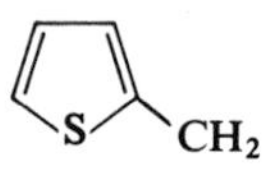 , $R_2 = CH_2CCl_3$, $R_3 = \overset{\overset{O}{\|}}{O}CCH_3$

(20d) $R_1 = $ 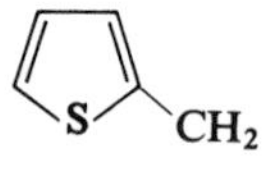 , $R_2 = C(CH_3)_3$, $R_3 = \overset{\overset{O}{\|}}{O}CCH_3$

Removal of the protective ester function of (20) gave a series of 7-acylamido-2-exomethylene-3-cephem-4-carboxylic acids (21).

Reduction of a mixture of α- and β-2-methyl cephalosporin sulfoxides with stannous chloride and acetyl chloride under the conditions described previously gave only the sulfide with an α-methyl group (22). The sulfoxide of the 2-β-methyl compound is inert to these conditions. This selective reactivity thus facilitated a simple chromatographic separation because of large differences in polarity between sulfoxide and sulfide. The C-2 methyl cephalosporins were also converted to the respective carboxylic acids (23), but no enhanced antibacterial activity was found.

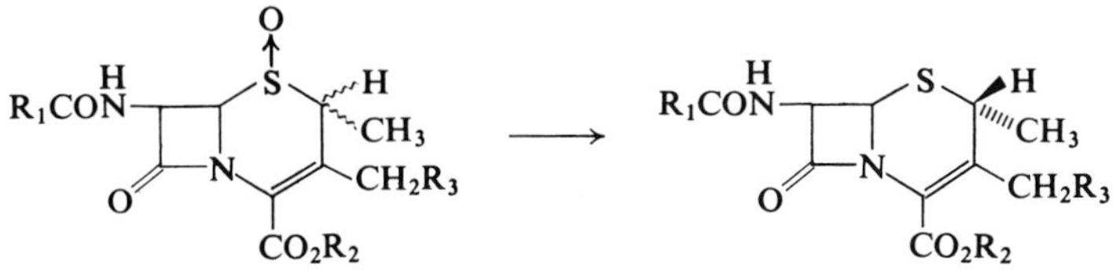

The exocylic methylene compound (16) also was found to undergo certain additional reactions. Bromine was added under mild conditions to give the dibromide (24). Amines or alcohols did not add to the double bond under the conditions studied.

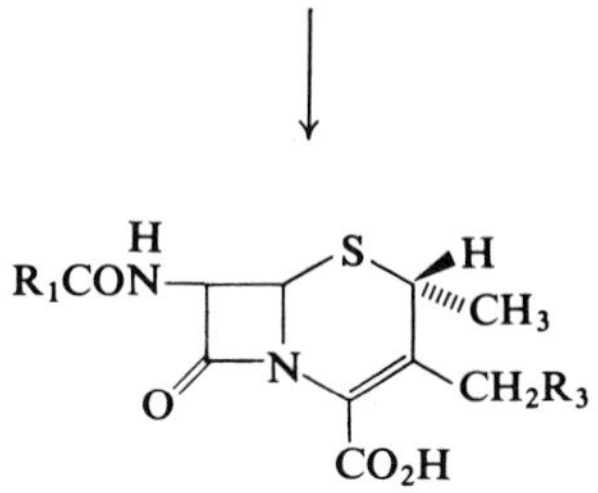

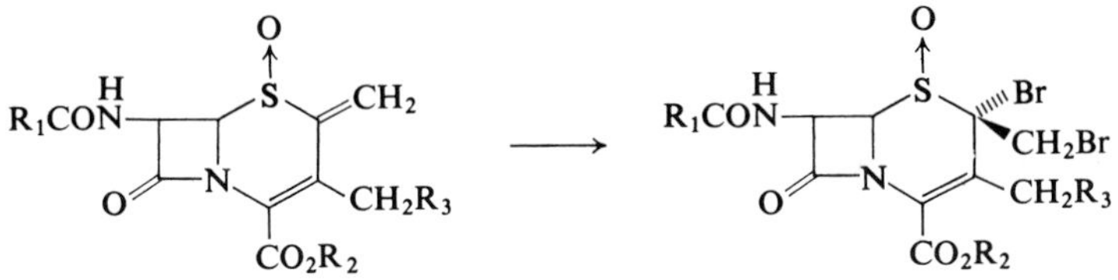

A mixture of C-2 epimers (25) resulting from the addition of thiols, at ambient temperature, to the 2-exomethylene compounds was described in a companion report (Kaiser et al., 1971).

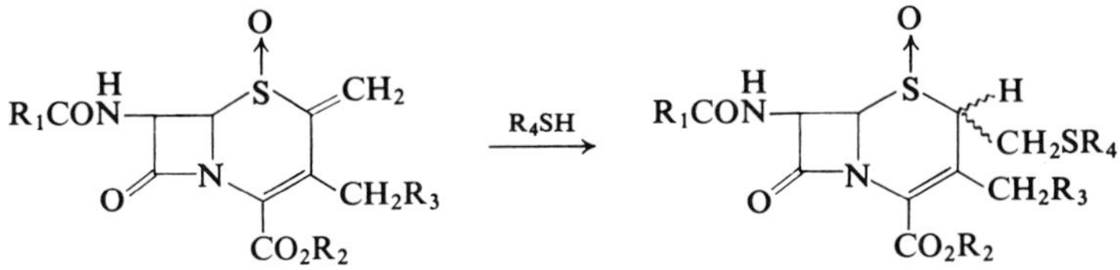

At −80°, however, thiols add stereospecifically to give the C-2 α-substituted product (26). Reduction of the C-2 α-substituted sulfoxide caused epimerization at C-2 and the sulfides (27) and (28) were obtained.

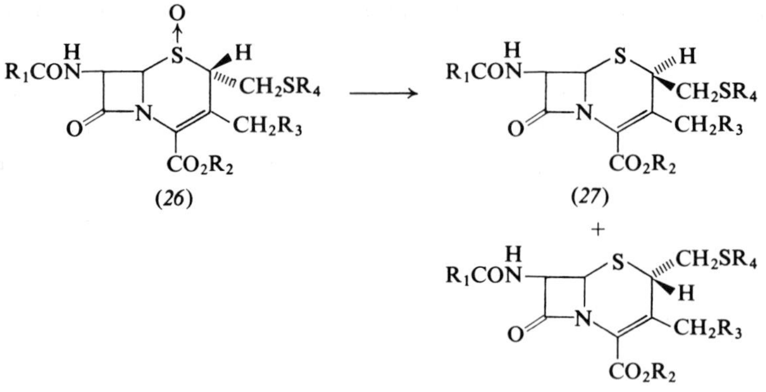

$R_1 =$ [thienyl]$-CH_2$, $R_2 = CH_2CCl_3$, $R_3 = OCCH_3$, $R_4 = p\text{-}BrC_6H_4$

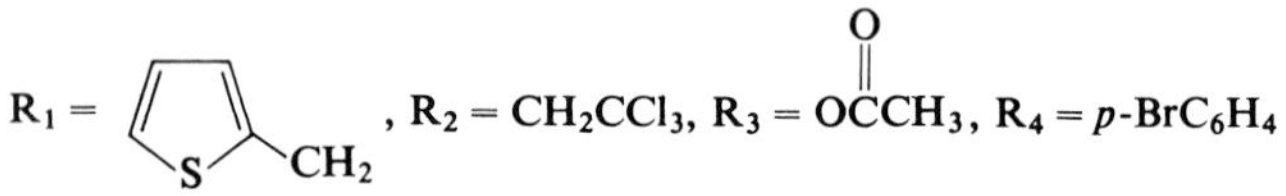

An attempt at separation of the epimeric sulfides gave only the 2-cephem derivative (29).

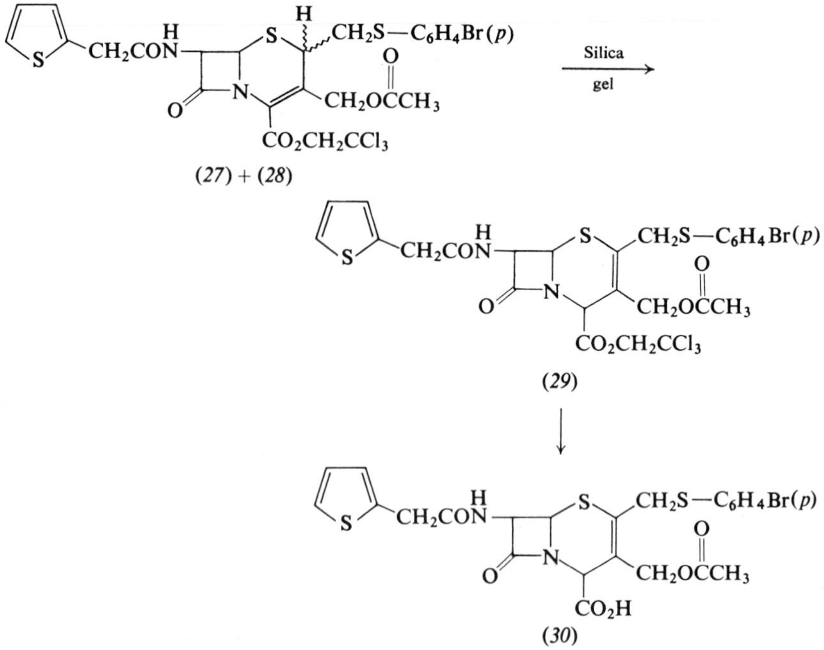

The carboxylic acid (30) resulting from removal of the trichloroethyl blocking group exhibited little antibiotic activity.

In sodium acetate–acetic acid solutions, the alkyl (aryl) thiomethyl sulfoxides (25) underwent facile dehydration to give the thiomethylene derivatives (31).

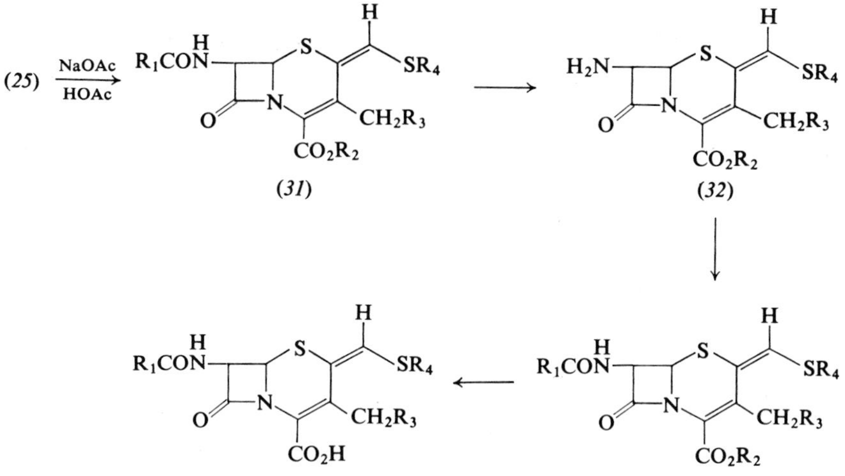

$(34a)$ $R_1 = C_6H_5OCH_2$, $R_3 = H$, $R_4 = p\text{-}BrC_6H_4$
$(34b)$ $R_1 = C_6H_5OCH_2$, $R_3 = H$, $R_4 = C_6H_5$
$(34c)$ $R_1 = C_6H_5OCH_2$, $R_3 = H$, $R_4 = C_6H_5CH_2$

$$(34d)\ R_1 = C_4H_3SCH_2,\ R_3 = O\overset{O}{\overset{\|}{C}}CH_3,\ R_4 = C_6H_5CH_2$$

$$(34e)\ R_1 = C_4H_3SCH_2,\ R_3 = O\overset{O}{\overset{\|}{C}}CH_3,\ R_4 = p\text{-}ClC_6H_4$$

$(34f)$ $R_1 = C_6H_5OCH_2$, $R_3 = H$, $R_4 = CH_3$
$(34g)$ $R_1 = C_6H_5OCH_2$, $R_3 = H$, $R_4 = CH_3CH_2$

$(34h)$ $R_1 = C_6H_5OCH_2$, $R_3 = H$, $R_4 =$

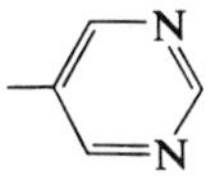

$(34i)$ $R_1 = C_6H_5OCH_2$, $R_3 = H$, $R_4 = m\text{-}CH_3O\overset{O}{\overset{\|}{C}}C_6H_4$
$(34j)$ $R_1 = C_6H_5OCH_2$, $R_3 = H$, $R_4 = p\text{-}BrC_6H_4$

$$(34k)\ R_1 = C_4H_3SCH_2,\ R_3 = O\overset{O}{\overset{\|}{C}}CH_3,\ R_4 = p\text{-}BrC_6H_4$$

The isomerically pure product was found to have the *cis* configuration (as shown) by the large nuclear Overhauser effects between the thio substituent and the 3-methylene group (Kaiser *et al.*, 1971) (see Chapter 8). Removal of the 7-acyl group via the imino ester (Chapter 2, Section II) provided a nucleus (*32*) which was reacylated with various activated carboxylic acids to give (*33*). The 4-carboxylate group was then converted to the carboxylic acids (*34*) which were tested for antibiotic activity. Most of these compounds exhibited gram-positive activity.

As part of a synthetic effort, another type of C-2 substitution was obtained with the 2-oxo compound (*35*). This synthesis is discussed in Chapter 6.

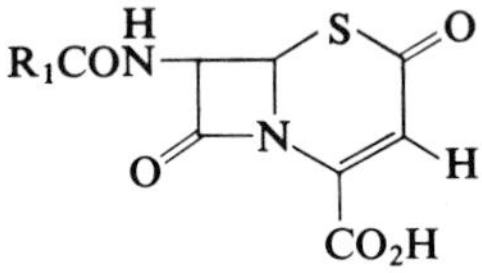

(*35*)

IV. Reactions of the Cephem Double Bond

A. Additions to the Cephem Double Bond

The 3-cephem double bond is tetrasubstituted, is α, β to a carboxyl group, and is part of an enamide system. The sum of electronic effects leads to an experimentally unreactive double bond, and relatively few addition reactions have been reported. Archer and Kitchell (1966) have described the addition of diazomethane to the double bond of compound (*36*) to give the pyrazoline (*37*). Electrophilic reagents such as bromine do not add to the double bond.*

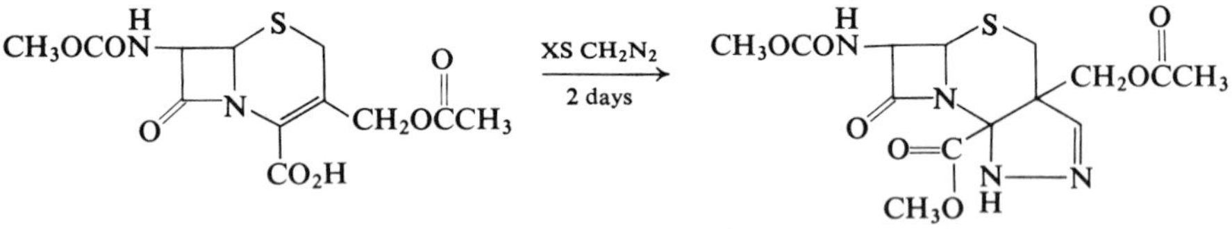

(*36*)   (*37*)

During a study of the displacement of the acetoxyl group of cephalosporanic acids with certain bidentate nucleophiles, Fazakerley *et al.* (1967) reported that the products did not exhibit ultraviolet absorption typical of 3-cephem compounds. An examination of the NMR spectrum showed a singlet (between

* Unpublished, R. D. G. Cooper.

4.5–5.0 ppm, depending upon the nucleophile) that was assigned to the C-4 proton. The conclusion was that cyclic compounds had formed. This led to structures (38)–(40) for products of the reaction of cephalosporanic acids with N,N-diethylthiourea, 2-pyridthione, and 2-thiouracil, respectively.

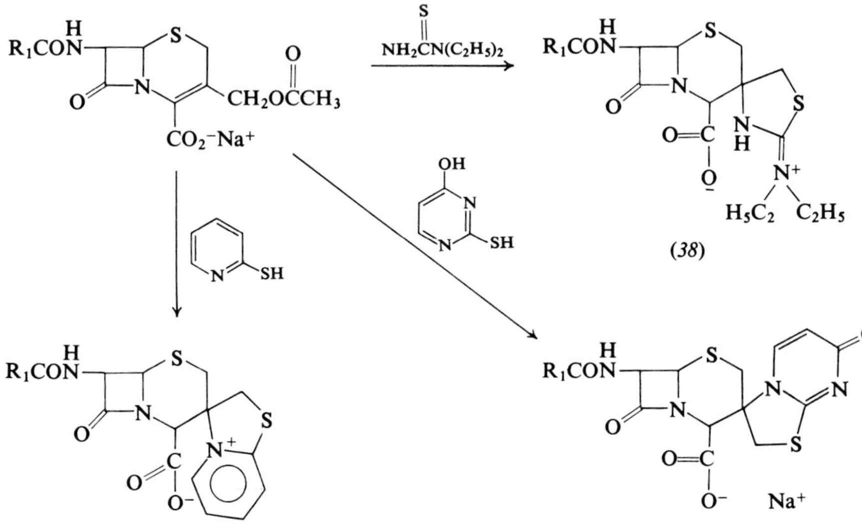

(38)

(39)

(40)

Isolated from the reaction of 2-pyridthione with the cephalosporanic acid was the intermediate C-3 methyl substituted derivative (41). Cyclization to compound (39) was found to occur under acidic conditions but was reversible in the presence of base. This delicately balanced equilibrium is also illustrated by the fact that thiourea and 2-pyrimidthione formed the C-3 methyl substituted derivatives but no cyclic products were found.

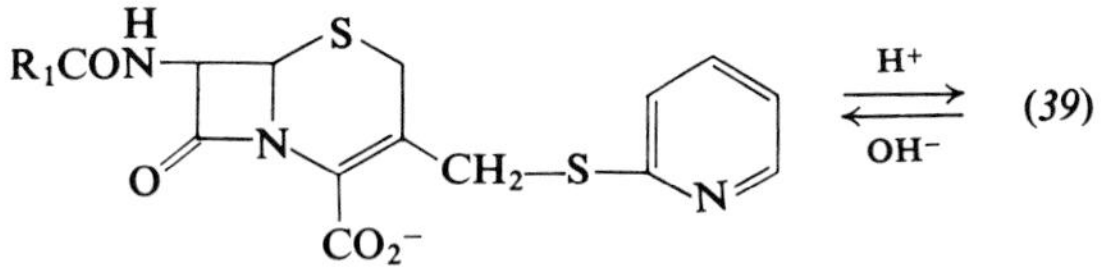

(41)

No other additions to the 3-cephem double bond have been reported. Daniels et al. (1970), Morin et al. (1969), and Barton et al. (1970), however, have isolated products from the rearrangement of penicillin sulfoxide esters which have either a 3-hydroxyl (42) or 3-acetoxyl group (43).

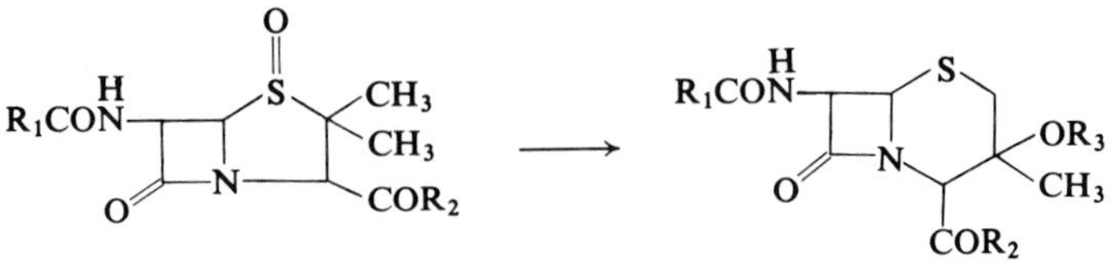

(42) $R_1 = C_6H_5CH_2$
$R_2 = NHC(CH_3)_3$
$R_3 = CCH_3$
         $\parallel$
          O

(43) $R_1 = C_6H_5OCH_2$
$R_2 = OCH_2C_6H_4NO_2(p)$
$R_3 = H$

These products are believed to be formed as the result of either the hydroxyl or acetoxyl group reacting with an intermediate carbonium ion and not as the result of addition to the double bond. When the compound (42) is heated or when (43) is heated with dehydrating agents, the corresponding 3-cephem compounds are formed.

Reduction of the 3-cephem double bond to the 3,4-dihydrocephalosporin compound has been reported (U.S. Patent 3,193,550). Cephalosporin C in the presence of platinum at 75° for 48 hours under 7200 lb of hydrogen pressure gave dihydrocephalosporin C (44). No stereochemistry or yield was reported for this compound.

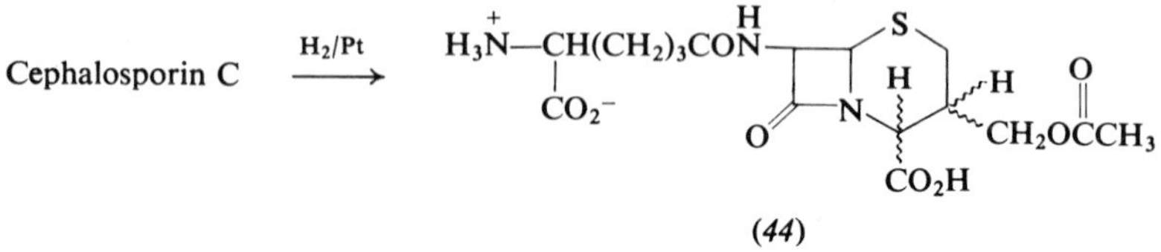

(44)

The only reported addition to the 2-cephalosporin double bond has been reduction of the methyl ester (45) to the cepham derivative (46), reported by Van Heyningen and Ahern (1968).

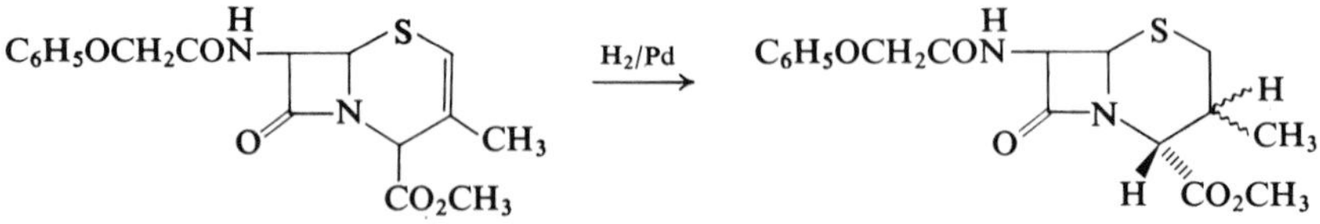

(45)   (46)

This reduction was carried out under considerably milder conditions (60°, 3 atm, 3 hours) than those described for reduction of the 3-cephem double bond. The cepham derivative (*46*) was subsequently degraded to the phenoxy-methyl desthiopenicillanate (*47*) which was identical to a degradation product of phenoxymethylpenicillin. This sequence constituted proof that the con-figuration of the C-4 proton of 2-cephem compounds is β and is identical to the configuration of the penicillins.

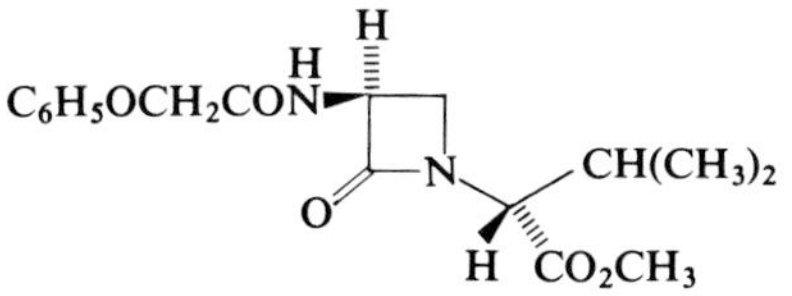

(*47*)

B. Isomerization of the Cephem Double Bond

Isomerization of the natural 3-cephem double bond to the 2-cephem posi-tion was first reported by Green *et al.* (1965) and Cocker *et al.* (1966). Although cephalosporin acids undergo a slow isomerization in pyridine (Cocker *et al.*, 1966), a much more facile double-bond isomerization occurs with an amine base when the carboxyl is esterified or otherwise blocked (i.e., mixed anhydride or chloride) (Cocker *et al.*, 1966; Chauvette and Flynn, 1966). The cephalo-sporanic acid, 3-acetoxymethyl-7-phenylacetamido-3-cephen-4-carboxylic acid, was converted to the 2-cephem analog in 50% yield in the pre-sence of acetic anhydride and pyridine by Cocker *et al.* (1966). 7-Acylamido-3-acetoxymethyl-3-cephem-4-carboxylic acid esters (*48*) are normally iso-merized to an equilibrium mixture, composed of a 7:3 ratio of 2-cephem to 3-cephem isomers. Morin *et al.* (1969) conjectured that the equilibrium com-position is largely determined by the size of the 3-methyl substituents. When $R_3 = H$ (*49*), the isomeric composition was found to be 3:7 2-cephem to 3-cephem.

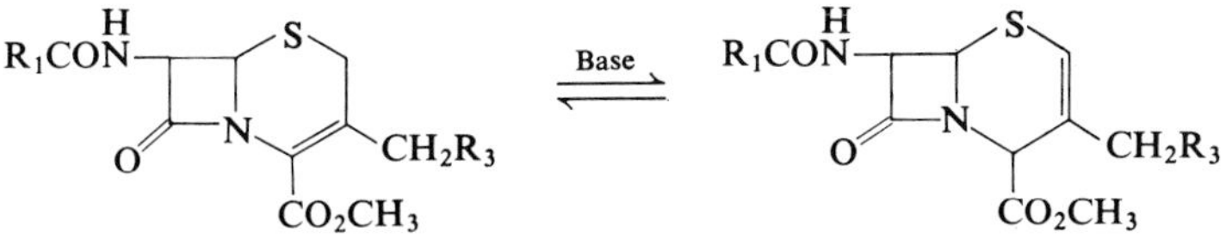

(*48*) $R_3 = OCCH_3$
(*49*) $R_3 = H$

The easily isomerized cephem double bond has been a significant hindrance to the preparation of isomerically pure compounds. Cocker *et al.* (1966)

attempted an acylation of 7-aminocephalosporanic acid in pyridine only to find a mixture of Δ^2 and Δ^3 cephalosporins as products. Chauvette and Flynn (1966) found mixtures of Δ^2 and Δ^3 cephalosporins were formed when the preparation of esters and amides of cephalosporin acids was attempted. Although the 2- and 3-cephem isomeric mixtures are sometimes separable, the ratio of isomers is not always the most desirable. For example (Woodward et al., 1966), in the total synthesis of cephalosporin C the 2-cephem compound (50) was isomerized to a mixture of one part 3-cephem to four parts 2-cephem and then separated by column chromatography.

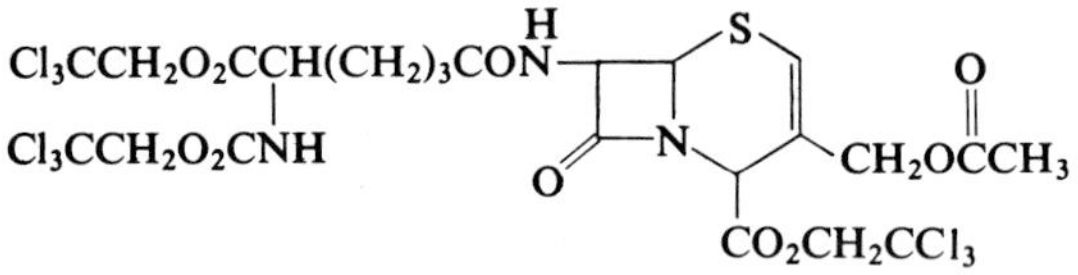

$Cl_3CCH_2O_2CCH(CH_2)_3CON$—
$Cl_3CCH_2O_2CNH$
CH_2OCCH_3
$CO_2CH_2CCl_3$

(50)

Base

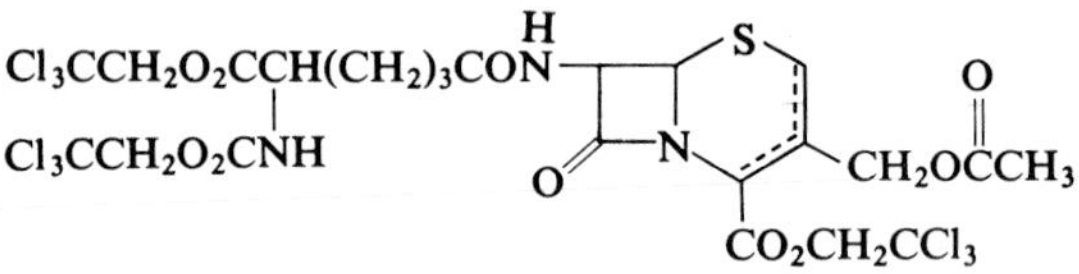

$Cl_3CCH_2O_2CCH(CH_2)_3CON$—
$Cl_3CCH_2O_2CNH$
CH_2OCCH_3
$CO_2CH_2CCl_3$

Chromatography

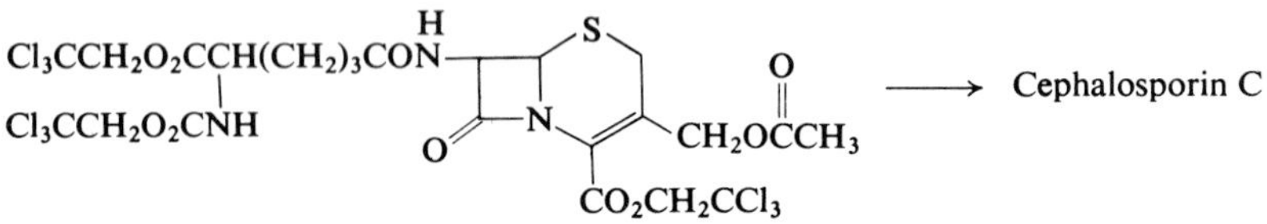

$Cl_3CCH_2O_2CCH(CH_2)_3CON$—
$Cl_3CCH_2O_2CNH$
CH_2OCCH_3
$CO_2CH_2CCl_3$

⟶ Cephalosporin C

As cephalosporin research developed, it became apparent that, because of the biological inactivity of Δ^2 cephalosporins (Cocker et al., 1965), an efficient method of isomer control was needed. The observation by Morin et al. (1969) that mild basic hydrolyses of 3-cephem carboxylic acid esters (51) gave only 2-cephem acids (apparently the Δ^3 acid is destroyed) provided part of the solution to the problem. Webber et al. (1969) chose these pure Δ^2 acids as a starting material for the functionalization of 3-methyl cephalosporins. Careful esterification of the 2-cephem acid (52) gave an ester [(53) $R_1 = C_6H_5OCH_2$, $R_2 = p\text{-}CH_3OC_6H_4CH_2$], which, when treated with N-bromosuccinimide, gave the 3-bromomethyl derivative (54).

During subsequent displacement of the bromide ion with acetate ion, the double bond was isomerized to give a mixture of Δ^2 and Δ^3 3-acetoxymethyl derivatives (55). In order to resolve the expected isomer problem, this mixture

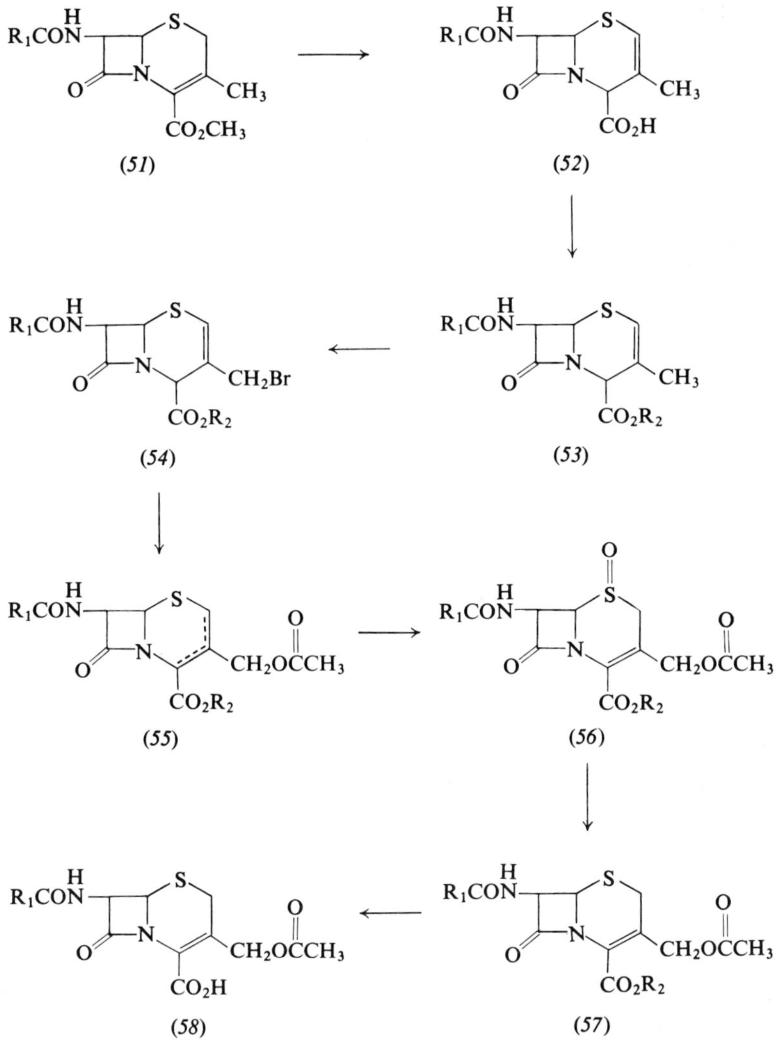

was oxidized to the sulfoxide (56). The fact that only the 3-cephem sulfoxide was isolated is consistent with the observation that β,γ-unsaturated sulfoxides are more stable than α,β-unsaturated sulfoxides (O'Connor and Lyness, 1964). The major difficulty of reducing the sulfoxide (56 → 57) was solved when an activating agent was introduced in the presence of the reducing agent. (See earlier discussion on sulfoxides in this chapter.) The remaining reaction of removing the ester protecting group was performed thus completing the transformation to give phenoxyacetamidocephalosporanic acid (58).

With the discovery of the 2 → 3-cephem conversion via oxidation to, and reduction of, cephalosporin sulfoxides, several reports have expanded the method's utility. An improved synthesis of 2-cephem esters was reported by Murphy and Koehler (1970). The 3-cephem-4-carboxylic acid was converted to the acid chloride (59) and then treated with a strong, tertiary amine base in the presence of an alcohol. The proposed intermediate ketene (60) then added the elements of the alcohol to give nearly isomerically pure 2-cephem ester (61).

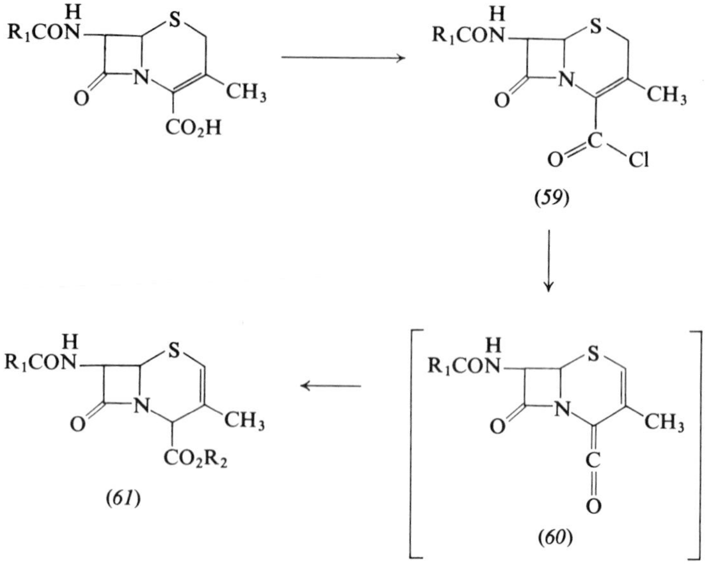

$$R_2 = CH_2C_6H_4OCH_3\ (p),\ C(CH_3)_3,\ CH_2C_6H_4NO_2\ (p),\ CH(C_6H_5)_2,\ \text{etc.}$$

Improved methods of oxidizing mixtures of cephem isomers to their 3-cephem sulfoxides and of reducing cephem sulfoxides have been extensively investigated by Kaiser et al. (1970) (discussed in Section IV,B). The overall process of functionalizing 2-cephem compounds and converting them to 3-cephem carboxylic acids by the oxidation–reduction sequence has been expanded by the work of Webber et al. (1971) and Kukolja (1970). The Webber et al. (1971) effort led to a series of 3-alkoxymethyl cephalosporins; whereas, Kukolja reported the preparation of 3-acyloxymethyl cephem acids (see later discussion in Section V,B). The reactivities of the functionalities and substituents of the various cephalosporins involved have limited the utility of this method.

V. Modifications at C-3

A. 3-Cephem Derivatives

Cephalosporins occurring naturally contain the 3-acetoxymethyl-3-cephem nucleus (62). The acetoxy group in this system has shown a surprising proclivity to be displaced by nucleophiles, leading to a host of 3-(substituted)methyl-3-cephem nuclei (63). An alternate nomenclature, using 3′, e.g., 3′-acetoxy

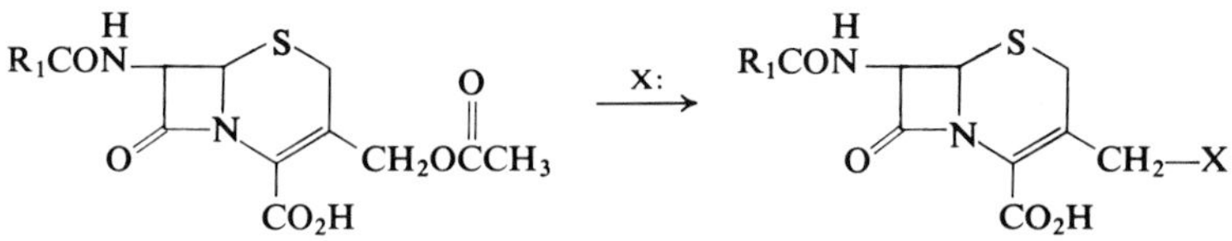

(62)   (63)

instead of 3-acetoxymethyl, although sometimes less cumbersome, has not found widespread acceptance and will not be used generally throughout this monograph. Therefore, this section will refrain from the use of the expression 3′ except where the alternative is prohibitively unwieldy. Additional modifications at the 3 position in the cephem nucleus have involved indirect, or formal, displacement of acetoxy facilitated by chemical manipulation of the S-1 oxidation state, 3′ functionality, double-bond position, and 4-carboxyl and 7-amino protection.

The ultimate goal in the preparation of new cephem nuclei has been to obtain 3-cephem derivatives for antibacterial testing. The discussion here will begin with an examination of the preparation and variety of three substituents on the 3-cephem nucleus, classified according to product type and not according to starting material. This approach has been deemed most desirable in an organizational sense. In general, because attention is focused on chemical manipulation of the substituent at the 3 position, discussion of the corresponding 7-acylamino group will be minimized. Those readers wishing a perspective of these two variations combined may consult Chapter 12, which discusses structure–activity relationships.

1. 3-METHYL COMPOUNDS

The 3-methyl-3-cephem or deacetoxycephalosporin compounds are now well known to be available from two sources.

Stedman *et al.* (1964) observed the hydrogenolytic removal of acetoxy from
7-aminocephalosporanic acid (7-ACA) in the presence of a palladium catalyst
to give the 3-methyl derivative, 7-aminodeacetoxycephalosporanic acid *(64)*
(7-ADCA). The process was also applied to cephalosporin C (U.S. Patent
3,124,576).

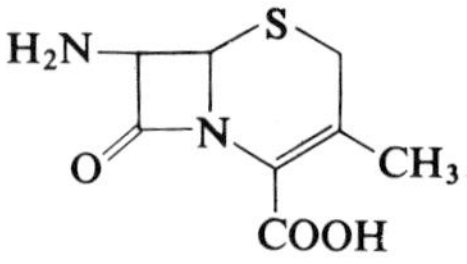

(64)

An alternative preparation of the deacetoxycephalosporin system is via the
penicillin sulfoxide ester rearrangement (U.S. Patent 3,275,626), which has
been reported in detail (Morin *et al.*, 1969) and is discussed elsewhere in this
monograph (Chapter 5). Significant improvements have been effected in the
original process (Neth. Patents 68,06532, 68,06533).

The significance of the deacetoxycephalosporin nucleus resides primarily
in its presence in the cephalosporin derivative cephalexin *(65)* (Ryan *et al.*,
1969; Chauvette *et al.*, 1971).

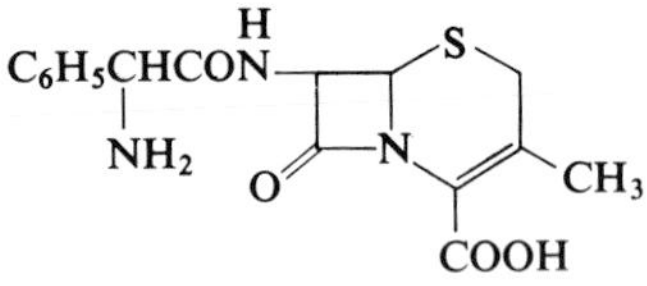

(65)

2. 3-HYDROXYMETHYL DERIVATIVES

The 3-hydroxymethyl-3-cephem* or deacetylcephalosporin-type compound was first observed as a minor component of cephalosporin C fermentation. Huber *et al.* (1968) demonstrated that although esterase activity exists in
this broth, deacetylcephalosporin C *(66)* did not result from this activity, nor
from direct biosynthesis, but probably from a nonenzymatic hydrolysis.

Jeffery *et al.* (1961) first observed the direct deacetylation of a cephalosporin,
in the conversion of cephalosporin C to *(66)*, using citrus acetyl esterase (U.S.
Patent 3,202,656). This enzyme has also been utilized in a more general application to cephem derivatives (U.S. Patent 3,459,746). Other esterases used for
deacetyl cephem preparation are those from *Schizomycetes* (U.S. Patent

* Such cephem acids have been assigned the trivial name cephalosporadesic acids (Van
Heyningen, 1965); this awkward name appears to have only slight advantage over more
systematic naming.

3,239,394), *Rhizobium* (U.S. Patent 3,436,310), and *Actinomycetes*, but especially *Bacillus subtilis* (U.S. Patent 3,304,236).

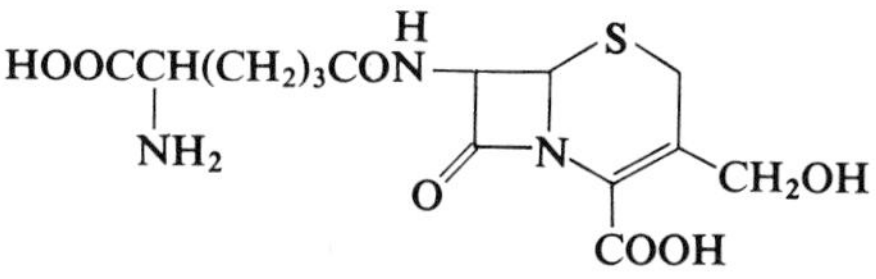

(66)

Although chemical deacetylation of a cephalosporin has been observed in the case of cephalosporin C sodium salt (pH 11) (Jeffery *et al.*, 1961), as these authors suggested, this conversion has no practical utility, being accompanied by extreme β-lactam destruction. Kukolja (1968) has reported an acidic hydrolysis of the acetoxy group in cephaloglycin to give either deacetylcephaloglycin (in poor yield) or cephaloglycin lactone, depending upon conditions. More recently, Neidleman *et al.* (1970) have observed hydrolytic ring opening of cephalothin lactone to provide deacetyl cephalothin. The low yield of this reaction (W. Germ. Patent 2000878) makes its practicality suspect.

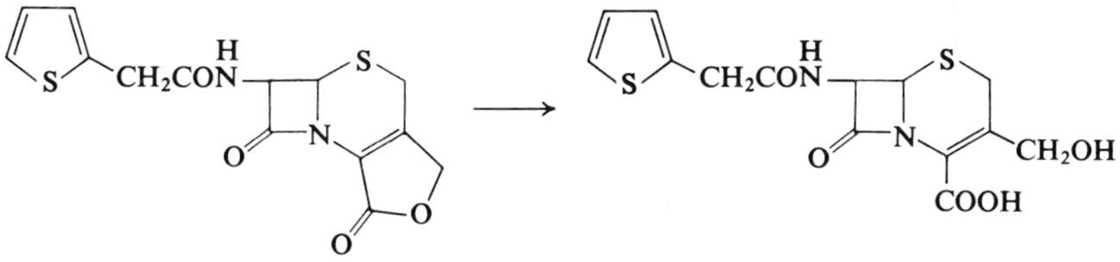

Like the 3-hydroxymethyl-3-cephem acids, the 3-hydroxymethyl-3-cephem esters are also inaccessible by direct chemical means from the acetoxy derivatives. Esters of this type have been prepared from the corresponding acids (U.S. Patent 3,532,694), however. The methods involved utilize primarily treatment with an aryldiazoalkane to give, e.g., (67). Additionally, reaction of the sodium salt of a deacetyl cephem acid with an aralkylhalide is mentioned. However, this reaction requires great care to prevent double-bond isomerization from occurring. Preparation of other esters of this type has been precluded by the problems of lactonization and double-bond isomerization (see Section VI). The lactonization reaction has been observed in the case of both acids and esters of the 3-hydroxymethyl-3-cephem series.

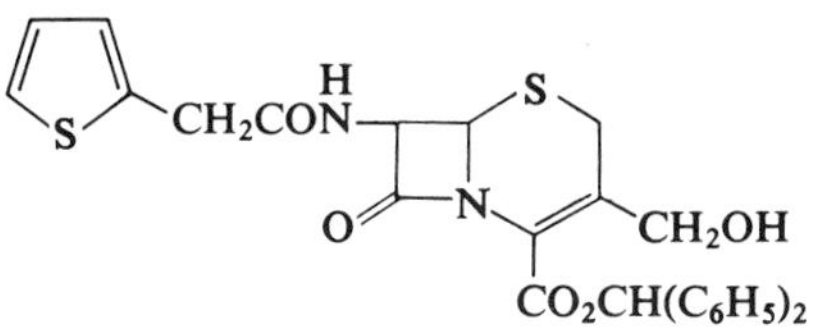

(67)

The 3-hydroxymethyl-3-cephem-1-oxide esters (W. Germ. Patent 1937015) appear to show a decreased tendency to lactonize as compared to the corresponding sulfide.

3. 3-ACYLOXYMETHYL SUBSTITUENTS

Compounds of type (*68*) (R_2 = H) are formally the result of replacement of acetyl in a cephalosporanic acid with the residue of another carboxylic acid.

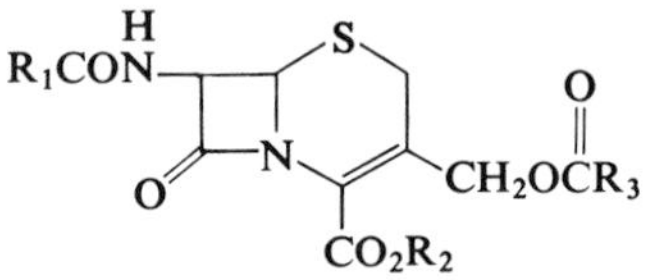

(*68*)

Attempted direct displacement of acetoxy with a carboxylate salt (Van Heyningen, 1965) has not been successful.

New 3-acyloxymethyl-3-cephem compounds have been prepared by acylation of the 3-hydroxymethyl derivatives discussed in Section V,A,2. Van Heyningen (1965), utilizing a Schotten–Baumann technique, was able to carry out acylations on deacetylcephalosporanic acids using some acid chlorides and sodium hydroxide in aqueous acetone. Aliphatic acid chlorides failed to react; they underwent hydrolysis. However, aryl and heterocyclic carboxylic acid chlorides were effective (U.S. Patent 3,445,463). Kukolja (1970) has reported the preparation of 3-(aliphatic)acyloxymethyl-3-cephem acids via their 2-cephem analogues (see Section V,B). Double-bond isomerization was effected by the technique described in Section II, i.e., oxidation and reduction at the sulfur atom.

.Perhaps the most general synthesis of 3-acyloxymethyl-3-cephem analogues involves the intermediacy of deacetyl esters [(*68*) R_2 = aralkyl] (as described in Section V,A,2). Acylations are carried out in organic solvent in the presence of an organic base using preferably an acid chloride, or alternatively, an anhydride (U.S. Patent 3,532,694). Using care in the reaction minimized lactonization or double-bond isomerization. Extension of this route (Belg. Patent 719,711) included acylation via a ketene (where pertinent) or active ester or azide, as well as carbodiimide condensation of a carboxylic acid and the deacetyl cephalosporin ester.

4. 3-CARBAMOYLOXYMETHYL SUBSTITUENTS

A variety of 3-(substituted)carbamoyloxymethyl-3-cephem acids (*69*) (sometimes referred to as O-deacetyl-O-carbamoyl cephalosporanic acids) are available by reacting deacetyl cephalosporin acids with isocyanates (U.S. Patents 3,355,452, 3,484,437; Belg. Patent 741,381).

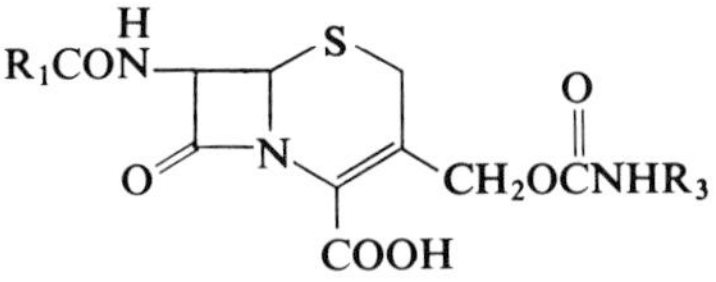

(69)

In these reactions as usually carried out, a salt of a 3-hydroxymethyl-3-cephem acid is dissolved or suspended in DMF in the presence of excess tertiary aliphatic amine. The isocyanate is added and subsequent work-up provides the carbamates. The substituent on carbamate nitrogen has included alkyl and substituted alkyl (with considerable emphasis on β-chloroethyl), aryl, acyl, and sulfonyl. No specific discussion or preparation of the cephalosporin primary carbamate (69) ($R_3 = H$) was included in this work, however, the α-amino adipoyl derivatives of the 3-carbamoyloxymethyl-3-cephem nucleus has been discovered in a fermentation (Nagarajan et al., 1971) (see Chapter 15).

5. 3-HALOMETHYL COMPOUNDS

3-Halomethyl-3-cephem derivatives (70) (X = Cl, Br, I) are useful as intermediates in the preparation of a wide variety of 3'-substituted cephem compounds. Chlorides and bromides have been prepared by a number of routes, but the iodides always are formed indirectly from the other halides.

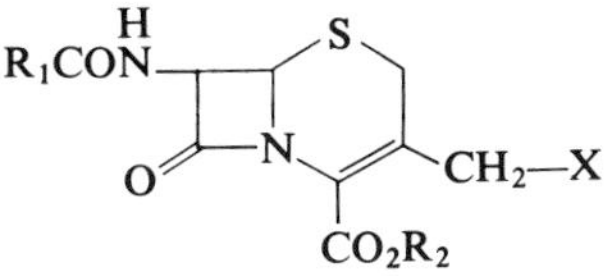

(70)

These 3-halomethyl cephem species both theoretically, and often practically, undergo more facile displacement than do the 3-acetoxymethyl analogues. The majority of work has been reported using cephem esters, ostensibly because 3-halomethyl-3-cephem-4-carboxylic acids might be expected to lactonize in neutral or basic medium.

The first report of a 3-halomethyl cephem derivative alluded to an N-bromosuccinimide (NBS) allylic bromination of a 3-methyl cephem phenacyl ester of type (71) (Belg. Patent 684,288). This conversion has not been substantiated and, in fact, has been observed to not take place with a number of different 3-methyl-3-cephem esters.* On the other hand, allylic bromination of a 3-methyl-3-cephem-1-oxide ester (72) using NBS and photochemical initiation does take place.† A discussion of the functionalization of

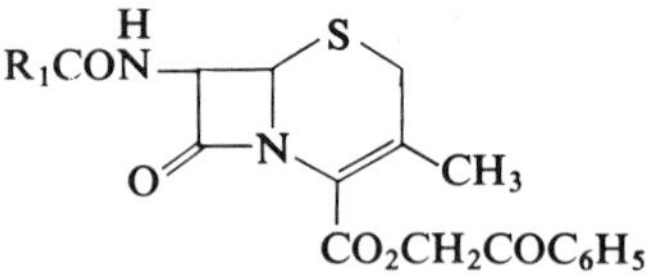

(71)

deacetoxycephalosporin using NBS is deferred to the 2-cephem discussion (Section V,B).

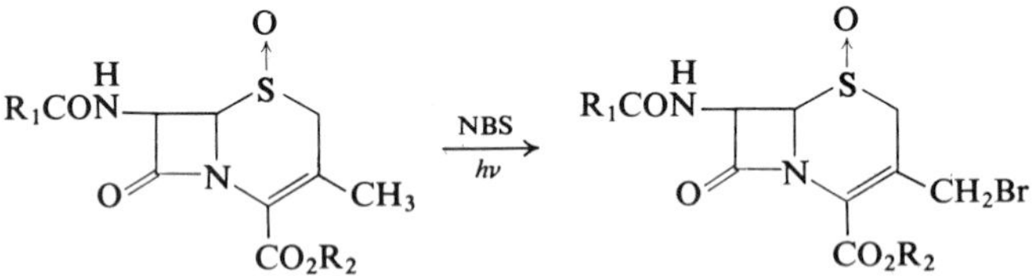

(72)

A Belgian patent (719,710) describes the preparation of 3-halomethyl-3-cephem esters, and their corresponding acids following deesterification. The deacetylcephalosporin benzhydryl esters discussed in Section V,A,2 were treated with reagents appropriate for incorporating halogen. The 3-chloromethyl cephem ester (70) (X = Cl) was prepared preferably with thionyl chloride or alternatively with an N,N-dialkyl (or diaryl) chlorosulfinamide or alkyl chlorosulfite. The bromo analogues of the latter two reagents, or optimally, phosphorous tribromide are used to prepare 3-bromomethyl cephem esters (70) (X = Br). Alkali metal iodide treatment of either cephem allylic chloride (70) (X = Cl) or bromide (70) (X = Br) provided the 3-iodomethyl cephem ester (70) (X = I).

A 3-bromomethyl-3-cephem ester or 1-oxide ester can be obtained by oxidation and reduction at sulfur (see Section II) of the Δ^2-allylic bromide to be discussed in Section V,B of this chapter or, on the other hand, by only oxidation of this bromide, respectively. The oxidation step is followed by a unique treatment with a weakly basic amine (e.g., dialkyl aniline) to insure complete double-bond isomerization to 3-cephem (C. F. Murphy and R. E. Koehler, unpublished).

Reaction of a 3-hydroxymethyl-3-cephem-1-oxide ester (73) with an

* Unpublished, R. D. G. Cooper, contrary to implication in Belg. Patent 684,288.
† Unpublished, R. D. G. Cooper.

appropriate phosphorous halide reagent also provides a choice of 3-halomethyl cephem derivatives (Belg. Patent 748,055). Reaction with phosphorous pentachloride or phosphorous pentabromide gives the corresponding 3-halomethyl sulfoxide in a typical alcohol to halide conversion. On the other hand, phosphorous trichloride or phosphorous tribromide converts alcohol sulfoxide (73) to the corresponding 3-halomethyl sulfide (70).

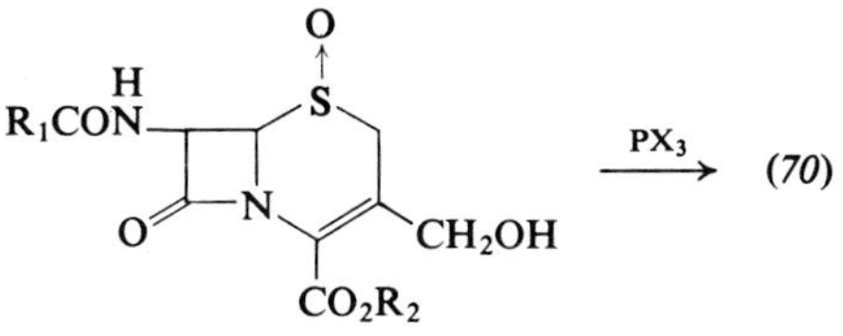

6. 3-Oxymethyl Ethers

The preparation of cephem 3-oxymethyl ethers occurred relatively late within the scope of cephalosporin research. This was undoubtedly a result of the fact that alcohols, unlike, for instance, many sulfur and nitrogen compounds, do not efficiently displace the acetoxy group from cephalosporins. Therefore, synthesis of the oxyethers awaited a more sophisticated level of cephem research.

A Belgian patent (719,710) allows a host of entries into the cephem 3-oxymethyl ether series. A second patent (Belg. Patent 719, 711) discusses this concept less thoroughly. These ether-forming reactions can be separated into two classes, i.e., those involving displacement of some group Y by the incoming alcohol residue (sometimes carried out on the cephem acid) and those involving condensation of a 3-hydroxymethyl cephem ester to generate an ether moiety.

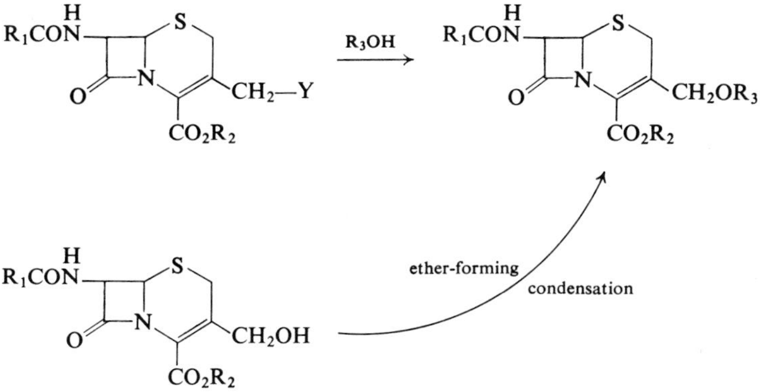

The displaceable group Y can be (a) acetoxy (not a preferred reaction), (b) a halogen (chloride, bromide, iodide), sometimes in the presence of mercuric nitrate, (c) an acetate residue appropriately substituted with at least one electron-withdrawing group, e.g., dichloroacetate, (d) benzoate, ring substituted with at least one electron-withdrawing group, (e) formate, (f) isothiocyanate, (g) and thiocarboxylate, thiocarbamate, or thioamide.

The ether-forming condensation reactions consist of either reaction with a diazo alkane or ortho ester in the presence of a Lewis acid, e.g., diazomethane plus boron trifluoride or methyl orthoformate plus perchloric acid, or alternatively, addition to ethyl vinyl ether in the presence of p-toluenesulfonic acid.

These patents state that one or more of the foregoing procedures can be used to prepare oxyethers from compounds of the type ROH, where R can be alkyl, alkenyl, alkynyl, a carbocycle, heterocycle, or aryl group, and various combinations and substitutions thereof.

Similar types of cephem 3-oxymethyl ether compounds are available from the corresponding 2-cephem ethers, discussed in Section V,B, via oxidation and reduction at sulfur (see Section II) (Neth. Patent 69,02013). The 3-alkoxy-methyl-3-cephem derivatives have been discussed in greater detail (Webber et al., 1971).

7. 3-THIOMETHYL DERIVATIVES

Numerous sulfur nucleophiles have been observed to displace the acetoxy group from cephalosporins. The facility of this type of reaction is unquestionably due to the high polarizability of the sulfur atom. Other examples exist of indirect replacement of the acetoxy group with sulfur species.

Thiols of various types in at least partly aqueous medium, under mildly basic conditions, displace acetoxy from cephalosporanic acids (Cocker et al., 1965) to give compounds of type (74). The phenomenon has been observed for thiophenols, heterocyclic thiols, and aliphatic thiols (U.S. Patent 3,278,531). Subsequently, specific extension to an important class of five-membered ring heterocyclic thiols was carried out (U.S. Patent 3,516,997). As discussed in Section IV, certain bidentate nucleophiles bearing an enolized thioamide (i.e., thiol) moiety react with cephalosporins to displace acetoxy and ultimately to provide a unique type of spiro derivative (Fazakerley et al., 1967).

Aliphatic and substituted aliphatic thiols smoothly replace many easily displaceable groups utilized in oxymethyl ether preparation (see Section V,A,6) such as dichloroacetoxy, halo, dinitrobenzoyloxy, and formyloxy (Belg. Patents 734,532, 734,533). The use of this indirect method of replacing an acetoxy moiety is far less significant with mercaptans than it is with alcohols.

Cocker et al. (1965) observed the displacement of the acetoxy function with sodium toluene-p-sulfinate to give a 3-sulfonylmethyl cephem derivative (75) ($R_3 = p$-toluene) (U.S. Patent 3,243,435). Magnesium methyl or propyl sulfinate also generate the sulfone species, which is alternatively said to be available via oxidation of the corresponding sulfoxide (76) (Belg. Patent 734,533). This sulfoxide species, on the other hand, can be prepared by oxidation of the sulfide (74) using chromium trioxide, benzoylperoxide, sodium periodate, peracetic acid, or oxygen. It is also claimed that indirect displacement of acetoxy, e.g., using 3-halomethyl derivatives, with a sulfenate salt yields a 3-sulfinylmethyl cephem species (76).

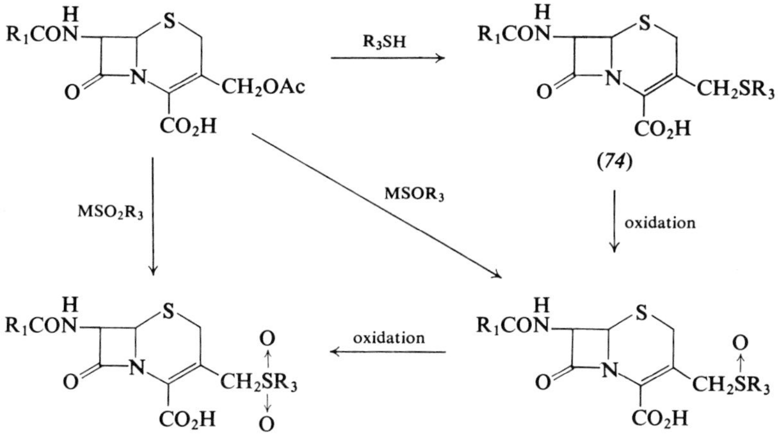

(74)

(75)

(76)

Probably the earliest report of acetoxy displacement from a cephalosporin by a sulfur moiety was the proposed formation of the Bunte salt (77) (Demain, 1963; Demain et al., 1963) as an explanation for increased antibacterial activity which was observed when cephalosporin C was reacted with sodium

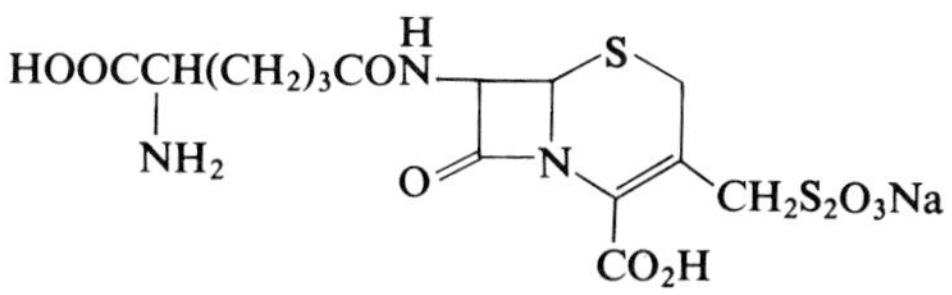

(77)

thiosulfate. It has been proposed that thiosulfate can react in this manner with a number of cephalosporin derivatives (U.S. Patent 3,278,531). Bisulfite and substituted thiosulfate are claimed to displace the acetoxy group, as do the thio- and dithioacids (U.S. Patent 3,243,435). Thiobenzoate displacement is particularly facile (Cocker et al., 1965) and leads to intermediate (78), which can conveniently be displaced by other nucleophiles (see Section V,A,8).

Thioamides and thioureas (U.S. Patent 3,278,531), especially thiourea itself (Cocker *et al.*, 1965), will displace the acetoxy group.

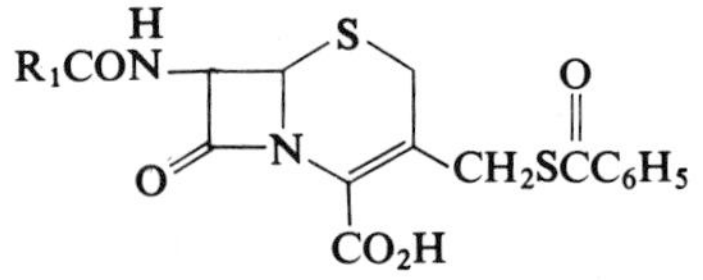

(78)

Van Heyningen and Brown (1965) observed the reaction of cephalosporanic acids with xanthates (U.S. Patent 3,446,803) to give compounds of type (79).

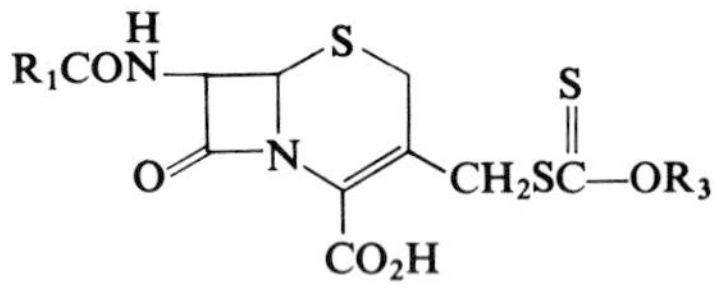

(79)

The ready displacement of an acetoxy group by a dithiocarbamate salt has been the subject of many patents (U.S. Patents 3,239,515, 3,239,516, 3,258,461, 3,431,259).

Van Heyningen and Brown (1965) described a number of these dithiocarbamates [of type (80)] in detail, including a dialkylamino-substituted series (U.S. Patent 3,239,515), emphasizing the piperazine dithiocarbamate analogs (U.S. Patent 3,239,516). Simple derivatives (U.S. Patent 3,258,461) have been claimed, and Cocker *et al.* (1965) have discussed in particular the dimethyldithiocarbamate (80) ($R_3 = R_4 = CH_3$). A novel cephalosporin dimer (81) has been reported based on the dithiocarbamate displacement (Jap. Patent 26105/69).

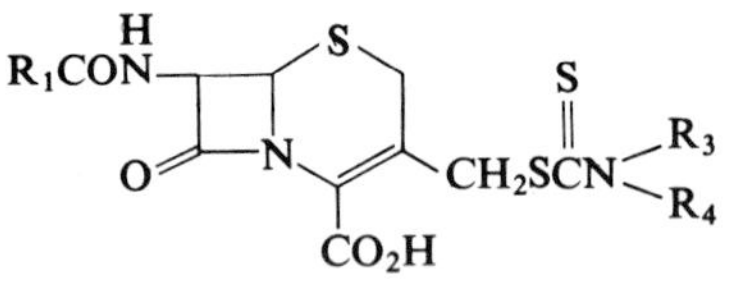

(80) 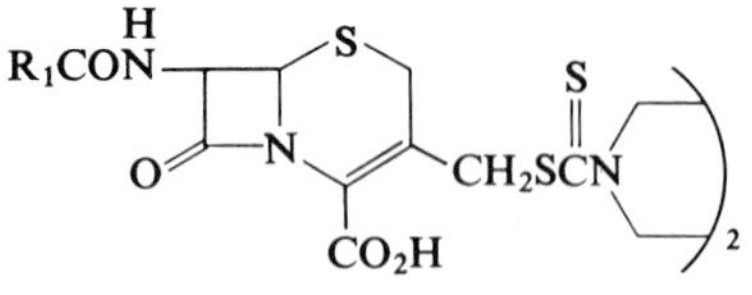   (81)

Discussion of mechanisms of displacement (including those by sulfur compounds) of acetoxy from cephalosporanic acids is presented in Section V,A,8.

8. 3-AMINOMETHYL DERIVATIVES

The first observation of acetoxy displacement from a cephalosporanic acid by a nitrogen nucleophile (in fact, by *any* nucleophile), namely, pyridine, resulted from the somewhat fortuitous overnight storage of cephalosporin C in a pyridine–acetate buffer (Abraham and Newton, 1958). These authors also observed an analogous reaction with nicotinic acid and nicotinamide. The product formed from pyridine, sometimes called cephalosporin C_A, has the betaine structure (82). This displacement was expanded to other cephalosporanic acid substrates (U.S. Patent 3,225,038) and resulted in the preparation of cephaloridine (83) (Spencer et al., 1967a) (see Chapter 12). Acetoxy displacement with a considerable number of substituted pyridines (Belg. Patents 641,338, 652,148; U.S. Patent 3,225,038) led to the corresponding cephem betaines, many of which have been described by Spencer et al. (1967b). These betaines are available in higher yield (than from simple acetoxy displacement) by displacement of some sulfur species, especially thiobenzoate, in the presence of a metal salt such as mercuric perchlorate (U.S. Patent 3,261,832).

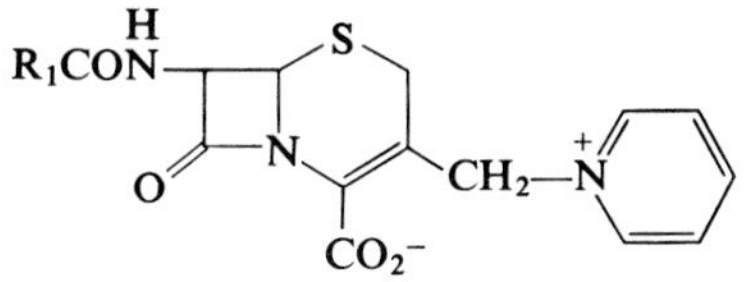

$$(82)\ R_1 = HO_2C—CH(CH_2)_3—$$
$$NH_2$$

$$(83)\ R_1 =$$

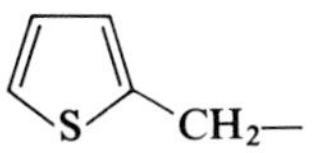

Taylor (1965) has proposed a mechanism for cephaloridine formation based on extensive experimental analysis. His comprehensive discussion has pertinence to the whole concept of acetoxy displacement (see below). Taylor concluded that low yields of cephaloridine were partially the result of product decay and nonspecific attack by pyridine on a dipolar carbonium ion intermediate. He calculated a maximum yield of betaine of 54% on the basis of rates of product formation and decomposition by pyridine and water. A similar calculation concerned with side reaction rates provided a limiting figure of 51% yield.

The addition of inorganic salts such as potassium thiocyanate or potassium iodide (U.S. Patent 3,270,012), leading to significant yield enhancement in the synthesis of cephaloridine, has been reported by Spencer et al. (1967a). The beneficial effect of the added salt may be, at least in part, the result of cephaloridine stabilization.

Other weakly basic heterocycles can be substituted for pyridine in the displacement of acetoxy from a cephalosporanic acid; these include quinoline, pyrimidines, pyrazoles, thiazoles, and triazoles (U.S. Patent 3,226,384), of which some have been discussed further by Hale *et al.* (1961), as well as imidazoles (U.S. Patent 3,228,934).

3-Azidomethyl-3-cephem acids (*84*) are available by acetoxy displacement from the corresponding cephalosporanic acids, upon treatment with azide ion in mildly basic aqueous medium (U.S. Patent 3,278,531). The reaction has been extended to a wide variety of cephalosporanic acid substrates (Neth. Patent 66,06820). The 3-azidomethyl moiety has been reduced to the 3-aminomethyl group (*85*) using tin and hydrochloric acid or catalytic hydrogenation, and the resulting primary amine has been acylated with phenoxyacetyl chloride (Cocker *et al.*, 1965). This reduction and acylation has been extended to produce a number of 3-acylaminomethyl cephem acids (*86*) (U.S. Patent 3,274,184) using acid chlorides, anhydrides, or a carboxylic acid with a carbodiimide; reaction of the primary amine (*85*) with isocyanates and isothiocyanates to give ureas and thioureas was also included in this work.

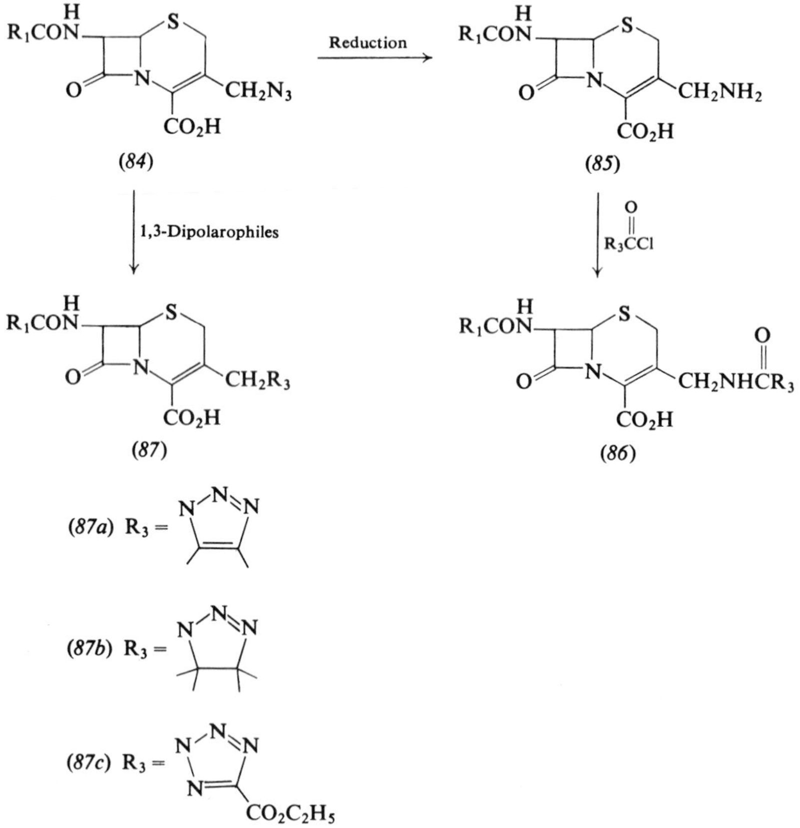

The 3-azidomethyl-3-cephem acids have reacted with 1,3-dipolarophiles to give heterocyclic derivatives (*87*) (Neth. Patent 67,17107). Acetylenes provided triazoles (*87a*), ethylenes gave triazolines (*87b*), and ethyl cyanoformate yielded a tetrazole (*87c*).

The 3-azidomethyl cephem acids have also been converted into lactams of type (*88*) (R_3 = H) via azide reduction and intramolecular cyclization (Neth. Patent 68,00751), presumably as relays for synthetic work described in Chapter 6.

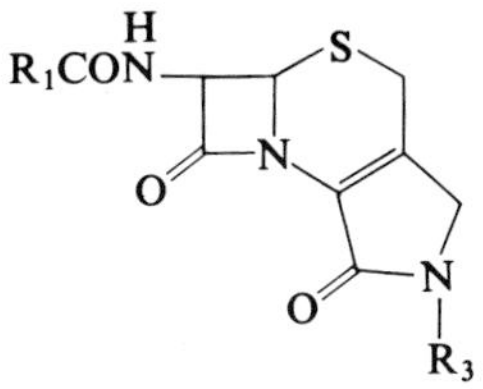

(*88*) 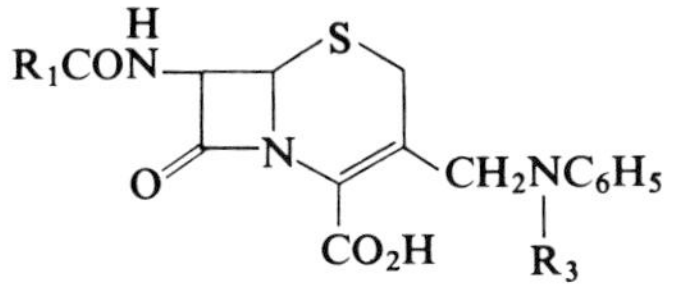   (*89*)

When cephalosporanic acids are treated with aromatic amines, acetoxy displacement occurs (U.S. Patent 3,278,531). Bradshaw *et al.* (1968) observed that lack of pH control in this reaction with aniline resulted in formation of the lactam (*88*) ($R_3 = C_6H_5$). If pH is maintained at 7.5, the secondary amine (*89*) (R_3 = H) is obtained. Reaction of sodium 7-phenylacetamido cephalosporanic acid with *N*-methylaniline, which precludes γ-lactam formation, caused diminished β-lactam destruction and produced the tertiary amine (*89*) ($R_3 = CH_3$).

The 3-isocyanatomethyl-3-cephem acid (*90*) is available in an indirect manner from a cephalosporanic acid by displacement on the 3′-dichloroacetoxy analog (Belg. Patent 719,711). This patent also suggests that the variety

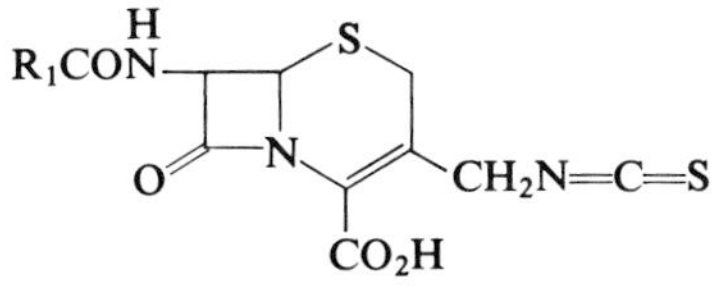

(*90*)

of good 3′-leaving groups discussed therein and enumerated in Section V,A,6, exemplified by halo, dichloroacetoxy, formyloxy, etc., can be displaced by a variety of nucleophilic nitrogen species in the general categories of tertiary amines, pyridines, and heterocyclic bases having more than one heteroatom. Specific examples given included thiazole and pyrazole displacements of dichloroacetoxy in aqueous acetone and pyridine displacement of a 3-chloromethyl cephem derivative.

A mechanism of acetoxy displacement from cephalosporanic acids has emerged from the observations of Cocker *et al.* (1965) and Taylor (1965). Some comments on pyridine-related displacements by the latter author have already been noted; the discussion below includes salient points of both of these papers.

It was noted that a number of sulfur and nitrogen nucleophiles replaced the acetoxy group from the 3-cephem nucleus, suggesting a common mechanism. However, these displacements were essentially inoperative on sulfoxides, methyl esters, and lactones; and oxygen nucleophiles do not readily displace acetate. Evolution of carbon dioxide during some displacements and various observations leading to the conclusion of an S_N1 displacement with leaving group solvation were important contributions to their mechanistic postulate. The intermediates indicated are implicated as contributing forms in the displacement, the dipolar allylic carbonium ion (*91*) being stabilized (with varying

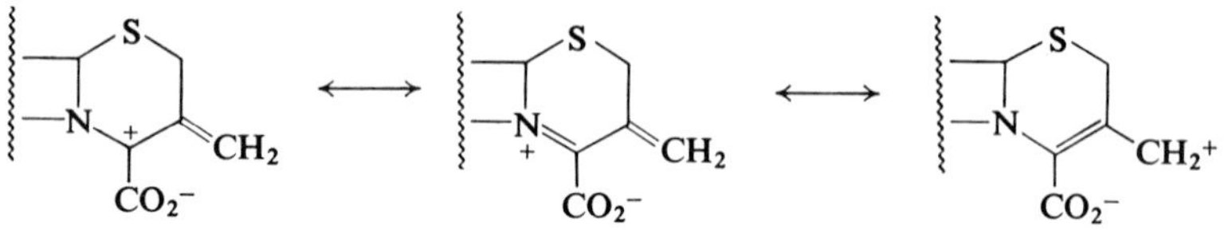

(*91*)

significance) by the resonance forms indicated. In order to include sulfur participation, the summarizing structure (*92*) has been invoked.

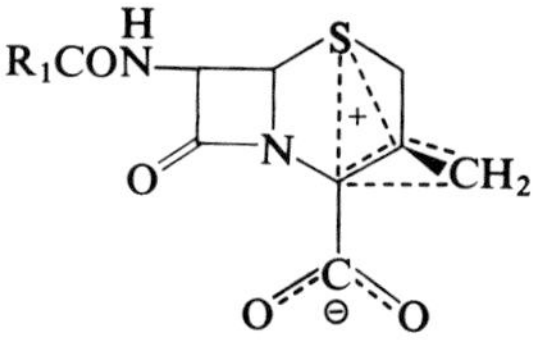

(*92*)

Lactone formation (see Section VI) might be an expected occurrence during acetoxy displacements with nitrogen and sulfur nucleophiles; however, its absence is consistent with the observed failure of oxygen nucleophiles to displace acetate, a phenomenon at least partially contributed to by anion solvation.

9. 3'-CARBON DERIVATIVES

Relatively few cephem derivatives have been discussed in which the acetoxy group in a cephalosporanic acid has been formally displaced by a carbon nucleophile. Even fewer examples are well documented.

The acetoxy was displaced from sodium 7-phenylacetamidocephalospora-nate by resorcinol in aqueous acetone to give (*93*) (Cocker *et al.*, 1965). These authors also found that the same substrate in aqueous acetone, with indole and *N*-methyl indole, gave (*94*) (R = H and R = CH$_3$, respectively). Paper chromatographic evidence suggested that an analogous derivative resulted from reaction with 2-methylindole but not with 3-methylindole.

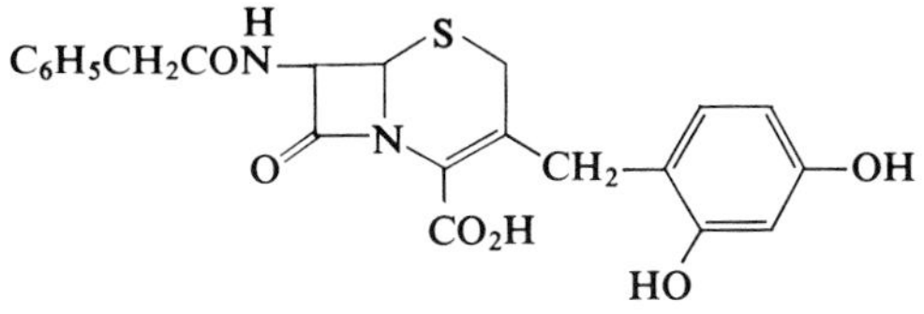

(*93*)

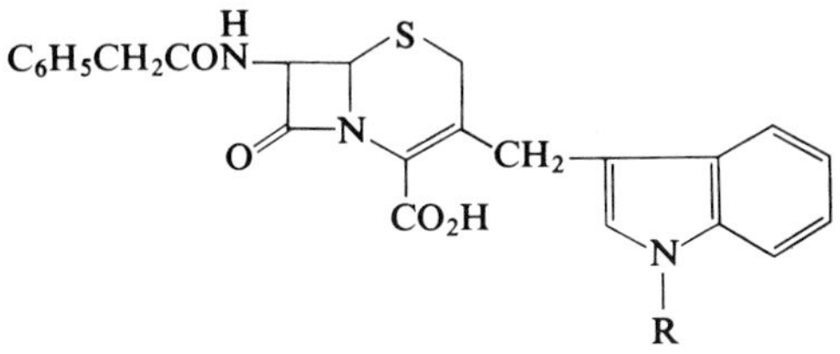

(*94*)

Pyrroles may also displace acetoxy from a cephalosporanic acid to give products assigned structure type (*95*) (U.S. Patent 3,278,531).

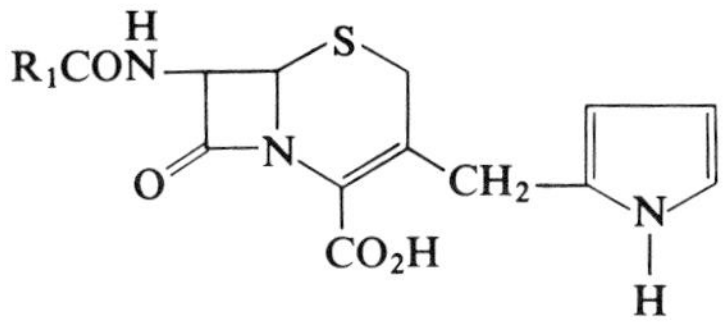

(*95*)

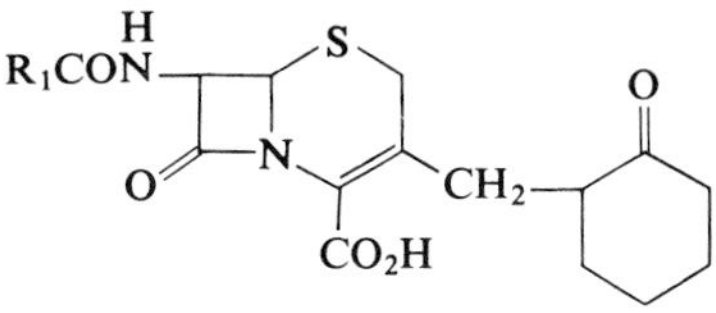

(*96*)

A 3-iodomethyl-3-cephem ester can apparently be reacted with the pyrrolidine enamine of cyclohexanone to give, after hydrolysis, the cephalo-sporin-alkylated cyclohexanone (*96*) (Belg. Patents 719,710, 719,711). The latter patent also suggests the possibility of reacting cephem derivatives having readily displaced groups, e.g., halo, dichloroacetoxy, formyloxy, isothio-cyanato, on the 3′ carbon with various vaguely outlined carbon nucleophiles such as pyrroles, indoles, "compounds giving stabilized carbanions," e.g., acetylenes and β-dicarbonyl compounds, and cyanide ion provided in some form. Further substantiation has not been forthcoming.

Finally, the 3-cyanomethyl-3-cephem nucleus (Webber and Vasileff, 1971) is available from the corresponding 2-cephem derivative, by oxidation and reduction at sulfur (see Section II). Its preparation is described in Section V,B (Neth. Patent 69,02013).

10. MISCELLANEOUS 3-SUBSTITUENTS

A few 3-derivatives of the 3-cephem system defy classification according to the organization set up for this discussion. Because of their uniqueness and in the interest of thoroughness, these derivatives will be briefly mentioned. The expanding frontiers of cephalosporin research bode well for growth of this category.

The 3-formyl-3-cephem ester (97) can be prepared by oxidation of the corresponding 3-hydroxymethyl derivative with chromium trioxide or manganese dioxide (Chamberlin and Campbell, 1967). It is claimed that the 3-formyl cephem species undergoes most of those reactions characteristic of an aldehyde group (U.S. Patent 3,351,596.)

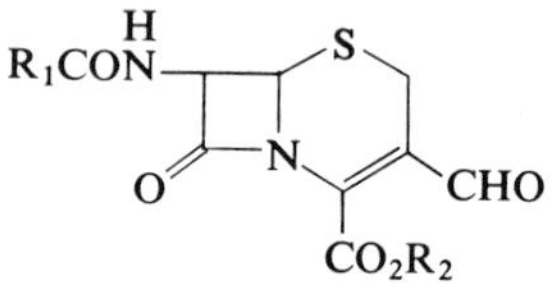

(97)

Displacement of acetate from a cephalosporanic acid by hydrogen phosphate ion (HPO_4^{--}) has been suggested (U.S. Patent 3,278,531), presumably to give (98).

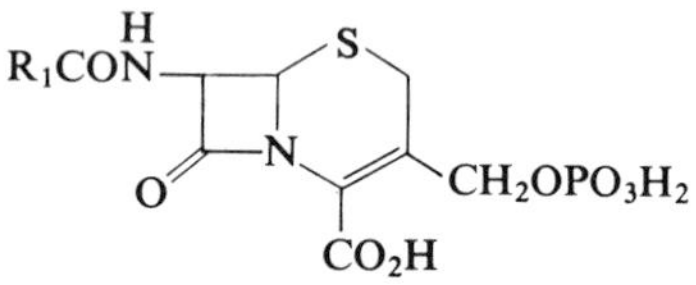

(98)

The preparation of a 3-cephem species bearing only a hydrogen at the 3 position has resulted from total synthetic efforts (Belg. Patent 742,934) (see Chapter 6).

B. 2-Cephem Derivatives

The variety of chemical manipulations of the 3-substituent in the 2-cephem series has been far less than that in the 3-cephem series. This is primarily due to the fact that the 2-cephem nucleus is neither naturally occurring nor biologically active to any significant degree. Much of the work to be discussed here is of a more recent nature. It could not have proceeded until 2-cephem compounds were available (chemistry discussed elsewhere in the chapter); further stimulation was derived from the practical isomerization of $\varDelta^2$ to $\varDelta^3$ systems which was discussed in Section II.

A majority of C-3 derivatives of the 2-cephem system has been derived from functionalization of the 3-methyl-2-cephem-4-carboxylate ester (99) series. The $\varDelta^2$-deacetoxycephalosporin ester (99) ($R_1 = C_6H_5OCH_2$) was converted to the corresponding allylic bromide (100) by treatment with N-bromo-succinimide (NBS), catalyzed by azobisisobutyronitrile, in hot carbon tetrachloride (Neth. Patent 69,02013).

(99)   (100)

When a p-methoxybenzyl ester was used, functionalization was not complete ($\approx 15\%$ deacetoxy remaining) due to attack of NBS at the benzylic methylene (Webber et al., 1969). Utilization of a t-butyl ester permitted an excess of brominating agent to bring about an essentially complete conversion to 3-bromo-methyl-2-cephem ester (100) (Webber et al., 1971).

Because of the importance of the NBS allylic bromination of deacetoxy-cephalosporin as an entry into a number of C-3 substituents, it seems appropriate here to discuss the vicissitudes of this reaction. On the one hand, there is the remarkable conversion and specificity in the $\varDelta^2$ series; on the other hand, this reaction fails to be useful in the $\varDelta^3$ (sulfide) series.* As a photochemically induced process, NBS allylic bromination can successfully functionalize a deacetoxycephalosporin sulfoxide ($\varDelta^3$),† as mentioned earlier in this chapter.

In the 3-methyl-2-cephem case, besides near quantitative conversion (95%+ by NMR analysis), the NBS functionalization shows significant selectivity. No observation has been made of attack at any position other than the 3-methyl except for very tenuous evidence for a 4-bromo-2-cephem minor constituent.‡ No 2-bromo-3-(exo)methylene species or product of its intermediacy is observed. Such a species might be anticipated if the selectivity of bromination

* Unpublished, R. D. G. Cooper.
† Unpublished, R. D. G. Cooper.
‡ In the purification of a 3-methoxymethyl-2-cephem ester a small amount of material was obtained whose NMR spectrum suggested a 2-methoxy-3-cephem structure, the product of allylic rearrangement and methanolysis of a 4-bromo-2-cephem species. Unpublished, J. A. Webber and R. T. Vasileff.

results from the superior allylic nature of the methyl group vinylogously alpha to the sulfur atom. An intermediate sulfonium exomethylene species might collapse with bromide to give the 2-bromo compound. This mechanism cannot be manipulated to give a 4-bromo cephem compound.

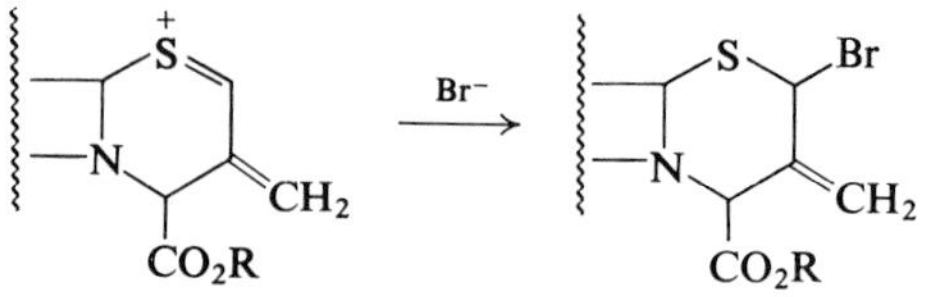

Given the successful functionalization in the 2-cephem series, why does it fail in the 3-cephem series? Simple crotonic esters (3-cephem is an analog) can be converted to allylic bromides by NBS. Although there may be steric crowding between the ester function and 3-cephem 3-methyl group, variation of ester bulk has no effect upon the result.*

The β-lactam nitrogen is uniquely attached to the double bond in the Δ^3 series but has no obvious electronic significance in Δ^2 derivatives. It has been suggested that the unshared electrons on this nitrogen atom participate in a conjugative sense with the 3-cephem double bond (Sweet and Dahl, 1970; see also, Section V,A,8 and Chapter 8). Such an effect is analogous to that of sulfur in 2-cephem derivatives, where this relationship is no liability to NBS functionalization.

A possible explanation for the apparently enigmatic NBS reactions is that in the 3-cephem series the C-2 allylic position is sufficiently activated (by being alpha to the sulfur atom) relative to 3-methyl to make a 2-bromo-3-cephem species the preferred product. This α-bromosulfide might then lead only to decomposition. In the 2-cephem series the alternate allylic position, C-4, may be unfavorable for functionalization due to steric reasons.

NBS bromination could be initiated by attack at sulfur.† In the Δ^3 series the resulting bromosulfonium intermediate could collapse via proton loss to give the 2-bromo species and decomposition as discussed above. If such attack by NBS prevails, selectivity in the Δ^2 case is a result of the significant decrease in

---

* Unpublished, R. D. G. Cooper.
† A suggestion of Professor Leo A. Paquette.

electron density at sulfur (see Section II) and the normal free-radical mechanism becomes dominant.

It would appear that photochemically induced allylic bromination of the deacetoxy sulfoxide* is the result of a different mechanism than for the sulfide because thermal initiation is ineffective for sulfoxides and photochemical initiation fails for Δ^3-sulfides.†

Phosphorous tribromide treatment of a 3-hydroxymethyl-2-cephem ester also provides the 3-bromomethyl cephalosporin (Belg. Patent 748,055).

The first observed displacement of the 3-bromomethyl-2-cephem species was with acetate ion to give a 3-acetoxymethyl moiety (Webber et al., 1969). Double-bond equilibration (see Section IV) due to the basicity of acetate ion was observed. Structural verification was based on comparison with an authentic Δ^2–Δ^3 equilibrium mixture (101) prepared by acetate treatment of known 3-acetoxymethyl-2-cephem ester. This result, together with NMR analysis of the allylic bromide (100) and other displacements to give pure Δ^2 species, minimized uncertainty concerning the positional integrity of the double bond in the NBS product.

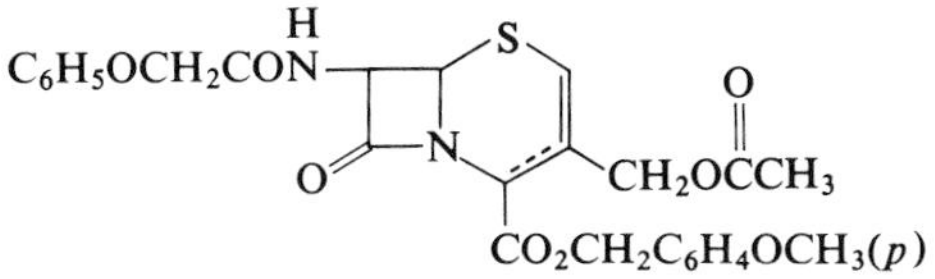

(101)

Derivatives of the 3-acetoxymethyl-2-cephem nucleus have been prepared from the naturally occurring Δ^3 isomer by double bond manipulation as described in Section IV,B and are intermediates in the Woodward et al. (1966) cephalosporin synthesis.

The Δ^2-allylic bromide (100) has been observed to undergo displacement by other good nucleophiles such as azide and thiocyanate as well as a variety of other species bearing nucleophilic nitrogen or sulfur atoms (Neth. Patent 69,02013). Of course, the most significant displacements of the Δ^2-allylic bromide are those which do not have an analogy in acetate displacement in the 3-acetoxymethyl-3-cephem series. For example, displacement of bromide from (100) by cyanide to give a 3-cyanomethyl-2-cephem ester (102) could be effected by using copper(I) cyanide in dimethyl sulfoxide (Webber and Vasileff, 1971). Sodium or potassium cyanide in any of a number of solvents led to extensive decomposition, while solvents other than dimethyl sulfoxide gave poor conversion. The conditions which employ copper(I) cyanide, often used to displace aromatic halogen, in dimethyl sulfoxide are apparently the optimum

---

* Unpublished, R. D. G. Cooper.
† Unpublished, R. D. G. Cooper and I. G. Wright.

compromise of solubility, nucleophilicity, and basicity which minimize β-lactam destruction while allowing bromide displacement to occur.

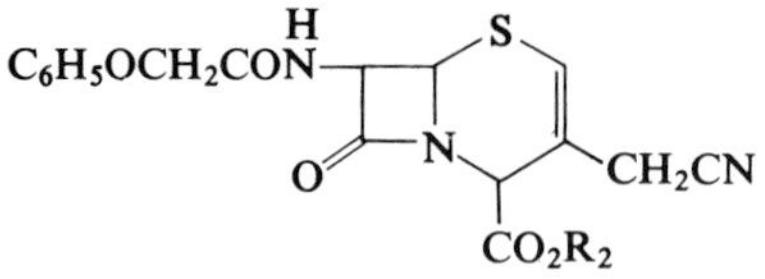

$C_6H_5OCH_2CON$ [structure] CH_2CN, CO_2R_2

(102)

$C_6H_5OCH_2CON$ [structure] CH_2OR_3, CO_2R_2

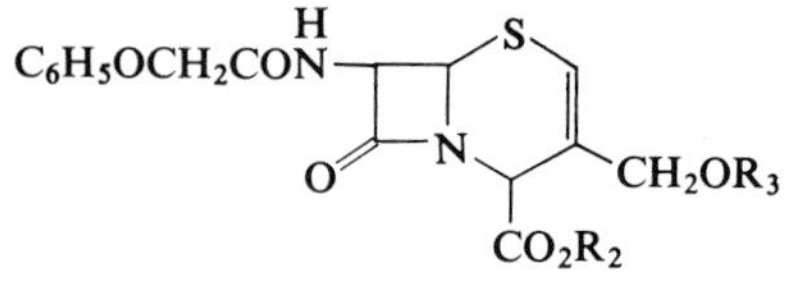

(103)

The dichotomy of displacement reactivity of the Δ^2 allylic bromide (100) is further illustrated by conversion to a 3-methoxymethyl-2-cephem ester (103) ($R_3 = CH_3$) (Webber et al., 1971). The replacement occurs nearly instantaneously in methanol without the need for base. Although methanol is a very nucleophilic alcohol, the replacement reaction was found to be general when the allylic bromide was dissolved in essentially any liquid alcohol (Neth. Patent 69,02013). Only the rate was affected. Because the Δ^2 allylic bromide (100) is a vinylogous α-bromo sulfide, the extreme solvolytic reactivity in an alcoholic medium seems reasonable. The Δ^2 bromide was, however, resistant to conversion to 3-alkoxymethyl derivatives when using a limited amount of an alcohol in an organic diluent together with an appropriate base.*

An analogous displacement, utilizing thiols which are better nucleophiles than alcohols, takes place at a reasonable rate even in an organic diluent (C. F. Murphy, R. E. Koehler, and C. W. Ryan, unpublished).

Although hydrolysis of allylic bromide (100) to a 3-hydroxymethyl-2-cephem-4-carboxylate ester (104) takes place under a variety of conditions, it is best carried out in a nonnucleophilic organic solvent containing 25–50% dimethyl sulfoxide and several equivalents of water (Neth. Patent 69,02013). These conditions give the highest yield and purest reaction product. An alkoxysulfonium intermediate which collapses with water to form the allylic alcohol (104) is postulated to explain the need for dimethyl sulfoxide.

[structure] CO_2R_2, CH_2—O—S^+Br^- with CH_3, CH_3 $\xrightarrow{H_2O}$ R_1CON [structure] CH_2OH, CO_2R_2

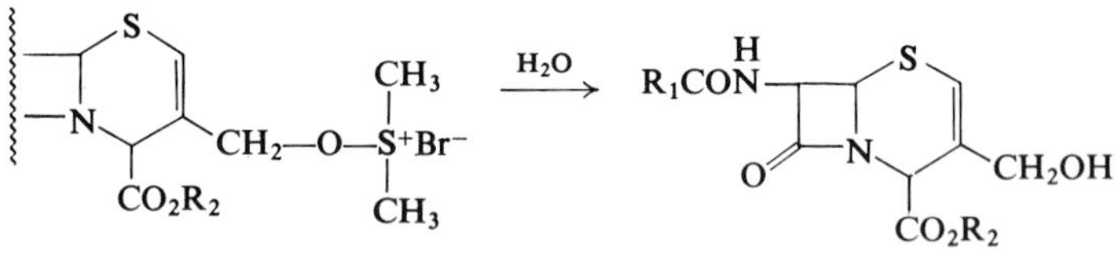

(104)

Other solvents which can generate analogous intermediates (e.g., dimethylformamide, N-methylpyrrolidone, hexamethylphosphoramide) perform less efficiently. If dimethyl sulfoxide is used as solvent in the hydrolysis reaction, uncharacterized side-reaction products are formed, possibly as a consequence

* Unpublished, J. A. Webber and R. T. Vasileff.

of allylic rearrangement to unstable 2-substituted species. An analogous [to (*104*)] type of Δ^2 allylic alcohol is an intermediate in the Woodward *et al.* (1966) cephalosporin total synthesis. The corresponding cephem acids (*104*) ($R_2 = H$) are available from the natural 3-acetoxymethyl-3-cephem nucleus (as ester) following tandem sodium hydroxide treatments.

3-Hydroxymethyl-2-cephem-4-carboxylic acids have been oxidized to the corresponding 3-formyl derivatives (*105*) ($R_2 = H$) by a number of oxidizing agents, dichlorodicyanoquinone being preferred (Neth. Patent 68,15631).

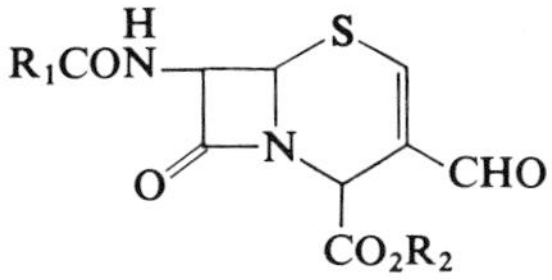

(*105*)

Of course, the Δ^2-aldehyde (*105*) (as trichloroethyl ester) was the preliminary β-lactam dihydrothiazine species obtained in the total synthesis of cephalosporin (Woodward *et al.*, 1966).

Δ^2-Deacetyl acids have been acylated with the appropriate acid anhydride in the presence of pyridine to yield aliphatic 3-acyloxymethyl-2-cephem acids (*106*) (Kukolja, 1970). This reaction does not provide lactone and is representative of the stability of Δ^2-deacetyl cephalosporin derivatives to lactonization.

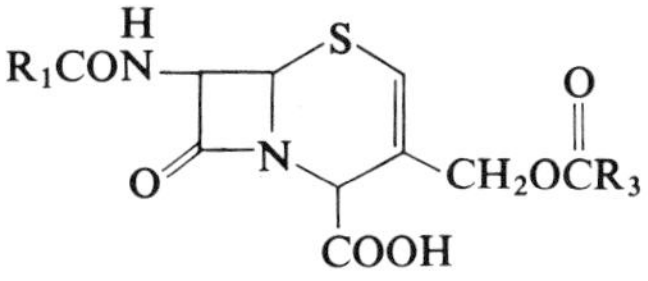

(*106*)

Cocker *et al.* (1966) have reported that the acetate group in 3-acetoxymethyl-2-cephem-4-carboxylic acids (*106*) ($R_3 = CH_3$) can be displaced by pyridine, thiourea, resorcinol, and by thiobenzoate, thiosulfate, *N,N*-dimethyldithiocarbamate, and azide ions. These displacements are apparently sluggish relative to those of Δ^3 analogs, and 3-hydroxymethyl compounds are observed as by-products. These authors also comment that the corresponding 2-cephem esters do not undergo direct acetoxy displacement.

VI. Modifications of the C-4 Carboxyl Group

The C-4 carboxyl group of cephalosporin compounds undergoes many reactions typical of the carboxylic acid function. However, complications such as steric hindrance (of the 3-methyl substituent), double-bond isomerization, and the highly reactive positions of the cephalosporin ring system frequently prevent high yields of the carboxylic acid reaction products.

A. Esterification

Although simple esters (such as methyl) of cephalosporin acids are easily prepared by reactions with corresponding diazoalkanes (Chauvette *et al.*, 1963), the lack of biological activity of such esters and difficulty in their removal has caused investigators to examine esters which can be used as protecting groups. The field of peptide chemistry has provided several such possibilities. Their selection, however, is limited by the ease of attaching and removing these groups. The cephalosporin esters must be formed under conditions which do not isomerize the double bond and must be removed by reagents compatible with cephalosporin compounds.

Phenyldiazomethane and diphenyldiazomethane have been found (Neth. Patent 64,01421) to react smoothly with cephalosporanic acids to give the corresponding esters. Thus, *N*-phthalimido cephalosporin C (*107*), when treated with excess diphenyldiazomethane, gave (*108*), an intermediate in the preparation of 7-aminocephalosporanic acid (see Chapter 2, Section II,A). The

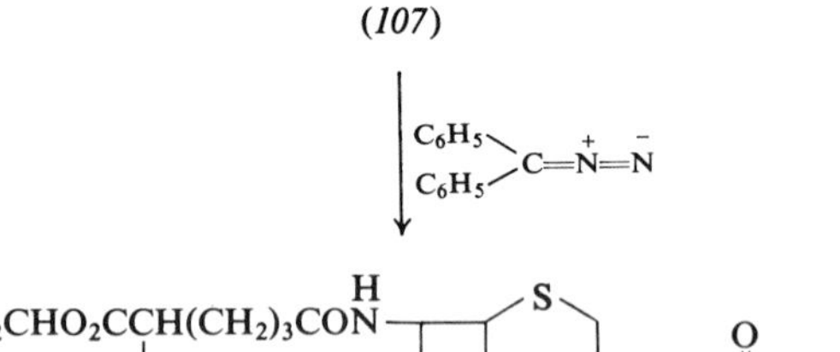

(*107*)

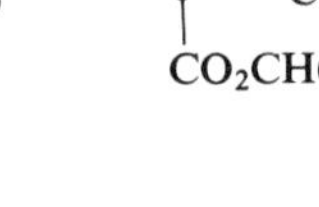

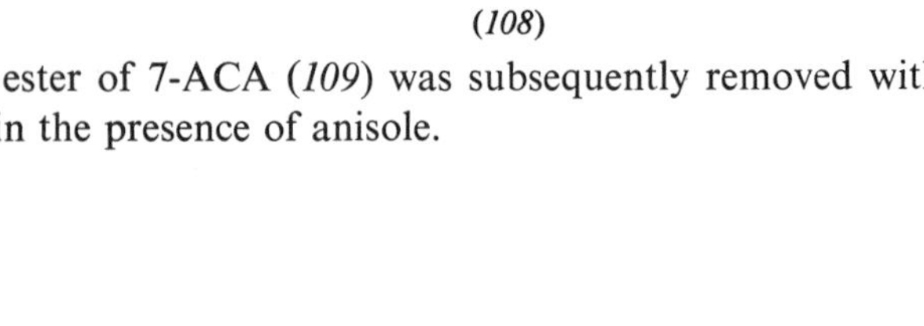

(*108*)

benzhydryl ester of 7-ACA (*109*) was subsequently removed with trifluoroacetic acid in the presence of anisole.

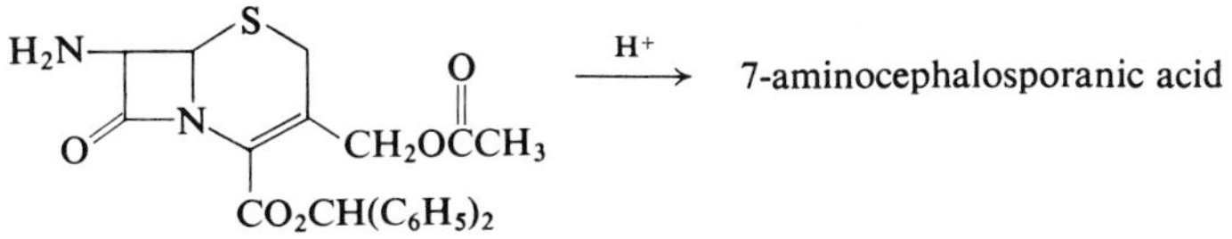

(109)

Tertiary-butyl esters have been used widely as protecting groups (Fieser and Fieser, 1967) and have found application in cephalosporin chemistry. Stedman (1966) has reported that 7-ACA and isobutene in dioxane–sulfuric acid react to give the 7-ACA t-butyl ester (110) in 52% yield. The ester was removed with neat trifluoroacetic acid. No double-bond isomerization was noted under the conditions described.

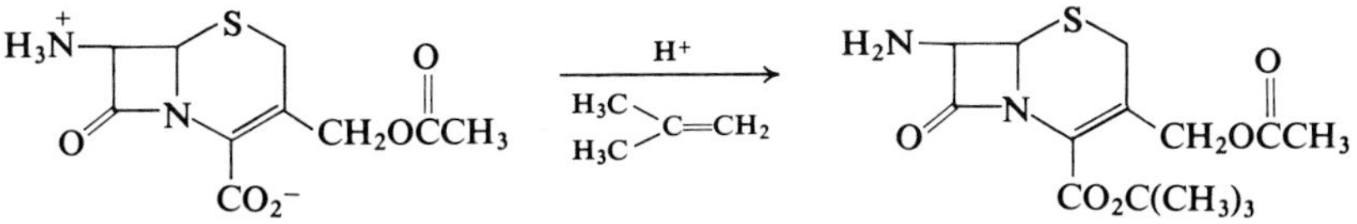

(110)

An example of the difficulty of preparing isomerically pure cephalosporin esters is found in experiments described by Chauvette and Flynn (1966). Cephalothin sodium salt, when reacted with activated alkylhalides generally gave a mixture of Δ^2 and Δ^3 esters (111). Occasionally, a single isomer could be isolated by crystallization but the yields were low. Phenacyl esters of cephalothin, however, have been prepared without isomerization in N,N-dimethylacetamide (U.S. Patent 3,284,451).

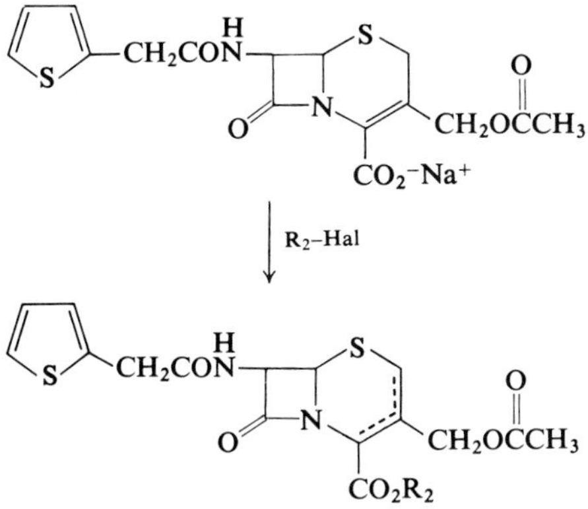

(111)

$\Delta^2 + \Delta^3$; $R_2 = CH_2OCH_3$, CH_2OCCH_3, $CH_2COC_2H_5$

Δ^3; $R_2 = CH_2COC_6H_5$

Another preparation of cephalosporin esters that has been used with success is the condensation of the cephem acid with an alcohol in the presence of a carbodiimide. Thus, *N*-hydroxyphthalimide (Chauvette and Flynn, 1966), anisylalcohol (Neth. Patent 64,10421), and 2,2,2-trichloroethanol (Kaiser *et al.*, 1970) react with cephalosporin acids in the presence of dicyclohexylcarbodiimide to give the corresponding esters [(*112*), (113) and (*114*), respectively].

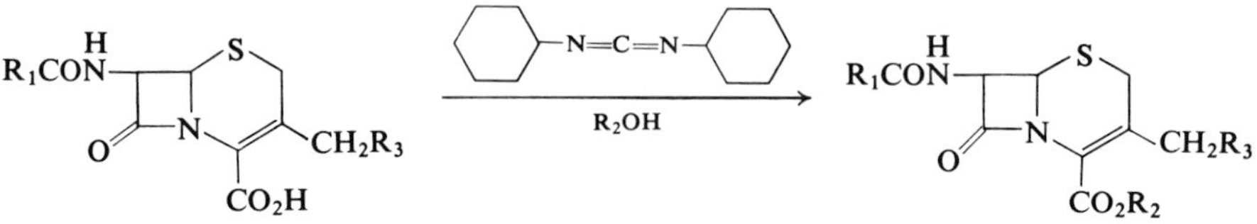

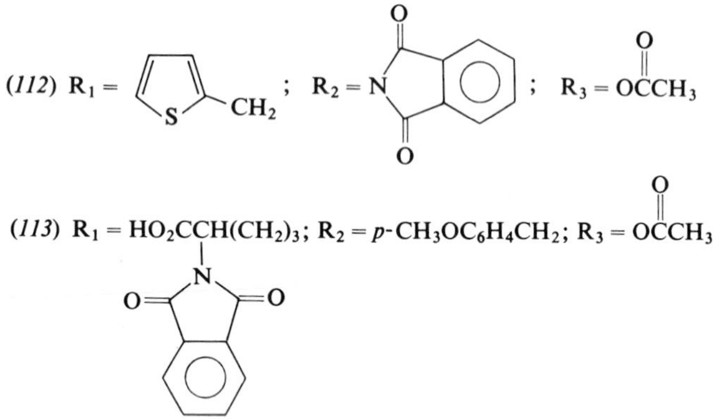

R₁CON
H
S
N
O
CH₂R₃
CO₂H
N=C=N
R₂OH
R₁CON
H
S
N
O
CH₂R₃
CO₂R₂

(112) R₁ =
S
CH₂
; R₂ = N
O
O
; R₃ = OCCH₃
O
(113) R₁ = HO₂CCH(CH₂)₃; R₂ = p-CH₃OC₆H₄CH₂; R₃ = OCCH₃
O
N
O
O

(*114*) $R_1 = C_6H_5OCH_2$; $R_2 = CH_2CCl_3$; $R_3 = H$

An alternative preparation of cephalothin esters (Chauvette and Flynn, 1966) involves the reaction of the mixed carbonic anhydride derived from cephalothin and isobutyl chloroformate. The mixed anhydride (*115*) was reacted with glycerol to give the desired ester (*116*). Unfortunately, the 3-cephem carboxylic acid ester was contaminated with the Δ^2-cephalosporin ester and the isobutyl ester derived from decomposition of the mixed anhydride.

In a report describing the functionalization of deacetoxy cephalosporins, Webber *et al.* (1969) prepared the 2-cephem carboxylic acid ester (*117*) in 90% yield using anisyl alcohol in the presence of *N*,*N*-dimethylformamide dineopentyl acetal (Brechbuhler *et al.*, 1965).

Δ^2-Cephalosporin esters have been prepared directly from the 3-cephem carboxylic acid chloride (*118*) by Murphy and Koehler (1970). This reaction served the twofold purpose of controlling the double-bond position (see discussion in Section IV,B) and providing good yields of 2-cephem carboxylic

(115)

(116)

(117)

acid esters. This method was especially useful for preparing esters that served as intermediate blocking groups for the carboxyl function.

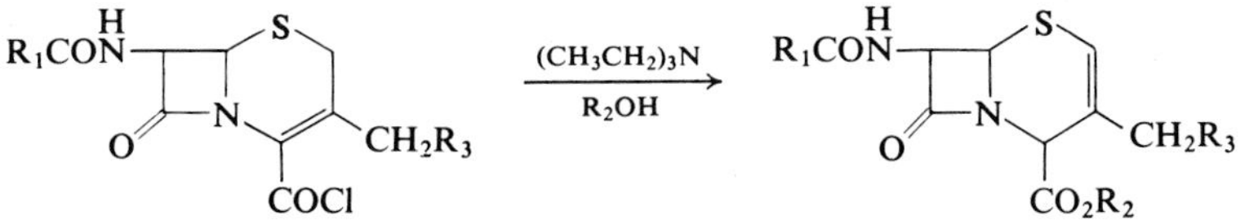

(118)   (119)

Tertiary esters (such as t-butyl) can be prepared by this reaction at ice temperature; however, to insure a high degree of isomer purity, primary esters are formed at dry ice–acetone temperatures.

B. Cephalosporin Lactone Formation

Cephalosporanic acids (120) when reacted in aqueous solutions have frequently led to lactone (121) formation (Chauvette and Flynn, 1966; Abraham and Newton, 1961; Green et al., 1965; Cocker et al., 1966). The variety of cephalosporin lactones reported would suggest that lactone formation is not dependent on the 7-amino substituent. Double-bond position is important, however, because Kukolja (1970) has shown the Δ^2-cephem compounds do not form lactones. Cephalosporin lactones are often insoluble in aqueous or organic solvents and are fairly stable. The lack of solubility has prevented extensive examination of their biological activities even though some lactones have antimicrobial and antibacterial activity (Chauvette et al., 1962).

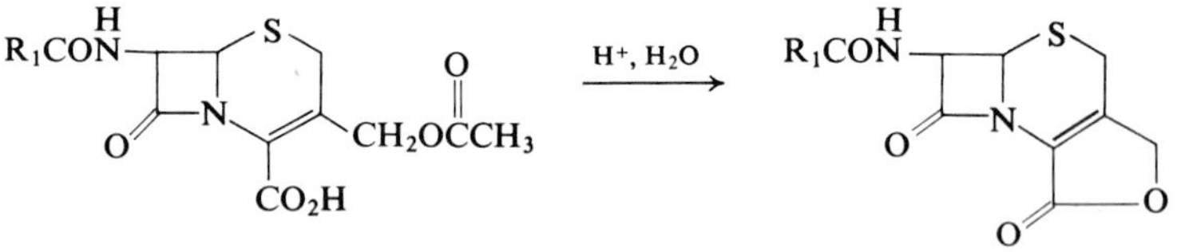

(120)   (121)

Although the synthesis of cephalosporin lactones has been the intermediate objective (see Chapter 6) for the synthesis of cephalosporin antibiotics (Heymes et al., 1966; Dolfini et al., 1969), opening of the lactone ring has presented considerable difficulty. Recently, Neidleman et al. (1970) have found that under carefully controlled conditions the lactone can be opened to the 3-hydroxymethyl derivative (see Section IV,A). This reaction was performed on a relatively small scale and is of questionable utility as a means for producing large quantities of antibiotics.

C. *Amides of Cephalosporin Acids*

The preparation of cephalosporin acid amides has been hindered by the same problem as the ester preparation, i.e., double-bond isomerization. Chauvette and Flynn (1966) reacted the *N*-hydroxyphthalimido ester of cephalothin (*122*) with glycine ethyl ester. The product isolated, however, was the 2-cephem amide (*123*).

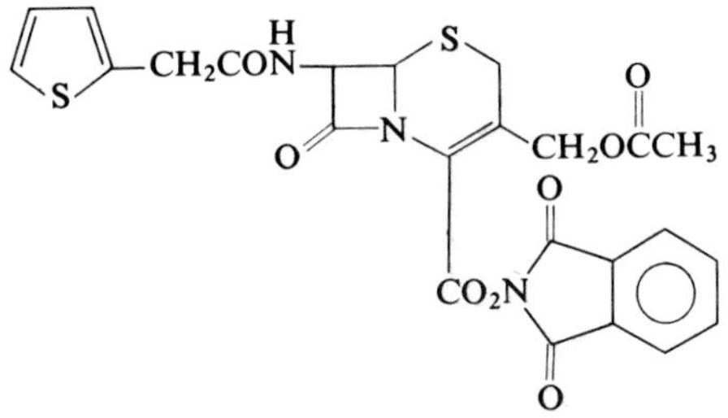
H
CH_2CON
S
N
O
O
CH_2OCCH_3
O
CO_2N
O
S

(*122*)

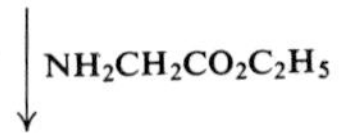
$NH_2CH_2CO_2C_2H_5$

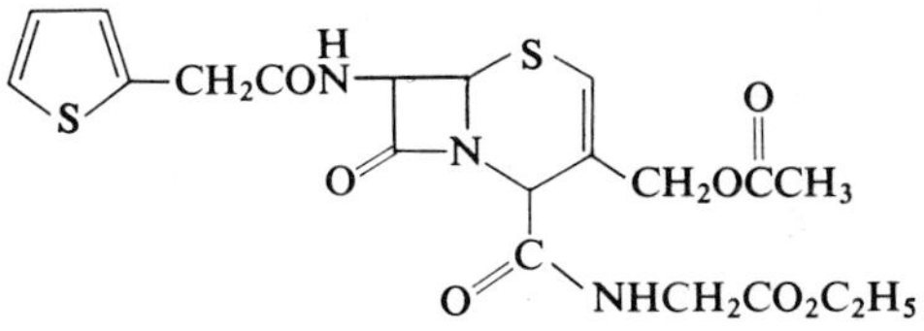
H
CH_2CON
S
N
O
O
CH_2OCCH_3
C
O
$NHCH_2CO_2C_2H_5$
S

(*123*)

Condensation of cephalothin with the *t*-butyl ester of alanine in the presence of *N*,*N*′-dicyclohexyocarbodiimide gave the 3-cephem amide (*124*), which was further converted to the acid (*125*). The products possessed only a low order of biological activity.

Cephalosporin carboxylic acids have also been converted to the saccharyl amide (*126*) as described in a Belgian patent (738, 929).

(124)

(125)

(126)

D. Other Reactions of the Cephalosporin Carboxyl Group

Several cephalosporin carboxylic acids have been treated with reagents to transform these groups into more effective acylating functions. The 3-cephem acid chlorides (Murphy and Koehler, 1970), prepared from the corresponding 3-cephem acid and oxalyl chloride with dimethylformamide catalysis, react with alcohol under mild conditions in the presence of tertiary amines to give 2-cephem esters. Mixed anhydrides prepared from cephalosporins and other carboxylic acid compounds are, in some cases, stable enough to be isolated (Chauvette and Flynn, 1966). These mixed anhydrides can be reacted with alcohols; however, unintentional double-bond isomerization sometimes occurs.

One of the most important reactions of the cephalosporin carboxyl group involves its temporary protection while other reactions are carried out. Protection of the carboxyl group has been especially important during removal of the 7-acyl side chain. Nitrogen-protected cephalosporin C (*127*), for example, reacts with trimethylsilyl chloride in the presence of a tertiary amine base to give the trimethyl silyl ester (*128*). The 7-acyl group is then removed via a phosphorous pentachloride process and the silyl ester removed during

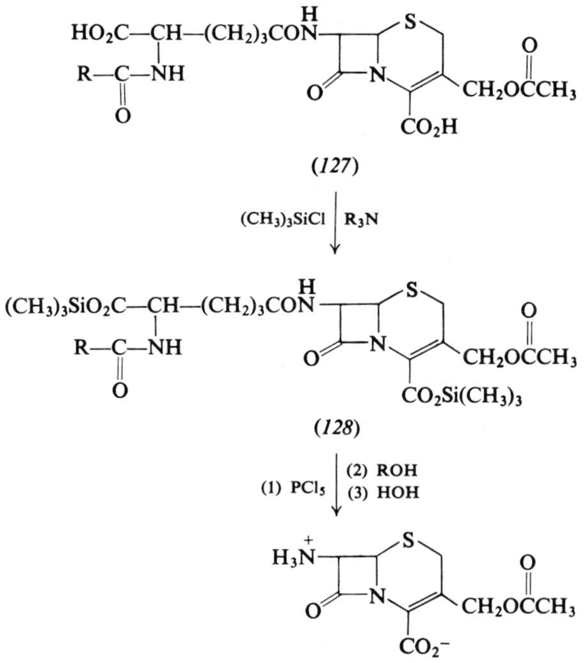

(*127*)

$(CH_3)_3SiCl$ | R_3N

(*128*)

(1) PCl_5 | (2) ROH
          | (3) HOH

hydrolysis to give 7-aminocephalosporanic acid (Belg. Patent 718,824) (see Chapter 2, Section II).

Similar silyl esters have been reported in a Belgium patent (719,712) and Netherlands patent (68,12413). Trimethyltin esters have been employed in an analogous manner in these patents.

References

Abraham, E. P., and Newton, G. G. F. (1958). *Ciba Foundation Symp. Amino Acids Peptides Antimetabolic Activity* p. 205.
Abraham, E. P., and Newton, G. G. F. (1961). *Biochem. J.* **79**, 377.
Archer, R. A., and Kitchell, B. S. (1966). *J. Org. Chem.* **31**, 3409.
Barton, D. H. R., Comer, F., Greig, D. G. T., Lucente, G., Sammes, P. G., and Wedgewood, W. G. E. (1970). *Chem. Commun.* 1059.
Belgium Patent 641,338.
Belgium Patent 652,148.
Belgium Patent 684,288.
Belgium Patent 718,824.
Belgium Patent 719,710.
Belgium Patent 719,711.
Belgium Patent 719,712.
Belgium Patent 734,532.
Belgium Patent 734,533.
Belgium Patent 738,929.
Belgium Patent 741,381.
Belgium Paent 742,934.
Belgium Patent 748,055.
Bradshaw, J., Eardley, S., and Long, A. G. (1968). *J. Chem. Soc. C* 801.
Brechbuhler, H., Buchi, H., Hatz, E., Schreiber, J., and Eschenmoser, A. (1965). *Helv. Chim. Acta* **48**, 1746.
Chamberlin, J. W., and Campbell, J. B. (1967). *J. Med. Chem.* **10**, 966.
Chauvette, R. R., Flynn, E. H., Jackson, B. G., Lavagnino, E. R., Morin, R. B., Mueller, R. A., Pioch, R. P., Roeske, R. W., Ryan, C. W., Spencer, J. L., and Van Heyningen, E. M. (1962). *J. Amer. Chem. Soc.* **84**, 3401.
Chauvette, R. R., Flynn, E. H., Jackson, B. G., Lavagnino, E. R., Morin, R. B., Mueller, R. A., Pioch, R. P., Roeske, R. W., Ryan, C. W., Spencer, J. L., and Van Heyningen, E. M. (1963). *Antimicrob. Ag. Chemother.* 687.
Chauvette, R. R., and Flynn, E. H. (1966). *J. Med. Chem.* **9**, 741.
Chauvette, R. R., Pennington, P. A., Ryan, C. W., Cooper, R. D. G., Jose, F. L., Wright, I. G., Van Heyningen, E. M., and Huffman, G. W. (1971). *J. Org. Chem.* **36**, 1259.
Cocker, J. D., Cowley, B. R., Cox, J. S. G., Eardley, S., Gregory, G. I., Lazenby, J. K., Long, A. G., Sly, J. C. P., and Somerfield, G. A. (1965). *J. Chem. Soc.* 5015.
Cocker, J. D., Eardley, S., Gregory, G. I., Hall, M. E., and Long, A. G. (1966). *J. Chem. Soc.* 1142.
Cooper, R. D. G., Demarco, P. V., Cheng, J. C., and Jones, N. D. (1969). *J. Amer. Chem. Soc.* **91**, 1408.
Cooper, R. D. G., Demarco, P. V., Murphy, C. F., and Spangle, L. A. (1970). *J. Chem. Soc. C* 340.

Daniels, C. J., Fisher, J. W., Foster, B. J., Gutowski, G. E., and Hatfield, L. D. (1970). Abstracts of 160th Nat. Meeting of the Amer. Chem. Soc., Chicago, Illinois, No. MEDI 001.

Demain, A. L. (1963). *Trans. N.Y. Acad. Sci.* **25**, 731.

Demain, A. L., Newkirk, J. F., Davis, G. E., and Harman, R. E. (1963). *Appl. Microbiol.* **11**, 58.

Dolfini, J. E., Schwartz, J., and Weisenborn, F. (1969). *J. Org. Chem.* **34**, 1582.

Fazakerley, H., Gilbert, D. A., Gregory, G. I., Lazenby, J. K., and Long, A. G. (1967). *J. Chem. Soc.* 1959.

Fieser, L. F., and Fieser, M. (1967). "Reagents for Organic Synthesis," p. 522. Wiley, New York.

Green, G. F. H., Page, J. E., and Staniforth, S. E. (1965). *J. Chem. Soc.* 1595.

Hale, C. W., Newton, G. G. F., and Abraham, E. P. (1961). *Biochem. J.* **79**, 403.

Heymes, R., Amiard, G., and Nomine, G. (1966). *C. R. Acad. Sci. Paris Ser. C* **263**, 170.

Huber, F. M., Baltz, R. H., and Caltrider, P. G. (1968). *Appl. Microbiol.* **16**, 1011. Japan Patent 26105/69.

Jeffery, J. D'A., Abraham, E. P., and Newton, G. G. F. (1961). *Biochem. J.* **81**, 591.

Kaiser, G. V., Cooper, R. D. G., Koehler, R. E., Murphy, C. F., Webber, J. A., Wright, I. G., and Van Heyningen, E. M. (1970). *J. Org. Chem.* **35**, 2430.

Kaiser, G. V., Ashbrook, C. W., Goodson, T., Wright, I. G., and Van Heyningen, E. M. (1971). *J. Med. Chem.* **14**.

Kukolja, S. (1968). *J. Med. Chem.* **11**, 1067.

Kukolja, S. (1970). *J. Med. Chem.* **13**, 1114.

Morin, R. B., Jackson, B. G., Mueller, R. A., Lavagnino, E. R., Scanlon, W. B., and Andrews, S. L. (1969). *J. Amer. Chem. Soc.* **91**, 1401.

Murphy, C. F., and Koehler, R. E. (1970). *J. Org. Chem.* **35**, 2429.

Nagarajan, R., Boeck, L. D., Gorman, M., Hamill, R. L., Higgens, C. E., Hoehn, M. M., Stark, W. M., and Whitney, J. G. (1971). *J. Amer. Chem. Soc.* **93**, 2308.

Neidleman, S. L., Pan, S. C., Last, J. A., and Dolfini, J. E. (1970). *J. Med. Chem.* **13**, 386.

Netherlands Patent 64,01421.

Netherlands Patent 66,06820.

Netherlands Patent 67,17107.

Netherlands Patent 68,00751.

Netherlands Patent 68,06532.

Netherlands Patent 68,06533.

Netherlands Patent 68,12413.

Netherlands Patent 68,15631.

Netherlands Patent 69,02013.

O'Connor, D. E., and Lyness, W. I. (1964). *J. Amer. Chem. Soc.* **86**, 3840.

Ryan, C. W., Simon, R. L., and Van Heyningen, E. M. (1969). *J. Med. Chem.* **12**, 310.

Spencer, J. L., Siu, F. Y., Jackson, B. G., Higgins, H. M., and Flynn, E. H. (1967a). *J. Org. Chem.* **32**, 500.

Spencer, J. L., Siu, F. Y., Flynn, E. H., Jackson, B. G., Sigal, M. V., Higgins, H. M., Chauvette, R. R., Andrews, S. L., and Bloch, D. E. (1967b). *Antimicrob. Ag. Chemother.* 573.

Stedman, R. J. (1966). *J. Med. Chem.* **9**, 444.

Stedman, R. J., Swered, K., and Hoover, J. R. E. (1964). *J. Med. Chem.* **7**, 117.

Sweet, R. M., and Dahl, L. F. (1970). *J. Amer. Chem. Soc.* **92**, 5489.

Taylor, A. B. (1965). *J. Chem. Soc.* 7020.

United States Patent 3,124,576.

United States Patent 3,193,550.
United States Patent 3,202,656.
United States Patent 3,225,038.
United States Patent 3,226,384.
United States Patent 3,228,934.
United States Patent 3,239,394.
United States Patent 3,239,515.
United States Patent 3,239,516.
United States Patent 3,243,435.
United States Patent 3,258,461.
United States Patent 3,261,832.
United States Patent 3,270,012.
United States Patent 3,274,184.
United States Patent 3,275,626.
United States Patent 3,278,531.
United States Patent 3,284,451.
United States Patent 3,304,236.
United States Patent 3,351,596.
United States Patent 3,355,452.
United States Patent 3,436,310.
United States Patent 3,431,259.
United States Patent 3,445,463.
United States Patent 3,446,803.
United States Patent 3,459,746.
United States Patent 3,484,437.
United States Patent 3,516,997.
United States Patent 3,532,694.
Van Heyningen, E. (1965). *J. Med. Chem.* **8**, 22.
Van Heyningen, E., and Brown, C. N. (1965). *J. Med. Chem.* **8**, 174.
Van Heyningen, E., and Ahern, L. K. (1968). *J. Med. Chem.* **11**, 933.
Webber, J. A., Van Heyningen, E. M., and Vasileff, R. T. (1969). *J. Amer. Chem. Soc.* **91**, 5674.
Webber, J. A., Huffman, G. W., Koehler, R. E., Murphy, C. F., Ryan, C. W., Van Heyningen, E. M., and Vasileff, R. T. (1971). *J. Med. Chem.* **14**, 113.
Webber, J. A., and Vasileff, R. T. (1971). *J. Med. Chem.* **14**, 1136.
West Germany Patent 1937015.
West Germany Patent 2000878.
Woodward, R. B., Heusler, K., Gosteli, J., Naegeli, P., Oppolzer, W., Ramage, R., Ranganathan, S., and Vorbruggen, H. (1966). *J. Amer. Chem. Soc.* **88**, 852.
Wright, I. G., Ashbrook, C. W., Goodson, T., Kaiser, G. V., and Van Heyningen, E. M. (1971). *J. Med. Chem.* **14**, 420.

Chapter 5

REARRANGEMENTS OF

CEPHALOSPORINS AND PENICILLINS

R. D. G. COOPER and D. O. SPRY

Strive not with your superiors in argument, but
always submit your judgement to others with modesty.

George Washington

I. Introduction

The chemistry, structure, and molecular modification of the penicillins was
the subject of a vast Anglo-American cooperative research effort in the years
during and following World War II. The results of this work are summarized in

a monograph published in 1949 (Clarke *et al.*, 1949). In 1959, the discovery of 6-aminopenicillanic acid (6-APA) (*1*) made possible the synthesis of new penicillins not previously available by fermentation procedures and spawned another decade of intensive world-wide research into the chemistry of this class of antibiotics.

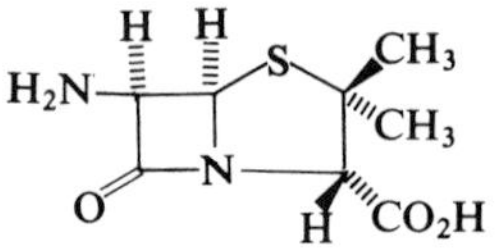

(*1*) 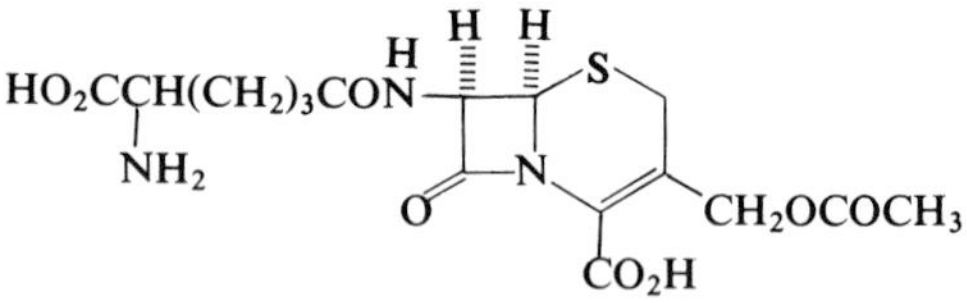   (*2*)

In 1955, a new antibiotic, cephalosporin C (*2*), was isolated by Newton and Abraham (1955) from the metabolism of *Cephalosporium acremonium*. Cephalosporin C, although it possessed antimicrobial activity of a relatively low order of magnitude, attracted interest because of its effectiveness against organisms which had become resistant to the penicillins. The investigation into the structure of the metabolite was successfully concluded in 1961 by employing both chemical (Abraham and Newton, 1961) and X-ray crystallographic procedures (Hodgkin and Maslen, 1961). The then obvious structural relationship between penicillin N (*3*) and cephalosporin C (*2*), which are both produced by the organism, suggested that there might be common intermediates in the biosynthetic pathway or, alternatively, that cephalosporin C is a metabolic transformation product of penicillin N.

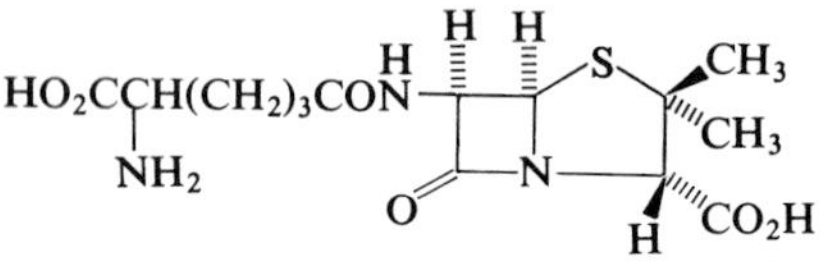

(*3*)

The enzymatic removal of the α-aminoadipoyl side chain from cephalosporin C (and also penicillin N) has been unsuccessful. Because the activity of cephalosporin C was insufficient to render it clinically useful, the problem of replacing the α-aminoadipoyl group with other acyl functions arose. Earlier, this approach had given rise to many semisynthetic penicillins of useful activity, and it was hoped to duplicate this success with the cephalosporins. Thus, the synthesis of 7-aminocephalosporanic acid (7-ACA) (*4*) in practical amounts became a major problem.

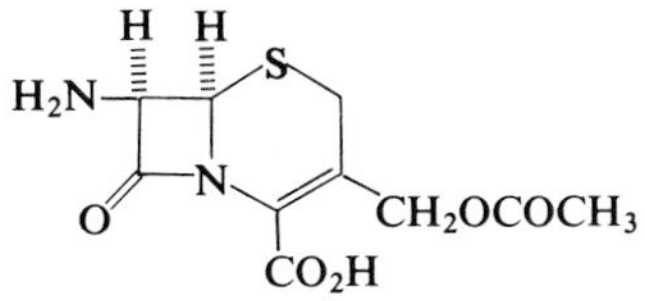

(4)

II. Synthesis of Cephalosporin from Penicillin via Intermediacy of Penicillin Sulfoxide

A. Rearrangements of Penicillin Sulfoxides

One attractive solution was the chemical transformation of a fermentation-produced penicillin into a cephalosporin, followed by enzymatic removal of the side chain. This approach assumed that a side chain which could be enzymatically cleaved in the penicillins could also be cleaved in the cephalosporins. In the chemical research of penicillin there was no evidence that it was possible to open the thiazolidine ring while keeping the more sensitive β-lactam function intact.

Morin and co-workers (1963) partially solved this problem when they converted a penicillin sulfoxide into a deacetoxycephalosporin. They reasoned that the transformation of a thiazolidine ring to a dihydrothiazine ring must involve an oxidative step; consequently, they oxidized the penicillin sulfur atom to the sulfoxide and then investigated the chemistry of the penicillin sulfoxide. The sulfoxide also had the advantage of increased acid stability. Although sulfoxides possessing an α-hydrogen atom normally undergo a Pummerer reaction to form the α-acetoxy sulfides, Morin et al. (1963, 1969a) found that the sulfoxide of methyl phenoxyacetamidopenicillanate (5) did not react to give the expected Pummerer product. Instead, on refluxing (5) in acetic anhydride they obtained a 2:1 mixture of two isomeric products, (6) and (7), in 60% yield. The structures, determined mainly by nuclear magnetic resonance spectroscopy evidence, were further reinforced by the fact that (7), when treated with base, eliminated acetic acid to give (8).

Compound (8) was also obtained in 10–20% yield by the rearrangement of (5) in xylene containing a trace of p-toluenesulfonic acid at 130°. In addition, Cooper et al. (1970a, b, c; Can. Patent 817,883; Chauvette et al., 1971) established that use of 5% acetic anhydride in dimethylformamide gave (8) in 60% yield as the only isolatable product.

Morin et al. (1969b) have shown that this type of abnormal 1,3 Pummerer rearrangement is also applicable to simpler cyclic sulfoxides. Rearrangement of the thiochromane sulfoxide (9) in refluxing acetic anhydride gave a 10:1 mixture of the two acetoxy derivatives, (10) and (11), whereas, in refluxing xylene containing p-toluenesulfonic acid, (9) gave the two olefins, (12) and (13).

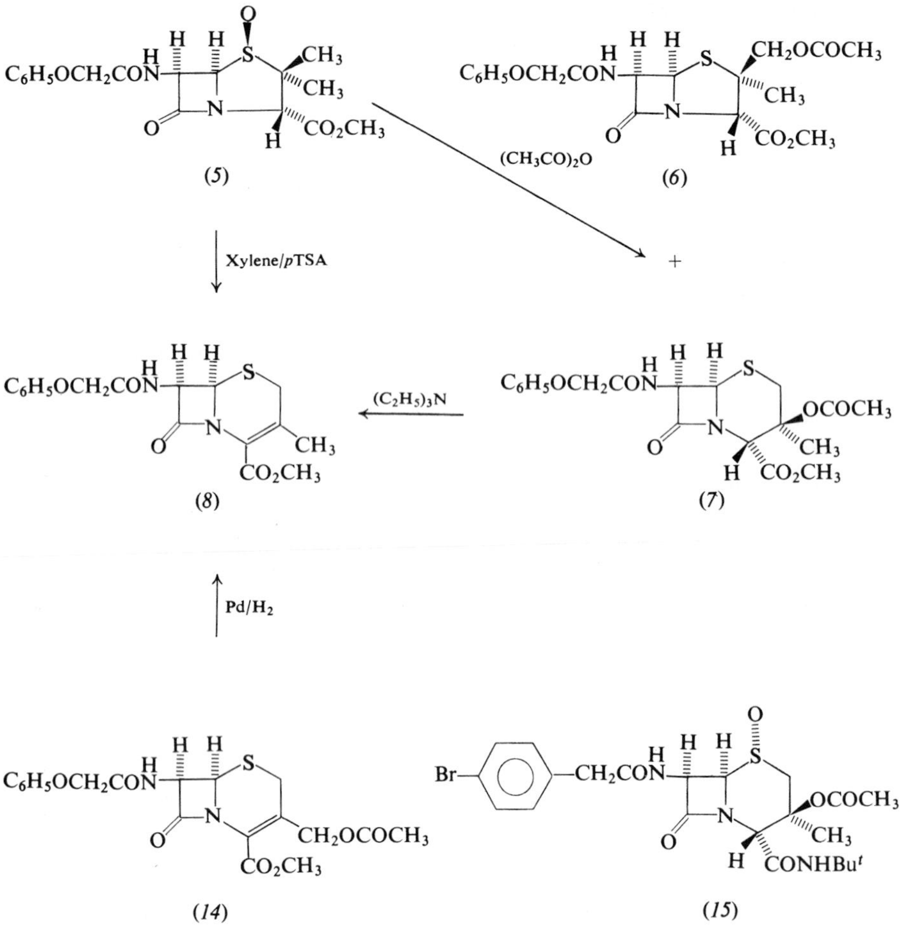

Hydrogenolysis of the phenoxyacetamidocephalosporin methyl ester (14) using a palladium catalyst also gave (8) and represented the first direct chemical correlation between these two series of antibiotics (Morin et al., 1963).

The configuration of (6) was assigned by Morin and co-workers by comparing its NMR spectrum with that of the methyl phenoxymethylpenicillanate and that of (7) as being the most probable one on mechanistic grounds. The latter has recently been proven by X-ray crystallographic investigation (Smart and

Rogers, 1970) of (*15*) which had been prepared by oxidation of the corresponding penicillin sulfoxide rearrangement product (Barton *et al.*, 1970a).

Morin *et al.* (1963, 1969a) found several other non-β-lactam-containing products were produced by the acid catalyzed rearrangement, these becoming

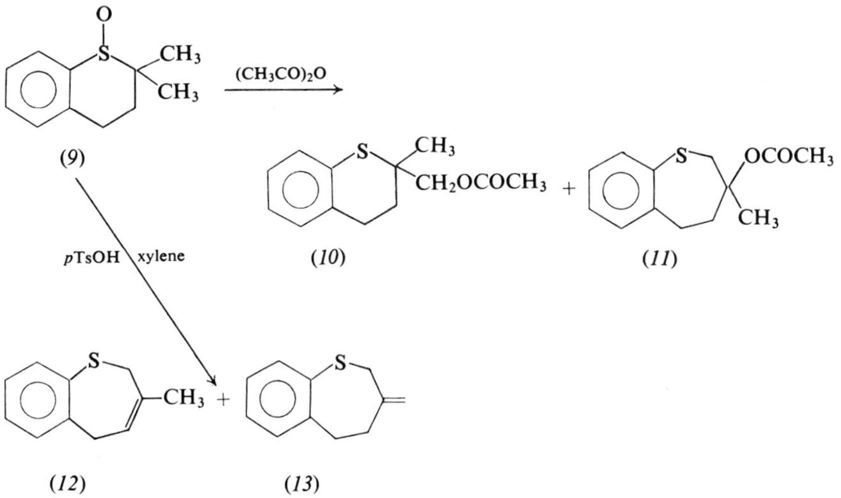

the major products under different reaction conditions. When the acetic anhydride and acid catalyzed rearrangement conditions were applied (Morin *et al.*, 1969a) to the penicillin sulfoxide acid (*16*), the decarboxylated compound (*17*) was the major product in both cases.

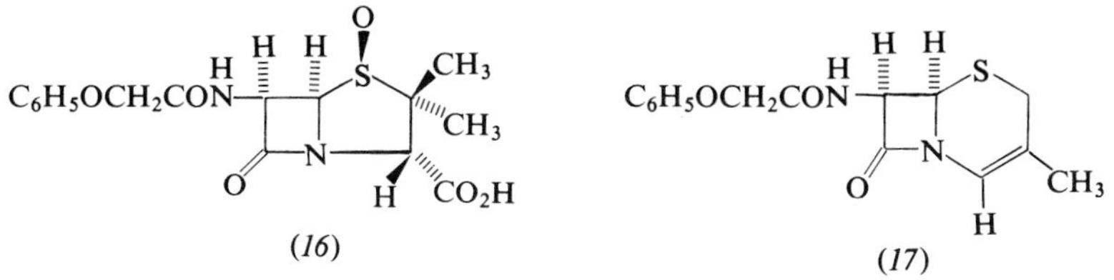

During an intensive investigation of the effect of solvents and diverse acidic catalysts on the rearrangement of (*18*), a new compound (*19*) was observed. This was obtained as the major rearrangement product if sulfuric acid was used, in dimethylformamide as solvent (Daniels *et al.*, 1970; Gutowski *et al.*, 1971b). The structure of (*19*) was based on NMR (Daniels *et al.*, 1970; Gutowski *et al.*, 1971b) and mass spectral data, together with its reaction with isopropenyl acetate to give the acetoxy derivative (*20*). Compound (*20*) was identical with the product obtained directly from (*18*) by treatment with acetic anhydride. Further stereochemical evidence was obtained (Gutowski *et al.*,

1971b) by the isolation of (*21*) during the chromatographic purification of (*19*) on silica gel.

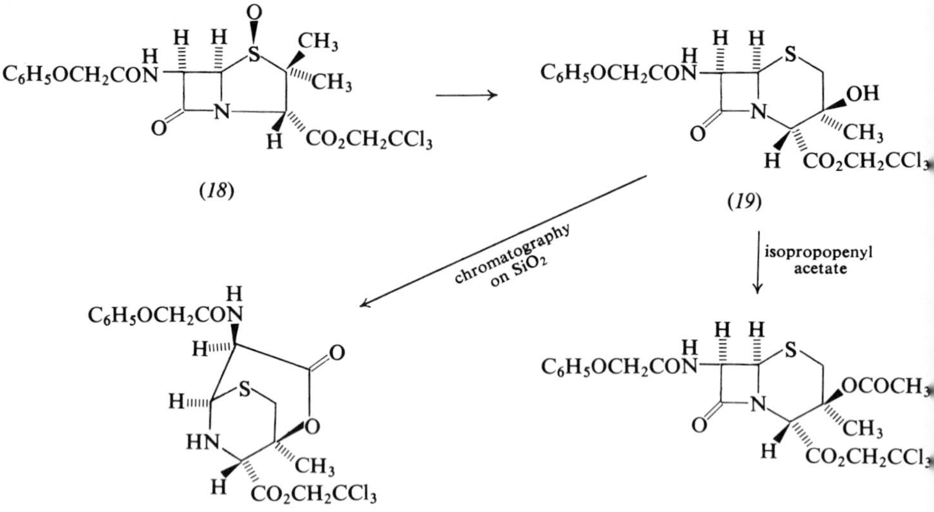

(*18*)

(*19*)

chromatography on SiO₂

isopropopenyl acetate

(*21*)

(*20*)

Three non-β-lactam-containing products (*22*, *23*, and *24*) were also isolated by Morin *et al.* (1969a), as minor components, from the acetic anhydride reaction of (*5*). Two of these components are closely related to products obtained by Leonard and Wilson (1964) via chlorination of the 1,4-thiazepine (*25*) and were assigned the isothiazoline structures (*26* and *27*).

Compound (*23*) was obtained more conveniently in 50% yield when the penicillin sulfoxide (*5*) was refluxed in pyridine. Indeed, in the preparation of

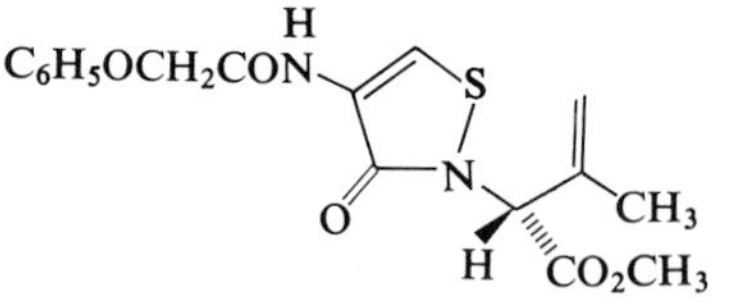

(*22*)

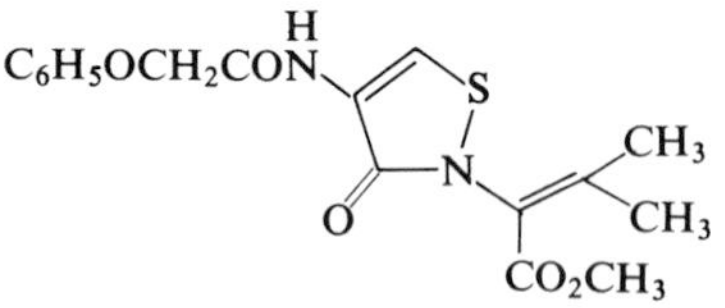

(*23*)

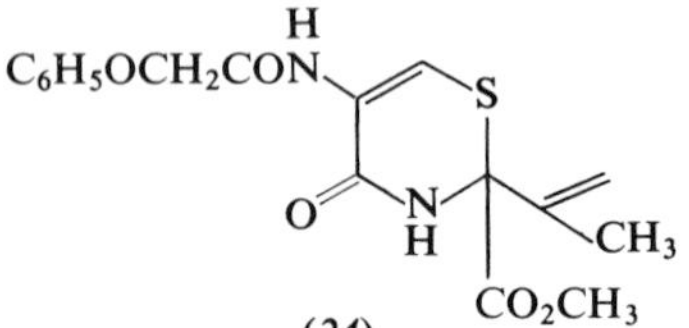

(*24*)

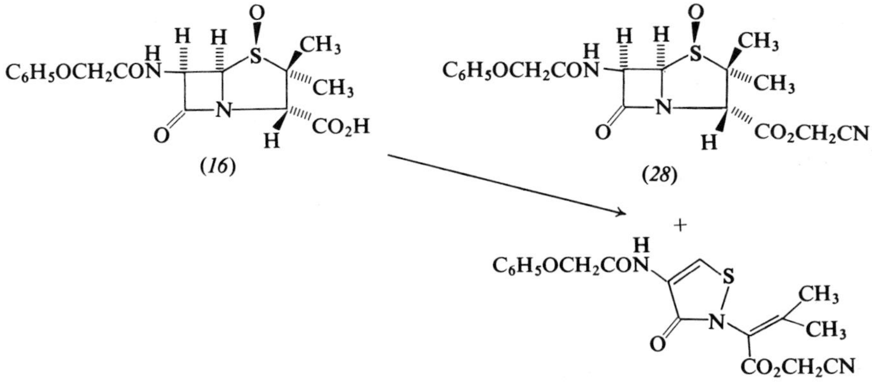

(16) → (28) + (29)

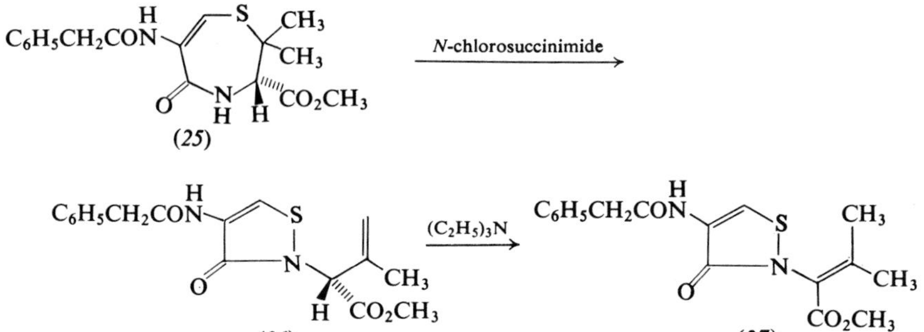

(25) →[N-chlorosuccinimide]

(26) →[(C₂H₅)₃N] (27)

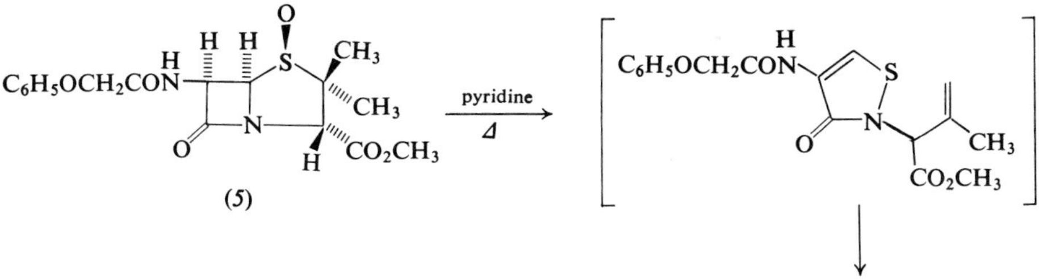

(5) →[pyridine, Δ] [(23)]

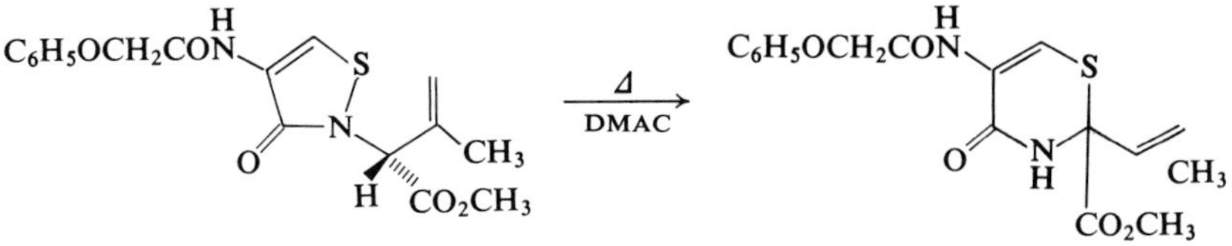

(22) →[Δ, DMAC] (24)

the cyanomethyl ester of the penicillin sulfoxide (*28*), rearrangement to the cyanomethyl ester (*29*) occurred, presumably due to the presence of triethylamine. The third component was assigned structure (*24*) on the basis of physical data. Additional experiments (Morin *et al.*, 1970) have indicated that (*24*) can be prepared by heating a solution of the isothiazolone (*22*) in dimethylacetamide (DMAC).

The ring expansion rearrangement of a penicillin sulfoxide into a Δ^3-deacetoxycephalosporin is an increase of one oxidation level to a system midway between the penam and cephem* systems. It also results in allylic activation of the second methyl group and a possible attractive conversion of penicillin to cephalosporin. Cooper and José (1970c) had shown that functionalization of the methyl group of a Δ^3-deacetoxycephalosporin could not be achieved by the normal free radical bromination procedures. These procedures resulted in initial attack at the C-2 position, causing extensive decomposition. However, reaction of lead tetraacetate in refluxing butanol on the deacetoxy-3-cephem ester (*30*) gave good yields of the 2-acetoxydeacetoxy derivative (*31*) (Cooper

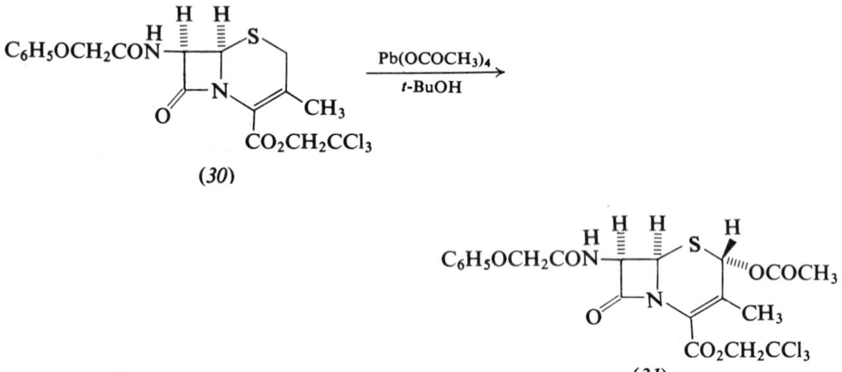

(*30*)

(*31*)

et al., 1970a) with no evidence of methyl group functionalization. Webber *et al.* (1969) solved this problem of attacking the methyl group by using a deacetoxy-2-cephem derivative (*32*). Previously, Morin *et al.* (1969a) had found that

* The nomenclature used is that suggested by Morin *et al.* (1962). This system is in accord with that generally accepted for the penicillins (Sheehan *et al.*, 1953).

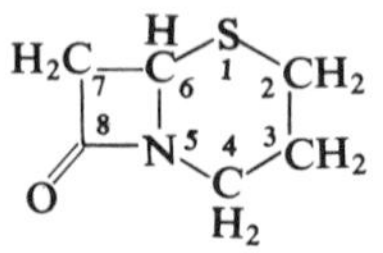

Cepham 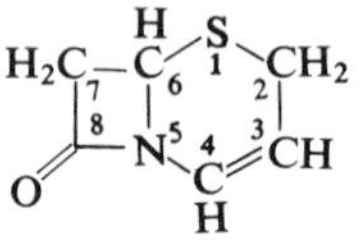   3-Cephem

attempted base hydrolysis of deacetoxy-3-cephem ester (*8*) gave good yields of Δ^2 acid (*33*). Webber converted this into the *p*-methoxybenzyl ester (*32*) by treatment with dimethylformamide, dineopentyl acetal, and *p*-methoxybenzyl

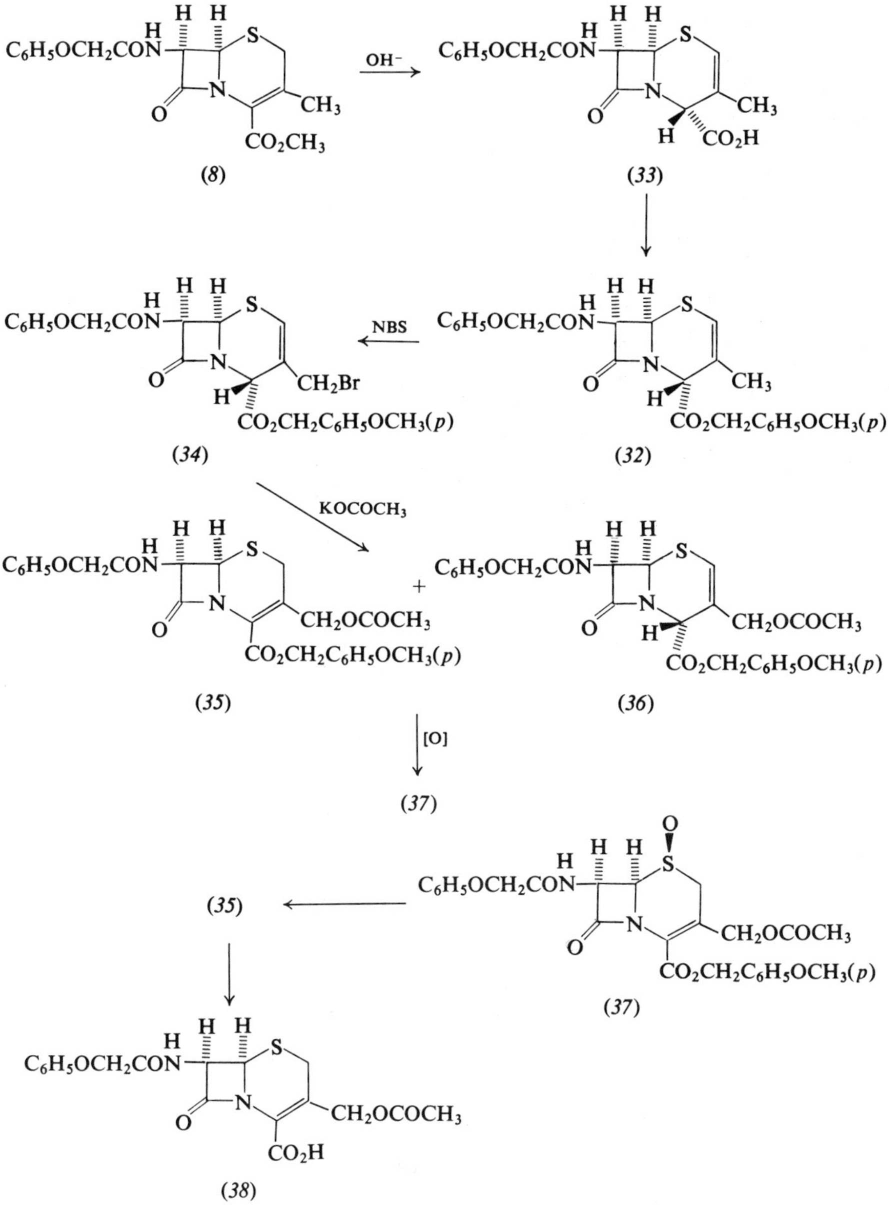

$C_6H_5OCH_2CON$ — ... CH_3
CO_2CH_3

(*8*)

$\xrightarrow{\text{OH}^-}$

$C_6H_5OCH_2CON$ — ... CH_3
H CO_2H

(*33*)

$C_6H_5OCH_2CON$ — ... CH_2Br
$CO_2CH_2C_6H_5OCH_3(p)$

(*34*)

$\xleftarrow{\text{NBS}}$

$C_6H_5OCH_2CON$ — ... CH_3
H $CO_2CH_2C_6H_5OCH_3(p)$

(*32*)

$\xrightarrow{\text{KOCOCH}_3}$

$C_6H_5OCH_2CON$ — ... CH_2OCOCH_3
$CO_2CH_2C_6H_5OCH_3(p)$

(*35*)

+

$C_6H_5OCH_2CON$ — ... CH_2OCOCH_3
H $CO_2CH_2C_6H_5OCH_3(p)$

(*36*)

(*37*)

$\downarrow$ [O]

$C_6H_5OCH_2CON$ — ... CH_2OCOCH_3
$CO_2CH_2C_6H_5OCH_3(p)$

(*37*)

(*35*) $\longleftarrow$

$\downarrow$

$C_6H_5OCH_2CON$ — ... CH_2OCOCH_3
CO_2H

(*38*)

alcohol. Reaction of (*32*) with *N*-bromosuccinimide in carbon tetrachloride, using azobisisobutyronitrile as a radical initiator, gave a product whose NMR was consistent with the assignment of structure (*34*). Immediate acetolysis of this bromination product with potassium acetate in acetone gave an isomeric mixture of 2- and 3-cephems (*35* and *36*), from which pure (*35*) was obtained by chromatography. A more attractive alternate procedure involved oxidation of the 2-cephem/3-cephem mixture with *m*-chloroperbenzoic acid, a process which had previously been shown (Kaiser *et al.*, 1970) to cause complete isomerization of a 2-cephem to a 3-cephem. Reduction of the 3-cephem sulfoxide (*37*) by acetyl chloride–sodium dithionite in dimethylformamide (Kaiser *et al.*, 1970) afforded (*35*) in 55% yield from (*33*). Removal of the ester protecting group with trifluoroacetic acid gave phenoxyacetamidocephalosporin (*38*). This represented the first synthesis of cephalosporin from penicillin.

Another alternate procedure developed by Cooper and José (1970c) involved conversion of (*30*) into the sulfoxide (*39*), followed by the functionalization of (*39*) using *N*-bromosuccinimide in refluxing methylene chloride containing a free radical initiator. Solvolysis to the acetoxy derivative (*41*) and reduction of

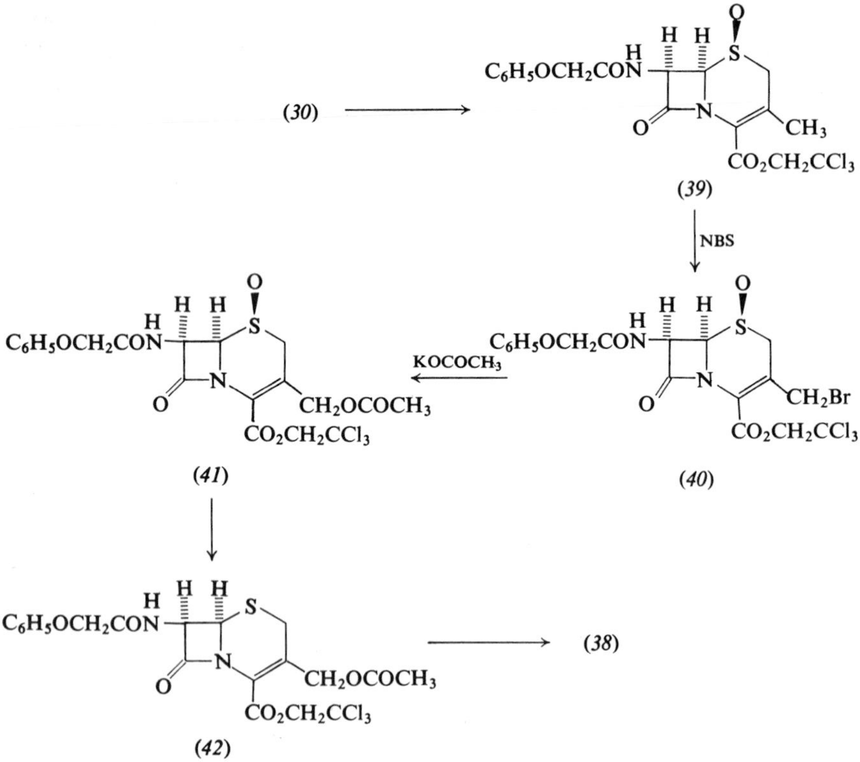

(*30*) $\longrightarrow$

$C_6H_5OCH_2CON$ ... S, N, O, CH_3, $CO_2CH_2CCl_3$

(*39*)

$\downarrow$ NBS

$C_6H_5OCH_2CON$ ... S, N, O, CH_2Br, $CO_2CH_2CCl_3$

(*40*)

$\xleftarrow{\text{KOCOCH}_3}$

$C_6H_5OCH_2CON$ ... S, N, O, CH_2OCOCH_3, $CO_2CH_2CCl_3$

(*41*)

$\downarrow$

$C_6H_5OCH_2CON$ ... S, N, O, CH_2OCOCH_3, $CO_2CH_2CCl_3$

(*42*)

$\longrightarrow$ (*38*)

the resulting sulfoxide (*41*) gave (*42*) from which the cephalosporin (*38*) was obtained by cleavage of the ester protecting group with zinc and acetic acid.

Attempts to complete the conversion of a penicillin into a cephalosporin by a ring expansion rearrangement of acetoxymethylpenicillin sulfoxide (*43*)

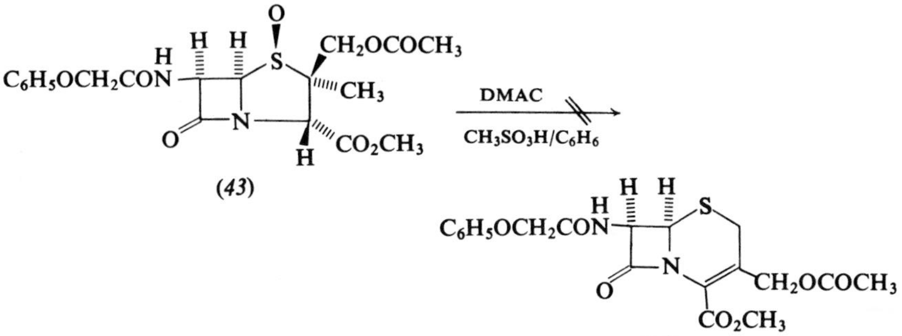

(*43*)

(*14*)

failed, probably due to the *cis* orientation of the sulfoxide bond and the acetoxymethyl group. However, studies on the thiochromane derivative (Spry, 1970b) showed that the sulfoxide (*44*) (sulfoxide bond and methylene acetoxy group are *trans*) rearranged upon heating in dimethylacetamide/toluene-methanesulfonic acid (conditions associated with ring expansion) to give a

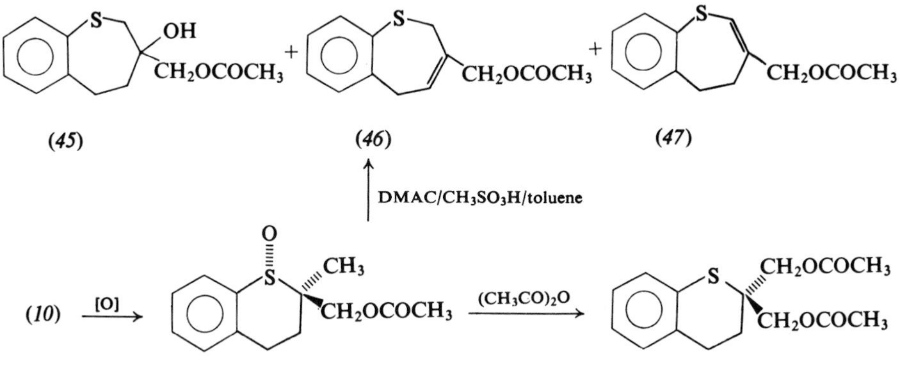

(*45*)   (*46*)   (*47*)

(*10*) → (*44*) → (*48*)

mixture of (*45*), (*46*), and (*47*). In refluxing acetic anhydride (non-ring expansion conditions) (*44*) gave the bisacetoxymethyl derivative (*48*). Oxidation of (*48*) with *m*-chloroperbenzoic acid gave the sulfoxide (*49*) which, under ring expansion conditions, gave (*50*) in moderate yield with no detectable amounts of ring expansion. Acetic anhydride rearrangement of (*49*) gave the triacetate (*51*) in high yield.

(*48*) (*49*)

83% (*51*) 37% (*50*)

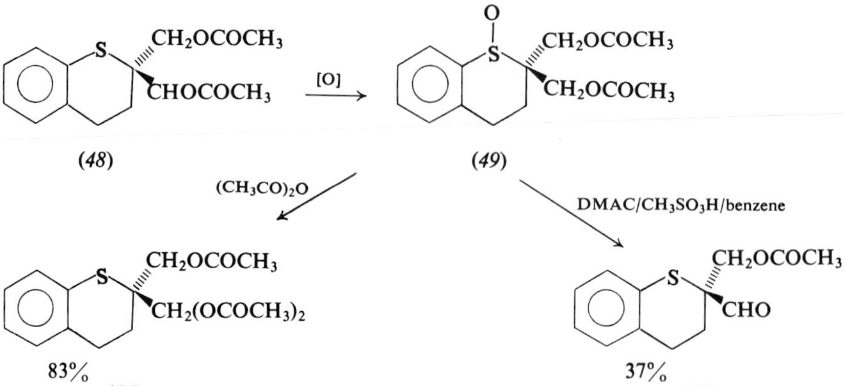

At that time no method was available for obtaining the penicillin isomers with the sulfoxide and acetoxymethyl group *trans* (*54*). Spry (1970a) then reported that rearrangement of methyl phthalimidopenicillanate (*R*)-sulfoxide (*52*) gave a mixture containing both the α-acetoxymethylpenicillin and the β-acetoxymethylpenicillin ester which, on oxidation with *m*-chloroperbenzoic acid, gave two (*R*)-sulfoxides (*53* and *54*).

(*52*) 10% (*53*) + 30–40% (*54*)

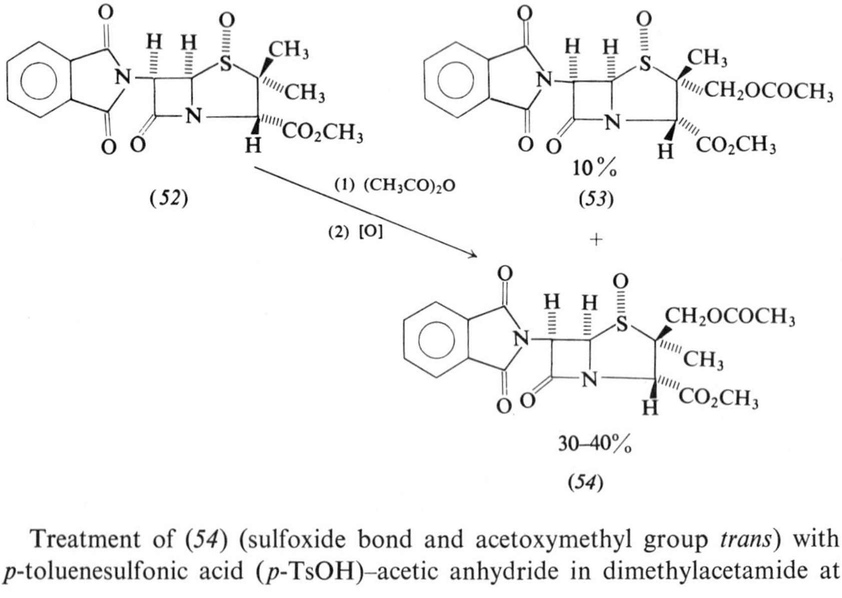

Treatment of (*54*) (sulfoxide bond and acetoxymethyl group *trans*) with *p*-toluenesulfonic acid (*p*-TsOH)–acetic anhydride in dimethylacetamide at

84° for 3 hours gave a mixture of cephalosporin (55) and 3-hydroxy-cephalosporin (56).

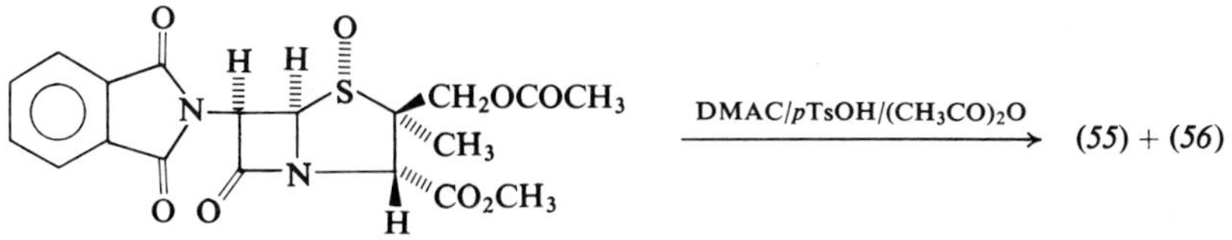

Further reaction of (56) under the rearrangement conditions caused partial dehydration to (55) which was identical to material prepared from 7-ACA. Application to the *p*-nitrobenzyl ester, removable by hydrogenolysis, and cleavage of the phthalimido group with hydrazine enabled Spry to evolve a synthesis of 7-aminocephalosporanic acid from 6-aminopenicillanic acid using two separate sulfoxide rearrangements. The formation of a cephalosporin by rearrangement of a compound possessing a sulfoxide group *trans* to the acetoxymethyl group appeared to be specific for imide-type side chains on the penicillins. Spry (1970a) overcame this problem by the photochemical epimerization of a penicillin sulfoxide, a reaction which had been previously discovered by Archer and Demarco (1969).

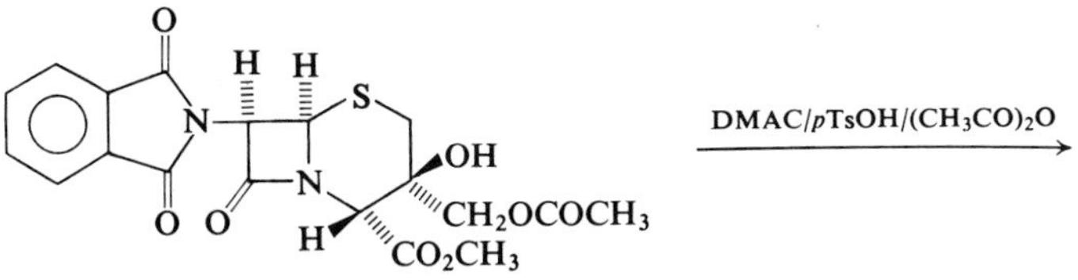

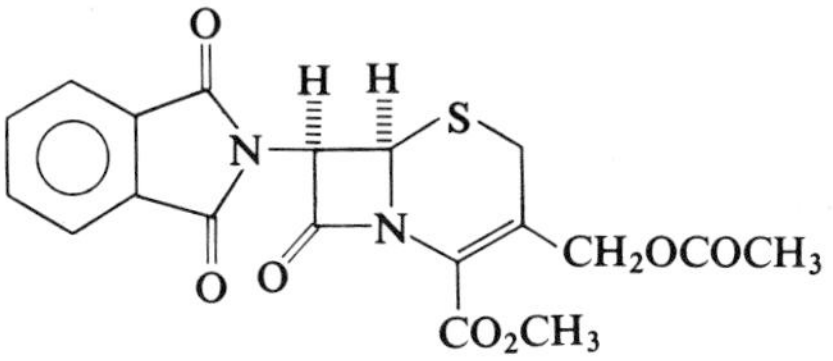

Reaction of methylacetamidopenicillanate (*S*) sulfoxide (57) with acetic anhydride gave the expected β-acetoxymethyl sulfide derivative (58), which on oxidation with *m*-chloroperbenzoic acid gave the sulfoxide (59). From the irradiation of (59) in acetone, a mixture of the four possible isomers, (59), (60), (61), and (62), was obtained. Spry (1970b) presented this observation as evidence that the mechanism of the photochemical epimerization of a penicillin sulfoxide involved S_1–C_2 homolytic cleavage to a diradical (63) followed by recombination. The diradical intermediate must also be sufficiently long lasting to allow rotation around the C_2–C_3 bond before recombination.

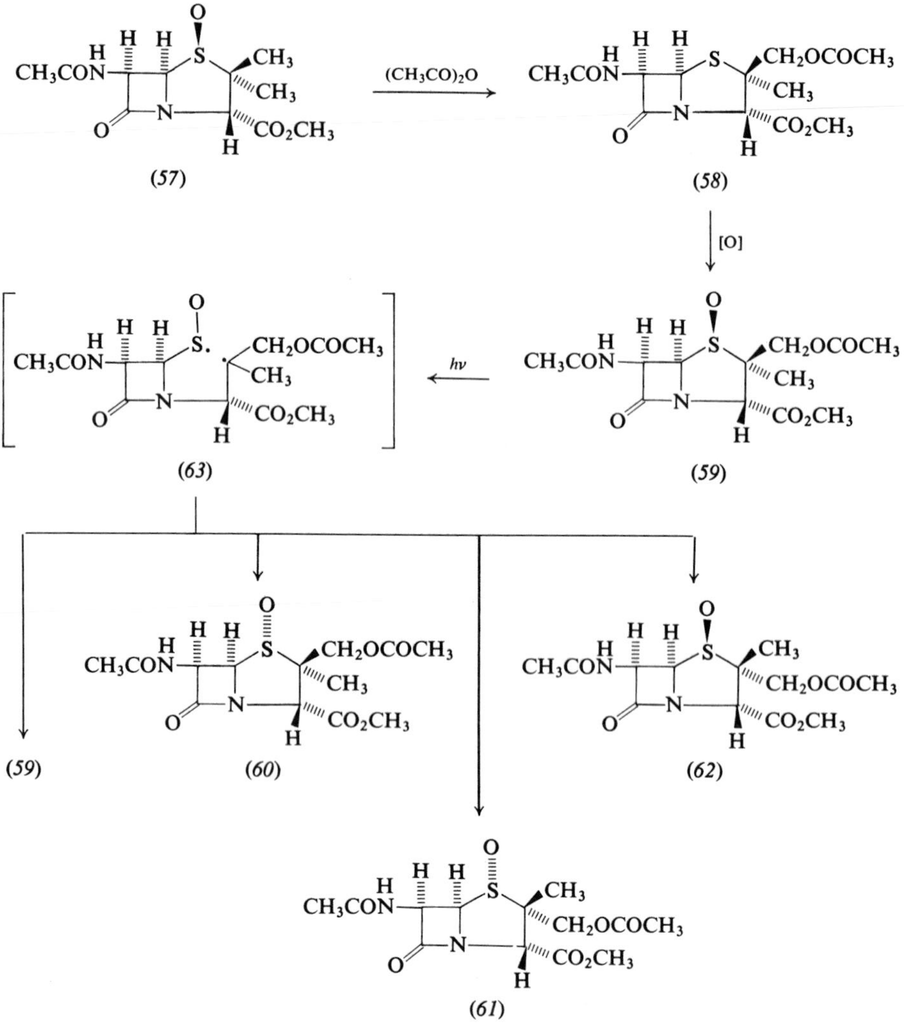

(57)

(58)

(63)

(59)

(59)

(60)

(62)

(61)

To circumvent the somewhat tedious photochemical procedure, together with the inherent separation problems, Spry (1970a, b) discovered that ozone oxidation of penicillin acids or esters gave a mixture of the two isomeric sulfoxides in high yield. Interestingly, this procedure led to no over oxidation of sulfoxide to the sulfone (see Table I).

It was also observed that the relative rates of reaction of the penicillins,

Table I

OXIDATION OF PENICILLIN DERIVATIVES WITH OZONE

Derivatives	Solvent	Yield sulfoxide	(S)/(R) ratio
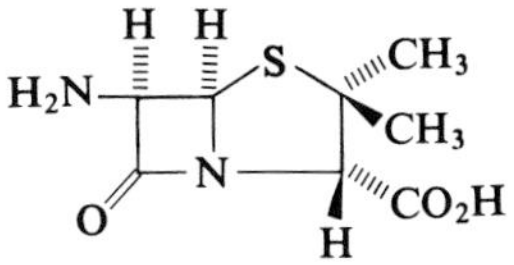	H_2O	100%	4/1
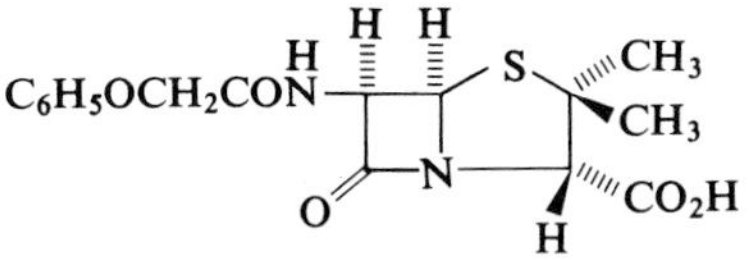	$H_2O/(CH_3)_2CO$	100%	1/1
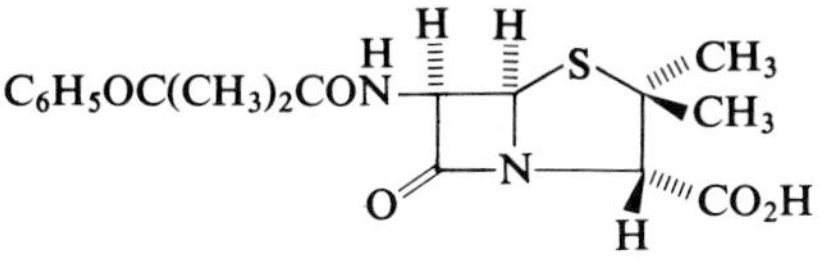	$H_2O/(CH_3)_2CO$	98%	1.4/1.0
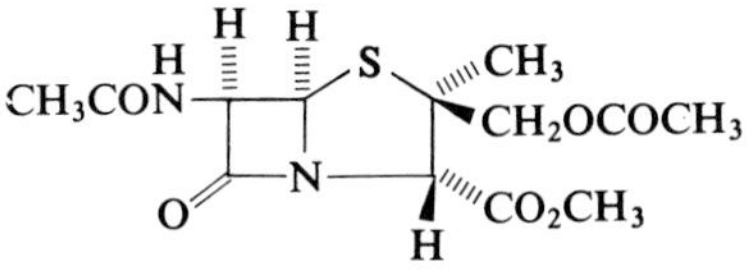	$H_2O/(CH_3)_2CO$	70%	1/2
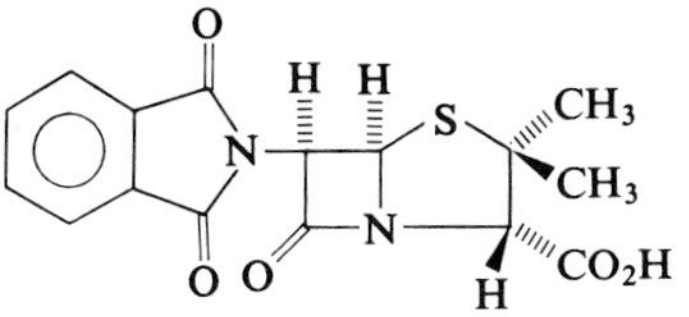	$H_2O/(CH_3)_2CO$	100%	only R

3-cephems, and cephams with ozone were considerably different, enough so that Spry (1970b) was able to partially ozonize a rearrangement mixture containing the acetoxymethyl penicillin and the acetoxycepham products and thus obtain, after column chromatography, pure acetoxymethylpenicillin. Prolonged ozonolysis of the purified acetoxymethylpenicillin (58) gave a mixture of sulfoxides (59) and (60) in the ratio (S/R) of 1:2. Spry (1970a) observed that mild thermal treatment of (60) in refluxing benzene for 30 minutes gave a smooth conversion to isomer (62) which, when treated with acetic anhydride/ methane-sulfonic acid in dimethylacetamide, gave a mixture of (64) and (65).

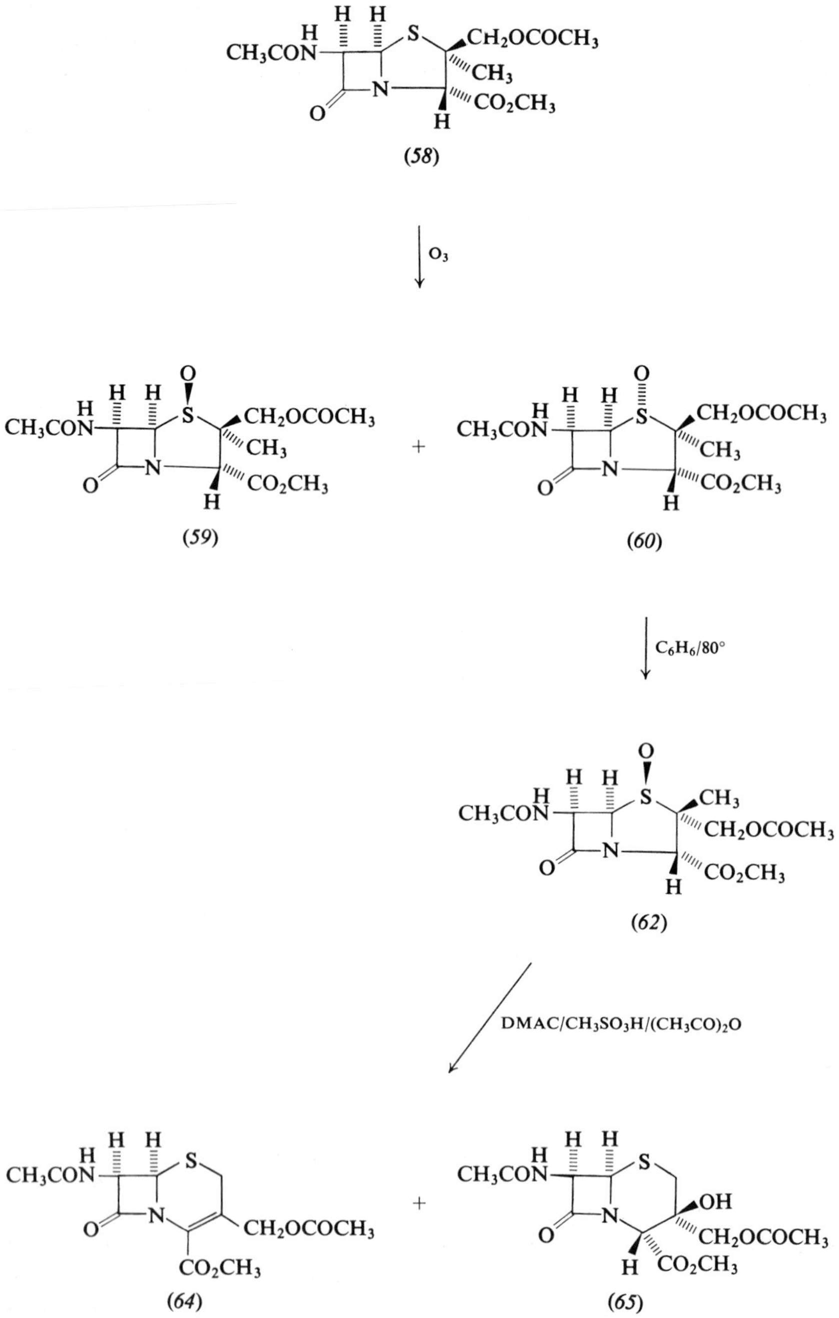

(58)

$\downarrow$ O$_3$

(59)   +   (60)

$\downarrow$ C$_6$H$_6$/80°

(62)

DMAC/CH$_3$SO$_3$H/(CH$_3$CO)$_2$O

(64)   +   (65)

Spry (1970b) applied the acetic anhydride rearrangement to the trichloroethyl ester (*18*) from which, after partial oxidation with ozone, the 2β-acetoxymethyl sulfide (*66*) was isolated. Cleavage of the ester group with zinc and acetic acid gave the 2β-acetoxymethylpenicillin (*67*). By substitution of isobutyric anhydride for acetic anhydride in the initial rearrangement, the 2β-isobutyroxymethylpenicillin ester (*68*) and hence the acid (*69*) could be obtained in similar manner. The activities of these penicillin derivatives is discussed in Chapter 12.

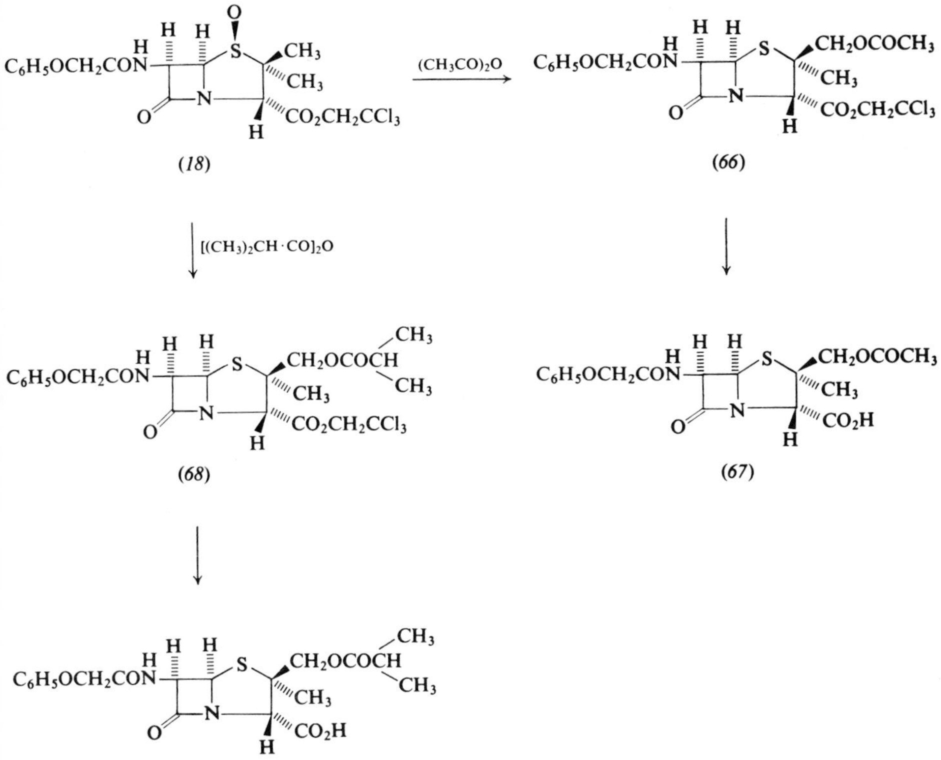

$C_6H_5OCH_2CON$ ... S ... CH_3 / CH_3 / $CO_2CH_2CCl_3$

(*18*)

$(CH_3CO)_2O$ →

$C_6H_5OCH_2CON$ ... S ... CH_2OCOCH_3 / CH_3 / $CO_2CH_2CCl_3$

(*66*)

$[(CH_3)_2CH \cdot CO]_2O$

$C_6H_5OCH_2CON$ ... S ... $CH_2OCOCH(CH_3)$ / CH_3 / $CO_2CH_2CCl_3$

(*68*)

$C_6H_5OCH_2CON$ ... S ... CH_2OCOCH_3 / CH_3 / CO_2H

(*67*)

$C_6H_5OCH_2CON$ ... S ... $CH_2OCOCH(CH_3)_2$ / CH_3 / CO_2H

(*69*)

An alternate procedure of converting a penam to a cephem was discovered by Cooper and José (1970a, b). It is based on the novel rearrangement of a penicillin sulfoxide (*18*) by treatment with a trialkylphosphite in refluxing benzene. A high yield of the new product (*70*) is obtained. Treatment of (*70*) with triethylamine [$(C_2H_5)_3N$] caused double-bond isomerization to (*71*) and vigorous base-catalyzed hydrolysis yielded dimethylpyruvic acid. Reaction of

(70) with acid or base caused rupture of the β-lactam ring to form the thiazoles (72) and (73).

A variation of the trimethylphosphite rearrangement was discovered by

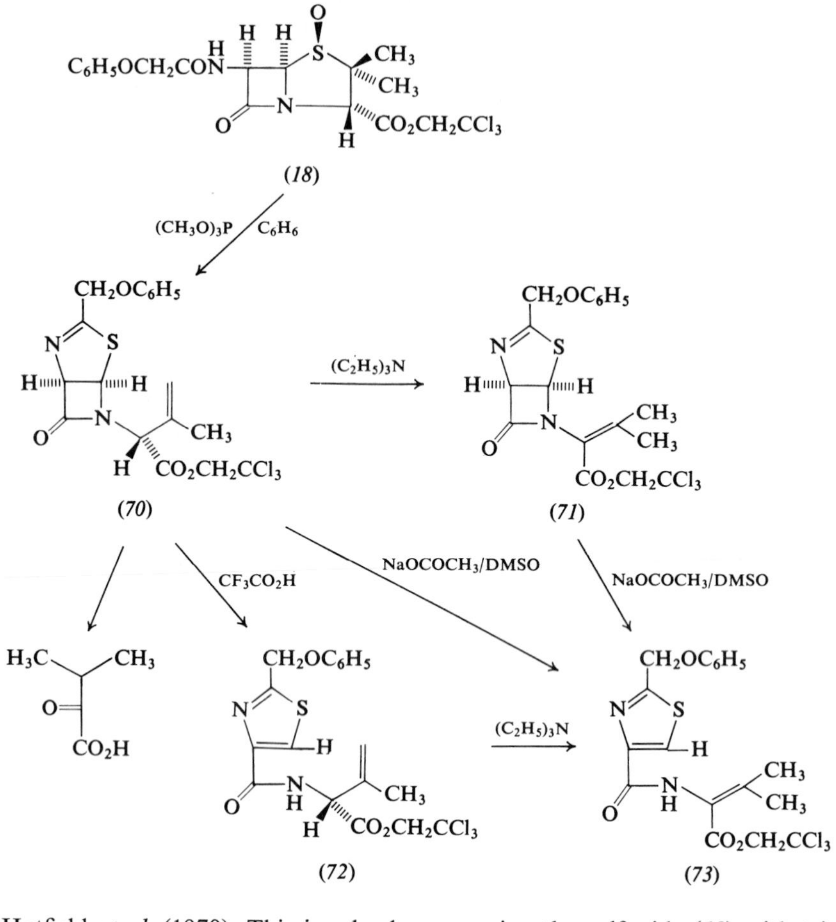

(18)

(70)   (71)

(72)   (73)

Hatfield *et al.* (1970). This involved rearranging the sulfoxide (18) with trimethylphosphite in the presence of acetic anhydride to form (70) in a limited yield, with the major product being the thioacetyl derivative (74).

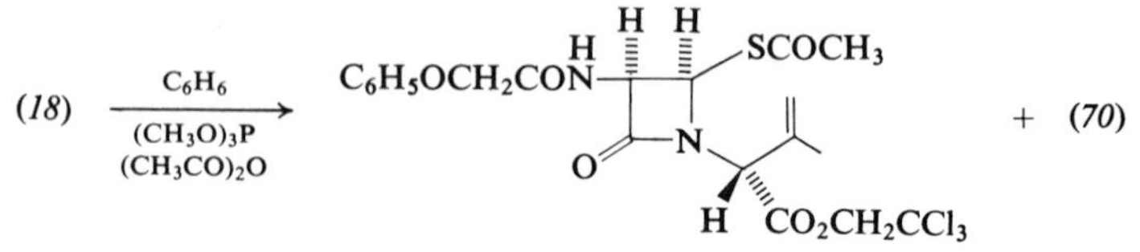

(74)

The formation of (70) obviously involved an internal condensation of the amido side chain. When this was either prevented [by use of the N-phthalimido derivative (75)] or sterically impeded [by use of the α,α'-dimethylphenoxy-methyl side chain (76)] then alternate products were formed (Cooper and José, 1970c) and shown to be the thioethers (77) and (78).

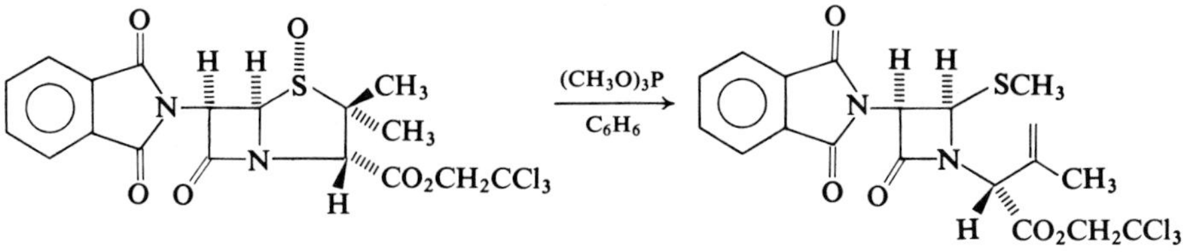

(75)

(77)

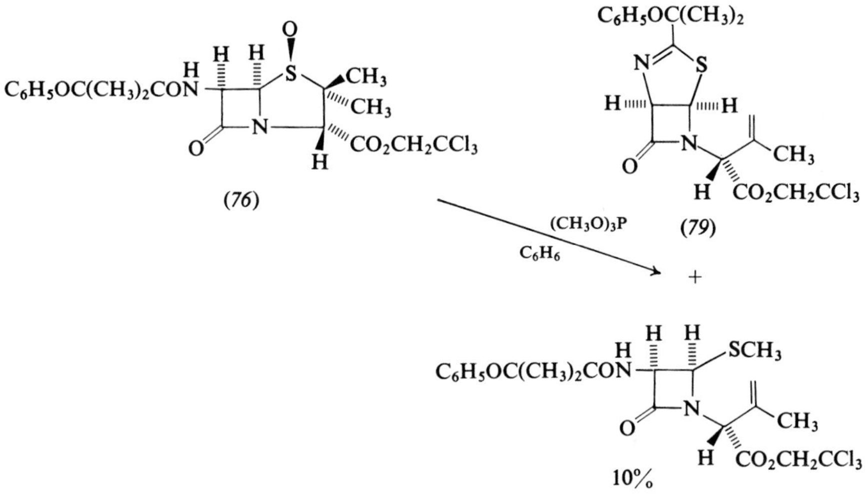

(76)

(79)

(78)

10%

Several minor products were also isolated from the rearrangement of (75) to (77). They contained phosphorous and were tentatively assigned structures (80) and (81). A related product (82) was also isolated from the reaction of (18) with dimethylphosphite.

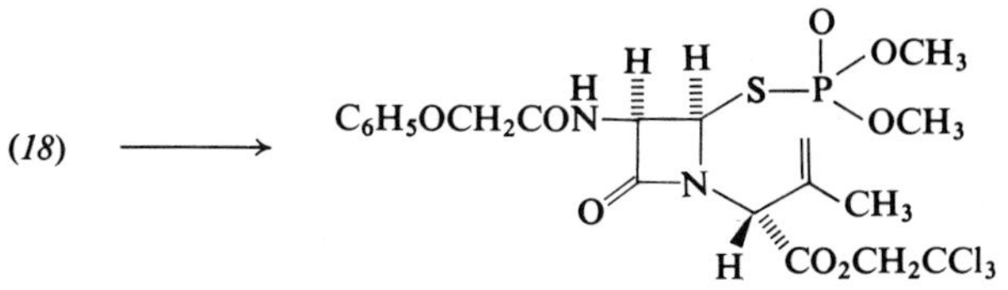

(18) ⟶

(82)

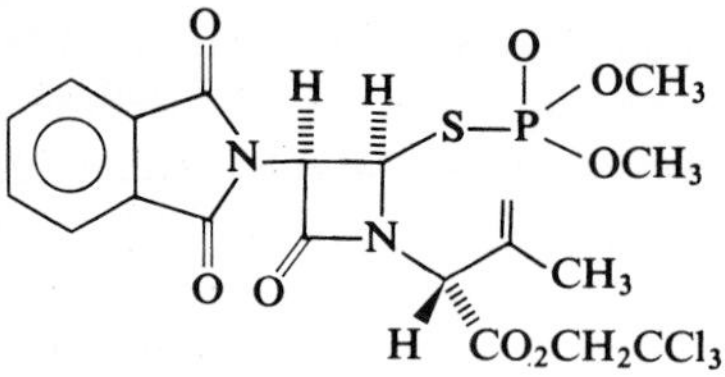

(80)

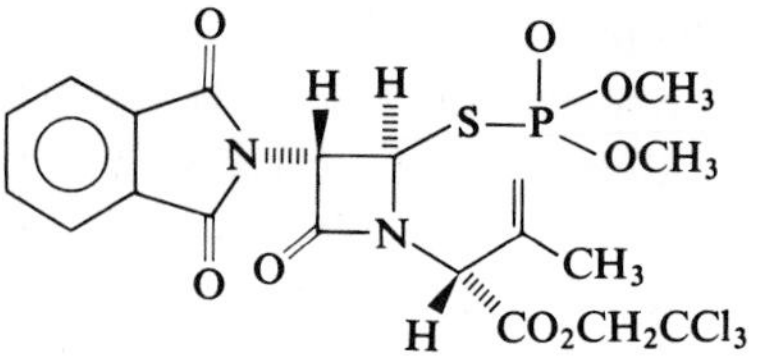

(81)

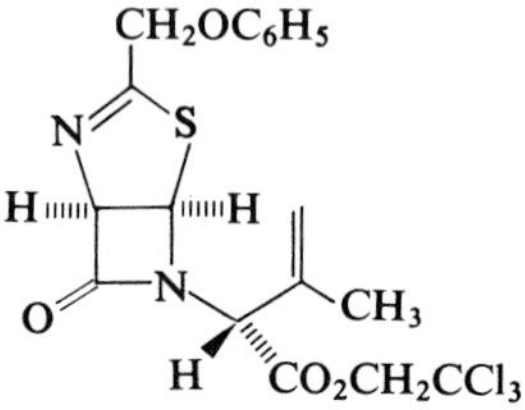

(70)

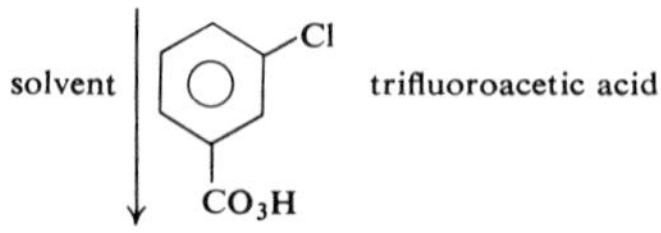

solvent   trifluoroacetic acid

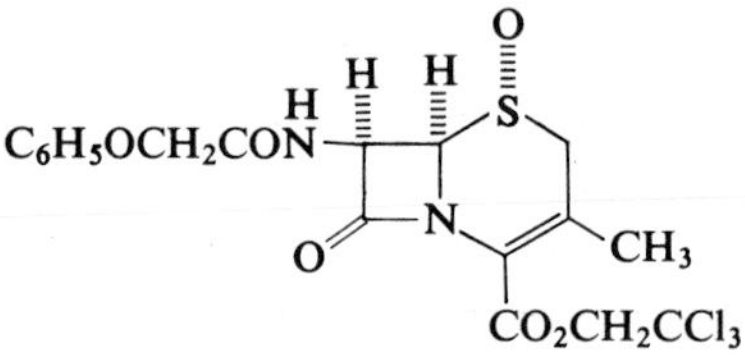

(85)

+

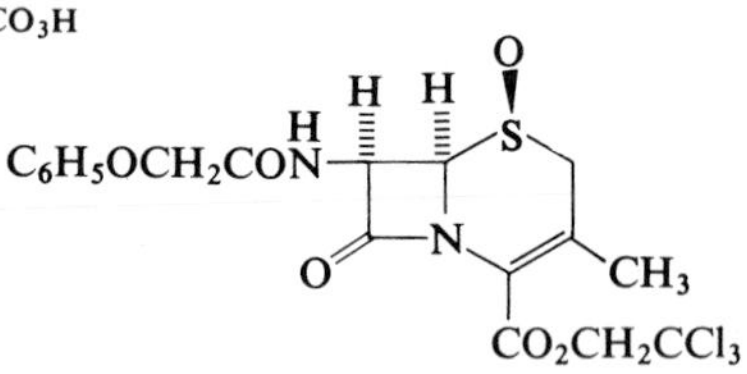

(39)

+

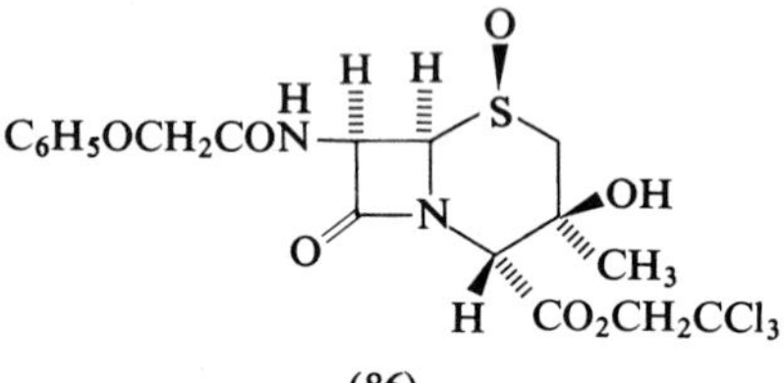

+

(86)

+

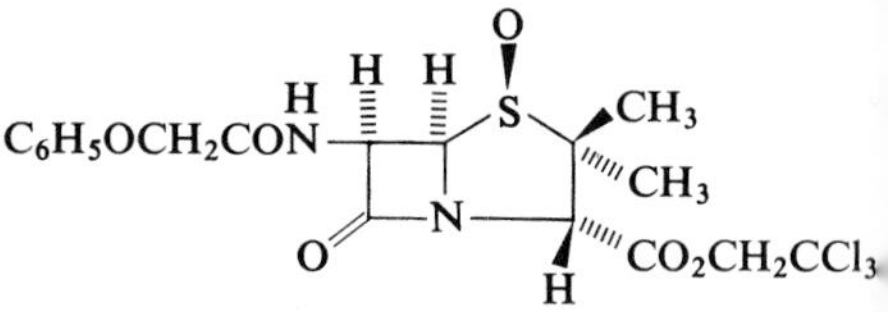

(18)

+

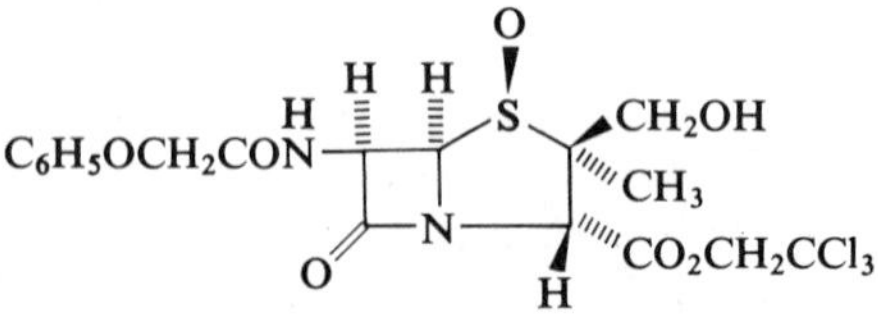

+

(83)

+

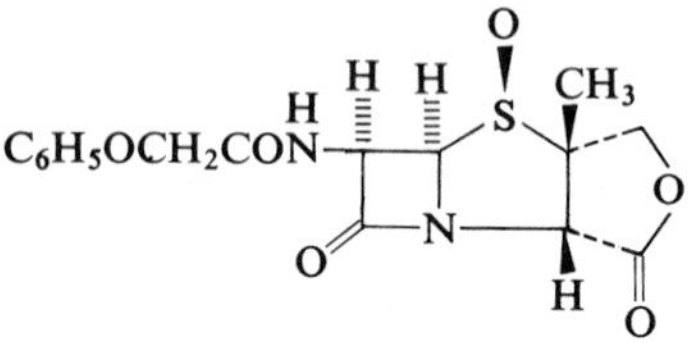

(84)

Cooper and José (1970b) reported that the carbon–carbon double bond of the β,γ-unsaturated ester system in (70) was resistant to electrophilic attack, being recovered unchanged after treatment with elemental bromine or permaleic acid in refluxing benzene. However, treatment with the peracid at room temperature in the presence of a catalytic amount of a stronger acid, e.g., trifluoroacetic acid, caused rearrangement to a mixture of products (18), (39), and (83)–(86); relative yields of the compounds depended on the solvent used.

B. Mechanism of Sulfoxide Rearrangement

In the rearrangement of the penicillin sulfoxide (5) to (6)–(8) as originally reported by Morin et al. (1963), the authors postulated the initial formation of a sulfenyl anhydride (87) followed by an intramolecular trans addition of the sulfenyl anhydride to the double bond through an episulfonium ion. The precedents considered operable were the thermal cis elimination of a sulfoxide to give an olefin (Kingsbury and Cram, 1960), and the addition of a sulfenyl halide to a double bond, postulated in 1946 as proceeding through an episulfonium ion (Fuson et al., 1946; Mueller, 1969).

In related experiments with benzothiazine derivatives, Morin and Spry (1970) obtained further evidence to corroborate this generalized mechanism. The rearrangement of (88) to the thiazolone (89) when treated with acetic anhydride, and conversion of the corresponding N-methyl derivative (90) to a mixture of (91)–(93), were explained by formation of sulfenyl anhydride intermediates (94) and (95).

In the original work of Morin and co-workers (1963), the products isolated from treatment with acetic anhydride, i.e., (6) and (7), possess a stereospecific introduction of the acetoxy group; no evidence for the presence of their isomers could be found. Morin et al. (1969a) postulated that, based on previously published information on the magnetic shielding effects of a sulfoxide group, the spatial arrangement of the sulfoxide bond was cis to the amido side chain. Cooper et al. (1969a) further investigated the structures of the penicillin sulfoxides via a detailed NMR study.

The oxidation of a penicillin derivative to its sulfoxide was first reported by Sykes and Todd (1949) who discovered, as part of the structural investigations on penicillin, that methyl benzylpenicillanate (96) could be oxidized to (97) by sodium metaperiodate.

Several other groups (Chow et al., 1962; Guddal et al., 1962; Essery et al., 1965) have reported on the oxidation of penicillin derivatives having various substituents at the 6 and 3 positions, and in no case did it appear that both isomers were obtained. Cooper et al. (1969a) also unsuccessfully attempted to obtain both isomers by varying the penicillin derivative and the oxidizing

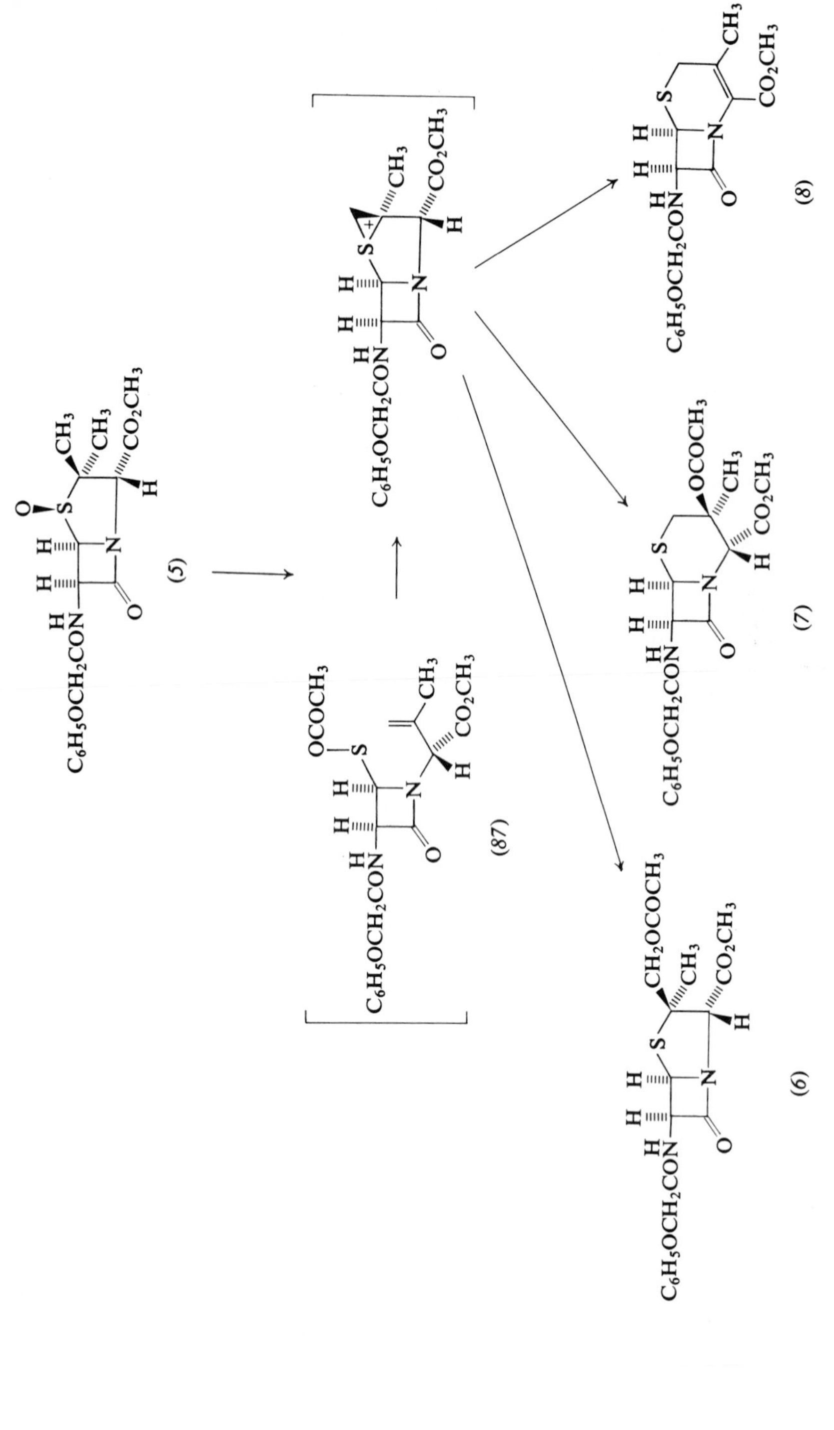

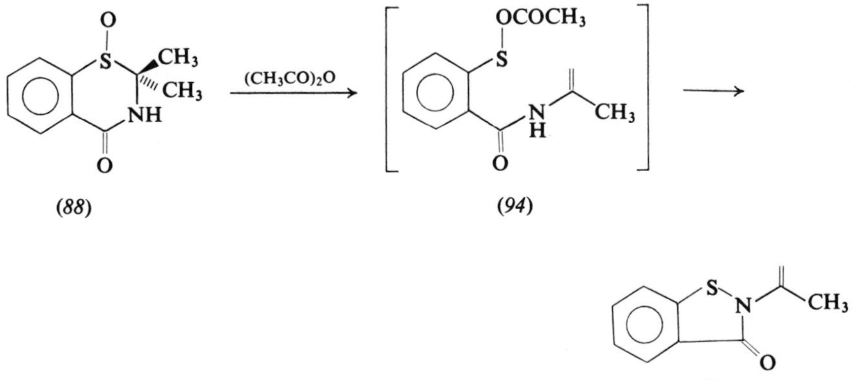

(88) (94) (89)

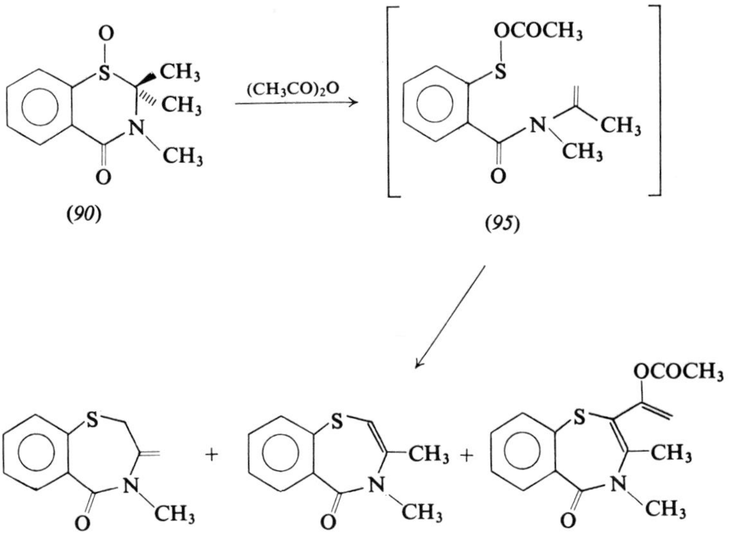

(90) (95) (91) (92) (93)

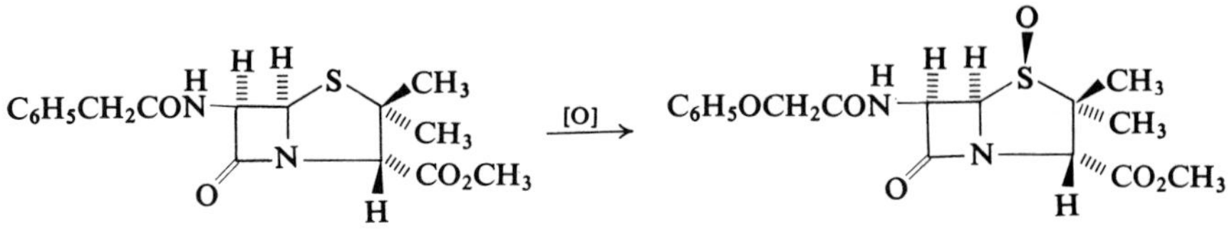

(96) (97)

conditions in preparative reactions. They also reported that attempts to epi-merize the sulfoxide of the phenoxymethylpenicillin sulfoxide ester (5) gave only recovered starting material or decomposition. These workers then under-took an extensive NMR investigation of phenoxymethylpenicillin sulfoxide methyl ester (5) and the sulfone methyl ester in which they observed the effects obtained by introducing one sulfur–oxygen bond (sulfoxide) and two sulfur–oxygen bonds (sulfone) into the penicillin molecule. The problem involved

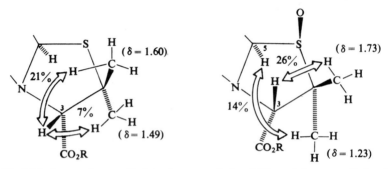

Fig. 1. Nuclear overhauser effects in phenoxymethylpenicillin and phenoxymethylpenicillin β-sulfoxide esters.

initially the assignment of the methyl group signals, which was solved by obser-ving the internal nuclear Overhauser effects (NOE's) (Fig. 1). The high field methyl signal was established as belonging to the α-methyl group.

The net aromatic solvent-induced shift Δ ($CDCl_3-C_6D_6$), which occurred when a sulfoxide bond was introduced into the molecule, was obtained by the expression $\Delta = \Delta_{S-O} - \Delta_S$, where $\Delta_{S-O} = J_{CDCl_3} - J_{C_6D_6}$ for the sulfoxide and $\Delta_S = J_{CDCl_3} - J_{C_6D_6}$ sulfide. The values which were obtained are shown in Table II (see also Chapter 8).

The two most pronounced shifts were those of the signals for the H_5 and α-methyl protons. A third technique used was measurement of the amide NH proton shift on changing from deuterochloroform to dimethylsulfoxide-d_6, a solvent known to hydrogen bond strongly to –OH and –NH groups and, consequently, to cause large downfield shifts. Whereas, in the sulfides, a shift of 1.21 ppm was observed, no effect was seen in the sulfoxide (*18*). From this observation it was concluded that a strong internal hydrogen bond existed. Geometrically, this was possible only with the sulfoxide bond in the *cis* or (*S*) configuration, a configuration supported by the solvent shift effects and by the qualitative and quantitative anisotropic shift studies (for further details see Chapter 8). Proof of stereochemistry was provided by an X-ray crystallo-graphic study by Jones and Cheng (Cooper *et al.*, 1969a) which brought to light the conformational differences of the thiazolidine ring between the sulfide

Table II

PROTON RESONANCE DATA AND BENZENE-INDUCED SOLVENT SHIFTS ($\Delta = J_{CDCl_3} - J_{C_6D_6}$) FOR SOME PHENOXYMETHYL PENICILLIN DERIVATIVES

Compound	Solvent	Resonance (ppm)				
		H_3	H_4	H_5	$2\alpha CH_3$	$2\beta CH_3$
Phenoxymethylpenicillin methyl ester	$CDCl_3$	4.47	5.58	5.74	1.49	1.60
	C_6D_6	4.39	5.11	5.54	1.13	1.20
	$\Delta_1 (J_{CDCl_3} - J_{C_6D_6})$	+0.08	+0.47	+0.20	+0.36	+0.40
Phenoxymethylpenicillin (S)-sulfoxide methyl ester (5)	$CDCl_3$	4.69	5.03	6.10	1.23	1.73
	C_6D_6	4.65	3.77	5.93	0.51	1.25
	$\Delta_1 (J_{CDCl_3} - J_{C_6D_6})$	+0.04	+1.26	+0.17	+0.72	+0.48
Phenoxymethylpenicillin trichloroethyl ester sulfone	$CDCl_3$	4.66	4.82	6.19	1.51	1.69
	C_6D_6	4.48	3.68	5.89	1.05	1.21
	$\Delta_1 (J_{CDCl_3} - J_{C_6D_6})$	+0.18	+1.14	+0.30	+0.46	+0.48
	$\Delta_{1s-o} - \Delta_{1s}$	-0.04	+0.79	-0.03	+0.36	+0.08

and sulfoxide (see Chapter 7). This conformational difference also explained the observed NOE differences in Fig. 1. In the (S) configuration the sulfoxide is the more sterically hindered since the oxygen is oriented towards the inside of the molecule. Cooper *et al.* (1969a) explained this as being due to reagent approach control brought about by hydrogen bonding of the peracid oxidizing agent to the amide side chain NH. This causes oxidation to occur from the side *cis* to the amido side chain. Alternatively, the control can be thermodynamic with the (S)-sulfoxide being more stable because of the amido-sulfoxide intramolecular hydrogen bond. In retrospect, it seems that both explanations could be correct, although the former is preferred. Oxidation of methyl phthalimido-penicillanate (*98*) with *m*-chloroperbenzoic acid (Cooper *et al.*, 1969b) gave only one sulfoxide (*52*) whose configuration could not be unequivocally assigned by NMR techniques used previously. Epimerization of (*52*) to the 6-epi derivative (*99*) gave a sulfoxide which was identical to one of the two sulfoxides (*99*) and (*100*) obtained by peracid oxidation of the 6-epi sulfide (*101*). The configurations of (*99*) and (*100*) were then deduced by study of the

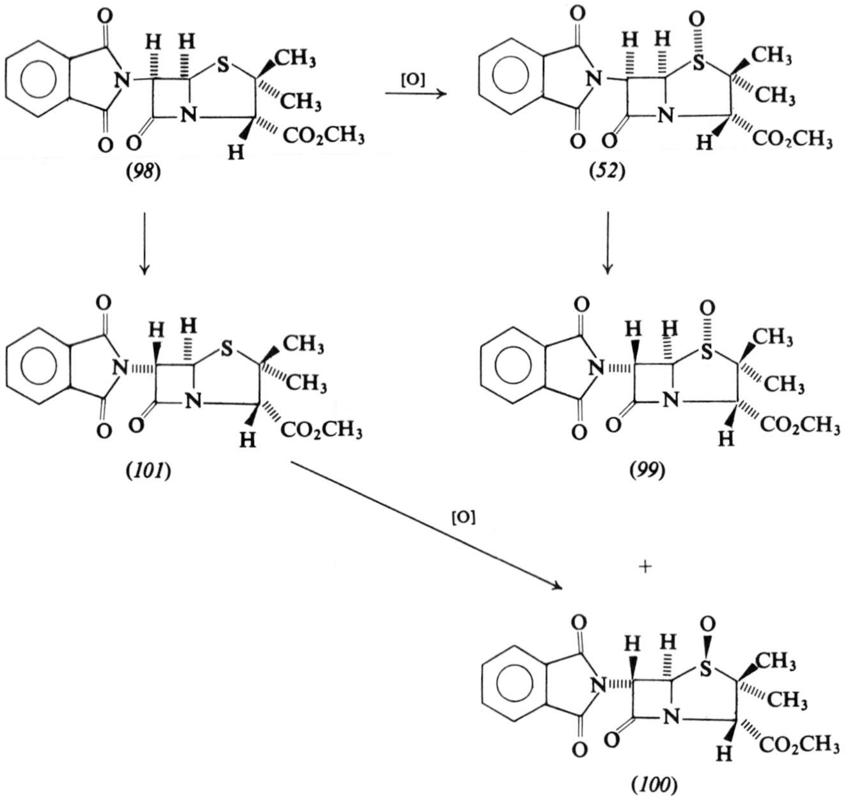

(98) [O]→ (52)

(101) (99)

[O]

+

(100)

aromatic-induced solvent shifts of their proton resonances in their NMR spectra.

The sulfoxide configuration of (52) was thus shown to be (R). In the absence of an amide NH, steric control becomes the major directing influence in the oxidation. Similar stereochemical conclusions concerning the sulfoxides were reached by Barton and co-workers (1969). They obtained the (S)-sulfoxide of methyl benzylpenicillinate (96) when using most oxidizing agents; their stereo-chemistry assignments were based on studies of benzene-induced solvent shifts and magnetic anisotropic properties. An exceptional result was obtained by the use of iodobenzene dichloride as the oxidizing agent, resulting in a 1:1 mixture of the two isomeric (S)- and (R)-sulfoxides (97) and (102) (Barton

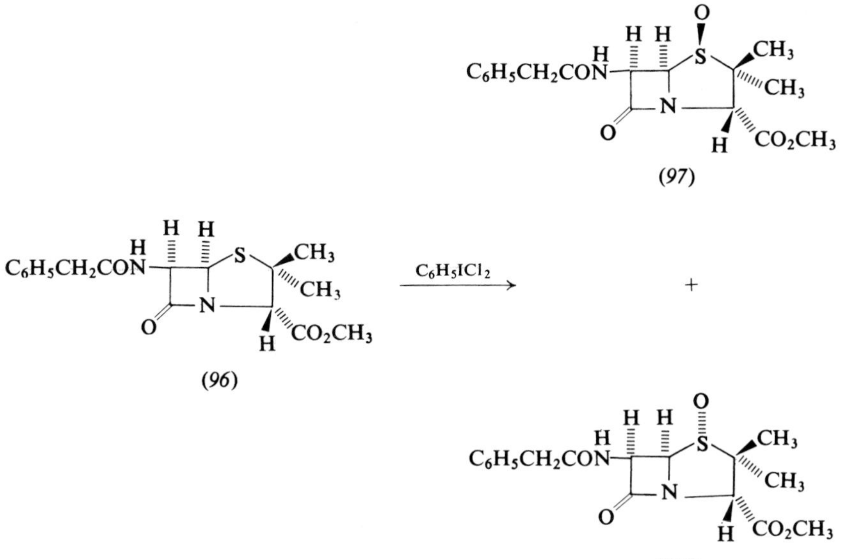

$$C_6H_5CH_2CON\text{—} \quad (97)$$

$$C_6H_5CH_2CON\text{—} \quad (96) \quad \xrightarrow{C_6H_5ICl_2} \quad +$$

$$C_6H_5CH_2CON\text{—} \quad (102)$$

et al., 1969). The (R)-sulfoxides (103) and (104) were also obtained from (5) and (57) by Archer and Demarco (1969), using an acetone-sensitized photo-chemical procedure and by Spry (1970a) using ozone as the oxidizing agent (see page 197).

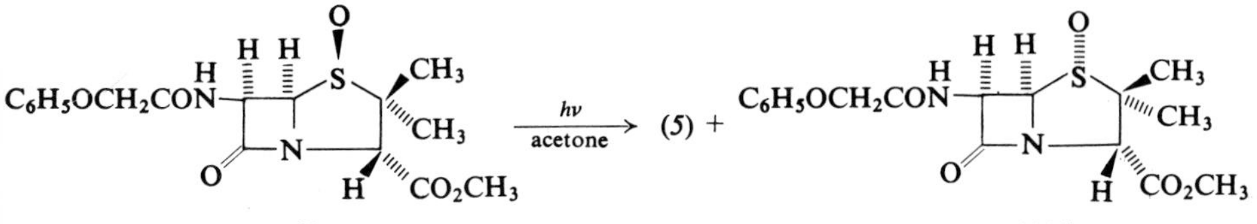

$$C_6H_5OCH_2CON\text{—} \quad (5) \quad \xrightarrow[\text{acetone}]{h\nu} \quad (5) + \quad C_6H_5OCH_2CON\text{—} \quad (103)$$

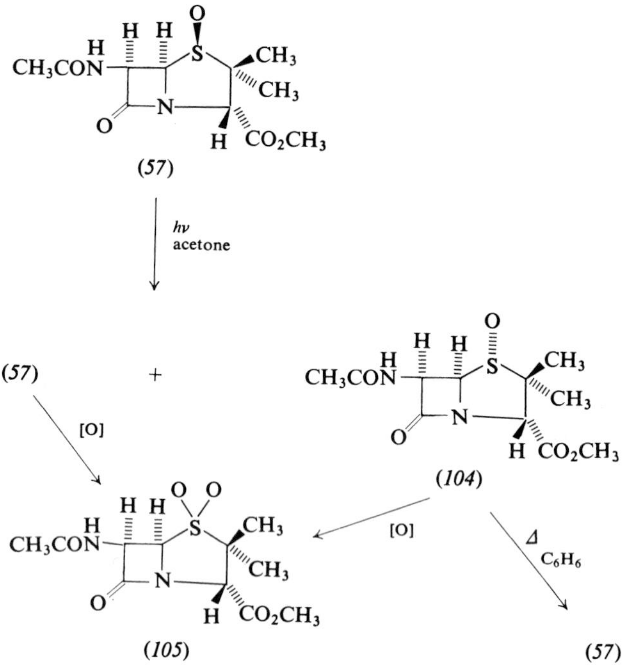

(57)

hν
acetone

(57)   +   (104)

[O]

(105)   [O]   Δ
C₆H₆

(57)

The structure of (104) was verified chemically by oxidation of both (57) and (104) to a common sulfone (105). Both Archer and Demarco (1969) and Barton et al. (1969) observed that (R)-sulfoxide was converted rapidly and in high yield to (S)-sulfoxide by refluxing a solution of the (R)-sulfoxide (104) and (102) in benzene. This result indicated a greater thermodynamic stability of the (S)-sulfoxide in instances where the amide side chain contains an NH group.

If the epimerization of (102) is carried out in deuterated tert-butanol, the resulting (S)-sulfoxide (97) contains deuterium located in the β-methyl group. A control experiment with the (S)-sulfoxide (97) gave no deuterium incorporation under identical conditions. The deuterium incorporation was postulated as occurring by hydrogen–deuterium exchange at the sulfenic acid stage.

Spry (1970a) described the rearrangement of a β-acetoxymethylpenicillin (R)-sulfoxide derivative (60) to the α-acetoxymethylpenicillin (S)-sulfoxide (62) which he explained as proceeding via the sulfenic acid followed by reclosure to the more thermodynamically stable (S)-sulfoxide.

The London group (Barton et al., 1970b) also later independently observed the thermal isomerization of the β-acetoxy-α-sulfoxide derivative (108) to the α-acetoxy-β-sulfoxide isomer (109). Both of these London publications (Barton et al., 1969, 1970b) report iodobenzene dichloride oxidation of the

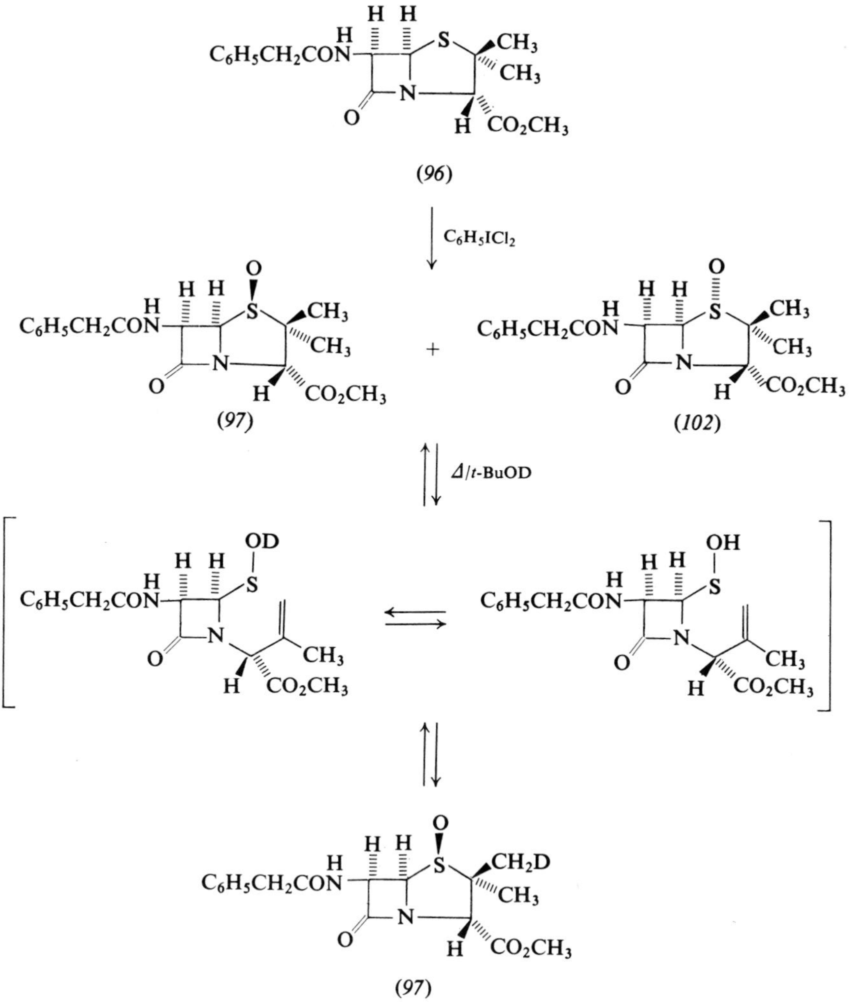

(96)

$C_6H_5ICl_2$

(97)   +   (102)

Δ/t-BuOD

(97)

benzylpenicillin derivatives (96) and (106) to a mixture of the α- and β-sulfoxides using iodobenzene dichloride in aqueous pyridine; however, no yields are reported, so its effectiveness in obtaining the elusive α-sulfoxides cannot be compared to the ozone procedure. Barton et al. (1970b), using the p-nitrobenzyl group as a removable ester function, reduced the α-acetoxymethyl-β-sulfoxide (110) to the sulfide (111) with phosphorous tribromide in dimethylformamide (DMF) and after subsequent hydrogenolysis, isolated the acid (112), a new type of penicillin derivative. Microbiological activity was reported for (112), but no comparison was made with benzylpenicillin (see Chapter 12).

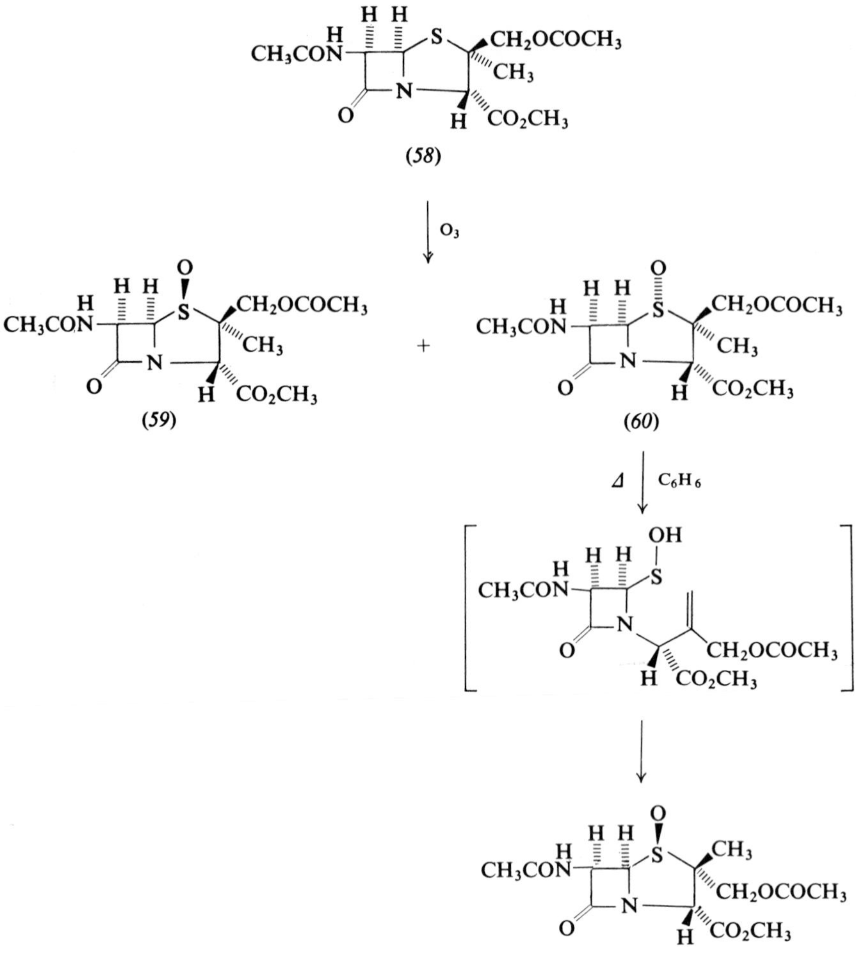

$$CH_3CON \overset{H}{-} \overset{\underset{\displaystyle H \ H}{|\ |}}{} S - CH_2OCOCH_3$$

(58)

$$\downarrow O_3$$

(59)   +   (60)

$$\varDelta \ | \ C_6H_6$$

(62)

Cooper (1970a) proposed that the conversion of the sulfoxide to a sulfenic acid (originally considered to be acid catalyzed) was a thermal six-electron sigmatropic rearrangement. The reaction was considered to be an allowable one since the orbitals on the hydrogen atom involved in the transfer were symmetrical (s orbital) and thus able to establish orbital overlap with the two p orbitals of the oxygen atom in the forward sense and with the π orbitals of the carbon–carbon double bond in the reverse sense. The epimerization of a sulfoxide by pyramidal inversion or homolytic scission–recombination has been reported (Rayner et al., 1968) to have energy requirements of greater than 35 kcal. mole^{-1}; whereas, the epimerization of the (R)-sulfoxides (102), (103), and

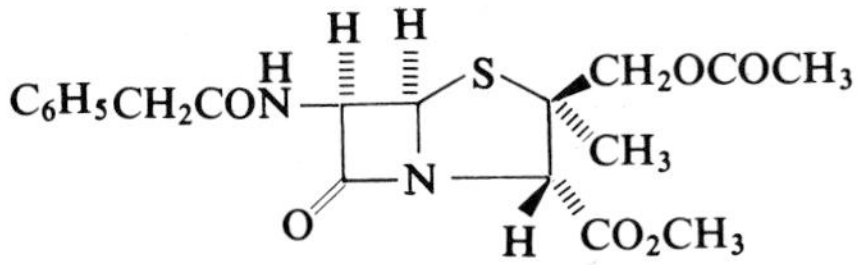

(*106*)

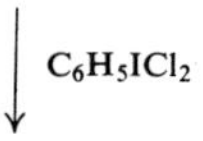

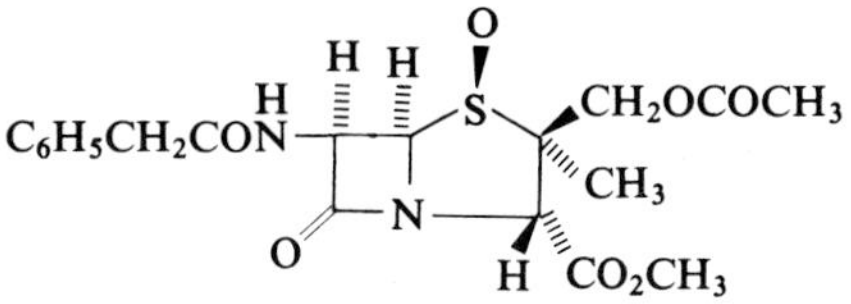

(*107*)

+

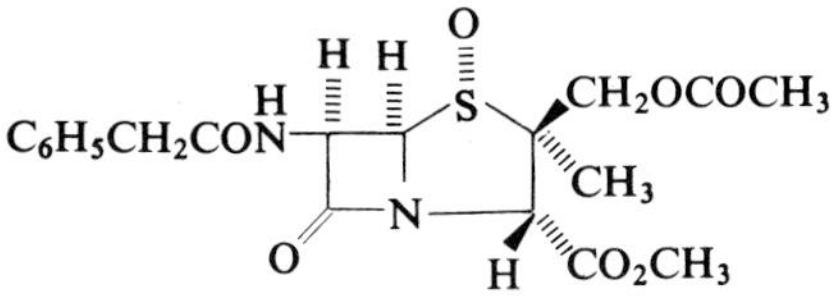

(*108*)

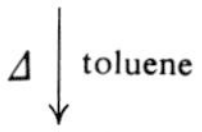

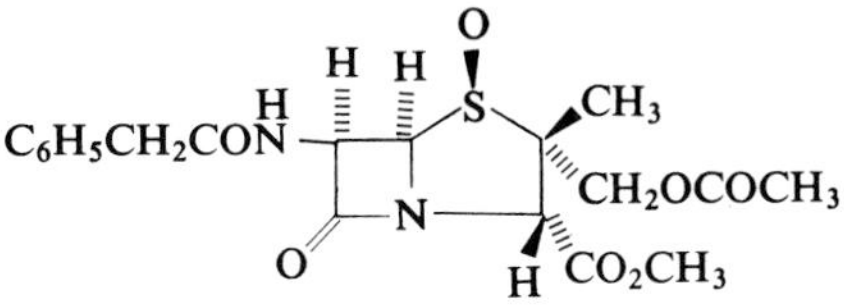

(*109*)

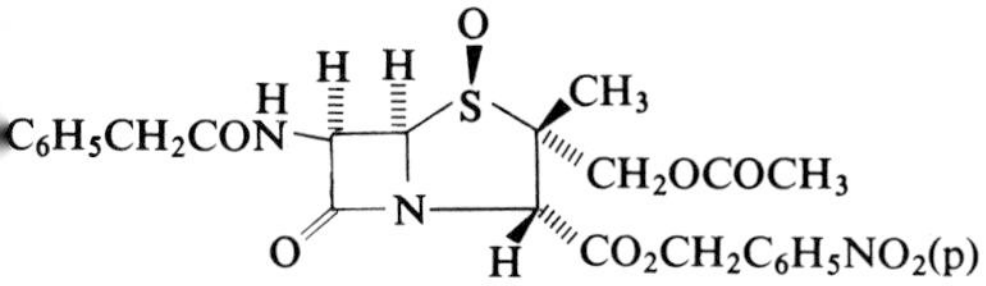

(*110*)

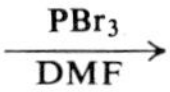

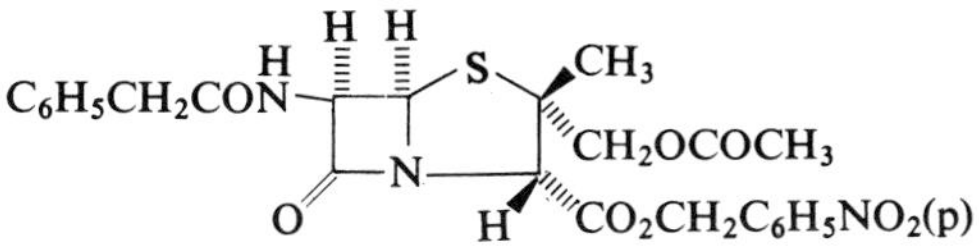

(*111*)

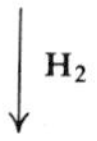

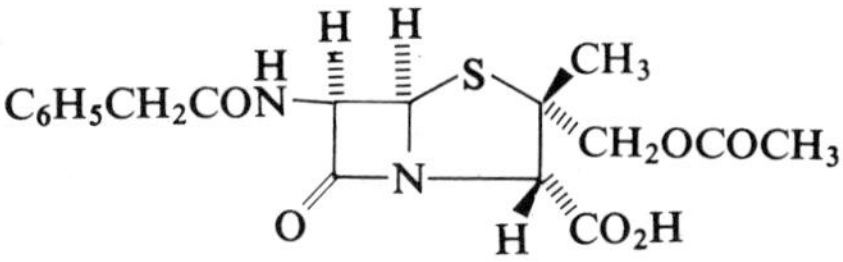

(*112*)

(*104*) into the (*S*)-sulfoxides was noted by Archer and Demarco (1969) and Barton *et al.* (1969) to occur in refluxing solvent at temperatures of less than 100°C. This ease of epimerization was explained by invoking the electrocyclic opening to a sulfenic acid, followed by reclosure to the thermodynamically stable sulfoxide (Barton *et al.*, 1970b; Spry, 1970a; Cooper and José, 1970a). When the side chain is a secondary amide, the (*S*)-sulfoxide is the more stable isomer due to intramolecular hydrogen bonding. An interesting example of this sulfoxide–sulfenic acid isomerization to give the thermodynamically stable products is provided by the work of Spry (1970b). He showed that methyl phthalimidopenicillanate (*R*)-sulfoxide (*52*) is the stable isomer for steric reasons in the absence of any intramolecular hydrogen bonding. However, methyl 6-epiphthalimidopenicillanate (*R*)-sulfoxide (*99*) on heating for 2 hours at 100°C gave an equilibrium mixture of (*S*)-sulfoxide (*100*) and (*R*)-sulfoxide (*99*) in the ratio 9:1.

(*99*)   (*100*)

1 : 9

The sulfenic acid was well implicated in the isomerization of a sulfoxide to the more stable configuration. Cooper (1970a) showed that the sulfenic acid could also be obtained from the thermodynamically more stable sulfoxides and that sulfoxide–sulfenic acid equilibrium is a thermal process. On refluxing a solution of the penicillin sulfoxide ester (*18*) in benzene containing a large excess of deuterium oxide for 24 hours, Cooper (1970a) showed that deuterium was incorporated into the β-methyl group (methyl group *cis* to the sulfoxide bond) (see Fig. 2). Similar treatment of the phthalimidopenicillin ester (*52*) gave deuterium incorporation only in the α-methyl group (methyl group *cis* to the sulfoxide bond).

The deuteration is remarkably stereospecific. Addition of the sulfenic acid to the double bond, on the basis of the postulated mechanism, would of necessity give deuterium in the methyl group *cis* to the sulfoxide bond. Since the sulfoxide stereochemistry is subject to thermodynamic control, the deuterated sulfoxide isomer obtained in each case is the more stable one.

Further trapping experiments on the sulfenic acid intermediate were reported by Barton *et al.* (1970b). In the presence of norbornadiene, generation of the sulfenic acid by refluxing the penicillin sulfoxide ester (*97*) in benzene caused formation of a new product (*113*) in good yield. Isomerization by

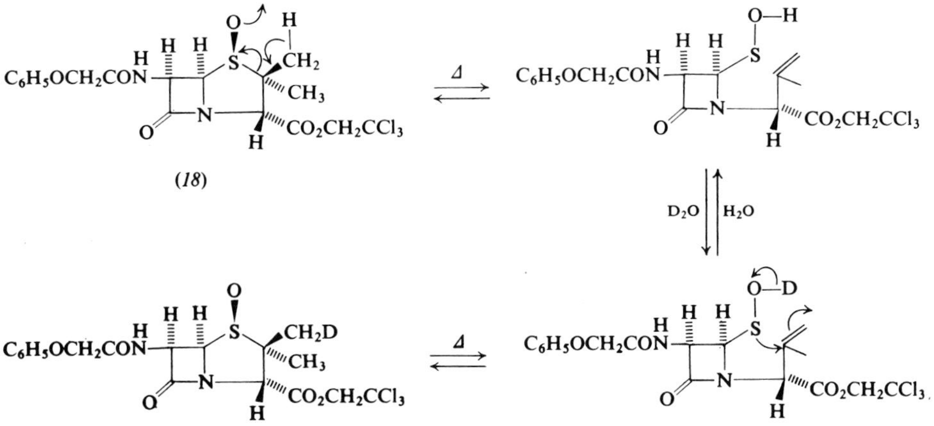

Fig. 2. Mechanism for deuteration of penicillin sulfoxide via a sulfenic acid.

triethylamine into the α,β-unsaturated ester (114) followed by reduction with phosphorous tribromide in dimethylformamide gave the sulfide (115). An alternative trapping experiment involved reaction of the sulfenic acid from (116) with dihydropyran in the presence of aluminum tribromide when, after treatment of the initial product (117) with triethylamine the crystalline sulfide

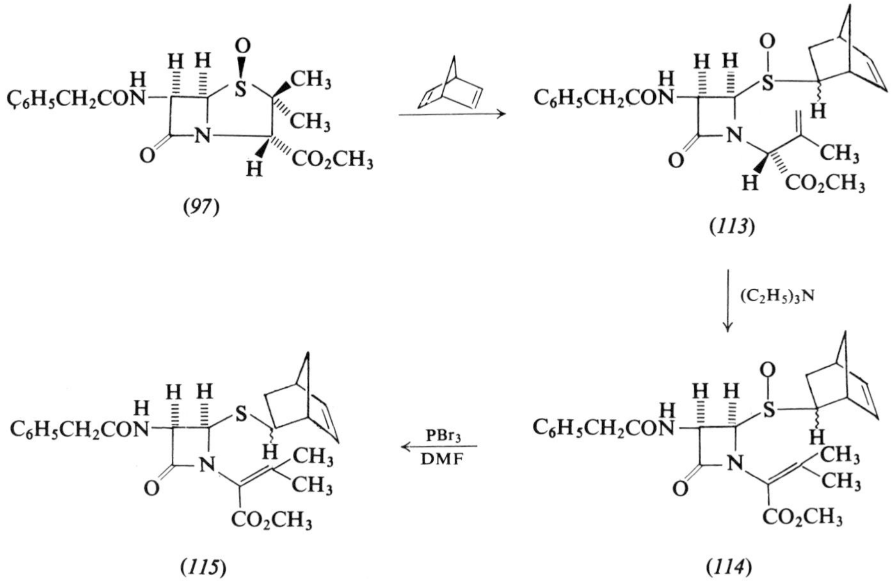

(*118*) was isolated. However, this latter reaction appears to be more rationally considered to proceed through a nucleophilic attack on the sulfenic acid (catalyzed by the Lewis acid) rather than an electrocyclic trapping reaction and, as such, has much in common with the reaction with acetic anhydride (see page 203).

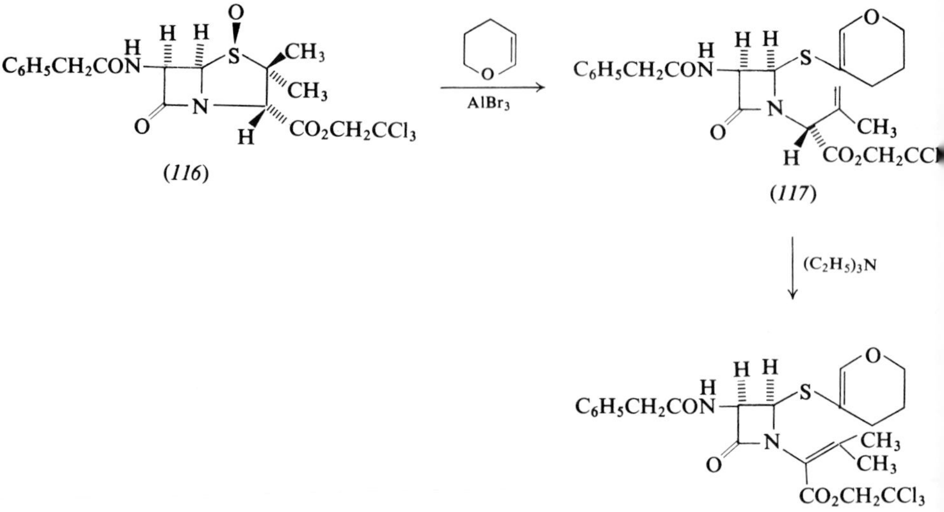

(*116*)

(*117*)

(*118*)

The involvement of sulfenic acid in the formation of the acetoxymethyl-penicillin and the 3-acetoxycepham during acetic anhydride catalyzed re-arrangement was indicated by reaction of the α-trideuteromethyl derivative (*119*) (Cooper *et al.*, 1970b) with acetic anhydride. Deuterium atoms in the resulting products were shown by NMR to be located as in (*120*), (*121*), and (*122*).

Whereas the original mechanistic proposals (Morin *et al.*, 1963, 1969a) offered a satisfactory explanation for the formation of an acetoxymethyl-penicillin and a 3-acetoxycepham, the explanation was inadequate to explain the observed stereospecificity of the acetic anhydride rearrangement of phenoxymethylpenicillin methyl ester (*S*)-sulfoxide (*5*) when only the 2β-acetoxymethylpenicillin (*6*) and the 3β-acetoxycepham (*7*) were isolated. Further experiments by Spry (1970a) showed that in the acetic anhydride rear-rangement of the phthalimidopenicillin sulfoxide ester (*52*), the stereospecific control was not operating as a mixture of the two 2-acetoxymethyl isomers (*123*) and (*124*) were observed (see p. 194). In the same experiment Spry (1970a) isolated the 3β-acetoxycepham (*125*); the 3α-isomer could not be found.

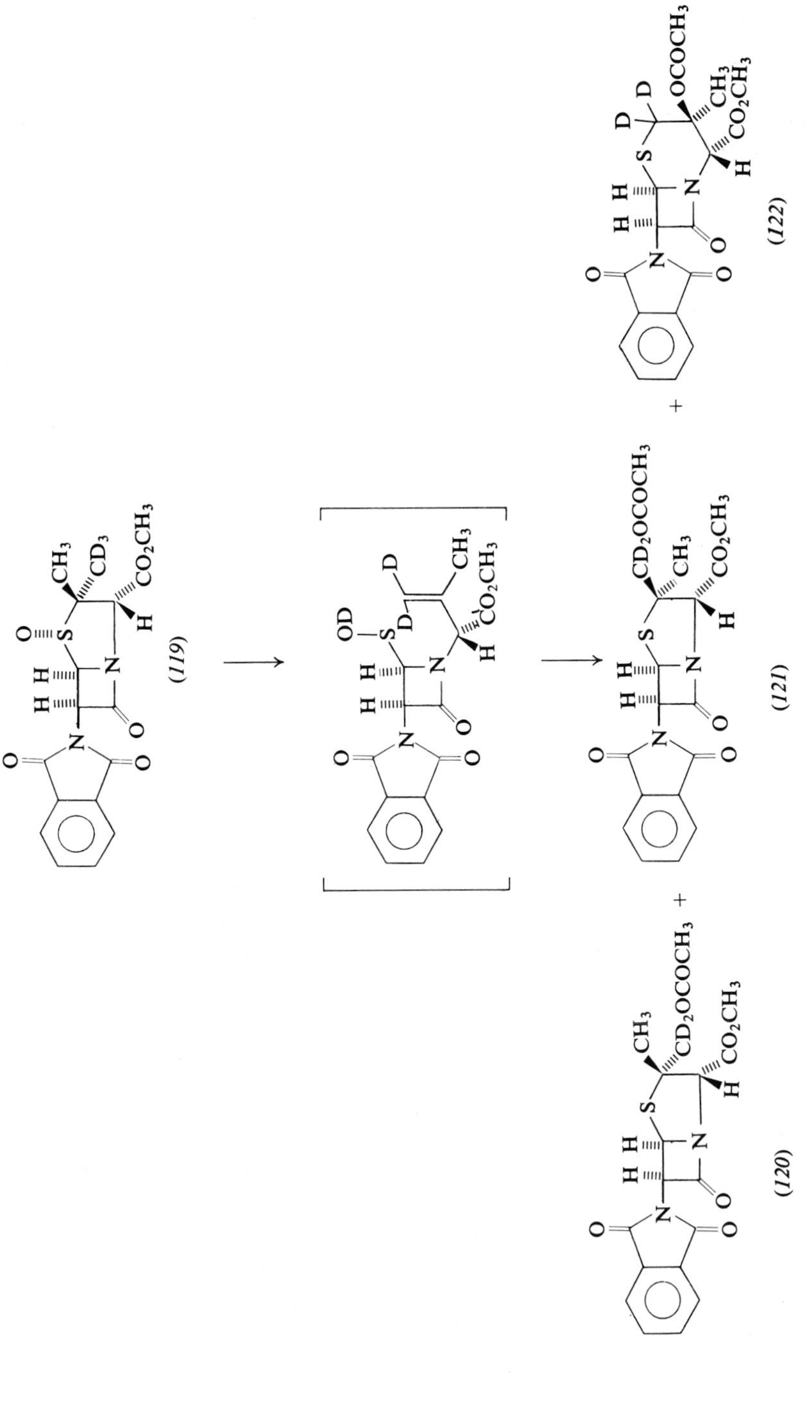

(119) (120) (121) (122)

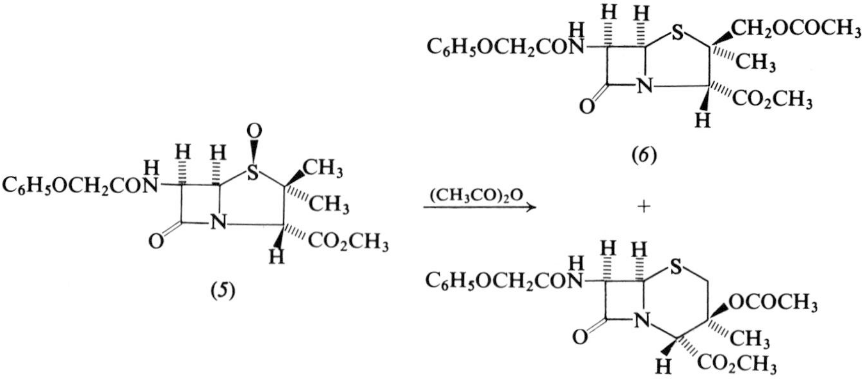

(6)

(5) $\xrightarrow{\text{(CH}_3\text{CO})_2\text{O}}$ +

(7)

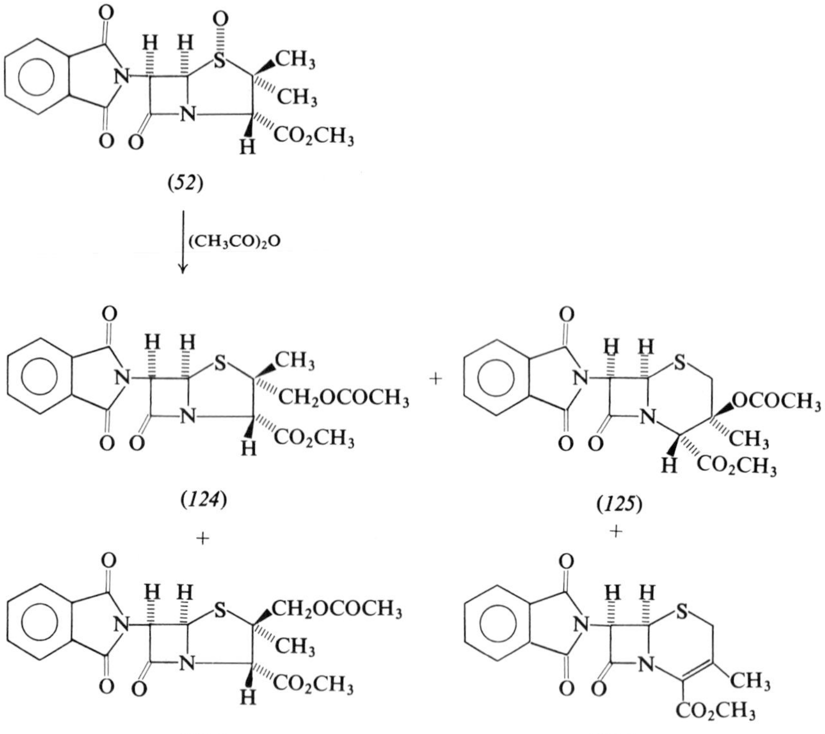

(52)

$\Big\downarrow$ (CH$_3$CO)$_2$O

(124)   +   (125)

+

(123)   (126)

Another anomaly was observed by Daniels *et al.* (1970) and Gutowski *et al.* (1971a), who found that the rearrangement of the phenoxymethylpenicillin (*16*) with sulfuric acid in dimethyl acetamide gave the 3-hydroxycepham (*127*) in approximately 47 % yield with the decarboxylated product (*17*) only present in trace amounts; whereas, a similar rearrangement using methanesulfonic acid instead of sulfuric acid gave the decarboxylated product (*17*) in 62 % yield and only a minor amount of the 3-hydroxycepham (*127*).

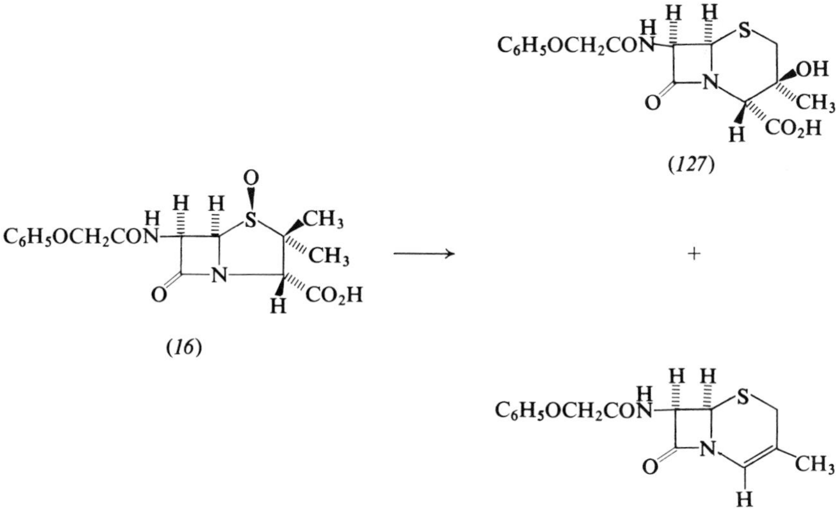

$C_6H_5OCH_2CON$

(*127*)

$C_6H_5OCH_2CON$

(*16*)

$\longrightarrow$

+

$C_6H_5OCH_2CON$

(*17*)

To account for these gaps in the mechanism as proposed by Morin *et al.* (1963), Cooper *et al.* (1970b) developed a somewhat more sophisticated argument based on the original proposals of Morin *et al.* (1963) but extended to explain more satisfactorily the stereochemical control (or lack of) in the reaction. They considered that the second stage after initial thermal ring opening of the sulfoxide to the olefin–sulfenic acid was the formation of a mixed anhydride derivative of the sulfenic acid with the reagent used (i.e., acetic anhydride, sulfonic acid, or sulfuric acid). The formation of this anhydride changed the electronic character of the sulfur atom from that of a reasonably good nucleophile in the sulfenic acid to that of an electrophile; as such, it was now able to undergo internal S_{N_2} displacement on the sulfur by the double bond. This step was assumed to be the key in controlling the product stereochemistry. The double bond approaches the sulfur orthogonally (at an angle of 180°) from the line of departure of the leaving group. Concurrent *trans* addition of the available anion (X) to the double bond results in an ion pair type of transition state which has the two possible geometries A and B in Fig. 3. The geometry of this transition state is controlled primarily by the preferred leaving direction of the group being displaced from sulfur. Formation of the sulfenic anhydride has

220   R. D. G. COOPER AND D. O. SPRY

given this leaving group a considerable steric requirement because, due to its
possible interaction with the β-amido side chain, it tends to leave from the α

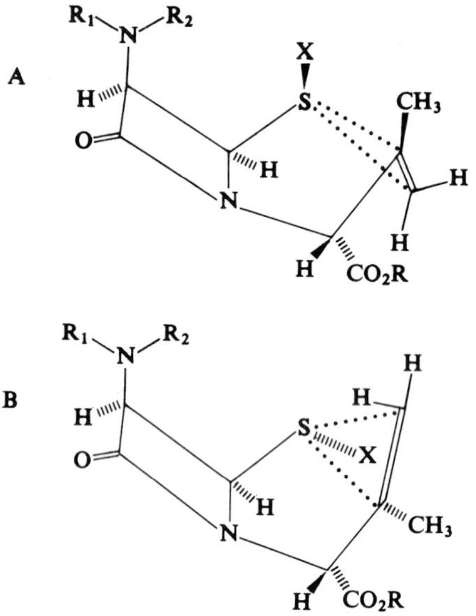

Fig. 3. Two possible transition states for the acid catalyzed rearrangement of penicillin sulfoxides.

face of the molecule, the double bond then approaching from the β face and the
transition state geometry B is the result. When X = –OCOCH₃ (Fig. 4),
collapse of the ion pair (geometry B) results in the observed β-acetoxymethylpenicillin ester and β-acetoxymethylcepham ester products. However, in the
case where a phthalimido side chain is present, examination of Dreiding models

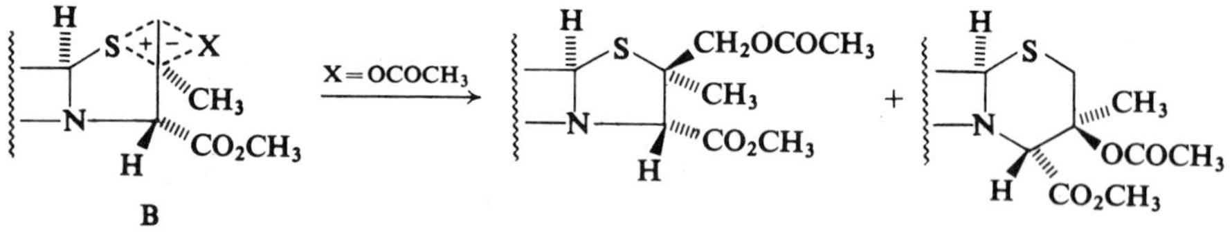

Fig. 4. Mechanism of product formation from transition state B in acid-catalyzed rearrangement of penicillin sulfoxide esters.

has shown a far greater steric interaction of the side chain, an effect previously
suggested by Cooper (1970a) to account for the lower activation energy of the
sulfoxide–sulfenic acid process for phthalimidopenicillin sulfoxide as compared to phenoxyacetamidopenicillin sulfoxide. This greater bulk establishes

steric repulsion between the β-phthalimido group and the orthogonal approach of the double bond from the β face of the molecule. Thus, two competing effects are operating, making possible some formation of a transition state with geometry A. Hence, the observation by Spry (1970a) that both β- and α-acetoxymethylphthalimidopenicillins could be obtained. That none of the corresponding 3α-acetoxycepham product was observed is not too unexpected since this compound if formed could undergo a facile *trans* elimination of acetic acid to the 3-cephem ester, a product which is observed to be formed (see Figs. 4 and 5).

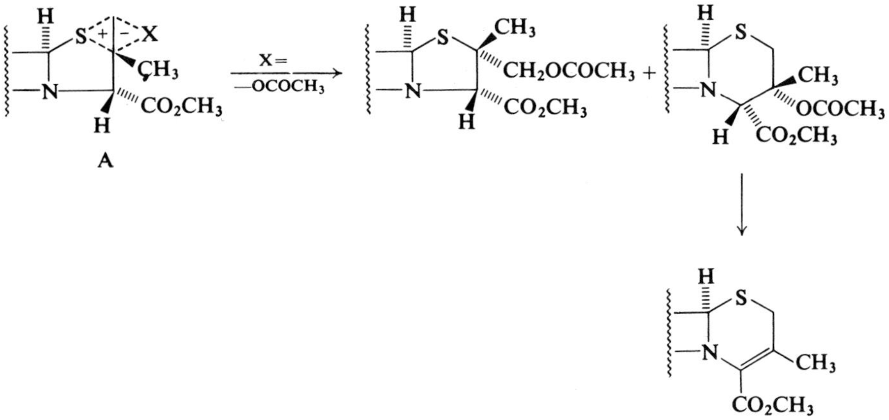

Fig. 5. Mechanism of product formation from transition state A in acid catalyzed rearrangement of penicillin sulfoxide esters.

When X $= -OSO_2CH_3$, the leaving group propensities are so much greater than those of an acetoxy group that elimination is facilitated, possibly by some type of internal *cis* elimination (Fig. 4), to give the observed 3-cephem products. When X $= -OSO_3H$, however, elimination could also occur, but now a second mode of fragmentation is possible. This mode involves internal collapse of the bisulfate group and produces the 3β-hydroxycepham ester. Relative amounts of the two possible products would be kinetically controlled.

Rearrangement of the penicillin sulfoxide acids was explained by considering the transition state (Fig. 6). When X $= -OSO_2CH_3$, the strength of its leaving group propensity establishes pathway A (Fig. 6), a *trans* elimination, as its sole mode of fragmentation to give the decarboxylated product. However, when X $= -OSO_3H$, the bisulfate group is a less effective leaving function and the relative kinetic rates of elimination versus fragmentation govern the products (pathway B). The major observed product was the 3β-hydroxycepham acid. Thus, the fragmentation mode of reaction could indeed be an effective competitive reaction for the loss of the bisulfate group.

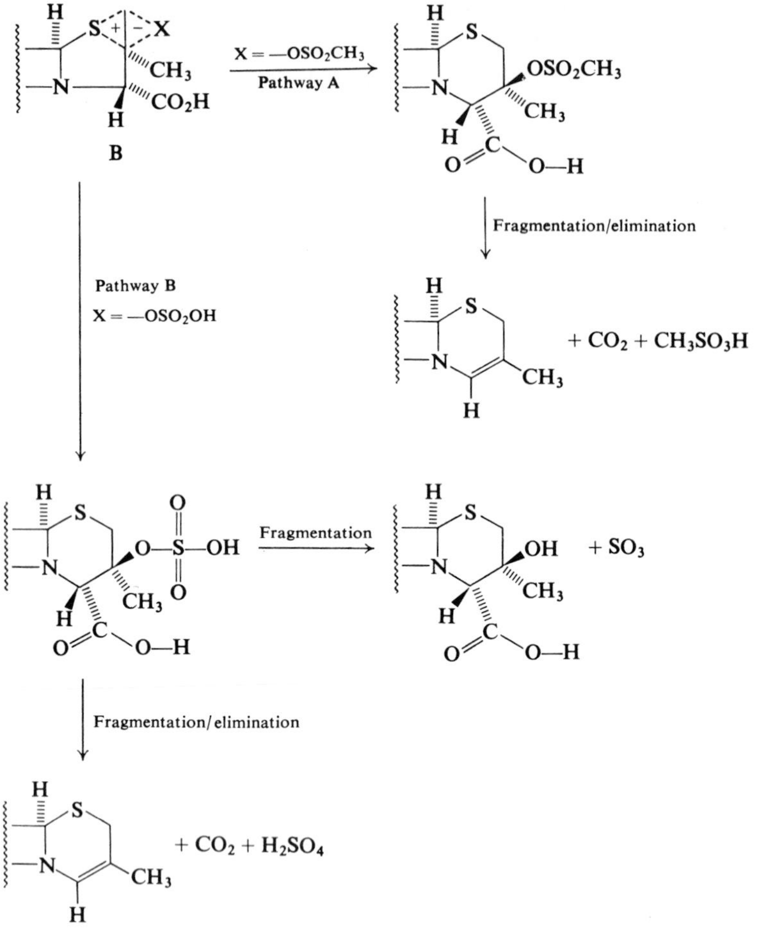

Fig. 6. Mechanism of product formation from transition state B in acid catalyzed rearrangement of penicillin sulfoxide acids.

The non-β-lactam products obtained from the treatment of penicillin sulfoxide ester with acetic anhydride were proposed by Morin et al. (1969a) as derived also from the sulfenyl anhydride (87) via displacement on sulfur by nitrogen to give initially the isothiazolone (22).

Double-bond isomerism of (22) would account for the second product (23). The third minor product was originally proposed as arising through the intermediate (87), followed by displacement on sulfur by the carbanion at C-3. More recent results (Morin et al., 1970) have shown that (22) can be converted to (24) by heating in dimethylformamide, thus indicating that elimination of

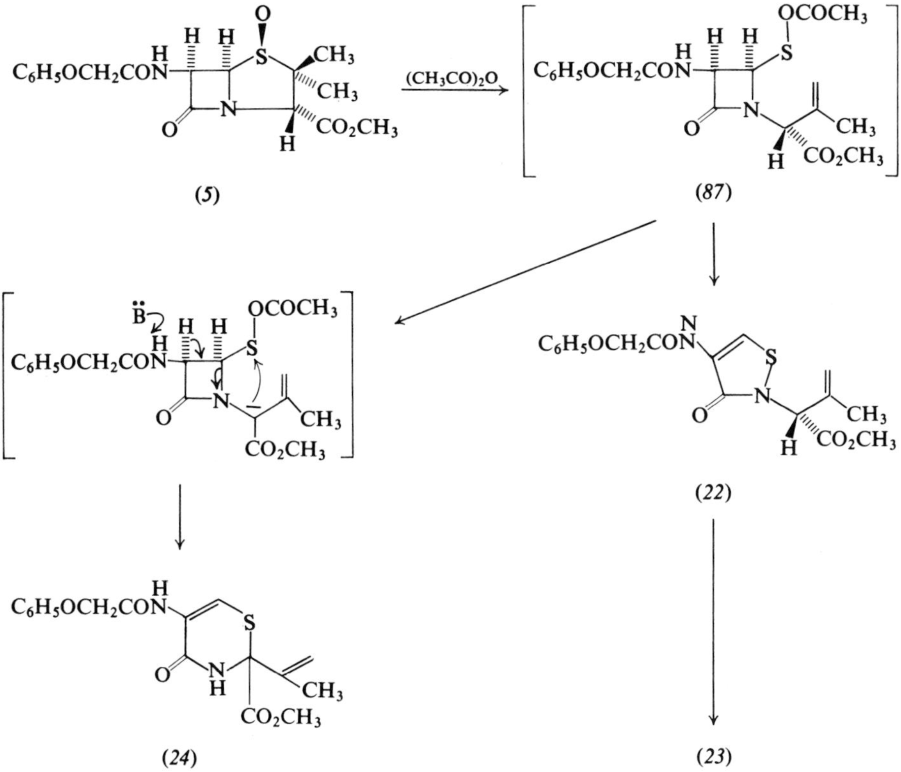

(5)   *(87)*

(22)

(24)   *(23)*

the thiol occurs, followed by Michael addition to the enamide system. The lack of optical activity of (24) suggested that the latter argument was valid.

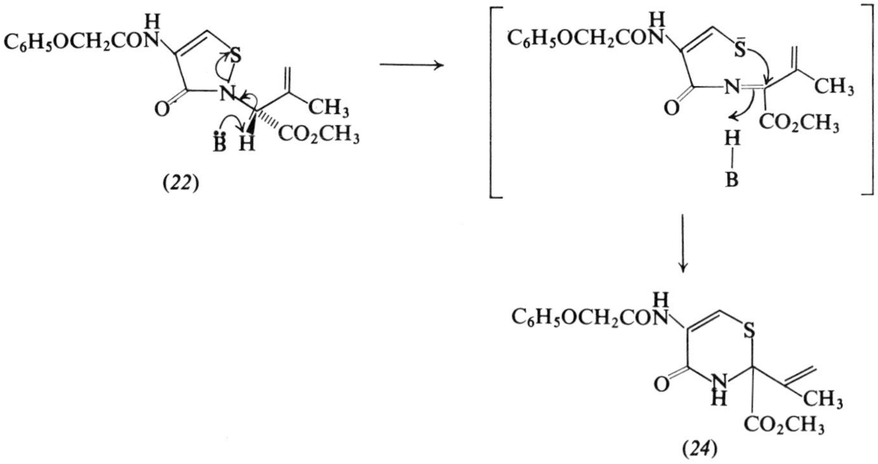

(22)

(24)

Because of the relatively low temperature needed for rearrangement to the isothiazolone, Cooper et al. (1970b) proposed an alternate pathway. This postulate, also recognized by Morin et al. (1969a) as being a possible explanation, involved an initial base-catalyzed β elimination of the sulfoxide to the thiazepine sulfoxide, which then thermally rearranged to the isothiazolone via a sulfenic acid. Attempts to isolate the sulfoxide (128) or observe by NMR the presence of a thiazepine sulfoxide in the reaction of (5) in deuteropyridine were unsuccessful, only (22) and (23) being observed. The reasons for not observing (128), however, could be kinetic if the rate of rearrangement of (128) to (22) exceeds its rate of formation.

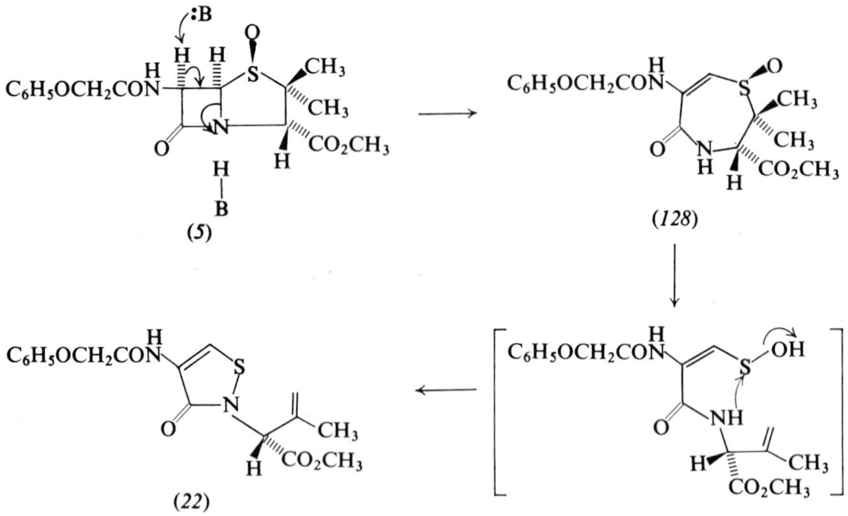

Oxidation of the thiazepine (25) with m-chloroperbenzoic acid gave a mixture of the two isomeric sulfoxides (129) and (130). The configuration of the sulfoxide bond of the two isomers was established by NMR solvent shifts. After being refluxed in acetone for 15 hours, the (S) isomer (129) was converted into the isothiazolone in 30% yield; the second isomer did not react. After 35 hours of refluxing, a 67% conversion of (129) into the isothiazolone was obtained, but the isomer (130) underwent no reaction. This conversion indicated a possible thiazepine sulfoxide intermediate in the isothiazolone (22) formation. Cooper et al. (1970b) assumed that the large reactivity difference between (129) and (130) could be explained by the different degrees of orbital overlap possible between the sulfoxide oxygen p orbitals and the methyl group hydrogen atom involved in the electrocyclic rearrangement. This overlap difference could result from possible changes in ring conformation with changes in the sulfoxide bond.

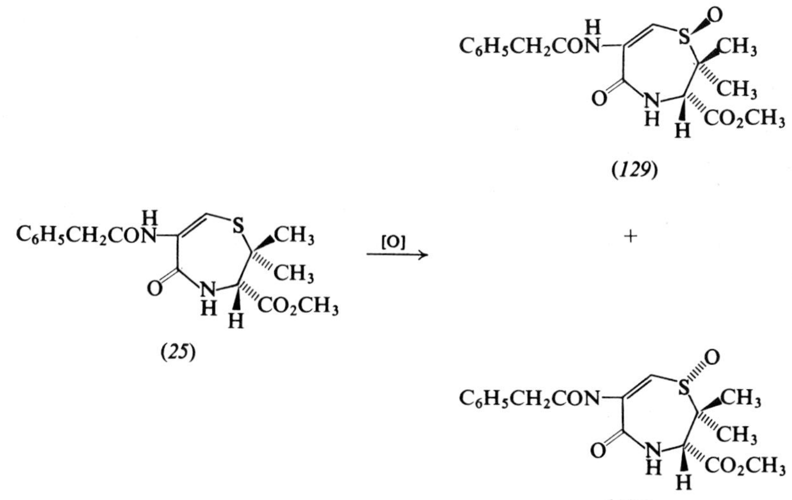

(129)

(25)

[O] →

+

(130)

In a related reaction reported by Leonard and Wilson (1964), the thiazepine (25) on treatment with N-chlorosuccinimide in refluxing chloroform gave the isothiazolone (26). It is interesting to speculate that this reaction has the same initial step as the sulfoxide rearrangement, viz., an electrocyclic rearrangement. Perhaps then, both reactions are just two examples of a more general reaction involving divalent sulfur when bonded to a more electronegative atom X, the driving force being the weakness of the S–X bond.

The mechanism for the rearrangement of penicillin sulfoxide with trimethylphosphite and trimethylphosphite/acetic anhydride was considered by both Cooper and José (1970a) and Hatfield et al. (1970) to be a reductive trapping of the intermediate sulfenic acid to a thiol or thiol type of intermediate. This then

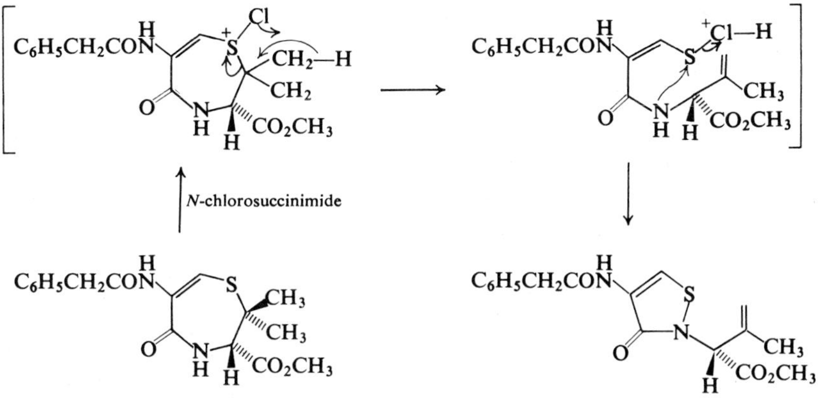

N-chlorosuccinimide

(25)

(26)

undergoes an intramolecular condensation with the secondary amide side chain to give (70) or acylation with acetic anhydride to give (74). The formation of the thioether derivative (77) was also rationalized (Cooper and José, 1970c) by alkylation of the intermediate thiol with trimethylphosphite. However, Hatfield and co-workers (1970) also postulated that the intermediate (131) could result directly from reaction of the sulfenic acid with trimethylphosphite. The analogy for this postulate was the known reaction of a trialkylphosphite with a dialkylperoxide when at low temperatures the essentially covalent tetraalkoxyphosphorous compound (132) could be observed (Denney and Relles, 1964).

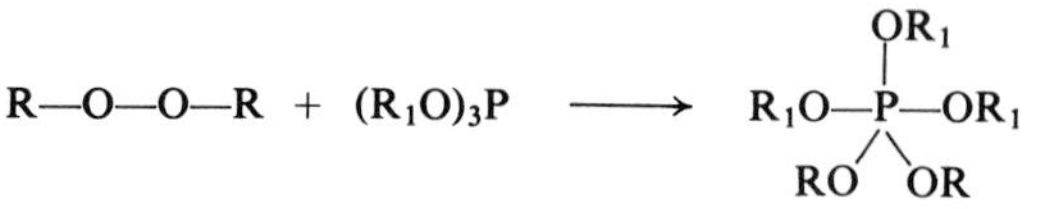

$$R-O-O-R + (R_1O)_3P \longrightarrow R_1O-\overset{\overset{\displaystyle OR_1}{|}}{\underset{\underset{\displaystyle RO\quad OR}{}}{P}}-OR_1$$

(132)

The isolation by Cooper and José (1970c) of the interesting phosphorous containing intermediates (80) and (81) can be considered as evidence for the initial existence of (131) which can then act as a source of the thiol anion by elimination of trimethylphosphate.

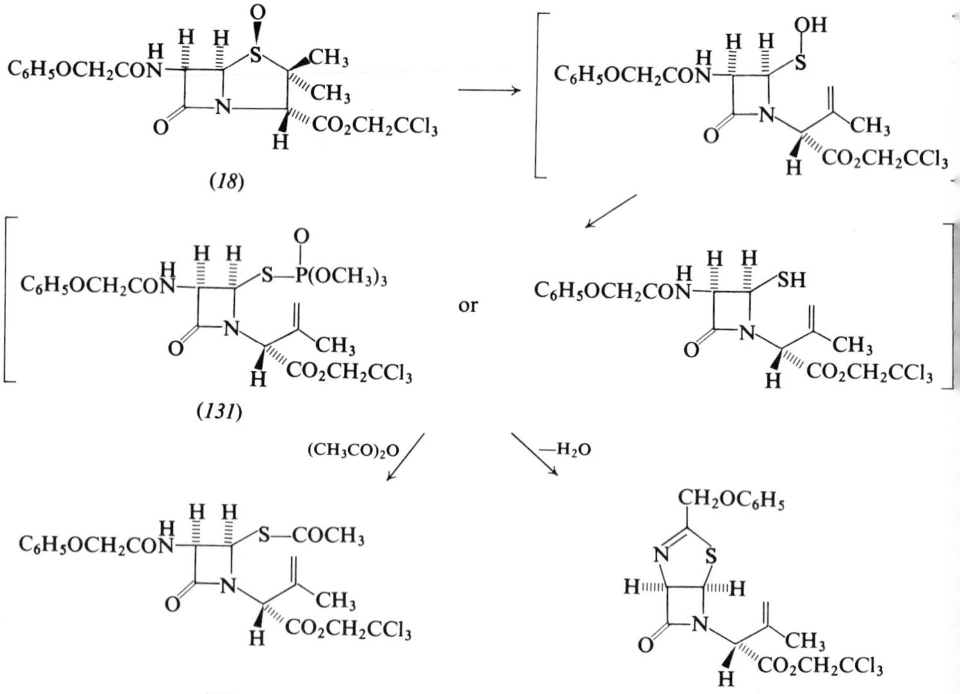

(18)

(131)

or

(74)

(70)

The reaction of (70) with peracids in the presence of trifluoroacetic acid was also considered to involve the sulfenic acid (Cooper and José, 1970c) formed by an acid catalyzed oxidative cleavage of the thiazoline ring. Protonation of the sulfenic acid and nucleophilic attack of the double bond on the sulfur atom gave an ion pair type of intermediate (133) analogous to that discussed previously on page 219 (Fig. 7).

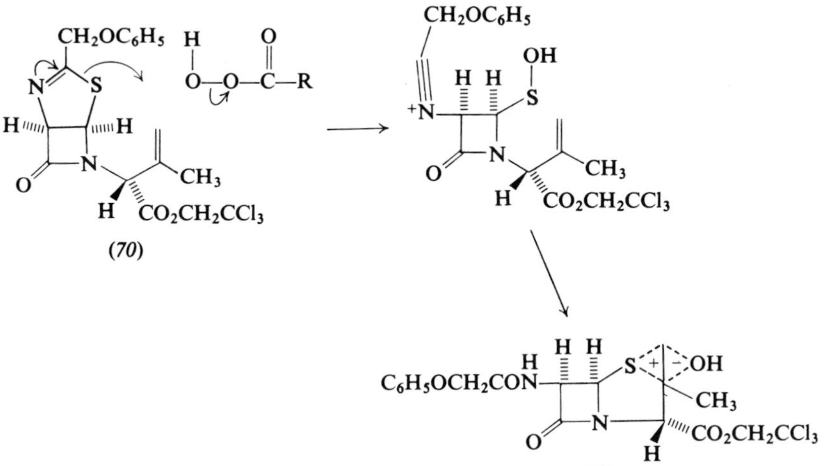

Fig. 7. Mechanism of synthesis of penams and cephems from a thiazoline–azetidinone.

The observed products (18), (83), (84), (39), (85), and (86), except for (18), can be derived from (133) followed by oxidation of the sulfides to the sulfoxides. Product (18), which was only observed in a nonpolar solvent (benzene) was derived from the electrocyclic reaction of the sulfenic acid with the double bond prior to protonation.

C. Synthesis of Cephalexin from Penicillin

The D-phenylglycyldeacetoxycephalosporanic acid (134) (cephalexin),* a derivative of 7-ADCA (135) and D-phenylglycine, has been shown to be a broad spectrum orally absorbed antibiotic (Wick, 1967; Wick and Boniece, 1967; Welles et al., 1968; Griffith and Black, 1968). A successful synthesis of (134) was developed by Ryan and co-workers (1969) by hydrogenolysis of 7-ACA (4) to 7-ADCA (135) followed by acylation of (135) with t-butoxycarbonyl protected D-phenylglycine. Removal of the protecting group

---

* Cephalexin is the generic name for 7-(D-2-amino-3-phenylacetamido)-3-methyl-3-cephem-4-carboxylic acid.

from (*136*) gave (*134*). An alternate route developed by the same authors involved prior acylation of 7-ACA (*4*) with *N-t*-butoxycarbonyl-D-phenylglycine followed by hydrogenolysis of the cephalosporin (*137*) to its deacetoxy derivative (*136*). However, both of these methods suffer from disadvantages of poor yield and the need for extravagant amounts of palladium catalyst in the hydrogenolysis step.

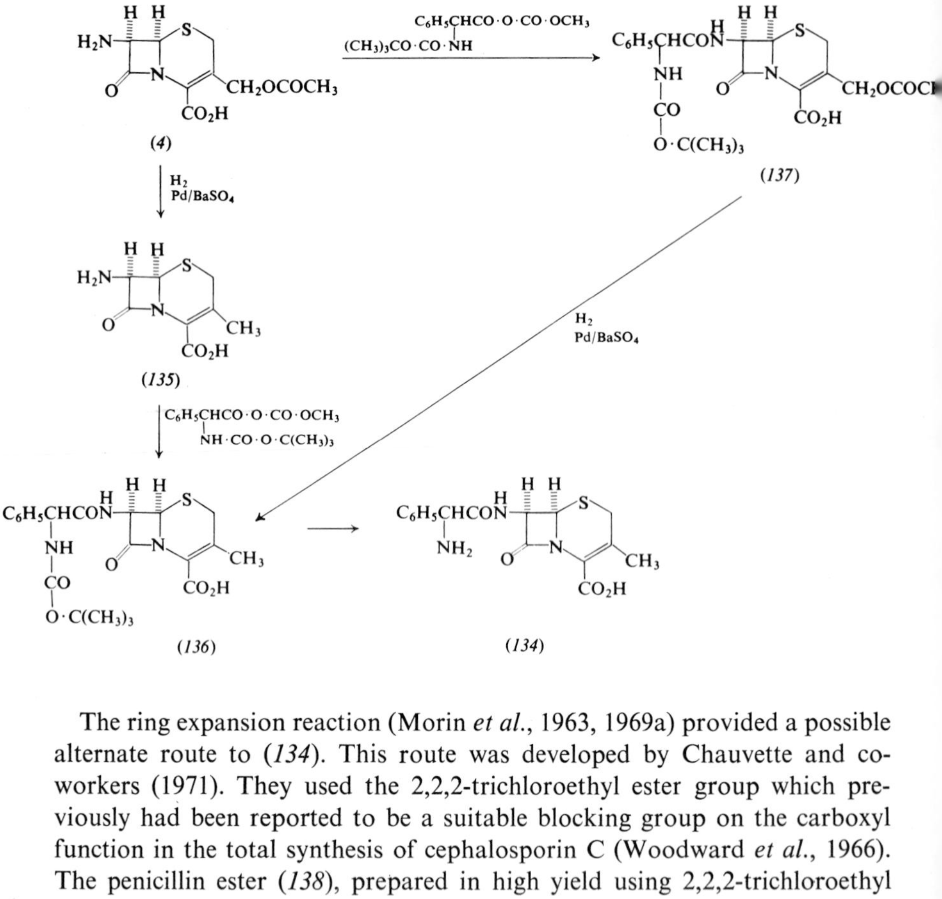

The ring expansion reaction (Morin *et al.*, 1963, 1969a) provided a possible alternate route to (*134*). This route was developed by Chauvette and co-workers (1971). They used the 2,2,2-trichloroethyl ester group which previously had been reported to be a suitable blocking group on the carboxyl function in the total synthesis of cephalosporin C (Woodward *et al.*, 1966). The penicillin ester (*138*), prepared in high yield using 2,2,2-trichloroethyl chloroformate, was oxidized by peracid to the sulfoxide (*18*). As originally conceived, the ring expansion reaction had the disadvantages of a low yield and the formation of non-β-lactam-containing side products. Exploration of the effects of solvents and various catalysts (Can. Patent 817,883; Chauvette *et al.*, 1971) showed that the most effective conditions for ring expansion used dimethylformamide as solvent with acetic anhydride or propane sultone as the other solvent. The phenoxyacetyl side chain of the deacetoxy-3-cepham product (30) from ring expansion was converted to the iminochloride with phosphorous pentachloride. Formation of the iminoether with methanol and subsequent acidic hydrolysis gave 7-aminocephalosporanic acid 2,2,2-trichloroethyl ester (139), isolated as the tosylate salt. The reported yield (Chauvette et al., 1971) of (139) from (18) was 60% overall.

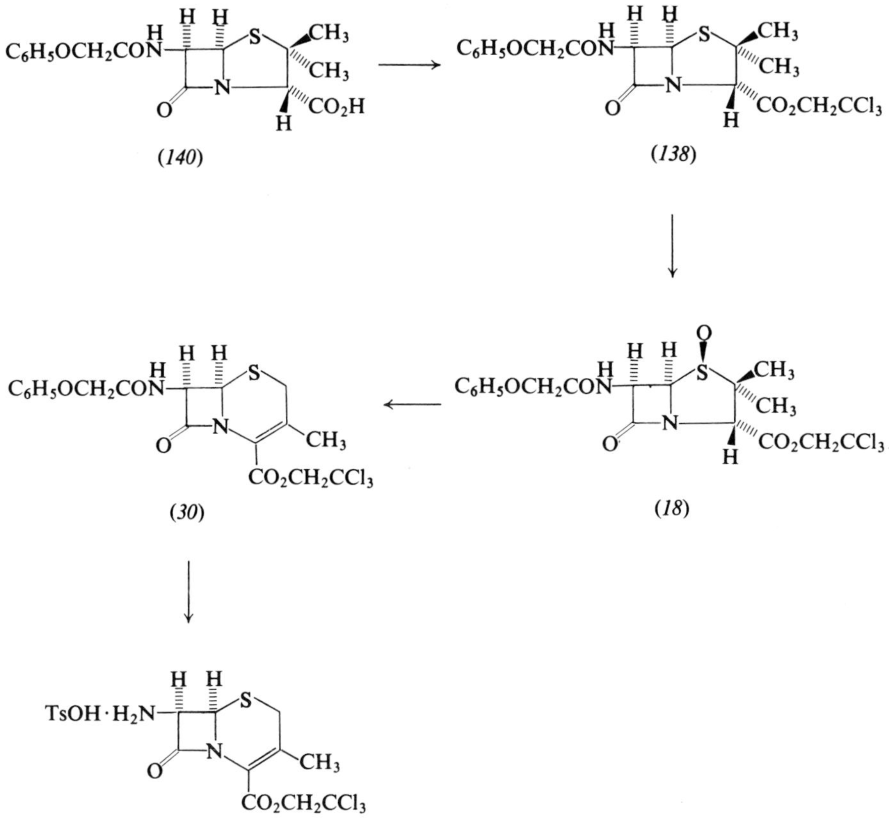

Reacylation of the free base of (139) with either N-2,2,2-trichloroethoxycarbonyl or N-butoxycarbonyl protected D-phenylglycine using a mixed anhydride technique with methyl chloroformate gave doubly protected cephalexin in nearly quantitative yield. Removal of the protecting groups from (141) yields 70% crystalline (134).

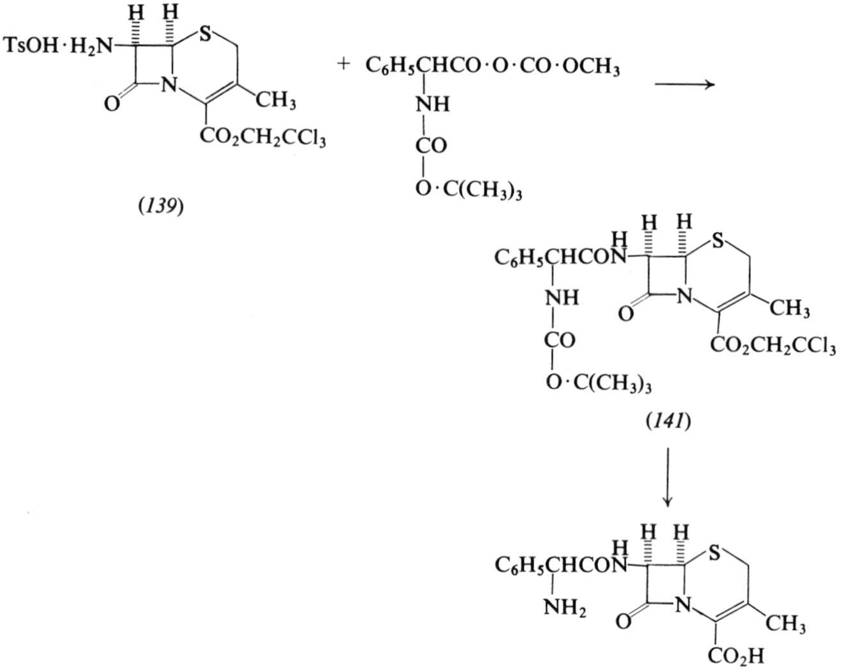

TsOH·H₂N — [structure with β-lactam ring, S, CH₃, CO₂CH₂CCl₃]

(139)

+ C₆H₅CHCO·O·CO·OCH₃   ⟶
        |
        NH
        |
        CO
        |
        O·C(CH₃)₃

C₆H₅CHCON — [structure with β-lactam ring, S, CH₃, CO₂CH₂CCl₃]
|
NH
|
CO
|
O·C(CH₃)₃

(141)

↓

C₆H₅CHCON — [structure with β-lactam ring, S, CH₃, CO₂H]
|
NH₂

(134)

III. Synthesis of Cephalosporin from Penicillin via an Azetidinone–Thiazolidine

In the total synthesis of cephalosporins by Woodward and co-workers (1966), the key intermediate was a thiazolidine–azetidinone (142) prepared by a somewhat lengthy procedure from L-cysteine. This same intermediate has now been synthesized by Heusler and Woodward (1970) from penicillin and represents another penam-to-cephem interconversion. An independent method of preparing related intermediates has also been developed recently by Cooper and José (1970c).

Sheehan and Brandt (1965) published a method of cleaving the thiazolidine ring of phthalimidopenicillin (143) between C-3 and the bridgehead nitrogen atom without rupture of the sensitive β-lactam moiety. This procedure utilized a Curtius rearrangement of the acyl azide (144) prepared by treatment of an activated ester [e.g., (145)] with sodium azide, to the isocyanate (146). This rearrangement was reported to be quite facile, proceeding in high yield at room temperature in 24 hours. Hydrolysis of (146) with tetrahydrofuran/dilute hydrochloric acid under conditions of high dilution gave the aldehyde (147).

The hydrolysis was accompanied by formation of urea (*148*), a problem which was somewhat alleviated when the high dilution technique was used. An alternate solution to this problem was developed by Heusler and Woodward (1970), who converted (*146*) to the carbamate (*149*) with 2,2,2-trichloroethanol, which on treatment with zinc and acetic acid gave the aldehyde in good yield.

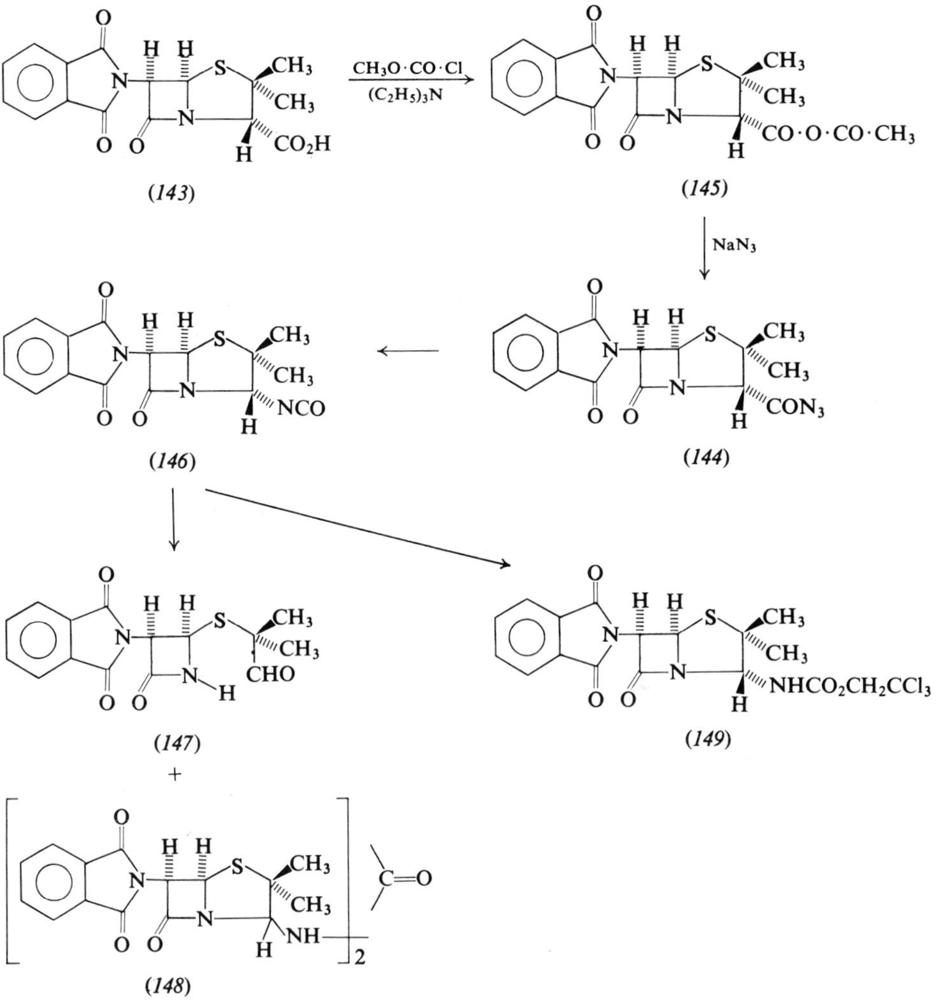

(*143*)　　　　　　　　　　　　　(*145*)

(*146*)　　　　　　　　　　　　　(*144*)

(*147*)　　　　　　　　　　　　　(*149*)

+

(*148*)

When repeating the above reaction sequence with phenoxymethylpenicillin (*140*), Heusler and Woodward (1970) observed that the product from cleavage of the carbamate (*150*) was no longer the expected aldehyde (*151*) but its tautomer, the carbinolamine (*152*). Further variation of the side chain showed a corresponding variation in the relative amounts of the two tautomeric forms. The position of equilibrium was believed to depend primarily on the size of the side chain R, the proportion of aldehyde increasing in the order R = $C_6H_5CH_2CONH-$; $C_6H_5OCH_2CONH-$; $\approx CCl_3CH_2OCONH-$; $<(CH_3)_3$-COCONH–; and

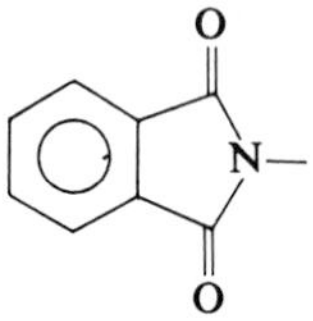

This was believed due to steric interaction of the large substituents with the β-methyl group of the thiazolidine ring. This interaction has previously been postulated as the reason for the lower activation energy in the equilibrium between penicillin sulfoxide and sulfenic acid in the case of the phthalimido side chain (see page 220).

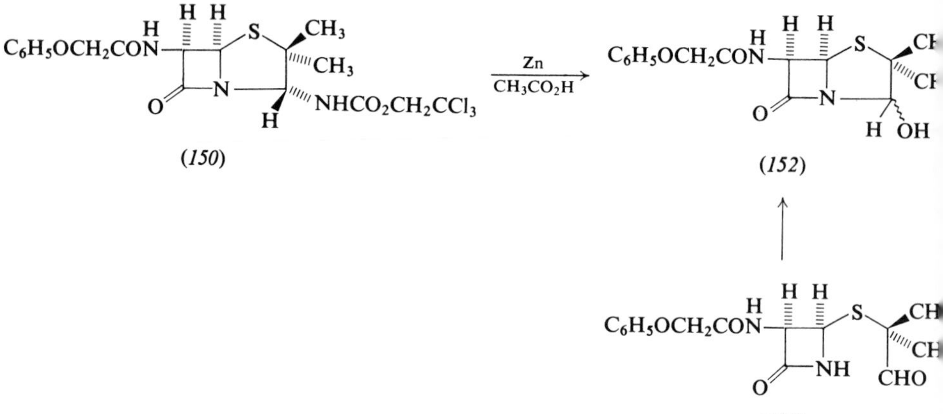

(150)   (152)

(151)

Reduction of the tautomeric mixture with sodium borohydride gave the alcohol (153) which on treatment with lead tetraacetate in benzene gave a complex mixture, from which the two acetoxy azetidinones (154) and (155) could be isolated. Also formed in 15% yield was the unstable acetoxy derivative (156) which rapidly lost the elements of acetic acid on warming to give the vinyl sulfide (157). An alternate method of preparing (157) without the complications of the side reactions was by the treatment of (152) with lead tetraacetate in benzene, when again the product (158) was unstable and facile elimination of acetic acid resulted in the N-formyl derivative (159) in good yield. Treatment with ammonium hydroxide in methylene chloride or, alternatively, decarbonylation with rhodium chloride–triphenylphosphine complex cleaved the *N*-formyl group to give (*157*).

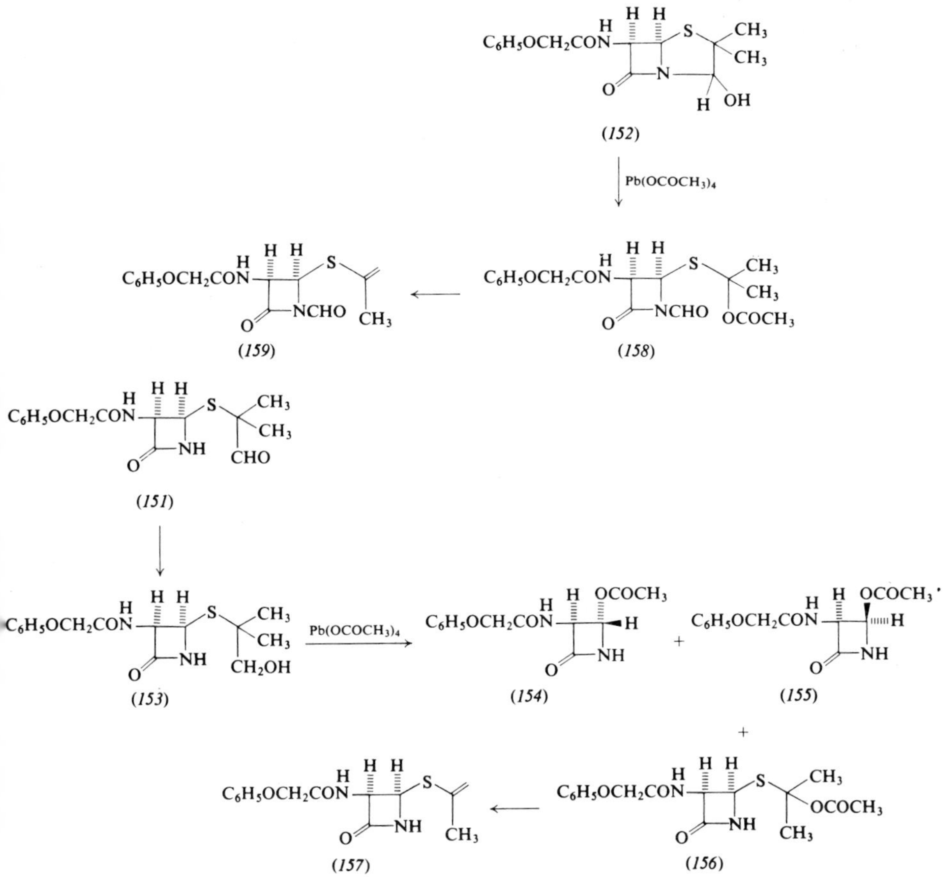

(*152*)

(*159*) ← (*158*)

(*151*)

(*153*) →[Pb(OCOCH₃)₄] (*154*) + (*155*)

+

(*157*) ← (*156*)

When the amide side chain is the *t*-butoxycarbonylamido group, treatment of the vinyl sulfide (*160*) with trifluoroacetic acid liberated the amino group. This immediately underwent an internal addition to the vinyl sulfide to give the thiazolidine–azetidinone (*161*).

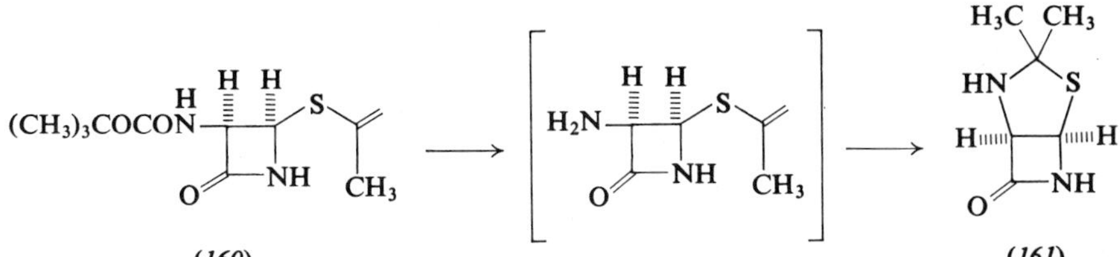

(*160*) → (*161*)

Protection of the thiazolidine nitrogen as the *t*-butoxycarbonyl derivative was accomplished in two stages by reaction first with phosgene to give the stable chlorocarbonyl derivative (*162*) followed by prolonged treatment with refluxing *t*-butanol to give the desired intermediate (*142*).

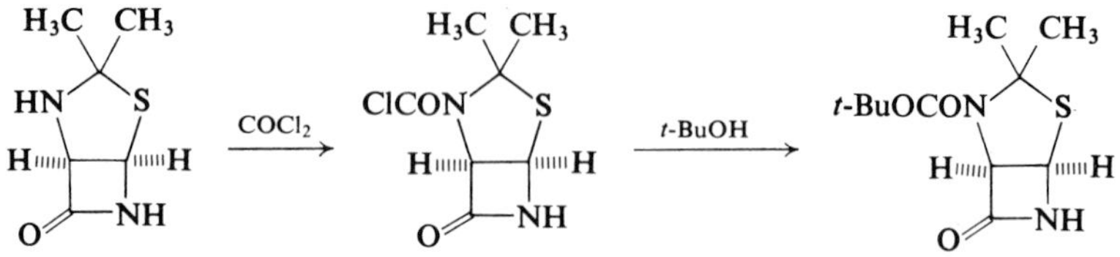

(*161*)   (*162*)   (*142*)

In an attempt to obtain the aminoaldehyde (*163*) by a much simplified procedure, diprotected carbamate (*164*) was treated with zinc/acetic acid and an unexpected product resulted. This initial product was probably (*163*); however, this then underwent an internal cyclization to (*165*). Further reduction of the imine to (*166*) followed by elimination of the thiol and recyclization gave the product (*167*), which was obtained in high overall yield. The *t*-butoxycarbonyl derivative of (*167*) was formed also by the route used for (*161*). This procedure

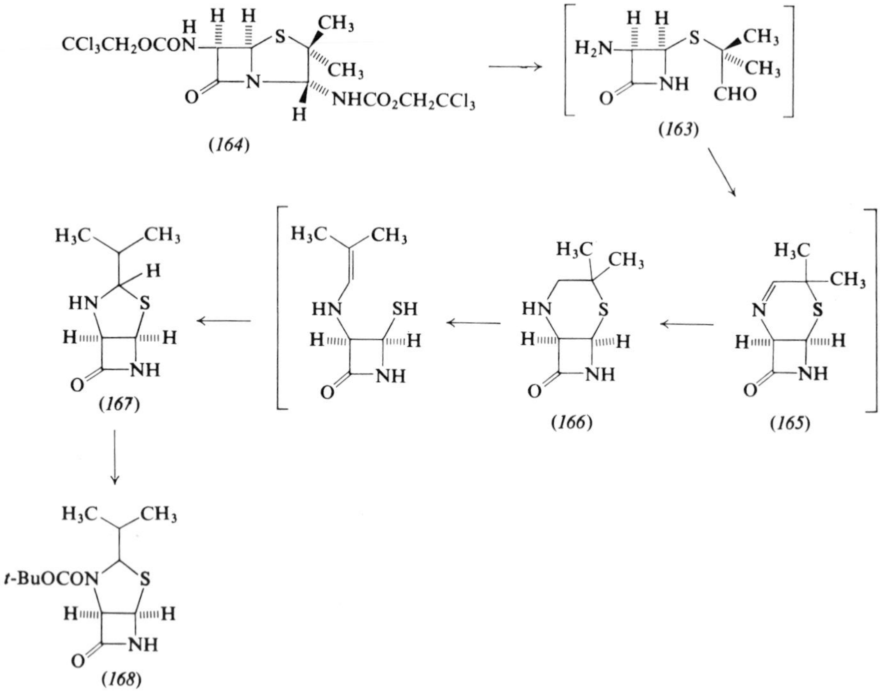

(*164*)   (*163*)

(*167*)   (*166*)   (*165*)

(*168*)

yielded a thiazolidine–azetidinone (*168*) from penicillin in good yield which presumably could also be used in the synthesis of cephalosporin.

An alternate procedure for the synthesis of (*167*) and related derivatives was developed by Cooper and José (1970c). This sequence was based on the thiazolines obtained by rearrangement of penicillin sulfoxide with trimethyl-phosphite. Treatment of phenoxymethylpenicillin sulfoxide (*16*) with tri-methylphosphite gave the thiazoline methyl ester (*169*) in high yield. Isomeri-zation of the double bond to (*170*) and ozonolysis in methylene chloride at −78°C resulted in (*171*) in high yield. Cleavage of the oxalyl side chain with sodium methoxide in methanol gave the thiazoline–azetidinone (*172*) in high overall yield from penicillin. Reduction with aluminum amalgam resulted in the thiazolidine (*173*). Application of this procedure to phenoxyisopropyl-penicillin (*174*) resulted in formation of (*167*), a compound previously pre-pared by Heusler and Woodward (1970).

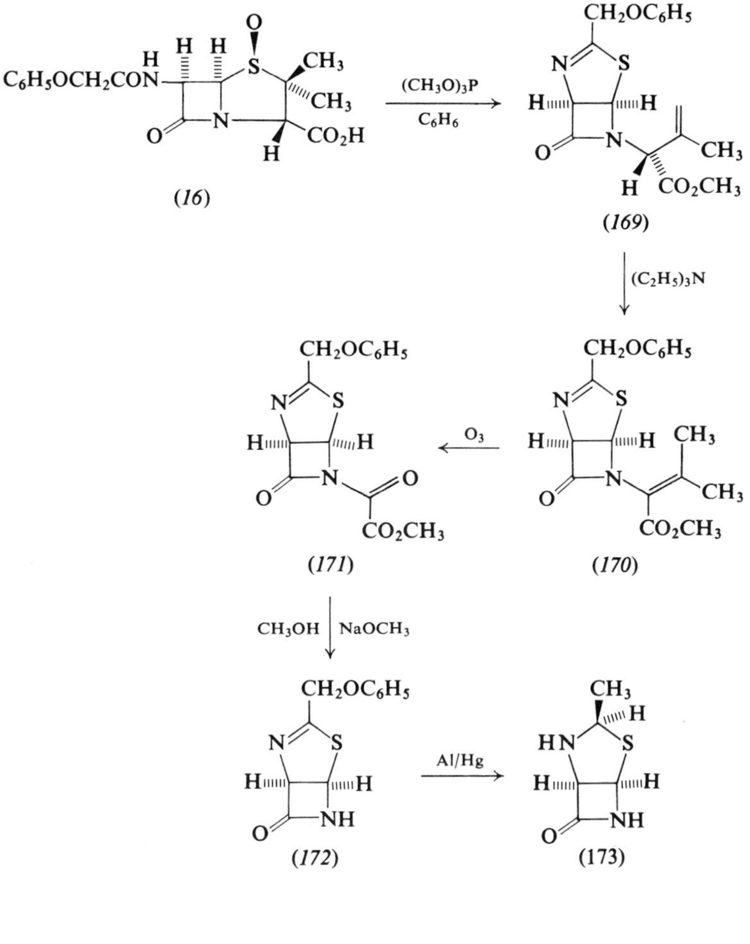

An alternate technique for the removal of the isopropylidene side chain resulted in a second method for the synthesis of (*172*) (Cooper *et al.*, 1969c). This method was based on the controlled hydrolysis of the acetoxy compound

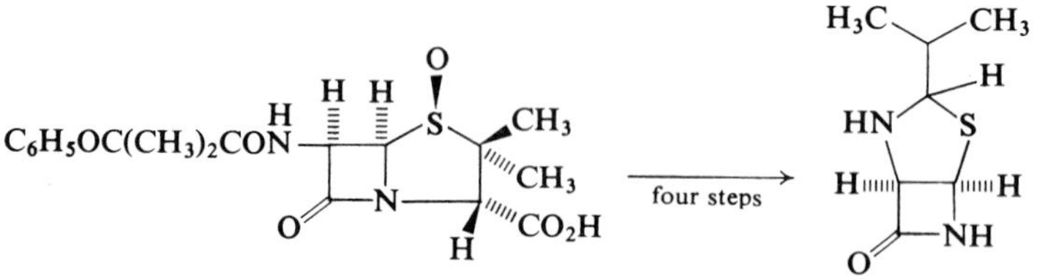

(*174*)   (*167*)

(*175*) to the carbinolamine (*176*) which fragmented to (*172*) and the C_4-unsaturated aldehyde. The acetate (*175*) could be prepared by reaction of either the alcohol (*177*) or acid (*178*), both prepared by the scheme shown below, with lead tetraacetate.

In addition to the application of (*142*) in the synthesis of cephalosporin, Heusler and Woodward (1970) have developed an elegant synthesis of modified β-lactam structures basically related to the cephem system using (*142*) as the key intermediate (see Chapter 6).

IV. Attempted Syntheses of Cephalosporin from Penicillanyl Alcohol

While investigating alternative approaches for the penicillin to cephalosporin conversion, Cooper and José (1970c) discovered two new rearrangements of the penicillin molecule. Stork and Cheng (1965) had shown, by using the bicyclic model compound (*179*), that it was possible to transform a thiazoline ring into the dihydrothiazine ring system (*180*) in excellent yields, giving rise to another possible method of converting penicillin into cephalosporin. The sequence would involve, first of all, obtaining the penicillin having the 2-methyl groups functionalized. Numerous approaches to the general problem of functionalization of isolated methyl groups have evolved in the last few years, mainly from the pioneering work of Barton and co-workers (1960); for a review of this work, see Sammes (1970). The general principle involved in this and parallel investigations was the generation of an alkoxy radical in the correct spatial relationship to the methyl group under attack. An intramolecular hydrogen radical abstraction by the alkoxy radical from the proximate methyl group, followed by reaction of an external radical with the methylene radical thus generated, gave the desired functionalization. Considering Dreiding models of penicillanyl alcohol (*181*), Cooper and José (1970c) reasoned that the

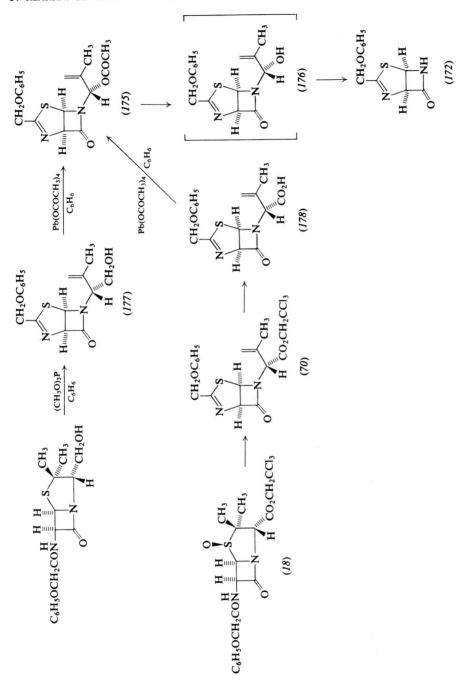

geometrical relationship between the alkoxy radical generated from the alcohol and the α-methyl group would be favorable for an intramolecular functionalization of this substituent. There are numerous methods reported in the literature for generation of the alkoxy radical from an alcohol. However, in this case

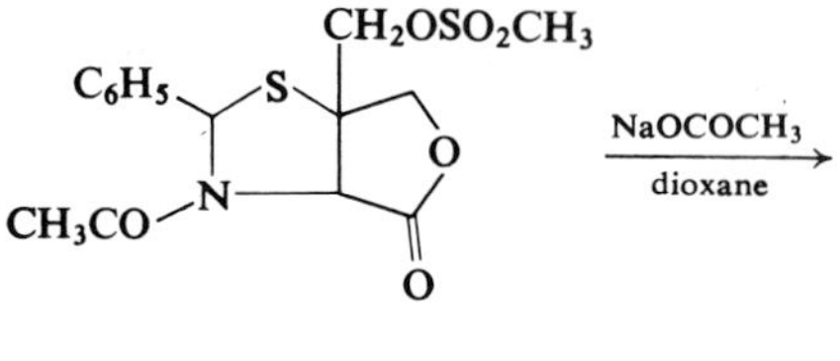

$$CH_2OSO_2CH_3$$

(179)   (180)

NaOCOCH₃ / dioxane

severe limitation is placed on the choice of methods due to the reactivity of the penicillin moiety. The method chosen was the use of lead tetraacetate, a technique used by Swiss workers (Heusler *et al.*, 1960; for a review of this technique, see Heusler and Kalvoda, 1964) with notable success in the steroid field. In applying this reaction to penicillin, Cooper and José (1970c) anticipated that complications concerning reaction of this reagent with the sulfur could arise since lead tetraacetate is known to oxidize sulfides to α-acetoxysulfides or sulfoxides under certain conditions. That this reagent did react with the sulfur atom was shown by the reaction of penicillin alcohol (181) with lead tetraacetate in benzene, when a smooth rearrangement to a new compound (182) (structure determined from spectral and NMR data) was observed. When the reaction was repeated on the phthalimidopenicillin derivative (183), they obtained the product (184) and a small yield of a second compound (185). They also observed that the thiazepine ring conformation as indicated by the

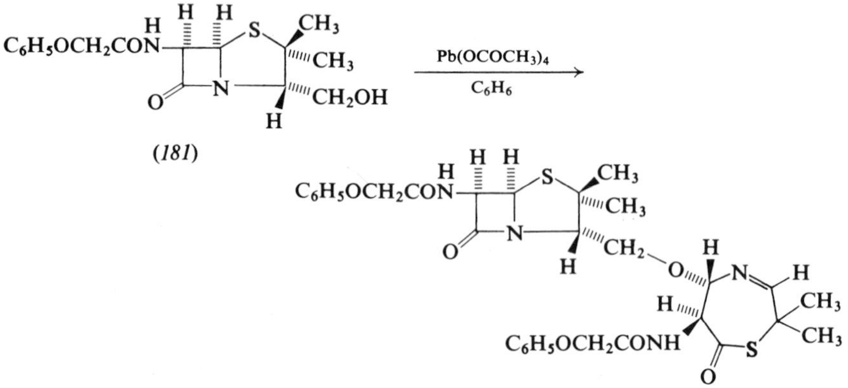

(181)

Pb(OCOCH₃)₄ / C₆H₆

(182)

vicinal hydrogen coupling constants changed markedly depending on the amide substituent. This was due to variation of the steric interaction between the amido side chain and the β-methyl groups (see, also, pages 220 and 232).

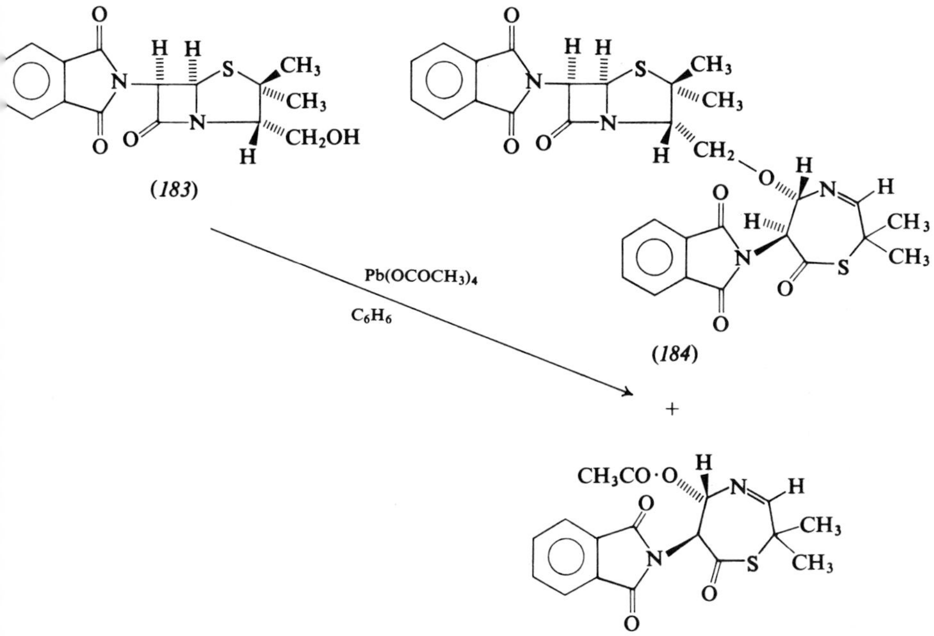

Reaction had indeed occurred at the postulated reaction site, the lead tetra-acetate complexing with sulfur and causing an S^{N_2} displacement reaction at C-5. The only displacing nucleophiles available in this system were the alkoxy group of a second molecule or, to a lesser extent, the acetoxy group. Attack by sulfur on the β-lactam carbonyl group, together with a concerted loss of formaldehyde, was proposed as a mechanism which explained the observed products (see Fig. 8).

In an attempt to prevent this interaction, these investigators oxidized the penicillanyl alcohol to its sulfoxide (186), which on treatment with lead tetraacetate/iodine in refluxing benzene gave a new rearrangement product. It was assigned the cyclic sulfinate structure (187). The same rearrangement also occurred with the phthalimidopenicillin derivative (188), with either lead tetraacetate and iodine or, alternatively, mercuric oxide and iodine. However, the product in this case (189) differed from (187) in the stereochemistry of the sulfoxide bond, (189) having the α configuration and (187) having the β configuration.

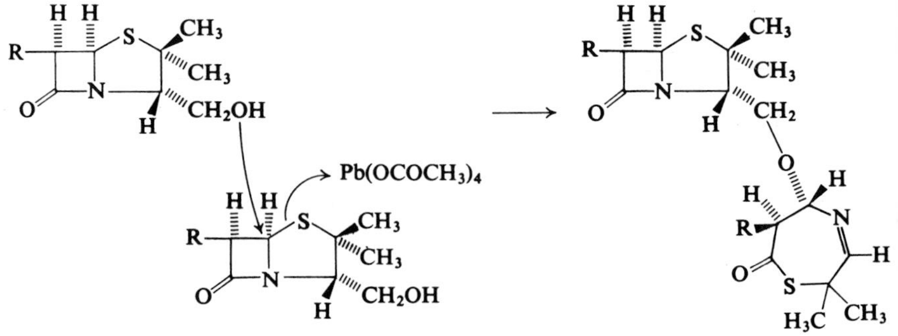

Fig. 8. Mechanism of reaction of penicillanyl alcohol with lead tetraacetate.

The reaction was proposed (Cooper and José, 1970c) to proceed through the sulfenic acid with the nucleophilic sulfur attacking the hypoiodite and displacing iodide ion. The configuration of the S–O bond of the sulfinate (*187*) was

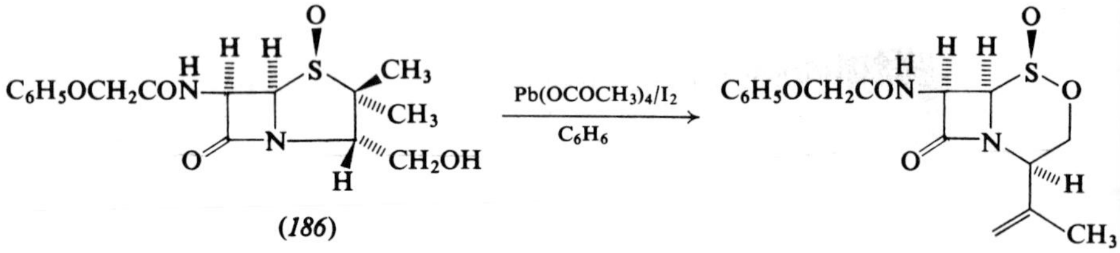

controlled by hydrogen bonding to the amido side chain such that (*187*) has the (*S*) configuration. When hydrogen bonding is absent, as in (*189*), the S–O bond configuration was sterically controlled, resulting in the (*R*) configuration.

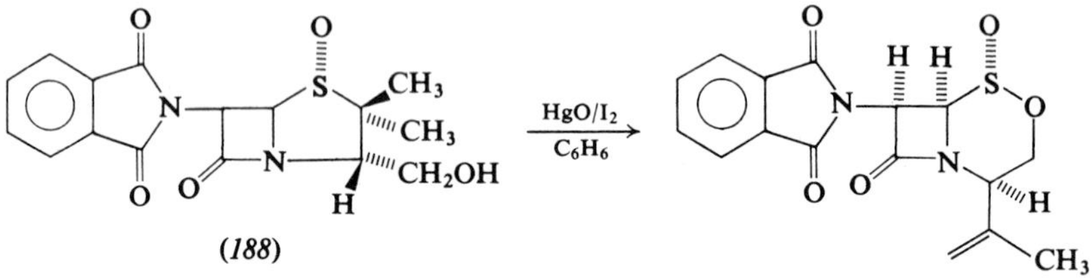

To confirm nucleophilic attack by the sulfenic acid sulfur atom on a suitable group at the three position, Cooper *et al.* (1970c) synthesized the diazoketone sulfoxide (*190*) by oxidizing the known sulfide precursor (Ramsey and Stoodley, 1969) with *m*-chloroperbenzoic acid.

Treatment of (*190*) in refluxing benzene with anhydrous copper sulfate gave isomeric sulfoxides (*191*) and (*192*). Both were oxidized by *m*-chloroperbenzoic acid to the same sulfone (*193*).

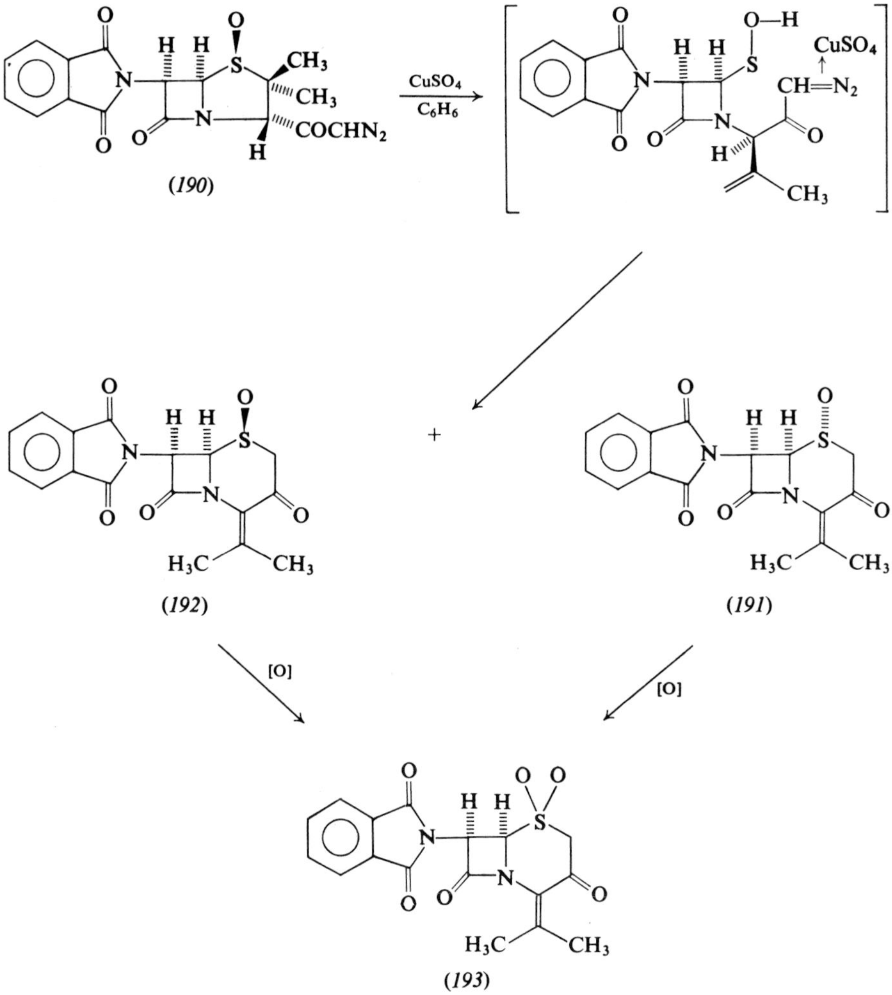

The isolated products were interpreted as further proof of the intermediacy of a sulfenic acid and of the nucleophilicity of the sulfur in the sulfenic acid.

The functionalization of the α-methyl group of a penicillin by internal radical abstraction suffers from the disadvantage of being a relatively high energy process. In such a reactive moiety as the penam system, it appeared that side reactions became too competitive to allow the desired reaction to proceed.

V. Attempted Syntheses of Cephalosporin from Anhydropenicillin

Wolfe and co-workers (1963, 1968) found that treatment of an activated ester derivative of penicillin [e.g., (*194*)] with excess triethylamine causes a rearrangement of the thiazolidine ring without concomitant rupture of the β-lactam ring. The product, obtained in yields of 20–30%, was assigned the structure (*195*) from NMR and IR spectral evidence. Because the rearrangement involved the loss of one molecule of water from penicillin, the product was named anhydropenicillin. In agreement with the designated structure, acetone was obtained on ozonolysis of (*195*), whereas no acetone could be detected on ozonolysis

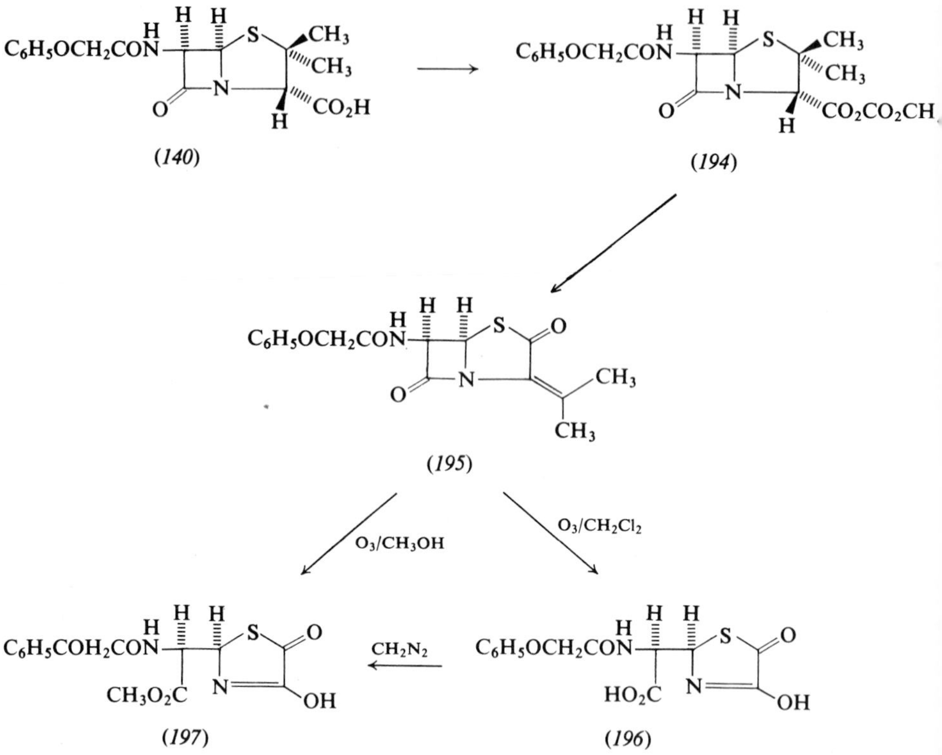

of the parent penicillin. Other investigators (Cooper, 1970b) found that the other product from ozonolysis in methylene chloride was the acid (*196*). Alternatively, use of methanol as solvent in the ozone reaction gave the ester (*197*), a compound also obtained by treatment of (*196*) with diazomethane.

Wolfe *et al.* (1963) suggested that rearrangement involves β elimination of the sulfur in a reverse Michael reaction, followed by recyclization of the intermediate thiol anion with the activated ester function (see Fig. 9).

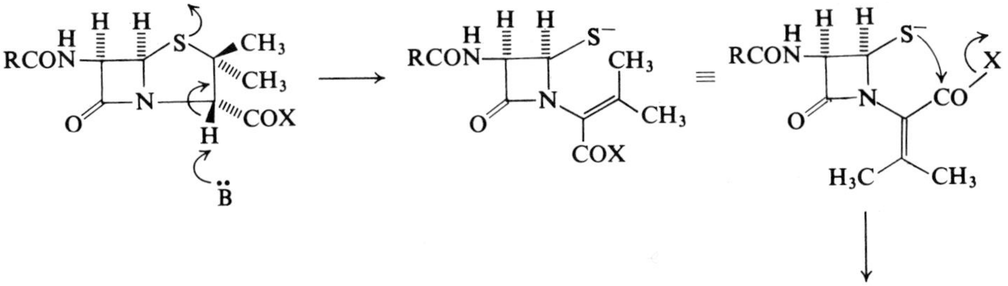

(*195*)

Fig. 9. Mechanism of rearrangement of penicillin to anhydropenicillin.

The anhydropenicillin rearrangement was also observed by Clayton (1969), using methyl 6,6-dibromopenicillanate (*198*) as the substrate. Besides the anhydropenicillin (*199*), a second derivative was isolated in 15% yield. This latter product was assigned the diester structure (*200*) and was rationalized as being formed by trapping of the intermediate sulfur anion by an intermolecular reaction with the ethoxycarbonyl group of a second molecule.

Further confirmation of the first part of this mechanism was obtained by Kukolja and co-workers (1969). They treated phenoxymethylpenicillin (*140*) with methyl chloroformate and triethylamine in dimethylformamide and obtained two new products (*201* and *202*).

The structure for (*201*) was established by consideration of its mass spectrum and NMR. Treatment of (*201*) with methanolic base caused hydrolysis of the oxazolone to the methyl ester (*203*), providing further evidence for the proposed structure. One fact of note in the IR spectrum was the existence of peaks at 1802 (sh) and 1776 cm^{-1}. Characteristic of 4-alkylidene-5(4)-oxazolones, these peaks can easily be confused with signals arising from a β-lactam carbonyl group. This confusion seems to have occurred with (*202*), which was recently identified (Kukolja *et al.*, 1969) as the symmetrical sulfide. This compound was found to be identical with the "dimer" obtained by Wolfe *et al.* (1963), which had been reported to contain a β-lactam based on IR evidence ($\nu = 1786$ cm^{-1}).

The anhydropenicillins are characterized by considerable stability and, in contrast to the penicillins, have the two methyl groups potentially activated by the double bond. Consequently, they are attractive intermediates for further transformations, in particular, the conversion of a penam to the 3-cephem

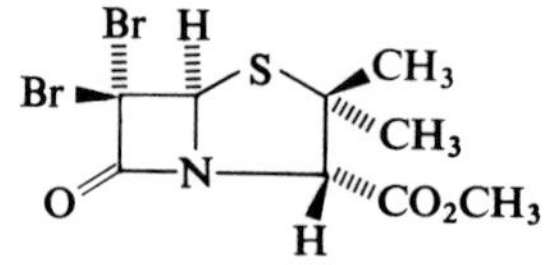

(198)

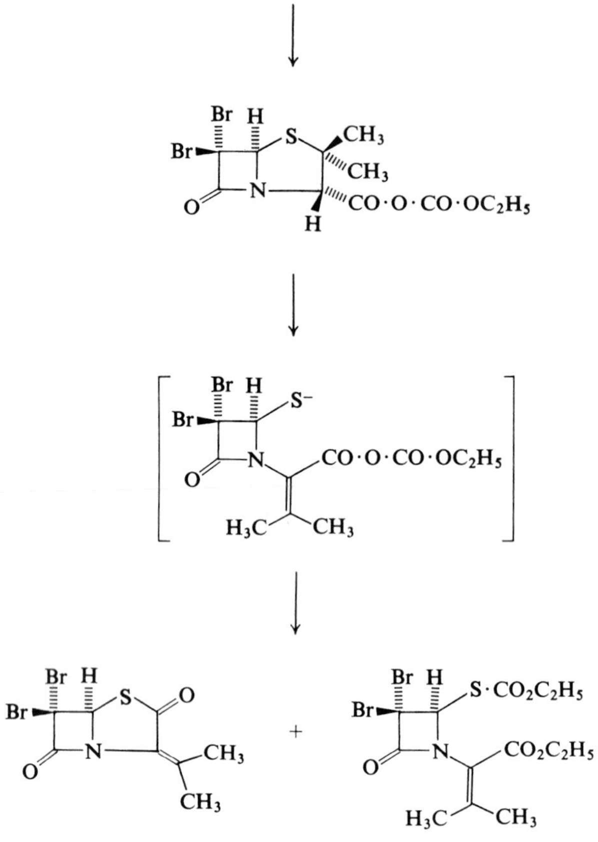

(199)   +   (200)

system. Wolfe and co-workers (1969a) found that the two allylic methyl groups were resistant to the action of both lead tetraacetate and selenium dioxide. Treatment of phenoxyethylanhydropenicillin (204) with mercuric acetate in refluxing benzene, however, gave a novel oxidative rearrangement to a product designated as anhydropenicillene. They suggested this product was a mixture of at least two of the three possible tautomeric structures (205), (206), and (207).

(201)

(203)

(202)

Anhydropenicillene was presumed to arise because of the presence of other more reactive sites of oxidation than the allylic methyl groups in the anhydropenicillin molecule (i.e., amide side chain, sulfur atom, and β-lactam nitrogen).

(204)

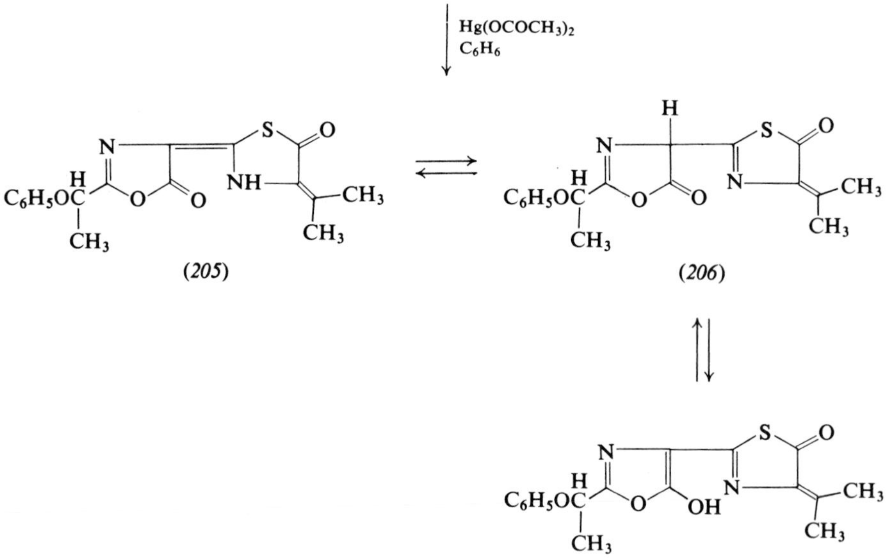

Hg(OCOCH₃)₂
C₆H₆

(205)   (206)

(207)

The initial reaction product of mercuric acetate with anhydropenicillin was found to be the mercury-containing dimer (208). Treatment of this dimer under the same reaction conditions failed to yield anhydropenicillene, indicating that (208) was the result of a side reaction and probably not an intermediate in the formation of (205). An alternate proposed pathway involved the intermediacy of (209), which was synthesized by treatment of anhydropenicillin (204) with boron trifluoride in methylene chloride. Reaction of (209) with mercuric acetate in benzene then yielded anhydropenicillene (205).

Wolfe and co-workers (1969b) succeeded in reversing the anhydropenicillin rearrangement; treatment of phthalimidoanhydropenicillin (210) with aqueous dimethylsulfoxide at pH 7.4 yielded 86 % (based on recovered starting material) of the penicillin (211).

Although protonation of the carbanion at C-3 in the Michael addition intermediate may result in the natural (D) configuration or its epimer, steric factors are most likely the controlling influences since only the penicillin with the natural configuration at C-3 was obtained from the reaction.

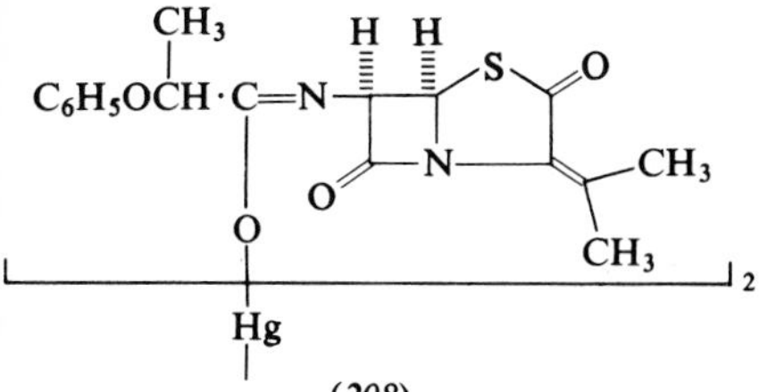

(208)

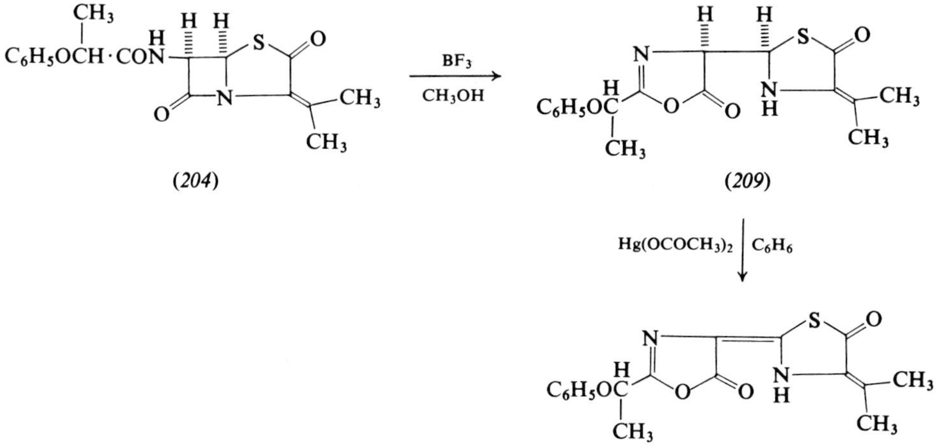

(204)
$\xrightarrow[\text{CH}_3\text{OH}]{\text{BF}_3}$
(209)

$\text{Hg(OCOCH}_3)_2 \mid \text{C}_6\text{H}_6$

(205)

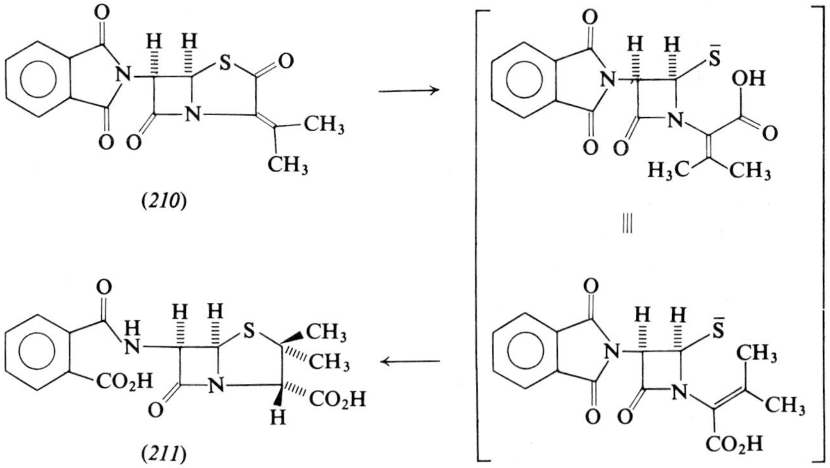

(210)

$\xrightarrow{\hspace{1cm}}$

|||

(211)

VI. Some Miscellaneous Reactions of β-Lactam Compounds

There are a few rearrangements of penicillin and cephalosporin which have been reported in the chemical literature which retain the β-lactam moiety intact and which have not been discussed elsewhere.

A. Reactions with t-Butylhypochlorite

One of the more interesting of these was reported in its original form by Sheehan (1964) and is the reaction of penicillin with t-butylhypochlorite. In the presence of a tertiary amine base the oxazolone (212) was isolated from the

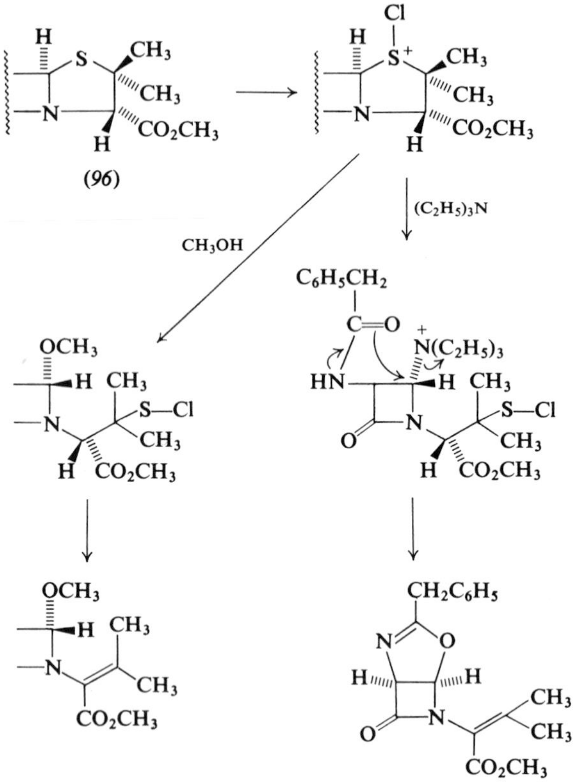

Fig. 10. Mechanism of reaction of penicillin with tert-butyl hypochlorite.

reaction of benzylpenicillin methyl ester (*96*). No experimental details or suggested mechanism was reported. Structural evidence was provided by the reduction of (*212*) to the desthiopenicillin derivative (*213*). More recently the same compound (*212*) was isolated by Barton *et al.* (1969) as a minor product of the oxidation of benzylpenicillin methyl ester (*96*) with iodobenzenedichloride. The most likely mechanistic pathway would appear to involve initial attack by positive chlorine on the sulfur atom followed by cleavage of the S–C-5 bond. Stabilization of the resulting carbonium ion can then be achieved by association of the triethylamine from the less hindered α-side of the molecule. Internal attack of the side chain on this carbonium ion gives the oxazolone (see Fig. 10). The stereochemical requirements of the internal attack of the amide oxygen preclude any direct displacement at C-5 and necessitate the postulation of an intermediate of inverted stereochemistry at C-5.

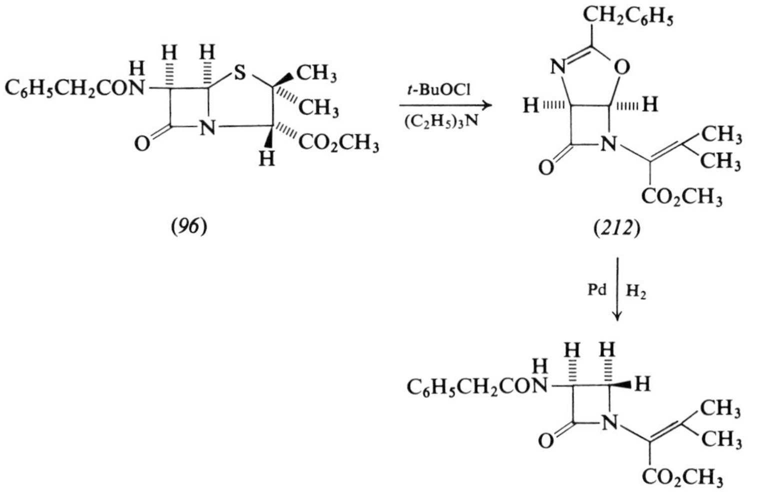

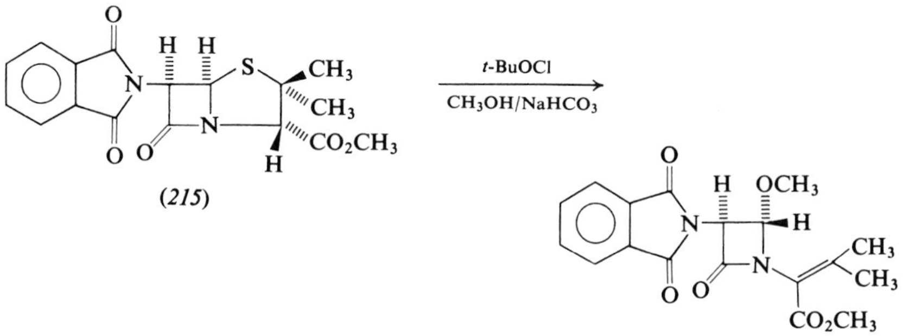

A direct displacement at C-5 can be achieved as evidenced by results of Spry (1970b) when, in the presence of an external nucleophile and in the absence of any possible amide side chain involvement, it was found possible to isolate the 5-methoxy derivative (*214*) by reaction of phthalimidopenicillin methyl ester (*215*) with *t*-butylhypochlorite in methanol.

B. Reactions of Penicillinyl Diazoketone

During work aimed at chemical modification of the functional centers of penicillin, Ramsey and Stoodley (1969) investigated rearrangements of the diazoketone (*216*). The preparation of (*216*) from phthalimidopenicillin (*143*) was achieved by treatment of either the acid chloride (*217*) (Kleiver *et al.*, 1966) or the active ester (*218*) (Daicoviciu and Postescu, 1967; Ramsey and Stoodley, 1969) with diazomethane. Irradiation of the diazoketone (*219*) in aqueous dioxane had been shown to give the homologous acid (*220*) in 19% yield (Kleiver *et al.*, 1966).

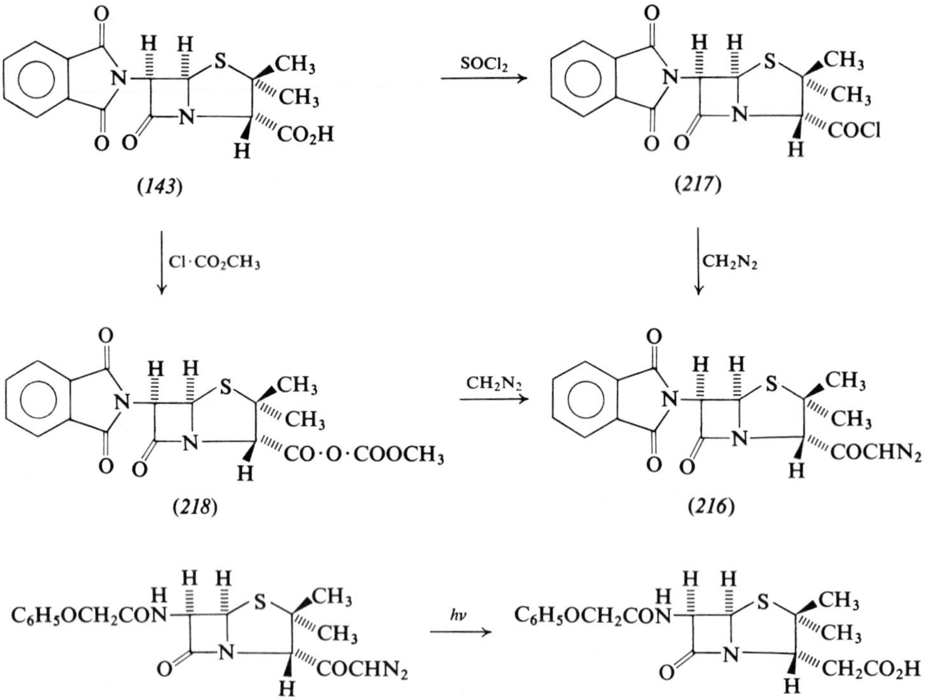

Ramsey and Stoodley (1969) found that irradiation of (216) gave the analogous homoacid (221) in 22% yield, together with a second acidic material (222) isolated as its methyl ester and shown to have structure (223). The origin of this second product presumably is from interaction of the bridgehead nitrogen with an intermediate oxocarbene (see Fig. 11).

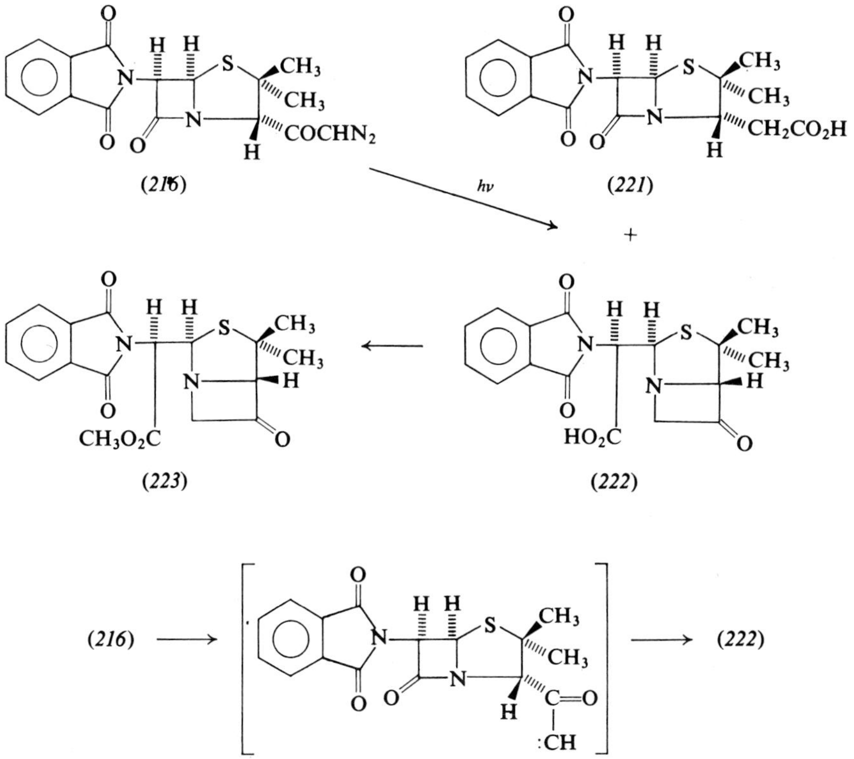

Fig. 11. Mechanism of rearrangement of penicillin diazoketone.

However, the chloroketone (224) rearranged to a new β-lactam-containing ring system (Ramsey and Stoodley, 1970) which the authors indicated possibly offered valuable entry to new types of cepham derivatives. The chloroketone (224) was obtained by treatment of the diazoketone (216) with hydrochloric acid in acetone. In the presence of triethylamine, (224) was quantitatively converted into a 2:3 mixture of two isomers, assigned structures (225) and (226). The two sulfoxides of (225) were shown previously (see page 241) to have been obtained from the corresponding diazoketone sulfoxide.

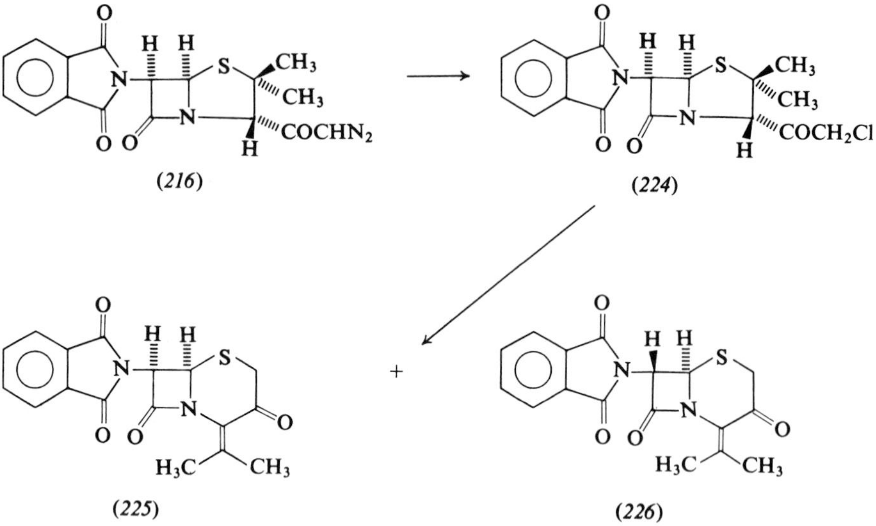

(216)   (224)

(225)   +   (226)

Acknowledgments

We wish to express our gratitude to Dr. R. B. Morin and Dr. L. D. Hatfield for helpful discussions concerning most of our own original work in this chapter, to Miss F. L. José for excellent experimental assistance, and to Mrs. P. Hager and Miss P. Guffin for careful patience in typing and proofreading the manuscript.

References

Abraham, E. P., and Newton, G. G. F. (1961). *Biochem. J.* **79**, 377.
Archer, R. A., and Demarco, P. V. (1969). *J. Amer. Chem. Soc.* **91**, 1530.
Barton, D. H. R., Beaton, J. M., Gello, L. E., and Pechet, M. M. (1960). *J. Amer. Chem. Soc.* **82**, 2640.
Barton, D. H. R., Comer, F., and Sammes, P. G. (1969). *J. Amer. Chem. Soc.* **91**, 1529.
Barton, D. H. R. Comer, F., Greig, D. C. T., Lucente, G., Sammes, P. G., and Underwood, W. G. E. (1970a). *Chem. Commun.* 1059.
Barton, D. H. R., Greig, D. C. T., Lucente, G., Sammes, P. G., Tayler, M. V., Cooper, C. M., Hewitt, G., and Underwood, W. G. E. (1970b). *Chem. Commun.* 1683.
Canada Patent 817,883.
Chauvette, R. R., Pennington, P. A., Ryan, C. W., Cooper, R. D. G., José, F. L., Wright, I. G., Van Heyningen, E. M., and Huffman, G. W. (1971). *J. Org. Chem.* **36**, 1259.
Chow, A. W., Hall, N. M., and Hoover, J. R. E. (1962). *J. Org. Chem.* **27**, 1381.
Clarke, H. T., Johnson, J. R., and Robinson, R. (1949). "The Chemistry of Penicillin." Princeton Univ. Press, Princeton, New Jersey.
Clayton, J. P. (1969). *J. Chem. Soc. C* 2123.
Cooper, R. D. G. (1970a). *J. Amer. Chem. Soc.* **92**, 5010.
Cooper, R. D. G. (1970b). Unpublished results.
Cooper, R. D. G., and José, F. L. (1970a). *J. Amer. Chem. Soc.* **92**, 2575.

Cooper, R. D. G., and José, F. L. (1970b). Abstracts of 160th Amer. Chem. Soc. Nat. Meeting, Chicago, Illinois, September 14–17.
Cooper, R. D. G., and José, F. L. (1970c). Unpublished results.
Cooper, R. D. G., Demarco, P. V., Cheng, J. C., and Jones, N. D. (1969a). *J. Amer. Chem. Soc.* **91**, 1408.
Cooper, R. D. G., Demarco, P. V., and Spry, D. O. (1969b). *J. Amer. Chem. Soc.* **91**, 1528.
Cooper, R. D. G., José, F. L., and Fukuda, D. S. (1969c). Unpublished results.
Cooper, R. D. G., Demarco, P. V., Murphy, C. F., and Spangle, L. A. (1970a). *J. Chem. Soc. C* 340.
Cooper, R. D. G., Hatfield, L. D., and Spry, D. O. (1970b). Unpublished results.
Cooper, R. D. G., José, F. L., and Shuman, R. (1970c). Unpublished results.
Daicoviciu, C., and Postescu, D. (1967). *Rev. Chim. (Sommaria)* **18**, 179.
Daniels, C. J., Fisher, J. W., Foster, B. J., Gutowski, G. E., and Hatfield, L. D. (1970). Abstracts of 160th Amer. Chem. Soc. Nat. Meeting, Chicago, Illinois, Sept. 14–17.
Denney, D. B., and Relles, H. M. (1964). *J. Amer. Chem. Soc.* **86**, 3897.
Essery, J. M., Dabado, K., Gottstein, W. J., Hullstrand, A., and Cheney, L. C. (1965). *J. Org. Chem.* **30**, 4388.
Fuson, R. C., Price, C. C., and Burness, D. M. (1946). *J. Org. Chem.* **11**, 475.
Griffith, R. S., and Black, H. R. (1968). *Clin. Med.* **75**, 11.
Guddal, E., Morch, P., and Tybring, L. (1962). *Tetrahedron Lett.* 381.
Gutowski, G. E., Foster, B. J., Daniels, C. J., Hatfield, L. D., and Fisher, J. W. (1971a). *Tetrahedron Lett.* 3433.
Gutowski, G. E., Daniels, C. J., and Cooper, R. D. G. (1971b). *Tetrahedron Lett.* 3429.
Hatfield, L. D., Fisher, J. W., José, F. L., and Cooper, R. D. G. (1970). *Tetrahedron Lett.* 4897.
Heusler, K., and Kalvoda, J. (1964). *Ang. Chem. Int. Ed.* **3**, 525.
Heusler, K., and Woodward, R. B. (1970). German Offenlegungsschift 1,935,607.
Heusler, K., Kalvoda, J., Meystre, C., Wieland, P., Anner, G., Wettsteen, A., Cainelli, G., Arigoni, D., and Jeger, O. (1960). *Experientia* **16**, 21.
Hodgkin, D., and Maslen, E. N. (1961). *Biochem. J.* **79**, 393.
Kaiser, G. V., Cooper, R. D. G., Koehler, R. E., Murphy, C. F., Webber, J. A., Wright, I. G., and Van Heyningen, E. M. (1970). *J. Org. Chem.* **35**, 2430.
Kingsbury, C. A., and Cram, D. J. (1960). *J. Amer. Chem. Soc.* **82**, 1810.
Kleiver, E. M., Senyavina, L. B., and Khokhlov, A. S. (1966). *Khun. Geterotsikl. Soedinenii* 702.
Kukolja, S., Cooper, R. D. G., and Morin, R. B. (1969). *Tetrahedron Lett.* 3381.
Leonard, N. J., and Wilson, G. E., Jr. (1964). *J. Amer. Chem. Soc.* **86**, 5307.
Morin, R. B., and Spry, D. O. (1970). *Chem. Commun.* 335.
Morin, R. B., Jackson, B. G., Flynn, E. H., and Roeske, R. W. (1962). *J. Amer. Chem. Soc.* **84**, 3400.
Morin, R. B., Jackson, B. G., Mueller, R. A., Lavagnino, E. R., Scanlon, W. B., and Andrews, S. L. (1963). *J. Amer. Chem. Soc.* **85**, 1896.
Morin, R. B., Jackson, B. G., Mueller, R. A., Lavagnino, E. R., Scanlon, W. B., and Andrews, S. L. (1969a). *J. Amer. Chem. Soc.* **91**, 1401.
Morin, R. B., Spry, D. O., and Mueller, R. A. (1969b). *Tetrahedron Lett.* 849.
Morin, R. B., McGrath, T., and Shuman, R. (1970). Unpublished results.
Mueller, W. H. (1969). *Ang. Chem. Int. Ed.* **8**, 482.
Newton, G. G. F., and Abraham, E. P. (1955). *Nature* **175**, 548.
Ramsay, B. G., and Stoodley, R. J. (1969). *J. Chem. Soc. C* 1319.
Ramsay, B. G., and Stoodley, R. J. (1970). *Chem. Commun.* 1517.
Rayner, D. R., Gordon, A. J., and Mislow, K. (1968). *J. Amer. Chem. Soc.* **90**, 4854.

254 R. D. G. COOPER AND D. O. SPRY

Ryan, C. W., Simon, R. L., and Van Heyningen, E. M. (1969). *J. Med. Chem.* **12**, 310.
Sammes, P. G. (1970). *Synthesis* **12**, 636.
Sheehan, J. C. (1964). *In* "Molecular Modification in Drug Design" (R. F. Gould, ed.), p. 15. Advan. in Chem. Ser. No. 45, Amer. Chem. Soc., Washington, D.C.
Sheehan, J. C., and Brandt, K. G. (1965). *J. Amer. Chem. Soc.* **87**, 5468.
Sheehan, J. C., Henery-Logan, K. R., and Johnson, D. A. (1953). *J. Amer. Chem. Soc.* **75**, 3293.
Smart, M. C., and Rogers, D. (1970). *Chem. Commun.* 1060.
Spry, D. O. (1970a). *J. Amer. Chem. Soc.* **92**, 5006.
Spry, D. O. (1970b). Unpublished results.
Stork, G., and Cheng, H. T. (1965). *J. Amer. Chem. Soc.* **87**, 3784.
Sykes, P., and Todd, A. R. (1949). *In* "The Chemistry of Penicillin" (H. T. Clarke, J. R. Johnson, and R. Robinson, eds.), pp. 156, 927, 946, 1008. Princeton Univ. Press, Princeton, New Jersey.
Webber, J. A., Van Heyningen, E. M., and Vasileff, R. T. (1969). *J. Amer. Chem. Soc.* **91**, 5674.
Welles, J. S., Froman, R. O., Gibson, W. R., Owen, N. V., and Anderson, R. C. (1968). *Antimicrob. Ag. Chemother.* 489.
Wick, W. E. (1967). *Appl. Microbiol.* **15**, 4.
Wick, W. E., and Boniece, W. S. (1967). *Proc. 6th Int. Congr. Chemother. Vienna* 717.
Wolfe, S., Godfrey, J. C., Haldrege, C. T., and Perron, Y. G. (1963). *J. Amer. Chem. Soc.* **85**, 643.
Wolfe, S., Godfrey, J. C., Haldrege, C. T., and Perron, Y. G. (1968). *Can. J. Chem.* **46**, 2549.
Wolfe, S., Ferrari, C., and Lee, W. S. (1969a). *Tetrahedron Lett.* 3885.
Wolfe, S., Bassett, R. N., Caldwell, S. M., and Nasson, F. (1969b). *J. Amer. Chem. Soc.* **91**, 7205.
Woodward, R. B., Heusler, K., Gosteli, J., Naegeli, P., Oppolzer, W., Ramage, R., Ranganathan, S., and Vorbrugge, N. (1966). *J. Amer. Chem. Soc.* **88**, 852.

Chapter 6

TOTAL SYNTHESES OF PENICILLINS

AND CEPHALOSPORINS

KARL HEUSLER

I. Introduction

A. General Considerations

In view of the highly efficient biosynthesis of penicillins and cephalosporins by microorganisms, a total synthesis of these antibiotics can hardly be expected to be of immediate practical importance. However, aside from the academic interest in a total synthesis of any natural product, there is an additional aspect which makes the chemical synthesis of the β-lactam antibiotics especially attractive. The microorganisms so far investigated are only capable of producing a limited number of structural variations, in fact, only penicillins and cephalosporin C. It is virtually certain that these two nuclei are not the only ones which can be used in the preparation of derivatives with antibacterial activity. Although intensive efforts have been and still are directed towards modifications of these nuclei, a much broader variability can be expected once compounds of this type are available by total synthesis. Thus, a more satisfactory answer to the complex question of structure–activity relationship can be expected from such studies.

The experiences gained so far seem to confirm the assumption that for antibacterial activity a β-lactam-containing bicyclic system with an acylated amino group α to the lactam carbonyl, stereochemically arranged as in the natural L-amino acids is essential. The presence of a free carboxyl function and of the sulfur atom *cis* oriented with respect to the acylated amino group also seems to be necessary, but not enough structural variations are known to establish these conditions with certainty. In this chapter only those synthetic approaches will be dealt with which have led to penicillins or cephalosporin or related compounds that at least show some antibacterial activity. The synthesis of inactive model compounds (lacking one or the other of the essential features) will not be discussed unless their preparation has a direct bearing on the synthesis of an active compound.

It is quite clear that the difficulty involved in the total synthesis of both penicillins and cephalosporins is not due to the size of these molecules (in terms of the total number of atoms) nor is the stereochemical problem one of major complexity: The penicillin nucleus contains three, the cephalosporin nucleus only two, asymmetric centers. It is rather the unusually high degree of substitution of the few carbon atoms, from which the skeleton is constructed, which poses a number of challenging problems to the synthetic chemist: Of the seven carbon atoms which constitute the penicillin nucleus (*1*), only the two carbon atoms of the methyl groups are not attached to any hetero atom. In the cephalosporins (*2*) this applies only to carbon atom 3, but this carbon is part of a reactive enamine system. Aside from the reactivity of the β-lactam structure, it is this unusually high substitution pattern which renders these antibiotics rather vulnerable to chemical attack.

(*1*)   (*2*)

B. Basic Concepts

Any synthesis of some potential practical importance must satisfy the following criteria:

1. It must be structurally specific, i.e., the synthetic plan should be such that no structural isomers are formed in any step.
2. It must be stereochemically specific, i.e., the desired stereoisomer should be formed exclusively (or at least as the major isomer) or else a step should be envisaged by which any undesired isomer is converted into the desired one.
3. Reaction conditions and reagents must be compatible with the stability of the intermediates or final products in order to avoid (partial) destruction of the synthetic material.

It is the last condition which in the early years of synthetic endeavor in the penicillin field influenced the planning profoundly. The instability of the (at the time) rather unusual β-lactam structure was considered to be the major reason for the extreme acid and base sensitivity of the penicillins. As a consequence of this assumption, all early synthetic attempts postponed the formation of this potentially dangerous structure as far as possible. However, as more information about β-lactams accumulated, it became clear that this structure in itself was only one of the factors contributing to the instability of the final product and—especially in the cephalosporins—certainly not the most important one. In recent years rearrangements and transformations of the penicillins and cephalosporins were discovered in which the β-lactam function could be preserved. These reactions are described in detail in earlier chapters.

It is, however, true that nucleophiles (such as alkoxides) do attack the β-lactam function quite readily, especially under basic conditions. Penicillins (1) are easily transformed into penicilloic acid derivatives (3) (Clarke et al., 1949).

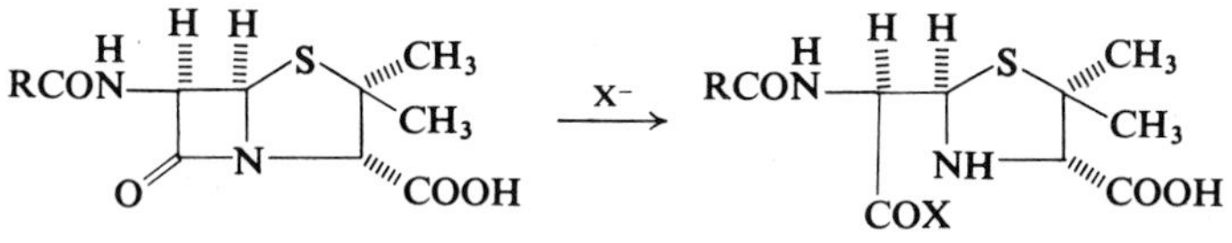

(1)   (3)

In the cephalosporin series it is possible to displace the acetoxy group of the 3-acetoxymethyl side chain without destruction of the β-lactam; opening of the four-membered lactam by base requires, however, rather severe conditions (Eggers et al., 1965; Hamilton-Miller et al., 1970).

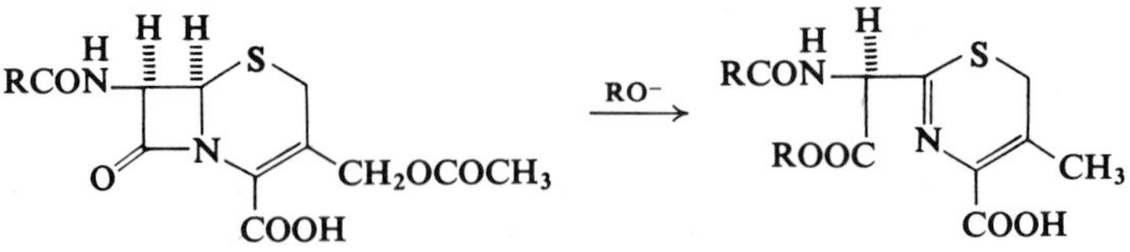

(2)   (4)

Towards acidic reagents the cephalosporin and penicillin nucleus is remarkably stable as long as the acylamino function at C-7 or C-6, respectively, is absent. The labilizing effect of this function is related to the fairly ready oxazolone formation and is especially important in the penicillin series because of its more reactive β-lactam. For this reason, and in order to be able to introduce at the end of a synthesis any desired acyl side chain, the attachment of this grouping should (and in fact was, in practically all synthetic schemes) be performed as one of the last steps.

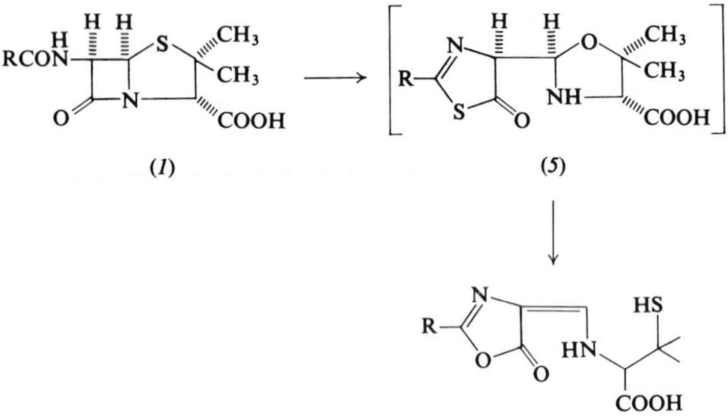

(1)   (5)

penicillenic acid

Another serious problem for any total synthesis is the presence of the free carboxyl function in both penicillins and cephalosporins, which seems to be essential for biological activity. It is often desirable or even mandatory to protect this function during synthetic operations. Since, however, the β-lactam is hydrolyzed faster by alkali than is an ester function,* only acid-sensitive protecting groups (such as *t*-butyl esters, benzhydryl esters, and the like) could be used in early synthetic schemes. Although hydrogenolysis of benzylic type esters is possible, the application of this method on a larger scale is impractical due to catalyst poisoning by the sulfur-containing substrates. A major advance

* This is not true in enzymatic hydrolysis (Snow, 1962).

was, therefore, the introduction of the trichloroethyl ester grouping by Woodward (Woodward, 1966; Woodward et al., 1966) which can be removed by mild reduction with zinc and acetic acid.

There are many ways in which the bicyclic ring system of penicillins and cephalosporins can be constructed. The structure of the nucleus can either be completed by formation of one particular bond or by a cycloaddition reaction. Some of the possibilities are schematically listed below, the arrow(s) indicating the bond(s) whose formation completes the synthesis of the bicyclic system.

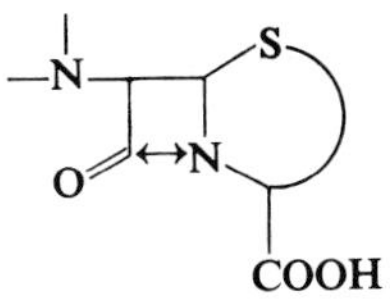

A 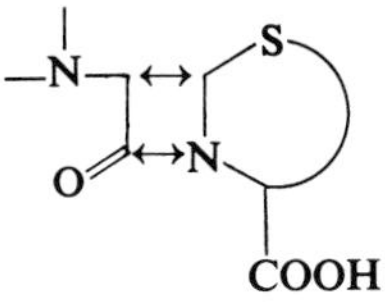   B 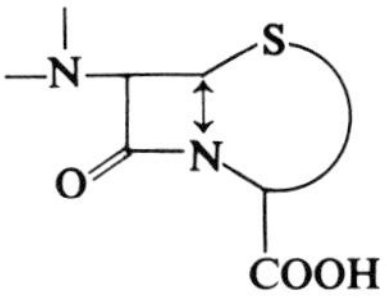   C

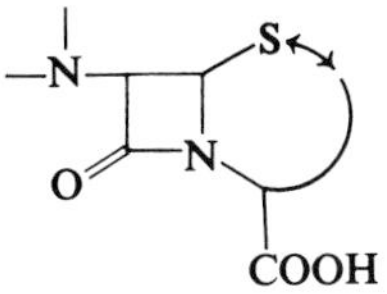

D 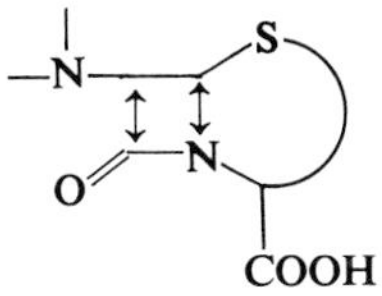   E 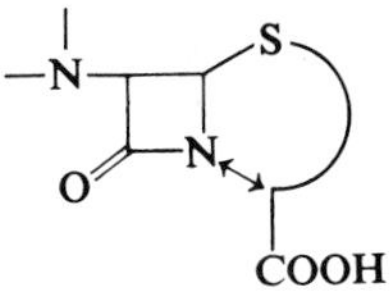   F

Not all of these possibilities have been realized, but attempts to use the synthetic schemes have been made. We shall discuss below these approaches in the order indicated, beginning with the "classical" approach of formation of the β-lactam amide bond as the last step in construction of the bicyclic nucleus (type A).

II. The Total Synthesis of Penicillin

A. Early Experiences

These experiments as well as Sheehan's first synthesis of penicillin (cf. below) were based on scheme A (above).

Since the carbon atom 5 of the penicillin nucleus represents a masked aldehyde function, it was considered a reasonable approach to use an aldehyde on the one hand, and a "masking" compound on the other hand, as the two building blocks.

The oxazolone structure (*6*) represents a protected form of an α-formyl-*N*-phenacetylglycine. The dimethylcysteine (*7*) (named penicillamine) can be

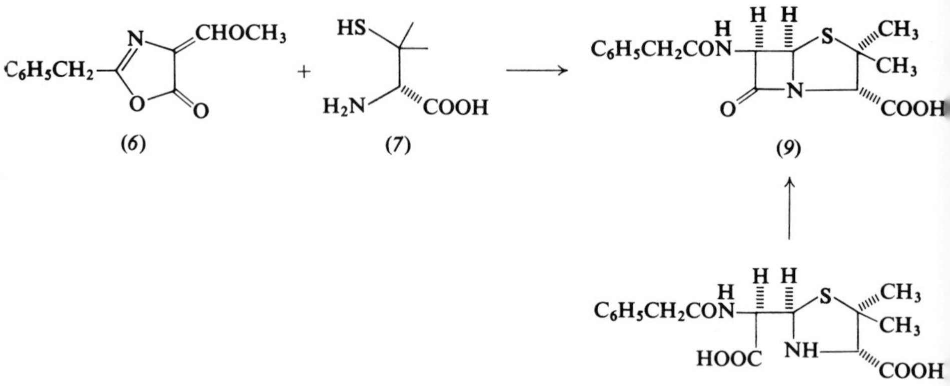

obtained from penicillin or synthesized from chloroacetylvaline (*10*) through the oxazolone (*11*) (Crooks, 1949).

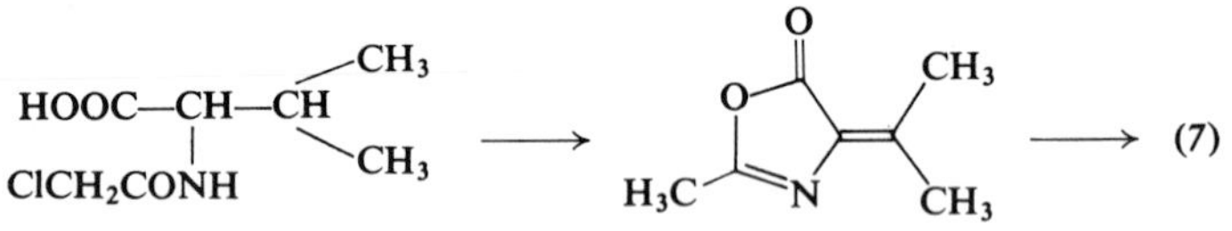

The above penicillin synthesis probably proceeds through an oxazolone of the type (*5*) and gives benzylpenicillin (*9*) only in very low yield (0.008%) (duVigneaud *et al.*, 1949; Folkers, 1956).

The cyclization of benzylpenicilloic acid (*8*) with phosphorous trichloride (Süs, 1951) also gives only traces of benzylpenicillin.

B. Sheehan's Penicillin Synthesis

The extensive studies of J. C. Sheehan at MIT were based on these early experiences. The developments, which by stepwise improvements led to the successful synthetic scheme, are described in a recent summary by Manhas and Bose (1969). The synthesis uses as starting material the enolized aldehyde (*12*) which was condensed with DL-penicillamine (or D-penicillamine) (Sheehan and Henery-Logan, 1957, 1959). This substance only contains one asymmetric center. In the condensation reaction two new centers are created (asterisks).

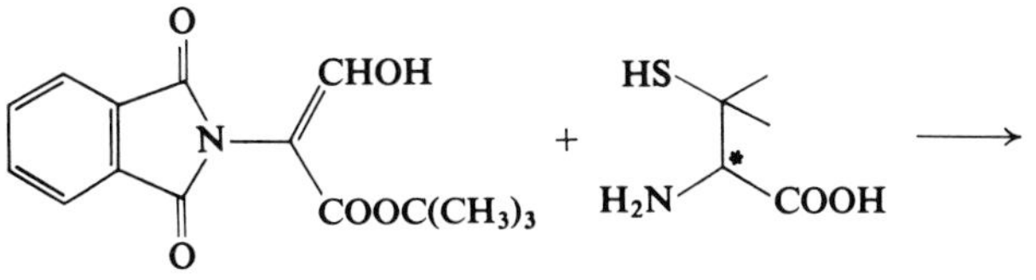

(12)　　　　　　　　　(7)

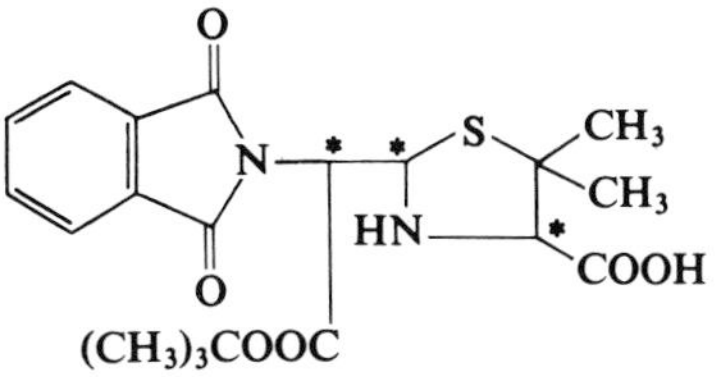

(13)

Only two of the four possible isomers were isolated, the α isomer in 24%, the γ isomer in 30% yield. Subsequent transformations established that the relative orientation of the groups in the α isomer corresponds to the one found in natural penicillin. Since it was likely that the crude mixture obtained did not correspond to the equilibrium mixture of the isomers and since, in principle, all the centers could be inverted either by deprotonation–protonation or elimination–addition, isomerization experiments were performed. Heating the γ isomer with pyridine did in fact produce an equilibrium mixture, from which additional α isomer could be obtained. Treatment of the isomers under acidic conditions (with concomitant cleavage of the t-butyl ester) at elevated temperature (Sheehan and Johnson, 1954) produced a third isomer (β isomer). The configurations of the β and γ isomers have not been established with certainty (Sheehan and Cruickshank, 1956).

Since the phthalimido group cannot be removed from a penicillin without destruction of the β-lactam function, the N-protecting group was removed at stage (13) by hydrazine treatment. From the α isomer of (13) the corresponding amino acid (14) was obtained in 82% yield.

(13) ⟶

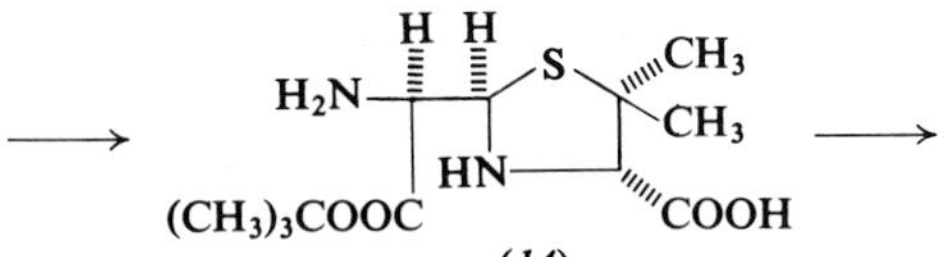

(14)

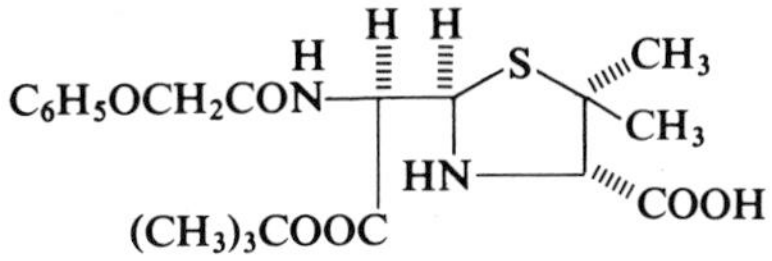

(15)

At this stage (*14*) any desired *N*-acyl group could be introduced, such as the phenoxyacetyl residue, and by mild acid treatment the *t*-butyl ester was cleaved to give the diacid (*16*) without any epimerization. All previous attempts to

(*15*) ⟶

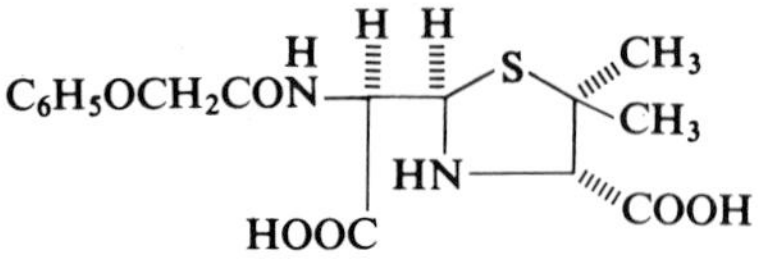

$$C_6H_5OCH_2CON-\underset{HOOC}{\overset{H}{\Big|}}...S...CH_3, CH_3, COOH$$

(*16*) ⟶

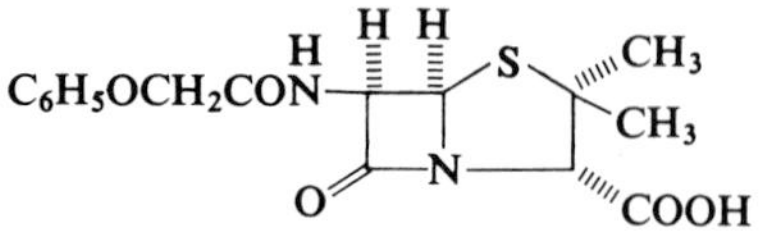

(*17*)

$$C_6H_5OCH_2CON-...O-N...S...CH_3, CH_3, COOH$$

cyclize acids of this type to penicillins had failed because under dehydrating conditions the acids readily formed oxazolones of structure (*5*). For this reason a number of N-protecting groups incapable of forming oxazolones were investigated by Sheehan (*N*-trityl, *N*-tosyl) (cf., for example, Bolhofer *et al.*, 1960). In these examples cyclization of the amino acids [related to (*16*)] by thionyl chloride could be effected very efficiently, but the breakthrough only occurred with the application of a carbodiimide for the ring closure. This reagent was introduced by Sheehan (Sheehan and Hess, 1955) for the formation of amide bonds from amines and carboxylic acids. The mono sodium salt of (*16*) could be cyclized to phenoxymethylpenicillin (*17*) in 5.4 % yield. Much more efficient was the cyclization of the *N*-trityl benzyl ester (*18*) with diisopropyl carbodiimide to (*19*) (67 %), from which by detritylation and hydrogenolytic removal of the benzyl group, 6-aminopenicillanic acid (*20*), was

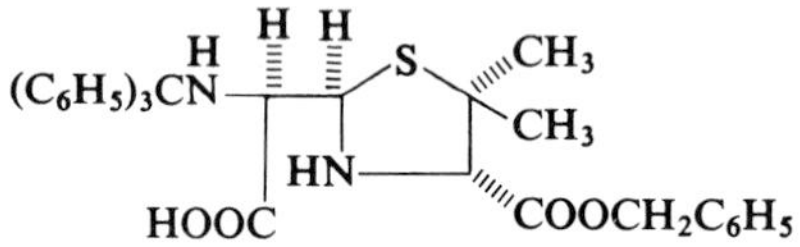

(*18*) 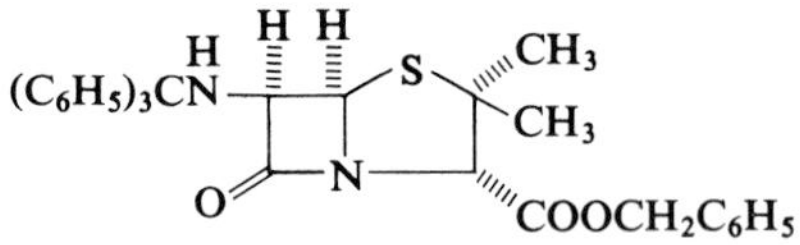   ⟶   (*19*)

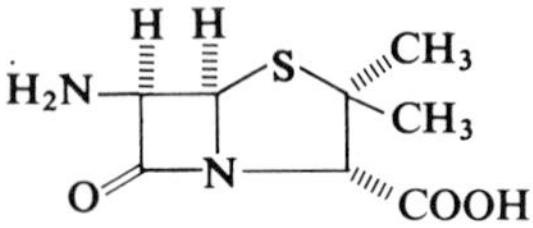

$$(C_6H_5)_3CN-...COOCH_2C_6H_5$$ $$(C_6H_5)_3CN-...COOCH_2C_6H_5$$

↓

(*20*)

$$H_2N-...O-N...S...CH_3, CH_3, COOH$$

obtained (Sheehan and Henery-Logan, 1962). From it, natural and semi-synthetic penicillins are accessible.

From the brilliant work of Sheehan's group a large body of experiences has evolved on which many further developments could be based. Notably, many different methods for the construction of β-lactams were investigated. One major drawback in Sheehan's scheme has been the lack of stereospecificity.

C. 6-Epipenicillanates

The cyclo-addition reaction between a Schiff's base and a ketene, first discovered by Staudinger (1907), to give a β-lactam was very early considered as a possibility for the synthesis of penicillins (Bachmann and Cronyn, 1949; Sheehan et al., 1950; Sheehan and Ryan, 1951). The appropriate thiazoline (22) (Bose et al., 1968) was easily accessible from DL-N-formylpenicillamine (21).

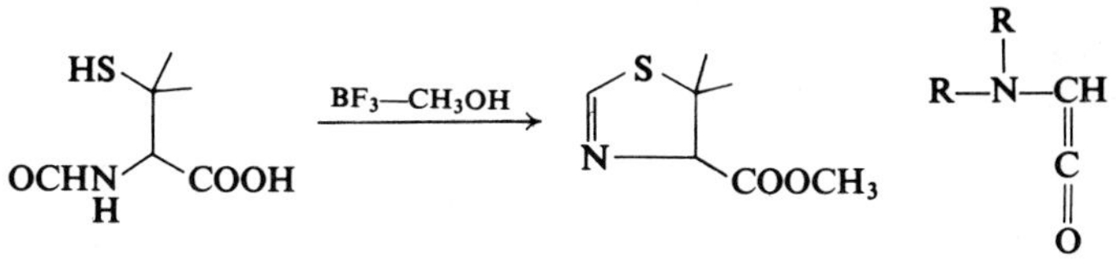

$$(21) \qquad (22) \qquad (23)$$

The second component had to be a protected amino ketene (23). Obviously, no simple acyl group could be used as a protecting function because of the well-known propensity of activated acylamino acid derivatives to form azlactones (24). The phthalimido-protecting group could be used for addition reactions (Bose, 1960), but its subsequent removal without destruction of the β-lactam was not feasible.

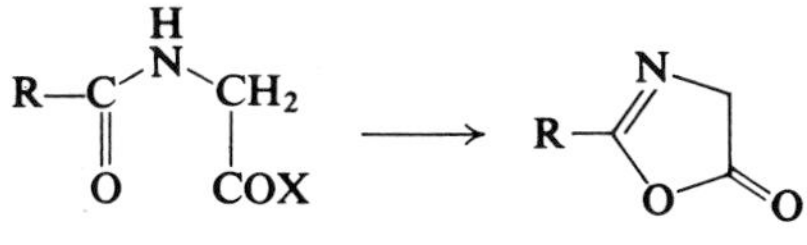

$$(24)$$

A very useful modification was introduced by Bose et al. (1968), who generated the azido ketene from azidoacetyl chloride (25) with triethylamine in the presence of the thiazoline (22).

The azido β-lactam was only formed in low yield. By catalytic reduction and acylation DL-methyl-6-epiphenoxymethylpenicillin was obtained. Assignment of the stereochemistry of the β-lactam substituents was based on NMR measurements.

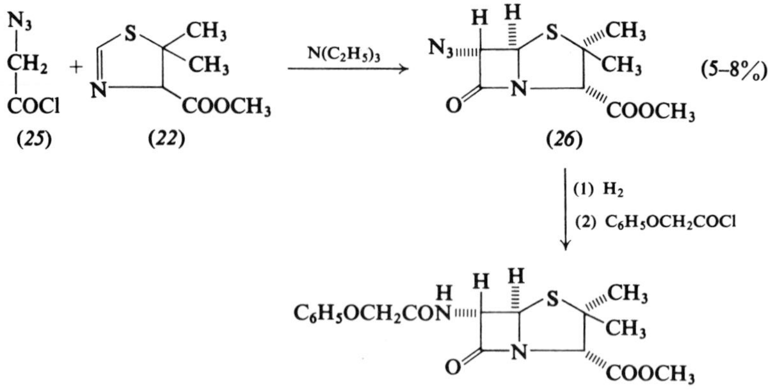

$$(25) \quad (22) \xrightarrow{\text{N(C}_2\text{H}_5)_3} (26) \quad (5\text{--}8\%)$$

$$\downarrow \begin{array}{l} (1)\ H_2 \\ (2)\ C_6H_5OCH_2COCl \end{array}$$

$$(27)$$

A number of methods for the epimerization of the C-6 center have recently been described and are discussed in Chapter 3. None of these methods is directly applicable to methyl 6-epiphenoxymethylpenicillin, but in principle, by an appropriate choice of both the amino- and the carboxyl-protecting groups, the epimerization and conversion of a 6-epipenicillin derivative into a penicillin could be effected.

D. Other Approaches

Although the structure of penicillin clearly suggested a biogenetic pathway using the amino acids cysteine and valine as precursors for the bicyclic nucleus, the order in which the various bonds are formed which connect the two amino acid parts in the final metabolic product is much less clear. If, however, a cysteinyl–valine derivative should be a precursor of penicillin, an attractive possibility would be the cyclization to a perhydrothiazepine followed by a transannular reaction to form the "strained" bicyclic penicillin nucleus.

The monocyclic analogs of benzylpenicillin and 6-aminopenicillanic acid (6-APA) (30) corresponding at both chiral centers to the natural penicillins were synthesized by Leonard and Ning (1966) from D-penicillamine (7) and appropriately substituted α-amino acrylates (28).

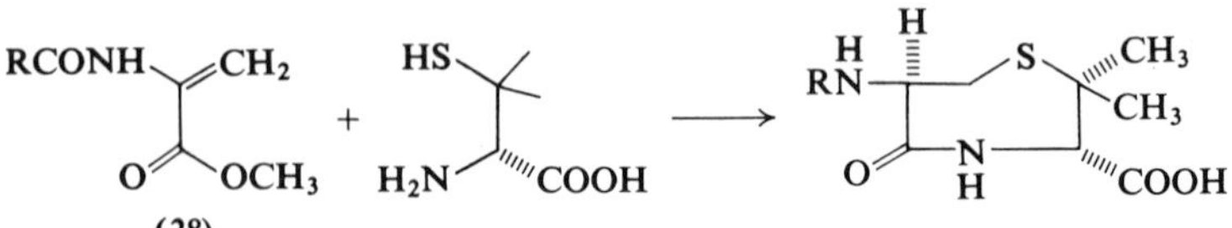

(28)   (7)   (30)

R = C$_6$H$_5$CH$_2$—   R = C$_6$H$_5$CH$_2$CO—

R = C$_6$H$_5$CH$_2$O—   R = H

The reaction produced two stereoisomers which were separated and the relative configurations of the two centers established.

Successful experiments to effect the transannular reaction *in vitro* or *in vivo* have so far not been reported. (For unsuccessful *in vitro* experiments, see Leonard and Wilson, 1964a, b; Sjöberg *et al.*, 1965.)

No synthesis of a penicillin using a preformed β-lactam ring has as yet been reported. In theory, a most attractive possibility appears to be the intramolecular Michael-type cyclization of a mercaptan of type (*31*).

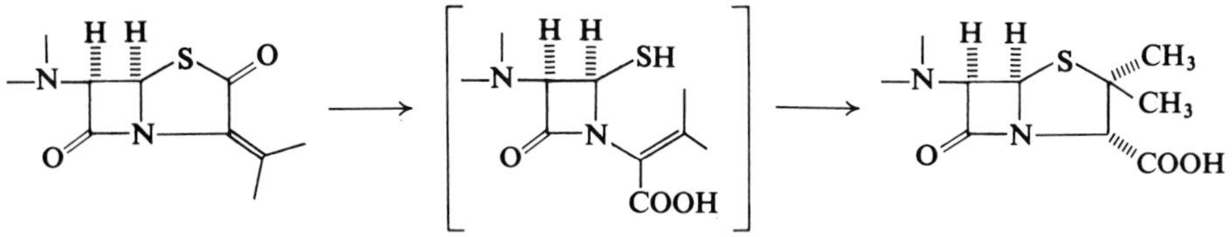

(*30a*)   (*31*)   (*32*)

Although the crucial step (*31* → *32*) has been realized in the conversion of anhydropenicillin (*30a*) back into penicillin (*32*) (Wolfe *et al.*, 1969), the total synthesis of (*31*) or a precursor thereof, which could give (*31*) under reaction conditions required for cyclization in the desired sense [to (*32*)], has not been reported. An intermediate of type (*31*) would be expected to have a very low stability indeed. Significantly, the conversion of (*31*) to (*32*) could only be successfully performed with an *N*-phthaloyl derivative in which the *N*-protecting group was able to provide some stabilization to the intermediate (*31*) by intramolecular participation.

III. The Total Synthesis of Cephalosporins

A. Cephalosporin Lactones and Lactams

In view of the success of Sheehan's work in the penicillin synthesis programs, efforts were initiated in a number of laboratories to adapt his plan to the synthesis of cephalosporins. Unfortunately, however, the analog of the penicillamine (*7*), the cephalosporamine (*33*) cannot be prepared by hydrolysis of a

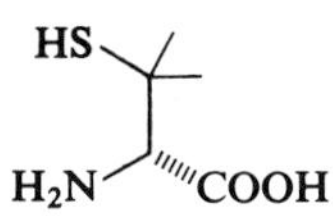

(*7*) 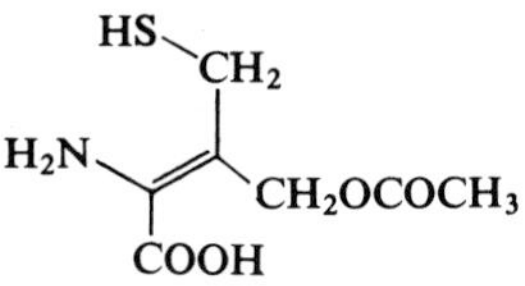   (*33*)

cephalosporin, nor would one expect to regard it as a stable compound. A certain stability could be conferred on a compound of this type by incorporating the enamine function into a five-membered lactone ring (34). But even the preparation of this compound met with difficulties and early attempts towards its synthesis (Galantay et al., 1964; Green et al., 1964; Barrett et al., 1964) failed or gave only trace amounts of the desired material.

HS—CH₂

H₂N

O   O

(34)

It was thus realized that only compounds in which the thiol group was protected could be used and two different protecting groups were applied, the acetyl group by the Roussel team (Fr. Patent 1365959; Heymes et al., 1966) and the trityl group by the Squibb team (Dolfini et al., 1969). The starting material for both groups was the condensation product (35) of pyruvic acid, formaldehyde, and dimethylamine, first prepared by Mannich and Bauroth (1924).

Displacement of the dimethylamino group by either thiolacetate [to (36)] or trityl mercaptan [to (37)] served to introduce the sulfur substituent. The completion of the skeleton required substitution of the hydroxyl by an amino group and condensation with the amino-substituted malonyl aldehyde–ester. The Squibb group performed these changes in two steps [(38) and (40)]*; whereas, the Roussel group used the aminomethylene glycine ester for the direct introduction of these two parts in one step (39 → 41). The protecting groups on the sulfur atom were removed in both cases by acid treatment. In the condensation reactions two adjacent asymmetric centers were introduced and (as in Sheehan's penicillin synthesis) no stereochemical selectivity was observed: Both the threo and the erythro forms of (41) were produced, the ratio in the Roussel synthesis being about 4:6.

The isomers of (41) could be separated, but Heymes et al. (1966) reported that, after removal of the phthaloyl group by hydrazinolysis, both threo and the erythro amino esters (42) gave the threo amino acid (43) on acid treatment. No rational explanation was put forward to explain the fact that the undesired erythro ester was converted essentially quantitatively into the threo acid, in which the stereochemical relationship of the two asymmetric centers corresponds to the one present in the natural cephalosporin. After protection of the primary amino function by the trityl group, ring closure of the β-lactam

* This compound (38) was also prepared by a very similar route by Reinhoudt et al. (1968) and the corresponding S-benzyl derivative was described by Green et al. (1964).

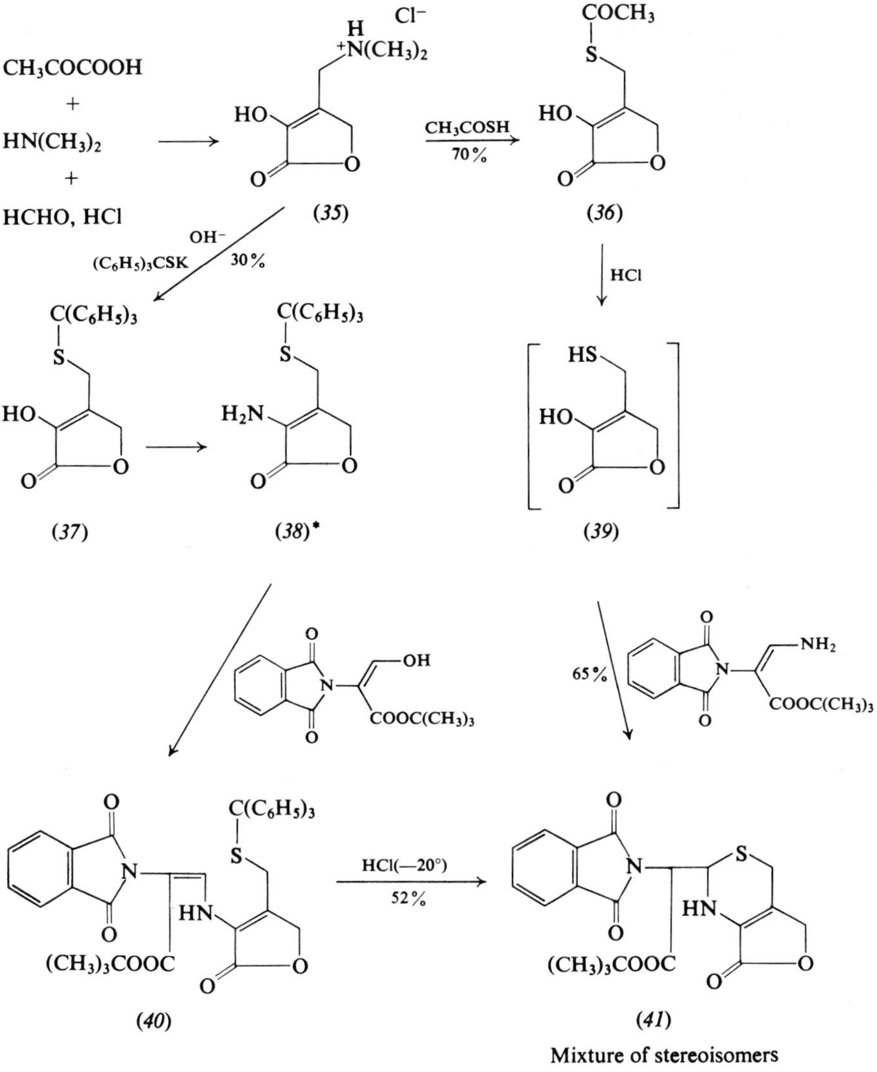

CH$_3$COCOOH

+

HN(CH$_3$)$_2$

+

HCHO, HCl

$\longrightarrow$

(35)

$\xrightarrow[70\%]{CH_3COSH}$

(36)

(C$_6$H$_5$)$_3$CSK   OH$^-$ 30%

HCl

(37) $\longrightarrow$ (38)*

(39)

65%

HCl(—20°)
52%

(40) $\longrightarrow$ (41)

Mixture of stereoisomers

ring with dicyclohexyl carbodiimide under carefully selected conditions proceeded in very satisfactory yield (70%), and after removal of the protecting group the amino lactone (46) was obtained.

This material could be resolved with (+)-tartaric acid (Nominé, 1971) and acylated with thienyl acetyl chloride to (47). The product was identical with a sample prepared from cephalothin, obtained from natural cephalosporin C, by comparison of its physical data and its antibacterial activity.

When the racemic *erythro* isomer was carried through to the above reactions, an isomer of (47) was obtained (with the amino and sulfur substituents on the

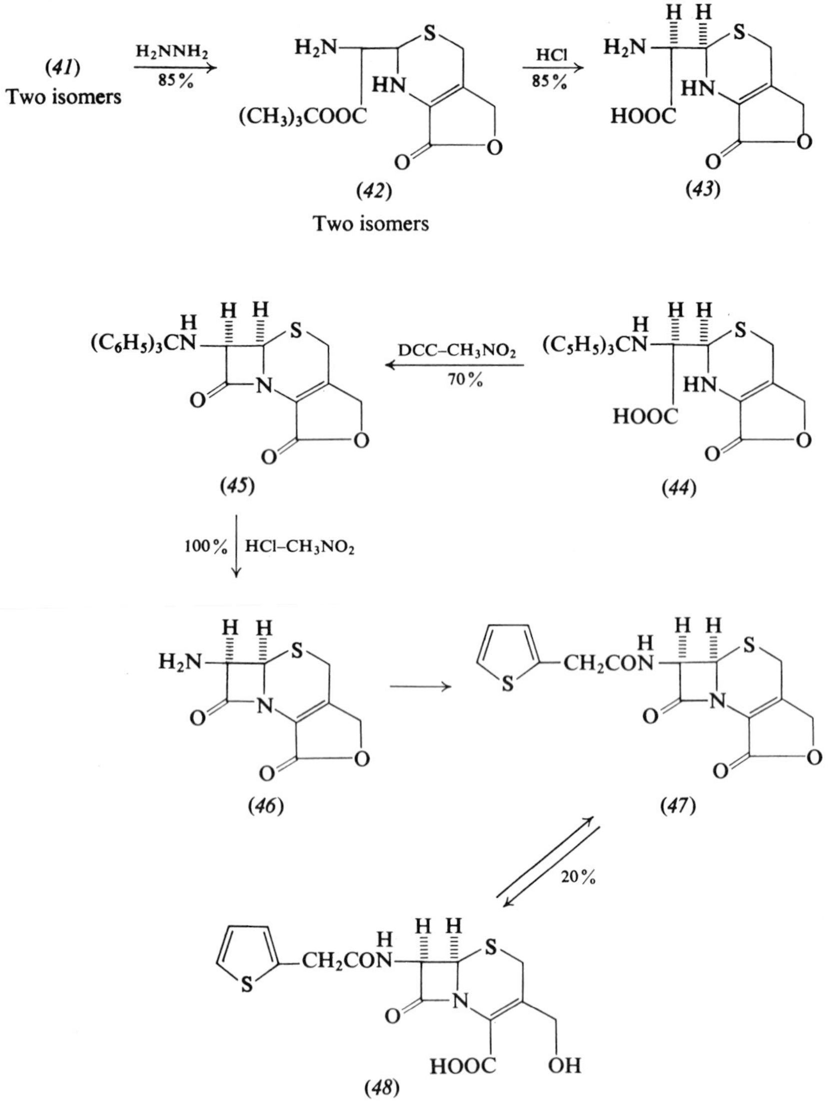

(41) Two isomers

(42) Two isomers

(43)

(44)

(45)

(46)

(47)

(48)

β-lactam *trans* to each other) which was found to be devoid of any antibacterial activity (Nominé, 1971).

Since the lactone in (47) is as stable as the β-lactam towards hydrolysis, selective hydrolytic opening of the former was difficult. Nevertheless, the

Squibb group (Neidleman *et al.*, 1970) succeeded in isolating about 20% of the hydroxy acid (*48*) from such experiments.

Recently, the French group (Nominé, 1971; Germ. Patent 1932504) prepared the lactam analog of (*36*) by the route indicated in the following flow sheet. This lactam (*54*) was carried through the same sequence of reactions as the corresponding lactone to give the amino lactam corresponding to (*45*). This material was resolved and thienyl-acetylated to (*55*). Again the product could be identified with a sample prepared from cephalothin via displacement of the acetoxy group with azide anion followed by reduction with tin and hydrochloric acid.

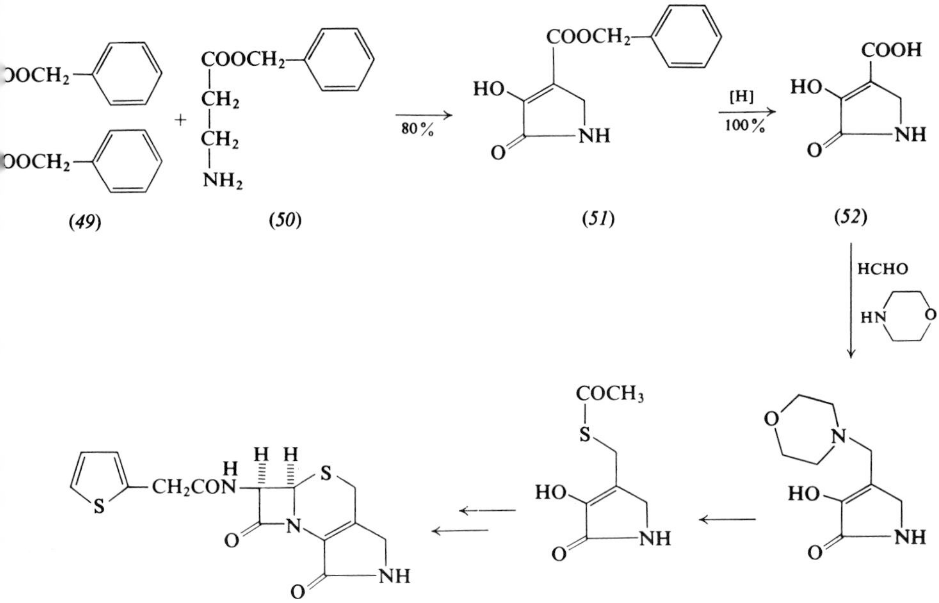

(*49*) (*50*) (*51*) (*52*)

(*55*) (*54*) (*53*)

The experiments described above demonstrate that Sheehan's penicillin scheme can indeed be adapted to the synthesis of cephalosporin analogs. The Roussel chemists have in fact developed the approach so efficiently that Mannich's dimethylaminomethyl lactone (*35*) can be converted into deacetyl 7-aminocephalosporanic acid lactone in well over 10% overall yield. This achievement represents a remarkable improvement over Sheehan's penicillin synthesis and is primarily due to the fact that by good fortune both the undesired and the desired isomer of the ester (*42*) can be converted into the desired acid (*43*) in high yield. This confers a high degree of overall stereospecificity to the scheme.

B. Woodward's Synthesis of Cephalosporin

An approach fundamentally different from the one used in the synthesis of penicillin was designed by Woodward in his total synthesis of cephalosporin which was first announced in his Nobel lecture in 1965 (Woodward, 1966; Woodward *et al.*, 1966). By using natural L-cysteine (*56*) as a starting material, no resolution step was necessary, and by protecting the various functional groups of this amino acid in a cyclic intermediate (*57*), complete stereochemical control in the introduction of the new asymmetric center was achieved. The introduction of the amino function designed to become the nitrogen atom of the β-lactam, however, required the development of a new substitution method. The problem was first solved in a thermal addition of dimethyl azodicarboxylate to the intermediate (*58*), which mechanistically involves a

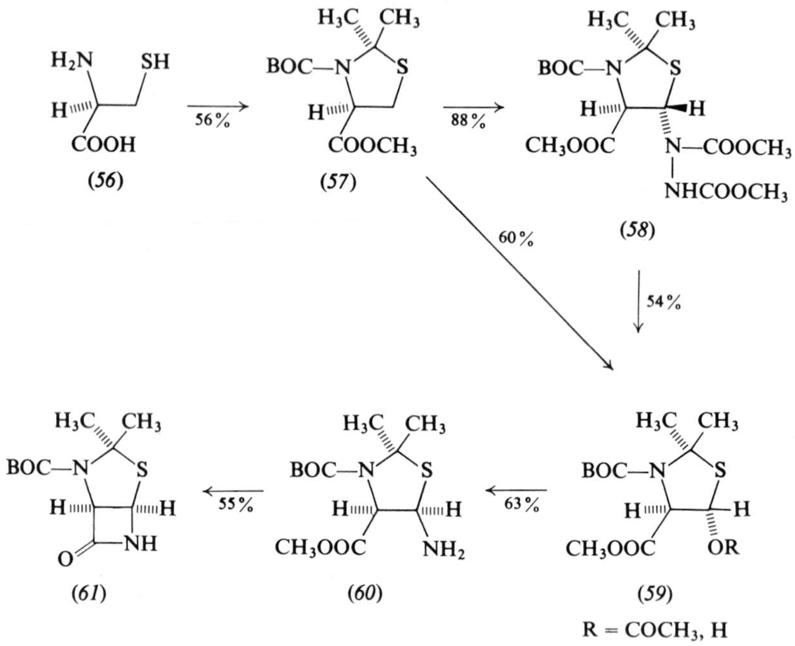

1,2 shift of the new substituent, which becomes first attached to the sulfur atom and, after a hydrogen transfer from carbon to nitrogen, moves to the desired carbon atom. An oxidative degradation of the hydrazo substituent in (*58*) by lead tetraacetate gave the acetoxy ester (*59*) (R = $COCH_3$) together with a small amount of its "*cis*" epimer. Transesterification with sodium acetate in methanol converts both isomers into the same hydroxy ester (*59*) (R = H).

The epimerization proceeds by a ring opening of (59) to a mercaptoaldehyde and recyclization to the more stable epimer of (59) (R = H). It was later discovered that the two acetates [(59) R = COCH$_3$, and its epimer] could also be formed directly from (57) by treatment with lead tetraacetate and *t*-butanol under irradiation with ultraviolet light (Heusler, 1967, 1968). The conversion of the "*trans*" hydroxy ester (59) (R = H) into the "*cis*" amino ester (60) followed conventional routes (through chloride or mesylate, displacement by azide and reduction). The complete retention of configuration in the thionyl chloride reaction and the complete inversion in the displacement reaction by azide is, however, noteworthy. Only reduction of the azido ester with alkaline stannite solution gave pure "*cis*" amino ester without any inversion to the thermodynamically more stable "*trans*" amino ester. The structure of (60), which was confirmed by a complete X-ray diffraction analysis, indicated a conformation of the functional groups eminently suitable for cyclization to the β-lactam (61). This reaction was eventually achieved by treatment of (60) with organo aluminum compounds such as triethyl aluminum.

The β-lactam (61) represents a key intermediate not only for the construction of cephalosporin; it is, in principle, a starting material for a wide variety of bicyclic structures related to both penicillins and cephalosporins (cf., below).

Although fairly labile to both acids and bases, the lactam (61) is thermally quite stable and its NH group readily combines with the strongly electrophilic center present in the dialdehyde (63) prepared from malondialdehyde and trichloroethyl glyoxylate via the aldol (62), Since (64) contains all the elements required for the construction of the additional dihydrothiazine ring, the N- and S-protecting group could now be removed by trifluoroacetic acid treatment, which also effected ring closure to the amino aldehyde (65a), which was acylated with thienyl acetyl chloride or a protected D-α-amino adipic acid to give (65b) or (65c). Reduction of the aldehyde function with diborane to (66a), followed by acetylation to (66b) and by pyridine-catalyzed equilibration, gave the protected cephalothin and cephalosporin C, respectively. The choice of the protecting group for the carboxyl function in (67a) was dictated by the acid and base sensitivity of the final product. The trichloroethyl group, which can be removed by zinc and aqueous acetic acid under mild conditions, served the purpose very efficiently and has since been used extensively, especially in the penicillin and cephalosporin field.

Due to the fairly large number of steps involved, the synthesis has limited practical importance. It provides, however, the basis for synthetic variations of cephalosporins and penicillins not accessible from natural sources. Experiments in this direction are described below. They have recently acquired additional importance through the fact that the key intermediate (61) of Woodward's synthesis can now also be prepared from 6-aminopenicillanic acid (Heusler and Woodward, 1970a).

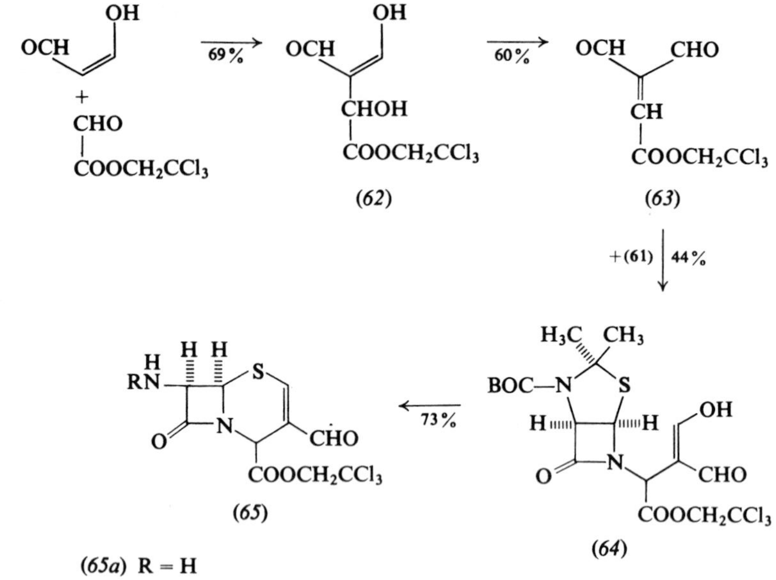

(62)

(63)

+(61) | 44%

(65)

(65a) R = H

(65b) R = [thiophene]—CH₂CO—

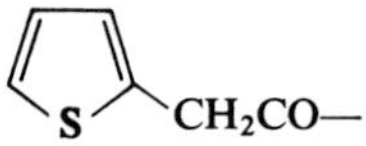

(65c) R = Cl₃CCH₂OOC(CH₂)₃—CH—CO—
 with NHCOOCH₂CCl₃

(64)

89%

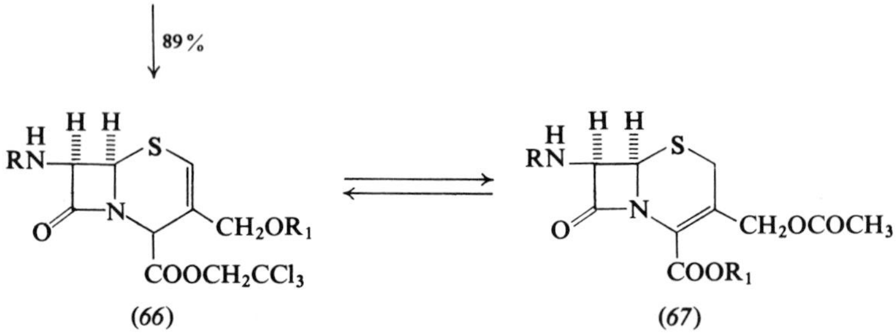

(66)

(66a) R₁ = H
(66b) R₁ = COCH₃

(67)

(67a) R₁ = CH₂CCl₃
(67b) R₁ = H

C. Various Attempts

Since a β-lactam can in principle be formed by a cyclo-addition reaction of an isocyanate to a (reactive) double bond, an intramolecular version of this reaction was considered as a possibility for a cephalosporin synthesis (Haefliger and Petrzilka, 1966).

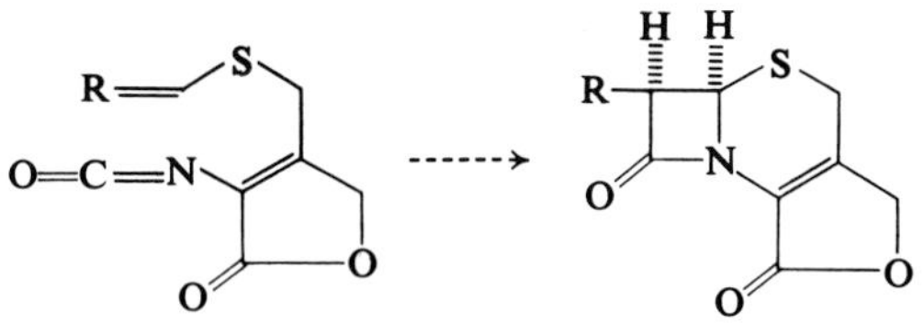

(68)   (69)

However, the precursor, the acid (70) proved to be too unstable to represent a useful intermediate for further transformation.

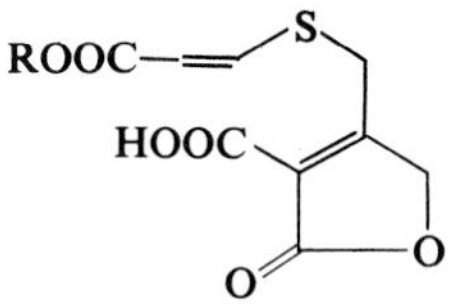

(70)

IV. Modified β-Lactam Antibiotics

Discovery of the cephalosporins and their powerful antibiotic activity has made it quite clear that this type of activity is not as strictly limited to a particular structural arrangement as one was led to believe in the early years of the penicillin era. A number of structural modifications (as opposed to functional modifications as in the "semisynthetic" penicillins) of both penicillins and cephalosporins were reported recently (and are described in detail in Chapters 4 and 5). In principle, a much wider structural variability could be expected from total synthesis. The number of biologically active compounds with a modified bicyclic structure prepared by total synthesis is still fairly small.

A suitable starting material appears to be the intermediate (61) of Woodward's total synthesis. In its N-protected form, (61), the most reactive center is the β-lactam nitrogen atom; whereas, in the deprotected form (71), the powerful nucleophilic character of the sulfur atom can be released.

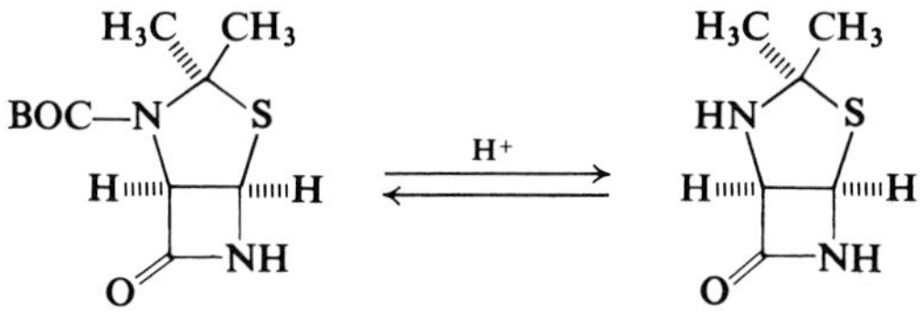

(61)   (71)

The β-lactam (61) reacted readily with glyoxylic esters to give, in an equilibrium reaction, two isomeric carbinolamide-type adducts (72) (Heusler and Woodward, 1970b) which could easily be isolated [R = C(CH₃)₃ or CH₂CCl₃]. The isomeric adducts gave, after conversion into a mixture of chlorides (73) and reaction with triphenylphosphine in the presence of base, a single, stable crystalline phosphorane (74). This phosphorane reacted readily with unhindered aldehydes (e.g., formaldehyde and straight-chain aliphatic aldehydes) or activated aldehydes (such as glyoxylic esters and α-keto aldehydes) but not with ketones. In these reactions both the "*cis*" and "*trans*" isomers (75) (with respect to the double-bond substituents) are formed.

The formaldehyde adduct (76) added mercaptans (or hydrogen sulfide) in a Michael fashion to form (77) (R = H or trityl). Removal of the *t*-butoxycarbonyl group, oxidation with iodine, and acylation with phenylacetyl chloride gave the two tetrahydrodithiazins (78), isomeric at the carbon bearing the carboxyl group (Woodward *et al.*, 1970a). Both isomers of (78) show some antibacterial activity *in vitro*. This activity is much increased in the unsaturated analog (81) (Woodward and Burri, 1970), which was produced when the mercaptan (77) (R = H) was alkylated with phenacyl bromide and, after removal of the *t*-butoxycarbonyl blocking group with acid, irradiated with UV light in the presence of pyridine (to promote a Norrish type II cleavage of the ketone and enolization of the resulting thioaldehyde). Final oxidation with iodine and acylation concluded the sequence.

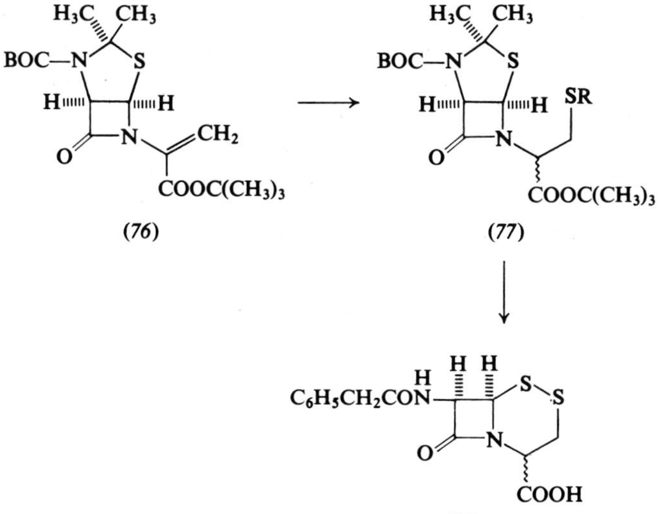

(76) → (77)

(78)

In the above reactions the sulfenyl iodide (formed from the mercaptan with iodine) functioned as an electrophile for the thiazolidine sulfur atom. Under appropriate conditions an activated carboxyl or a protonated ketonic function can serve the same purpose.

The product (82), formed from the phosphorane (74) (R = CH$_2$CCl$_3$) and t-butyl glyoxylate (cis and trans isomer), could be hydrogenated catalytically

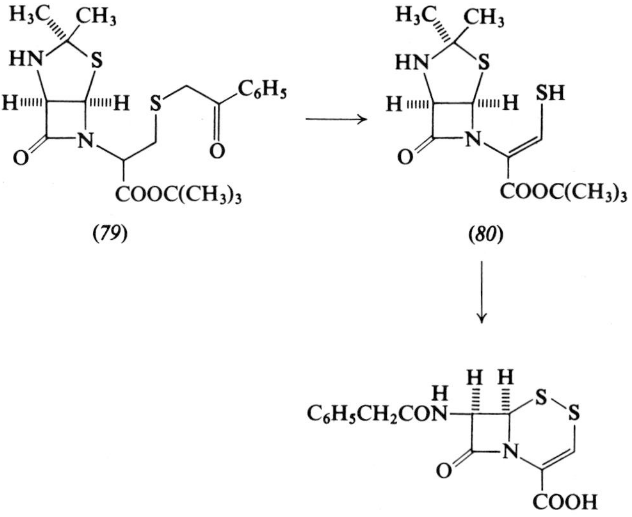

(79) → (80)

(81)

or with cobalt tetracarbonyl hydride to two stereoisomeric dihydro derivatives (*83*) which could be separated. The isomer whose stereochemistry corresponded to the orientation of the carboxyl group in penicillin* was first treated with a mixture of trifluoroacetic acid and trifluoroacetic anhydride, then with acetic anhydride and gave the trifluoroacetamidothiolactone (*84*), which only showed a low order of antibacterial activity *in vitro* (Woodward *et al.*, 1969).

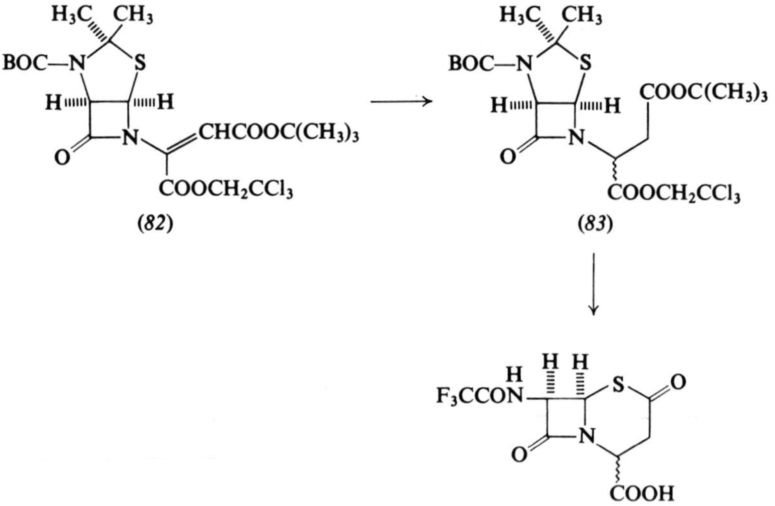

(*82*) → (*83*)

(*84*)

A greatly increased activity against gram-positive bacteria was, however, found in a series of compounds (Woodward *et al.*, 1968, 1970b) prepared from the phosphorane (*74*) (R = *t*-butyl) and various α-keto aldehydes. The con-

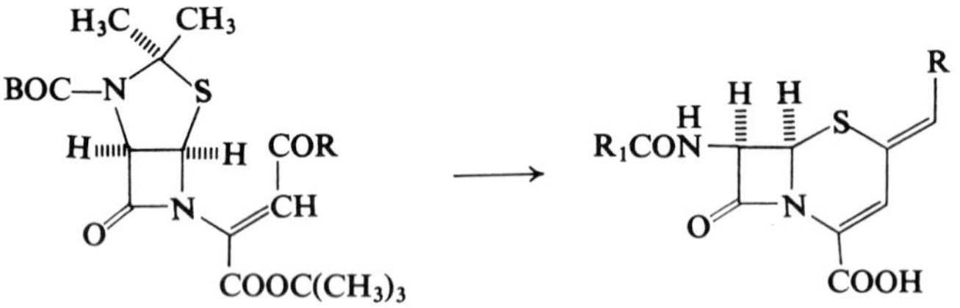

(*85*) → (*86*)

---

* The configuration was established by degradation of the final product (84) to D-aspartic acid, unpublished experiments by Dr. P. Bollinger, Woodward Research Institute, Basel, Switzerland.

densation reaction gave the ketoesters (85) (R = C_2H_5, $CH_2C_6H_5$, etc.) in the form of their cis and trans isomers.

Treatment of the "trans" isomer [$COOC(CH_3)_3$ and COR trans] with trifluoroacetic acid, followed by acylation (e.g., by phenylacetyl chloride) gave the final product (86). Since under the influence of UV light an equilibrium between the cis and trans forms of (85) is established, a possibility for the conversion of cis-(85) into trans-(85) exists. The α-keto aldehydes required were readily prepared from the diazo ketones (87) via the phosphazines (88) (cf., Bestman et al., 1959) and nitrosating cleavage.

$$R—CH_2COCHN_2 \longrightarrow R—CH_2—COCH{=}N—N{=}P(C_6H_5)_3$$

$$(87) \qquad\qquad\qquad (88)$$

$$\downarrow$$

$$R—CH_2—COCHO$$

The substituents R were varied considerably; various alkyl and haloalkyl as well as a number of substituted phenyl derivatives were prepared. Some of the compounds of type (86) showed activities against staphylococci in vitro comparable to or better than penicillin, but their in vivo activity was lower. No clear correlation of structure and activity could be established.

The reactivity of the sulfur atom in the deprotonated derivative (71) could be demonstrated by oxidation with iodine in benzene (Woodward et al., 1967, 1970c) which via the Schiff's base salt (89) gave, after acylation, the disulfide (90).

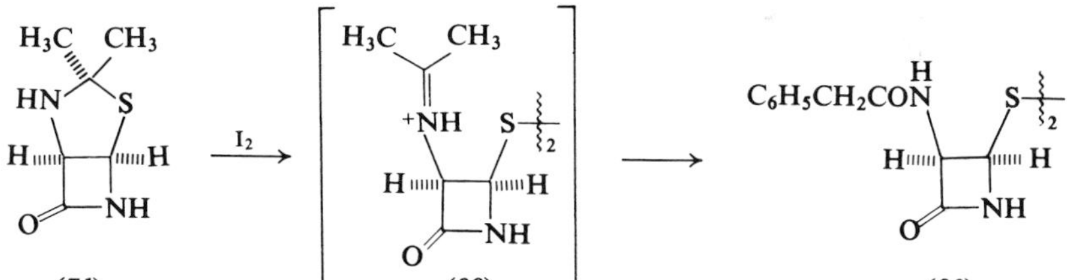

Although a number of analogs of cephalosporin have now been prepared by total synthesis, it is already clear that still more information is needed before the various structural features required for high or more specific activity, increased stability against degrading enzymes, and in vitro and in vivo activity can be defined. But it also becomes clear that total synthesis can contribute significantly towards this goal.

References

Bachmann, W. E., and Cronyn, M. W. (1949). *In* "The Chemistry of Penicillin" (H. T. Clarke, J. R. Johnson, and R. Robinson, eds.), p. 856. Princeton Univ. Press, Princeton, New Jersey.

Barrett, G. C., Eggers, S. H., Emerson, T. R., and Lowe, G. (1964). *J. Chem. Soc.* 788.

Bestmann, H. J., Buckschewski, H., and Leute, H. (1959). *Chem. Ber.* **92**, 1345.

Bolhofer, W. A., Sheehan, J. C., and Abrams, E. L. A. (1960). *J. Amer. Chem. Soc.* **82**, 3437.

Bose, A. K. (1960). *Org. Syn.* **40**, 82.

Bose, A. K., Spiegelmann, G., and Manhas, M. S. (1968). *J. Amer. Chem. Soc.* **90**, 4506.

Clarke, H. T., Johnson, J. R., and Robinson, R. (1949). "The Chemistry of Penicillin." Princeton Univ. Press, Princeton, New Jersey.

Crooks, H. M. (1949). *In* "The Chemistry of Penicillin" (H. T. Clarke, J. R. Johnson, and R. Robinson, eds.), p. 455. Princeton Univ. Press, Princeton, New Jersey.

Dolfini, J. E., Schwartz, J., and Weisenborn, F. (1969). *J. Org. Chem.* **34**, 1582.

duVigneaud, V., Carpenter, F. H., Holley, R. W., Livermore, A. H., and Rachele, J. R. (1949). *In* "The Chemistry of Penicillin" (H. T. Clarke, J. R. Johnson, and R. Robinson, eds.) p. 1018. Princeton Univ. Press, Princeton, New Jersey.

Eggers, S. H., Kane, V. V., and Lowe, G. (1965). *J. Chem. Soc.* 1262.

Folkers, K. (1956). *In* "Perspectives in Organic Chemistry" (Sir A. Todd, ed.). Wiley (Interscience), New York.

French Patent 1365959.

Galantay, E., Engel, H., Szabo, A., and Fried, J. (1964). *J. Org. Chem.* **29**, 3560.

German Patent 1932504.

Green, D. M., Long, A. G., May, P. J., and Turner, A. F. (1964). *J. Chem. Soc.* 766.

Haefliger, W., and Petrzilka, T. (1966). *Helv. Chim. Acta* **49**, 1937.

Hamilton-Miller, J. M. T., Richards, E., and Abraham, E. P. (1970). *Biochem. J.* **116**, 385.

Heusler, K. (1967). *Chimia* **21**, 557.

Heusler, K. (1968). *In* "Topics in Pharmaceutical Sciences" (D. Perlman, ed.), Vol. I, p. 33. Wiley (Interscience), New York.

Heusler, K., and Woodward, R. B. (1970a). German Offenlegungsschrift 1935607.

Heusler, K., and Woodward, R. B. (1970b). German Offenlegungsschrift 1935970.

Heymes, R., Amiard, G., and Nominé, G. (1966). *C. R. Acad. Sci. Paris* **263**, 170.

Leonard, N. J., and Ning, R. Y. (1966). *J. Org. Chem.* **31**, 3928.

Leonard, N. J., and Wilson, G. E. (1964a). *Tetrahedron Lett.* 1465.

Leonard, N. J., and Wilson, G. E. (1964b). *J. Amer. Chem. Soc.* **86**, 5307.

Manhas, M. S., and Bose, A. K. (1969). "Synthesis of Penicillin, Cephalosporin C and Analogs." Dekker, New York.

Mannich, C., and Bauroth, M. (1924). *Ber. Dtsch. Chem. Ges.* **57**, 1108.

Neidleman, S. L., Pan, S. C., Last, J. A., and Dolfini, J. E. (1970). *J. Med. Chem.* **13**, 386.

Nominé, G. (1971). *Chimie Therapeut.* **6**, 53.

Reinhoudt, D. N., Tan, H. S., and Beyerman, H. C. (1968). *Rec. Trav. Chim.* **87**, 1153.

Sheehan, J. C., and Cruickshank, P. A. (1956). *J. Amer. Chem. Soc.* **78**, 3677, 3680, 3684.

Sheehan, J. C., and Henery-Logan, K. R. (1957). *J. Amer. Chem. Soc.* **79**, 1262.

Sheehan, J. C., and Henery-Logan, K. R. (1959). *J. Amer. Chem. Soc.* **81**, 3089.

Sheehan, J. C., and Henery-Logan, K. R. (1962). *J. Amer. Chem. Soc.* **84**, 2983.

Sheehan, J. C., and Hess, G. P. (1955). *J. Amer. Chem. Soc.* **77**, 1067.

Sheehan, J. C., and Johnson, D. A. (1954). *J. Amer. Chem. Soc.* **76**, 158.

Sheehan, J. C., and Ryan, J. J. (1951). *J. Amer. Chem. Soc.* **73**, 1204.

Sheehan, J. C., Buhle, E. L., Corey, E. J., Laubach, G. D., and Ryan, J. J. (1950). *J. Amer. Chem. Soc.* **72**, 3828.

Sjöberg, B., Thelin, H., Nathorst-Westfelt, L., van Tamelen, E. E., and Wagner, E. R. (1965). *Tetrahedron Lett.* 281.

Snow, G. A. (1962). *Biochem. J.* **82**, 6P.

Staudinger, H. (1907). *Liebigs Ann.* **356**, 51.

Süs, O. (1951). *Ann.* **571**, 201.

Wolfe, S., Bassett, R. N., Caldwell, S. M., and Wasson, F. I. (1969). *J. Amer. Chem. Soc.* **91**, 7205.

Woodward, R. B. (1966). *Science* **153**, 487.

Woodward, R. B., and Burri, K. (1970). Unpublished results.

Woodward, R. B., Heusler, K., Gosteli, J., Naegeli, P., Oppolzer, W., Ramage, R., Ranganathan, S., and Vorbruggen, H. (1966). *J. Amer. Chem. Soc.* **88**, 852.

Woodward, R. B., Gosteli, J., Ranganathan, S., and Scartazzini, R. (1967). Unpublished results.

Woodward, R. B., Ernest, I., Burri, K., Friary, R., Haviv, F., Paioni, R., and Syhora, K. (1968). Unpublished results.

Woodward, R. B., Bollinger, P., Nadelson, J., and Wenger, R. (1969). Unpublished results.

Woodward, R. B., Burri, K., and Oppolzer, W. (1970a). Unpublished results.

Woodward, R. B., Ernest, I., Burri, K., Friary, R., Haviv, F., Paioni, R., and Syhora, K. (1970b). Unpublished results.

Woodward, R. B., Gosteli, J., Ranganathan, S., and Scartazzini, R. (1970c). Unpublished results.

Chapter 7

CHEMICAL AND BIOLOGICAL ACTIVITY: INFERENCES FROM X-RAY CRYSTAL STRUCTURES

ROBERT M. SWEET

I. Introduction

A. X-Ray Crystallography as a Tool

X-Ray crystal structure analysis played an important part in the initial characterization of the molecular structures of both the penicillin and the cephalosporin antibiotics. In each case, first with benzylpenicillin (Crowfoot *et al.*, 1949) and then with cephalosporin C (Hodgkin and Maslen, 1961) the crystal structure appeared in the literature simultaneously with the structure determined by chemical means. Also, in each case, Dorothy Crowfoot Hodgkin directed the X-ray work. The penicillin structure and the knowledge which came with it of the detailed conformation around the β-lactam had a profound effect on the ideas about β-lactam chemistry which developed after this time. As time has progressed and experimental techniques have improved, the information about molecular structure ultimately available to the crystallographer has become increasingly accurate. Now, one can regularly examine systematically the structures of similar compounds in order to rationalize differences in chemical properties in terms of small structural changes. This chapter is an attempt to make this sort of systematic examination of known penicillin and cephalosporin crystal structures as well as those of some analogs. Comparisons among these molecules give definite indications of the relations between structure and chemical or biological activity.

B. The Biological Mode of Action*

As these antibiotics are biologically active, we shall discuss briefly the evidence pertaining to their mode of biological action and shall show the constraints this mechanism places on the molecules involved. We shall then examine in detail the molecular structures available and, finally, rationalize observed activity phenomena in terms of these structures.

To begin, let us consider the proposed mechanism for the biological activity of these antibiotics. Early experiments showed that one of the final steps in bacterial cell wall synthesis is the three-dimensional cross-linking of peptidoglycan strands (Tipper and Strominger, 1965; Wise and Park, 1965). In this step the enzyme peptidoglycan transpeptidase cleaves the C-terminal D-alanine residue from a short peptide chain which terminates with D-ala-D-ala and replaces it with a particular free amino group which is part of an adjacent peptidoglycan strand. Workers first demonstrated that the cell walls of *Staphylococcus aureus* grown in the presence of benzylpenicillin contained a

---

* Brief portions of this section are reprinted by permission from Sweet and Dahl (1970).

larger amount of D-alanine (Wise and Park, 1965; Tipper and Strominger, 1965) and had more of the proper free amino groups (Wise and Park, 1965) to indicate that less of this transpeptidation occurs than in cells grown in its

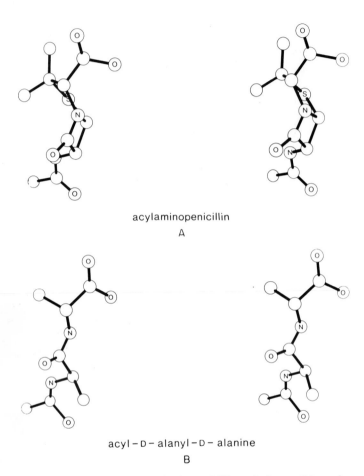

acylaminopenicillin

A

acyl – D – alanyl – D – alanine

B

Fig. 1. Stereoscopic drawing of an acylaminopenicillin and of a possible conformation of acyl-D-alanyl-D-alanine, designed to follow closely the dipeptide backbone of the penicillin.

absence. Direct evidence for the inhibiting effect the penicillin and cephalosporin antibiotics have on this transpeptidation was obtained by Strominger and co-workers (Izaki *et al.*, 1966, 1968; Strominger *et al.*, 1967), who demonstrated that, in a cell-free, particulate enzyme preparation from *Escherichia coli* acting on monomeric precursors of the bacterial cell wall, an insoluble product was formed along with release of half of the total D-alanine. The cross-linking of the monomers by transpeptidation seemed to be occurring. Conversely, in the presence of various penicillins or of the cephalosporin antibiotic, cephalothin, a soluble product was formed with no release of D-alanine. Normal transpeptidation was inhibited. Finally, Tipper and Strominger (1968) demonstrated by pulse-labeling experiments with cultures of *S. aureus* that this transpeptidation is, in fact, the terminal step in the synthesis of the cell wall and that this step is inhibited by several penicillins and cephalothin.

What, then, does this well-defined mechanism have to do with the molecular structure of the antibiotic? Earlier, Tipper and Strominger (1965) suggested that penicillin has a conformation equivalent to one which can be adopted by D-ala-D-ala. The reader can judge for himself whether or not this seems reasonable. Figure 1 shows drawings made from accurate molecular models of 6-acylaminopenicillanic acid and of acyl-D-ala-D-ala in which the peptide chain was made to look as much like the penicillin model as possible. The transpeptidase presumably recognizes the penicillin molecule as its substrate and becomes irreversibly acylated by the antibiotic when the amide link in the β-lactam ring, analogous to the peptide bond in D-ala-D-ala, is cleaved. Thus, further cross-linking by that particular enzyme molecule is prevented. The growing bacterial cell wall eventually loses the structural strength necessary to contain the endoplasm, and the bacterium bursts.

C. The Role of Structural Chemistry

With this clear picture of the action of these antibiotics in mind, a short list can be prepared of chemical and structural characteristics which the antibiotic molecule must have in order to be effective and the ways that systematic crystallographic studies will give information about these characteristics can be discussed. First, as the antibiotic apparently is involved in the competitive inhibition of an enzymic reaction, its shape must be such that it will be mistakenly recognized by the transpetidase enzyme as a normal substrate. We shall examine the molecular conformation of antibiotic molecules in the region of the labile lactam amide bond to see how they compare and shall contrast these molecular forms to a similar compound which is not biologically active. Second, the antibiotic must contain a bond analogous to the D-ala-D-ala peptide bond which is at least as easily hydrolyzed as the normal peptide link. Various physical evidence will show us that, in the case of active β-lactam antibiotics, the lactam amide bond has less multiple bond character from amide resonance than do normal amide bonds. And finally, the inhibition of the enzyme must be irreversible. The enzyme effects the hydrolysis of an amide bond, thus acylating itself. During normal transpeptidation a free amino group removes the acylating agent from the enzyme, thus forming a new peptide bond. In the case of acylation by a β-lactam antibiotic, removal of the acyl group by free amine must be prevented. This is accomplished by the fact that the leaving group from the original bond cleavage must remain nearby since it is part of a cyclic amide, and it thus sterically blocks further reaction.

D. The Structures

We now have an idea of the sort of structural information which may be useful as we attempt to explain chemical or biological activity in terms of molecular structure. Let us keep these things in mind as we examine the information available from crystal structure analyses of assorted β-lactam compounds. The specific molecular structures which will be discussed are as follows. Several structural studies have been carried out to a high degree of accuracy on penicillins (1), derivatives of 6-aminopenicillanic acid. These are

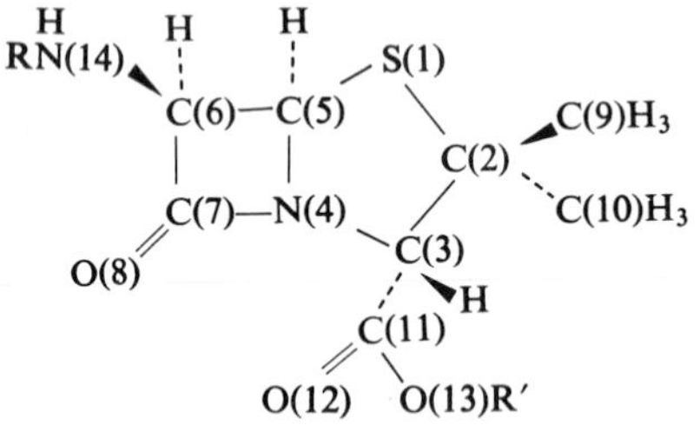

(1)

penicillin V (pen V), which is (2), investigated by Abrahamsson and co-

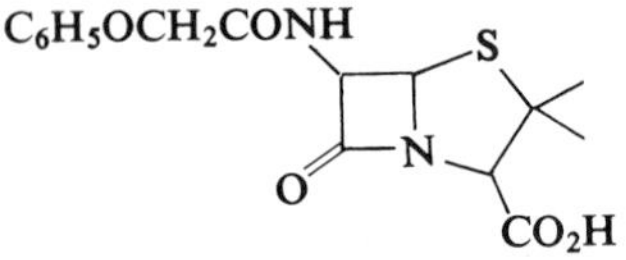

(2)

workers (1963), ampicillin trihydrate (3), studied by James and associates

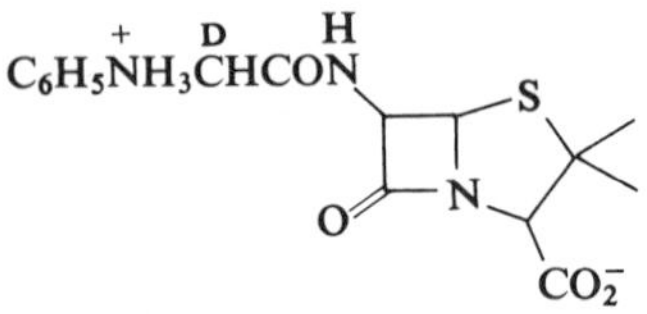

(3)

(1968), and 6-aminopenicillanic acid (6-APA), which is (*1*) where R = R′ = H, studied by Diamond (1963). Other penicillin crystal structures have been investigated, but their results will be quoted sparingly if at all because the data are either less accurate or unavailable. These are benzylpenicillin (pen G), which is (*4*), investigated initially by Crowfoot and co-workers

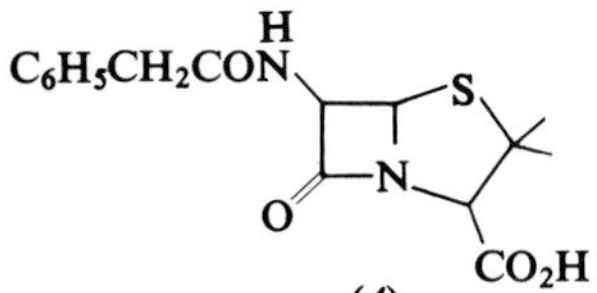

(*4*)

(1949) and refined subsequently by others (Pitt, 1952; Vaciago, 1960), phenoxymethylpenicillin sulfoxide methanolate (*5*), studied by Cooper and associates

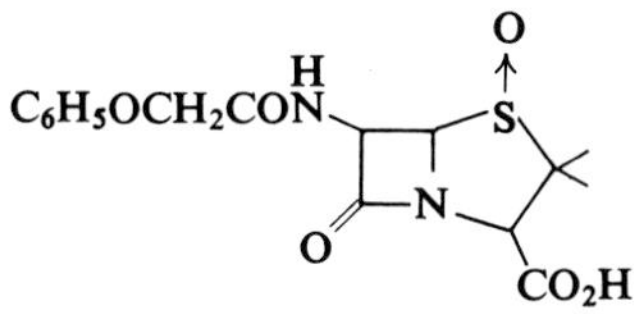

(*5*)

(1969), 6-(*N*-benzylformamido)penicillanic acid (*6*) (Hunt and Rogers, 1964),

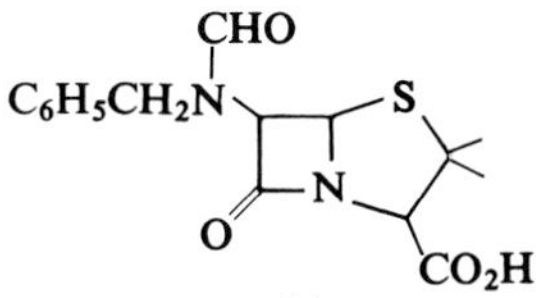

(*6*)

and hetacillin (*7*) (Hardcastle *et al.*, 1966).

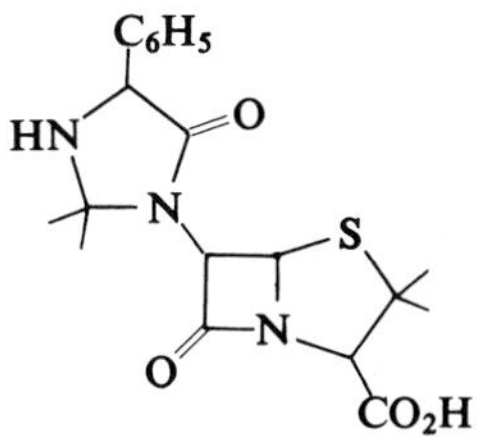

(*7*)

There are two accurately determined 3-cephem structures, derivatives of 7-ACA, 7-aminocephalosporanic acid, which is (*8*) where R = R′ = H and R″ = $OCOCH_3$. These are cephaloridine hydrochloride monohydrate (*9*)

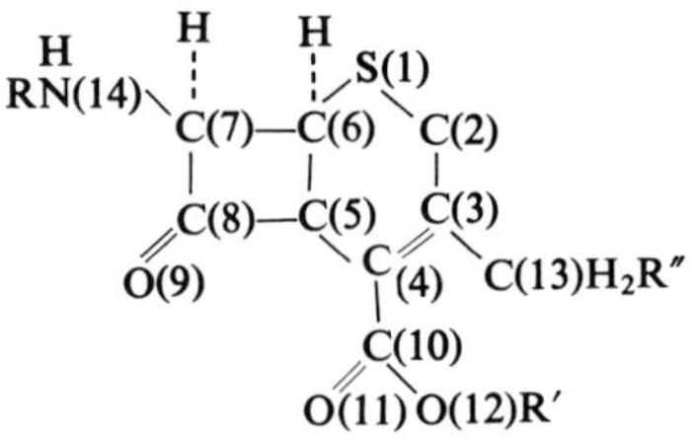

(8)

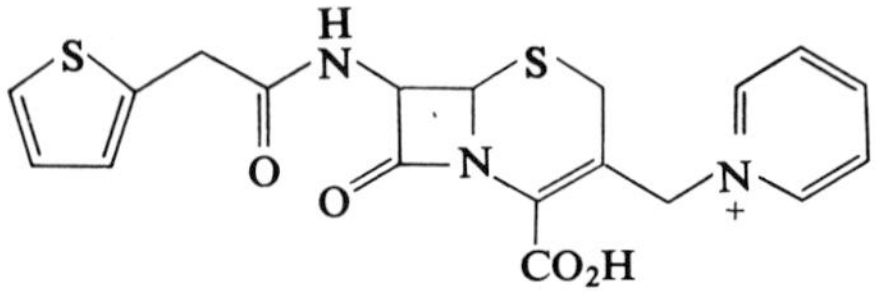

(9)

(Sweet and Dahl, 1969; 1970) and cephalosporin C_c (ceph C_c) (*10*), the

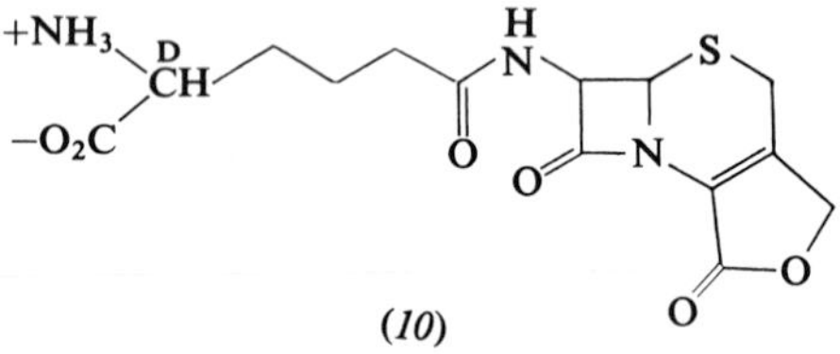

(*10*)

deacetyl lactone of cephalosporin C (Diamond, 1963). Other 3-cephem structures which are available but which have less accurate results are cephalosporin C (*11*) (Hodgkin and Maslen, 1961), cephaloglycin acetic acid hydrate

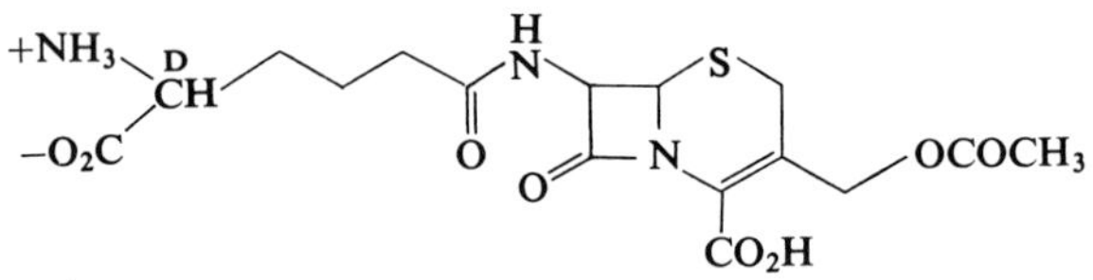

(*11*)

(*12*) (Sweet and Dahl, 1970), and 7-bromoacetamidocephalosporanic acid

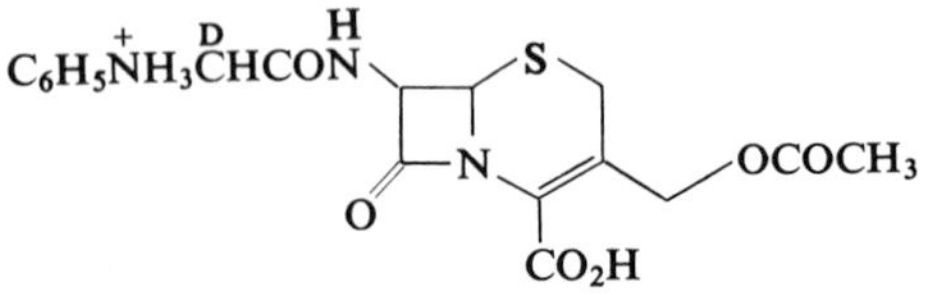

(*12*)

(7-BrAc-ACA) (*13*), examined crystallographically by Gougoutas (1970). As

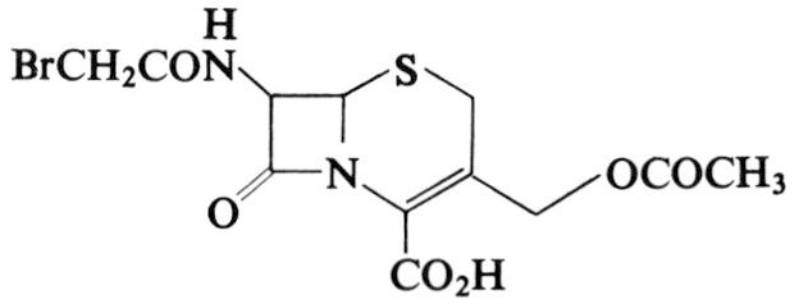

(*13*)

part of a systematic study of these β-lactam compounds, it could be instructive to examine several β-lactam-containing molecules with structures similar to the antibiotics but with enough differences to render them biologically inactive. Fortunately, there are four such compounds for which the crystal structures are well determined. These are anhydro-α-phenoxyethylpenicillin (an-pen) (*14*) prepared initially by Wolfe and co-workers (1968) and investigated crystal-

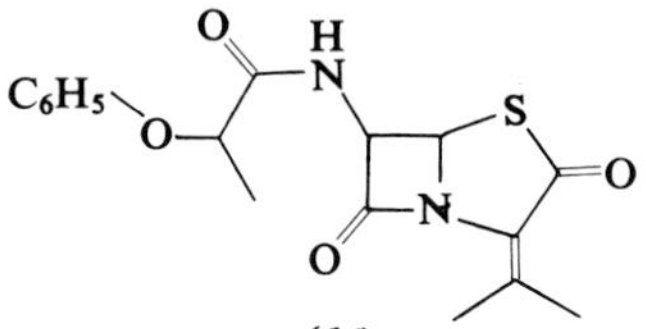

(*14*)

lographically by Simon and Dahl (1970), phenoxymethyl-Δ^2-deacetoxyl-cephalosporin (2-cephem) (*15*) (Sweet and Dahl, 1970), a synthetic β-lactam

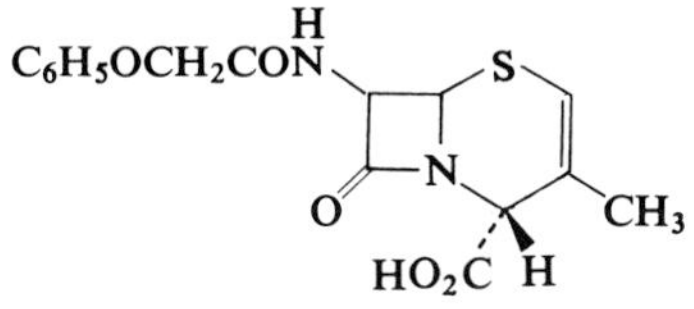

(*15*)

compound (syn-ceph) (*16*), similar in structure to the cephalosporins, the

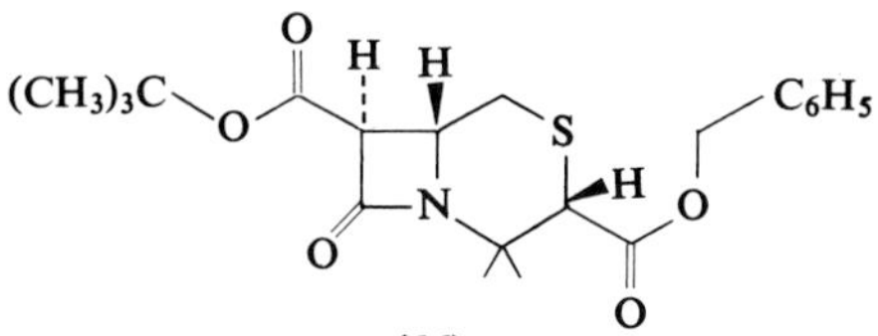

(*16*)

crystallography of which was done by Kalyani and Hodgkin (1970), and a synthetic fused β-lactam–thiazolidine system (syn-pen) (*17*) with a different

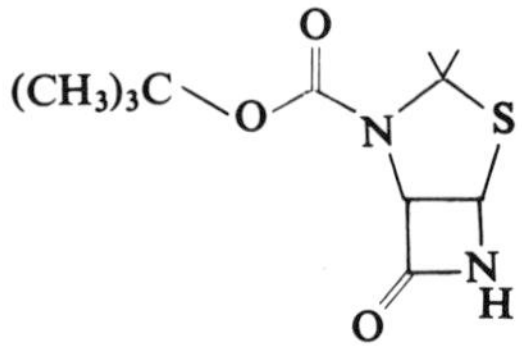

(17)

ring fusion from penicillins, examined by Gougoutas (1970). An additional
β-lactam compound for which a crystal structural analysis has been carried out
by Parthasarathy (1970) is (18).

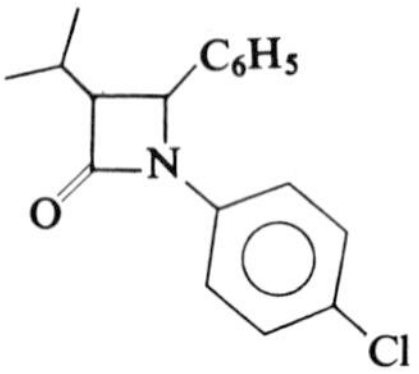

(18)

II. Crystallographic Results

A. Introduction

In a review of this sort, the reader should have access to as large a body of
experimental data as possible, within the limits of journalism, in addition to the
analyses of the reviewer. Although the printing of all the available data is
clearly impractical, a comprehensive set of bond lengths and angles for the
available β-lactam antibiotic structures is listed in Table I. The atom numbering
system used is consistent with (1) and (8). The molecular parameters listed are
confined to the region of the penicillanic acid or cephalosporanic acid ring
system. Table II contains bond lengths and angles for only the β-lactam region
of the four available penicillin or cephalosporin analogs which have no biological activity. The convention that will be in use throughout this chapter
with regard to standard errors of parameters is that, unless stated otherwise,
the standard deviation of the least significant figures of a parameter is shown
in parentheses following the parameter.

Table I

Molecular Parameters for Some Penicillanic and
Cephalosporanic Acid Derivatives[a]

Penicillanic acid interatomic distances (Å)			
	6-APA[b]	Pen V[c]	Ampicillin[d]
S(1)–C(2)	1.859(10)	1.87[e]	1.855[f]
S(1)–C(5)	1.822(10)	1.82	1.791
C(2)–C(3)	1.575(14)	1.57	1.573
C(3)–N(4)	1.445(11)	1.46	1.463
N(4)–C(5)	1.450(13)	1.52	1.470
N(4)–C(7)	1.392(13)	1.46	1.360
C(5)–C(6)	1.554(13)	1.58	1.554
C(6)–C(7)	1.520(15)	1.55	1.540
C(7)–O(8)	1.228(14)	1.21	1.198
C(2)–C(9)	1.547(15)	1.51	1.529
C(2)–C(10)	1.502(14)	1.58	1.514
C(3)–C(11)	1.527(12)	1.54	1.538
C(11)–O(12)	1.273(11)	1.35	1.240
C(11)–O(13)	1.230(12)	1.21	1.245
C(6)–N(14)	1.474(12)	1.44	1.420
N(14)–CO	—	1.37	1.341
C=O	—	1.29	1.226
CO–C$_\alpha$	—	1.49	1.512

Penicillanic acid bond angles (deg)			
	6-APA[b]	Pen V[c]	Ampicillin[d]
C(2)–S(1)–C(5)	95.6(5)	96[e]	89.8[f]
S(1)–C(2)–C(3)	105.7(6)	105	104.2
C(9)–C(2)–C(10)	111.2(8)	112	110.8
C(2)–C(3)–N(4)	106.0(7)	104	105.3
C(2)–C(3)–C(11)	111.8(7)	113	114.6
N(4)–C(3)–C(11)	109.8(7)	114	113.3
C(3)–N(4)–C(5)	118.0(7)	120	117.8
C(3)–N(4)–C(7)	132.5(8)	129	127.7
C(5)–N(4)–C(7)	93.5(7)	88	93.4
S(1)–C(5)–N(4)	103.4(6)	103	103.7
S(1)–C(5)–C(6)	120.2(7)	122	118.4
N(4)–C(5)–C(6)	88.1(7)	92	88.4
C(5)–C(6)–C(7)	84.6(7)	83	83.6
C(5)–C(6)–N(14)	118.4(8)	115	118.2
C(7)–C(6)–N(14)	117.3(8)	115	114.6
N(4)–C(7)–C(6)	91.7(8)	96	93.1
N(4)–C(7)–O(8)	131.7(10)	128	132.3
C(6)–C(7)–O(8)	136.4(10)	136	134.5

Table I —*continued*

Penicillanic acid bond angles (deg)			
	6-APA[b]	Pen V[c]	Ampicillin[d]
C(3)–C(11)–O(12)	116.1(8)	115	117.4
C(3)–C(11)–O(13)	118.2(8)	122	116.6
O(12)–C(11)–O(13)	125.7(9)	122	126.0
C(6)–N(14)–CO	—	125	123.3
N(14)–C=O	—	125	124.5
N(14)–CO–C_α	—	120	113.8
C_α–C=O	—	116	121.6

Cephalosporanic acid bond lengths (Å)		
	Cephaloridine[g]	Ceph C_c[b]
S(1)–C(2)	1.817(7)	1.802(11)
S(1)–C(6)	1.787(6)	1.798(12)
C(2)–C(3)	1.501(8)	1.486(19)
C(3)–C(4)	1.360(8)	1.329(19)
C(3)–C(13)	1.500(9)	1.476(19)
C(4)–N(5)	1.393(8)	1.419(14)
C(4)–C(10)	1.514(9)	1.459(18)
N(5)–C(6)	1.463(7)	1.479(14)
N(5)–C(8)	1.382(9)	1.385(13)
C(6)–C(7)	1.567(9)	1.535(15)
C(7)–C(8)	1.499(10)	1.527(15)
C(7)–N(14)	1.440(8)	1.442(10)
C(8)–O(9)	1.214(8)	1.209(15)
C(10)–O(11)	1.183(8)	1.188(21)
C(10)–O(12)	1.304(8)	1.358(18)
N(14)–CO	1.352(8)	1.332(11)
C=O	1.224(8)	1.245(11)
CO–C_α	1.528(10)	1.489(10)

Cephalosporanic acid bond angles (deg)		
	Cephaloridine[g]	Ceph C_c[b]
C(2)–S(1)–C(6)	94.4(3)	96.9(5)
S(1)–C(2)–C(3)	115.7(5)	113.0(9)
C(2)–C(3)–C(4)	123.1(6)	124.0(11)
C(2)–C(3)–C(13)	114.5(5)	128.6(13)
C(4)–C(3)–C(13)	122.4(6)	107.2(12)
C(3)–C(4)–N(5)	120.3(5)	125.6(11)
C(3)–C(4)–C(10)	126.0(6)	110.0(11)
N(5)–C(4)–C(10)	113.4(5)	124.3(11)
C(4)–N(5)–C(6)	126.3(5)	119.5(9)
C(4)–N(5)–C(8)	130.4(5)	130.5(10)
C(6)–N(5)–C(8)	94.0(5)	93.7(7)

	Cephalosporanic acid bond angles (deg)	
	Cephaloridine[g]	Ceph C_c[b]
S(1)–C(6)–N(5)	110.7(4)	111.9(7)
S(1)–C(6)–C(7)	116.5(4)	114.5(7)
N(5)–C(6)–C(7)	86.7(4)	86.6(8)
C(6)–C(7)–C(8)	85.5(5)	86.1(7)
C(6)–C(7)–N(14)	120.4(5)	121.0(11)
C(8)–C(7)–N(14)	116.3(6)	115.6(8)
N(5)–C(8)–C(7)	92.4(5)	90.3(8)
N(5)–C(8)–O(9)	131.1(6)	132.1(9)
C(7)–C(8)–O(9)	136.3(6)	137.5(9)
C(4)–C(10)–O(11)	120.9(6)	132.1(13)
C(4)–C(10)–O(12)	113.4(6)	107.7(13)
O(11)–C(10)–O(12)	125.7(6)	120.0(12)
C(7)–N(14)–CO	121.6(6)	122.6(8)
N(14)–C=O	123.4(6)	119.3(7)
N(14)–CO–C_α	114.2(6)	116.7(7)
C_α–C=O	122.2(6)	123.8(7)

[a] The atomic numbering is consistent with (1) and (8).
[b] Diamond (1963).
[c] Abrahamsson et al. (1963).
[d] James et al. (1968).
[e] The estimated standard deviations for pen V are σ(S–C) = 0.016 Å, σ(C–O, N) = 0.018 Å, σ(C–C) = 0.021 Å, and for bond angles, σ = 1.5°.
[f] Standard deviations for ampicillin bond lengths and angles are roughly 0.007 Å and 0.4°, respectively.
[g] Sweet and Dahl (1970).

Table II

NONANTIBIOTIC β-LACTAM BOND LENGTHS AND ANGLES

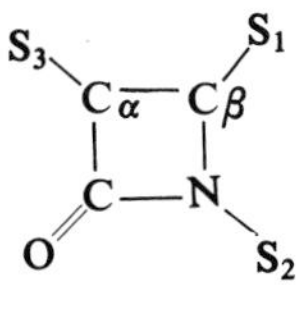

	An-pen[a]	2-Cephem[b]	Syn-ceph[c]	Syn-pen[d]
	β-Lactam interatomic distances (Å)			
N–C	1.415(7)	1.339(7)	1.355(6)	1.337[e]
N–C_β	1.466(6)	1.453(7)	1.483(6)	1.500
N–S_2	1.431(7)	1.449(7)	1.461(6)	—

Table II —*continued*

	An-pen[a]	2-Cephem[b]	Syn-ceph[c]	Syn-pen[d]
C–O	1.183(6)	1.223(7)	1.202(6)	1.201
C–C_α	1.527(8)	1.536(8)	1.545(7)	1.559
C_α–C_β	1.562(7)	1.551(9)	1.552(7)	1.565
C_α–S_3	1.435(6)	1.438(7)	1.489(7)	1.460
C_β–S_1	1.790(6)	1.795(7)	1.510(7)	1.757

β-Lactam interatomic angles (deg)

	An-pen[a]	2-Cephem[b]	Syn-ceph[c]	Syn-pen[d]
C–N–C_β	93.4(4)	95.6(4)	95.6(3)	96[e]
C–N–S_2	124.8(5)	136.7(5)	136.2(4)	—
C_β–N–S_2	116.6(4)	127.0(5)	126.6(3)	—
N–C–O	131.2(5)	133.2(6)	134.4(5)	133
N–C–C_α	91.9(5)	92.2(5)	91.8(4)	93
C_α–C–O	136.9(6)	134.5(6)	133.8(5)	135
C–C_α–C_β	85.4(4)	84.2(5)	85.6(4)	85
C–C_α–S_3	115.5(4)	119.2(5)	114.9(4)	117
C_β–C_α–S_3	118.7(4)	121.1(5)	121.8(4)	108
N–C_β–C_α	88.6(4)	87.4(4)	86.9(3)	86
N–C_β–S_1	107.3(4)	110.4(4)	112.8(4)	117
C_α–C_β–S_1	121.0(4)	115.8(4)	115.8(4)	108

[a] Simon and Dahl (1970).
[b] Sweet and Dahl (1970).
[c] Kalyani and Hodgkin (1970).
[d] Gougoutas (1970).
[e] Standard deviations for syn-pen bond lengths and angles are roughly 0.015 Å and 1.0°, respectively.

B. Comparison of Bond Lengths and Angles

Upon examination of the molecular parameters in Table I for the penicillanic acid structures listed, one can see that the molecular nuclei of these molecules are not identical, but there is some similarity. Although one could propose a reasonably consistent average model for the penicillanic acid molecular nucleus from these bond length and bond angle values, there is clearly a degree of freedom in the detailed conformation the penicillin molecule can adopt. In the case of the two cephalosporanic acid derivatives listed, however, the agreement between molecular parameters is remarkable. Most of the large differences in bond lengths and all of the large differences in bond angles seem to pertain to the lactone fused at positions 3,4 in ceph C_c (*10*).

C. Molecular Conformation

1. INTRODUCTION

Bond strain within the sulfur-containing and the β-lactam rings places rather firm restrictions on the conformations of the fused-ring penicillin and cephalosporin systems. A convenient technique for the description of molecular conformation in addition to the listing of interatomic distances and angles is the calculation of the best mean plane through specific sets of atoms and the examination of the distances these and other atoms lie from this plane. Various aspects of molecular conformation in the cephalosporins and penicillins will now be discussed in terms of appropriate mean plane calculations. Obvious features to be considered in turn are the thiazolidine ring in penicillins, the dihydrothiazine ring in cephalosporins, the β-lactam ring, and the amide link exocyclic to the β-lactam.

2. THE THIAZOLIDINE OF PENICILLINS

The thiazolidine ring, constrained by the β-lactam, can adopt one of two conformations to assure that the substituents at C(2) and C(3) do not eclipse one another. These are (*19*), with α-CH$_3$ equatorial, β-CH$_3$ axial, and α-CO$_2$H axial, or (*20*) with α-CH$_3$ axial, β-CH$_3$ equatorial, and α-CO$_2$H equatorial (Cooper *et al.*, 1969).

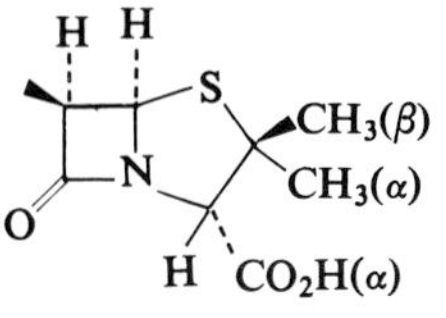

(*19*) 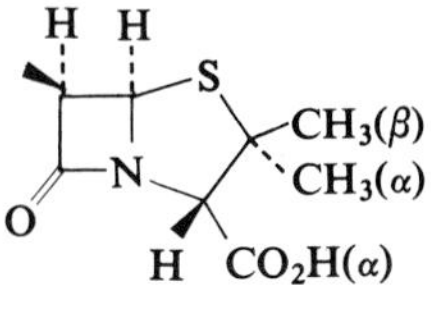   (*20*)

Pen G, the nucleus of which is shown in Fig. 2A, has conformation (*19*) and ampicillin, Fig. 3, is (*20*). In order to realize this steric necessity, each penicillin thiazolidine ring exists with four of its atoms nearly coplanar and with the fifth atom out of this plane. The particular atom which is out and the direction of its deviation correlates with the conformation of the ring substituents as follows—where up or down indicates toward or away from the β-lactam, respectively—for type (*19*):

6-APA	N(4) up
Pen V	C(3) down
Pen G	C(3) down

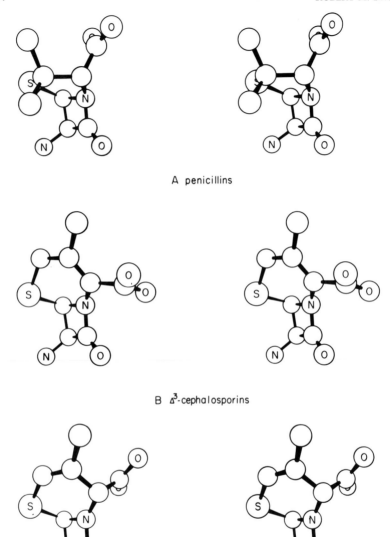

A penicillins

B Δ³-cephalosporins

C Δ²-cephalosporins

Fig. 2. Stereoscopic views of the solid state conformations of the molecular nuclei of the penicillins, the biologically active Δ³-cephalosporins, and the biologically inactive Δ²-cephalosporins. [Reprinted by permission from Sweet and Dahl (1970).]

and for type (*20*):

Ampicillin	S(1) up
Pen sulfoxide	S(1) up

The most obvious systematic difference between the bond lengths and angles of type (*19*) and type (*20*) molecules is that in 6-APA and pen V the C–S–C angle is 96° while in ampicillin it is 90°. All other bond lengths and

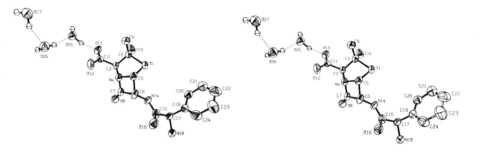

Fig. 3. Stereoscopic view of the molecular conformation of ampicillin trihydrate. (Drawing courtesy of Dr. M. N. G. James.)

angles compare within one or two standard deviations. In the thiazolidine ring ·of syn-pen (*17*) the two atoms held in common with the β-lactam are essentially coplanar with the nitrogen and sulfur atoms; the fifth atom in the ring is out of this plane.

3. THE DIHYDROTHIAZINE OF CEPHALOSPORINS

The dihydrothiazine ring in the 3-cephem can be described as having five of its six atoms lying roughly in a plane with the sixth, the sulfur atom, out of this plane. In ceph C_c (*10*) and cephaloridine (*9*) the root mean square (rms) deviation of atoms C(2), C(3), C(4), N(5), and C(6) from their best plane is 0.04 and 0.05 Å and the distance from this plane to the sulfur atom, S(1), is 0.87 and 0.90 Å, respectively. In each case the atoms involved in the C(2)=C(3) double bond are nearly coplanar but are twisted to form a right-handed screw with a displacement of about 5°.

4. THE β-LACTAM

An important consideration related to the chemical and biological activity of these compounds is the coplanarity of the β-lactam nitrogen atom with its three substituents. The presence of amide resonance in the β-lactam depends upon this coplanarity, and when it is absent this electron delocalization is diminished. This degree of planarity can be expressed in at least two ways. One can tabulate the perpendicular distance from the nitrogen atom to the plane of its substituents and the sum of the bond angles about this atom. These values appear in Table III for several compounds. Rather clearly, systems such as the 2-cephem (15) and syn-ceph (16) with relatively less bond angle strain in the sulfur-containing ring have a more nearly planar lactam nitrogen atom. Presumably in syn-pen (17) the hydrogen atom on the lactam nitrogen is free to lie in the plane of this atom and its other two substituent atoms.

A further characteristic of the β-lactam ring is the degree of coplanarity of its atoms. In general, the four atoms involved in the amide link, N(4), C(6), C(7), and O(8) for the penicillins (1) and N(5), C(7), C(8), and O(9) for the cephalosporins (8), are more nearly coplanar than are the four atoms in the ring. Also in general, the β-carbon atom in the ring, C(5) in (1) and C(6) in (8), is displaced from the plane of the amide link toward the sulfur atom. The net effect seems to be a bending of the lactam oxygen up toward the sulfur atom. This apparently systematic distortion of the β-lactam ring extends to non-antibiotic β-lactams as well, but only to those which are β-substituted with sulfur. This same bending of the lactam carbonyl group toward the sulfur atom is observed in an-pen, 2-cephem, and syn-pen. In syn-ceph and Parthasarathy's compound (18), however, which have no sulfur atom bonded directly to the β-lactam ring, the four-membered rings are planar within experimental error. The rms deviation of the four atoms in the lactam amide from their best plane and the distance from this plane of the fourth atom in the ring are shown in Table III for several compounds.

5. THE EXOCYCLIC AMIDE

The amide group exocyclic to the β-lactam is present in nearly all of the biologically active penicillanic and cephalosporanic acid derivatives. The four atoms of the amide link, C_α–CO–N, are uniformly planar for the examples studied and the carbon atom which is in the β-lactam ring and is bonded to the amide nitrogen atom is usually reasonably close to this plane. All available evidence indicates that this amide grouping adopts a conformation which minimizes interaction between the amide carbonyl and the rest of the molecule.

Table III

STRUCTURAL CHARACTERISTICS OF β-LACTAM IN SOME PENICILLINS AND CEPHALOSPORINS

The $\overset{C}{\underset{\underset{O}{\parallel}}{C}}-N$ fragment

Compound	Planarity of nitrogen atom		The 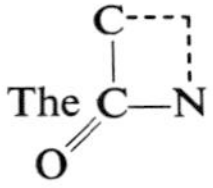 C—C(=O)—N fragment		N–CO bond length (Å)	C=O bond length (Å)
	Sum of bond angles about nitrogen (deg)	Distance of N atom from plane of three substituents (Å)	RMS dev. of four atoms from best least-squares plane (Å)	Distance of fourth ring atom from plane (Å)		
Pen V	337(2)	0.40	0.003	0.166	1.46(2)	1.21(2)
Ampicillin	339(1)	0.38	0.010	0.282	1.360(7)	1.198(7)
6-APA	343(2)	0.32	0.015	0.326	1.392(13)	1.228(14)
Ceph-C$_c$	345(2)	0.32	0.004	0.357	1.385(13)	1.209(15)
Cephaloridine	350.7(8)	0.24	0.015	0.287	1.382(9)	1.214(8)
An-pen	334.8(8)	0.42	0.005	0.168	1.415(7)	1.183(6)
2-Cephem	359.3(8)	0.06	0.002	0.145	1.339(7)	1.223(7)
Syn-ceph	358.4(8)	0.10	0.002	0.010	1.355(6)	1.202(6)
Syn-pen	—	—	0.007	0.149	1.337(15)	1.201(15)

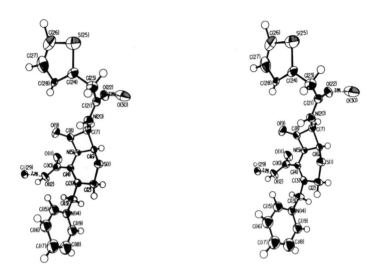

Fig. 4. Stereoscopic view of the molecular conformation of cephaloridine hydrochloride monohydrate. [Reprinted by permission from Sweet and Dahl (1970).]

This conformation is shown for ampicillin, cephaloridine, and the 2-cephem in Figs. 3–5, respectively. The observed extremes of torsion about the C(lactam)–N(amide) bond are illustrated in the cases of ampicillin (Fig. 3) and the 2-cephem (Fig. 5).

D. Intramolecular Interactions in the Side Chain

The antibiotics pen V (*2*), ampicillin (*3*), and cephaloglycin (*12*) are more acid-stable than most other penicillins and cephalosporins, a desirable

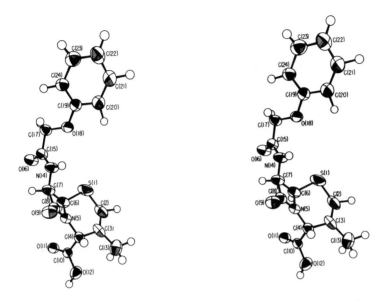

Fig. 5. Stereoscopic view of the molecular conformation of phenoxymethyl-Δ^2-deacetoxyl-cephalosporin (2-cephem). [Reprinted by permission from Sweet and Dahl (1970).]

property for compounds to be administered orally. Abrahamsson *et al.* (1963) and James *et al.* (1968) mentioned this fact in their investigations of pen V and ampicillin, respectively. In all three of these compounds, the exocyclic amide is α substituted with an electron-withdrawing group. Although some workers speculated (Abrahamsson *et al.*, 1963) that internal hydrogen bonding contributed to the acid stability, there is no systematic solid state evidence to support a particular type of interaction. The interaction (*21*) in pen V is probably not a hydrogen bond, no such interaction exists in the side chain of ampicillin (*22*) and Fig. 3, and the interaction in cephaloglycin (*23*) and Fig. 6 is quite different from that in pen V. The short $\overset{+}{CO\cdots NH_3^-}$ distance of 2.81(4) Å in the side chain of cephaloglycin (*23*) indicates a strong interaction which is possibly

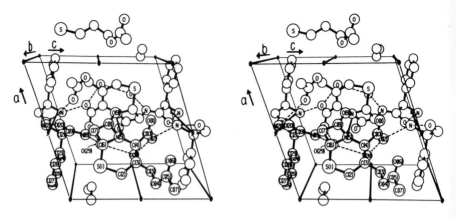

Fig. 6. Stereoscopic view of the molecular packing and conformation of cephaloglycin. [Reprinted by permission from Sweet and Dahl (1970).]

part electrostatic and part hydrogen bonding. The absence of this interaction in the identical side chain of ampicillin may be due to packing constraints within the crystal. In any event, the observed acid stability is probably due to a resistance to protonation caused by inductive effects in (21) and by electrostatic ones in (22) and (23).

(21)

(22)

(23)

E. Molecular Packing in the Crystal

Hydrogen bonding occurs quite regularly as part of the packing mechanism of these compounds in the solid state. The carboxyl or carboxylate group is involved in at least one hydrogen bond in every structure published where that group was present. Both the nitrogen atom and the carbonyl oxygen atom of the exocyclic amide regularly take part in hydrogen bonding, as do primary amines. The zwitterionic structures show an exceptionally large amount, as is illustrated by the particularly intricate net of hydrogen bonds in the cephaloglycin structure (Fig. 6). Four of the structures, ceph C (*11*), ceph C$_c$ (*10*), the 2-cephem (*15*), and apparently 7-BrAc-ACA (*13*) experience peptide-like hydrogen bonding (*24*) between the exocyclic amide groups of adjacent molecules. It is interesting to note that in no case studied does an active cephalosporin or penicillin antibiotic experience a hydrogen bond involving either the

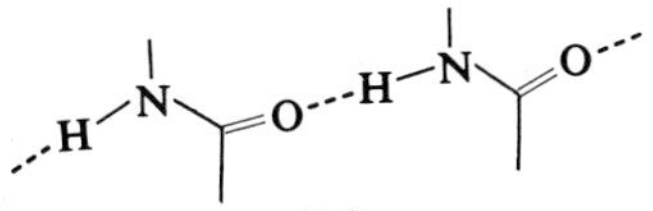

(*24*)

nitrogen or the oxygen atom of the β-lactam ring. At the same time, the 2-cephem structure shows an H bond of the type C=O · · · H–O– linking the lactam carbonyl oxygen atom to a carboxyl OH.

In general, these molecules pack, as expected, with polar regions together and with nonpolar regions together, as, for example, in the cephaloglycin packing, as shown in Fig. 6. Several of the available structures contain phenyl rings as substituents. An extraordinary variety of interactions among these aromatic groups is observed. In ampicillin there is no close contact among phenyl groups. In pen V and cephaloglycin, two such symmetry-related rings face each other in sandwich fashion with ring planes approximately parallel at roughly van der Waals distance. In syn-ceph, potassium pen G, and the 2-cephem structure, symmetry-related phenyl rings lie with ring planes oblique to one another, the edge of one near the face of another. Symmetry-related phenyl rings in sodium pen G pack with nonparallel rings in contact edgewise.

F. In Defense*

Those who would speculate that the molecular conformations of these molecules determined in the solid state have, at best, a vague relationship to their solution conformations, should be made aware of the recent structural investigation of phenoxymethylpenicillin sulfoxide (*5*). Cooper and co-workers (*1969*) have used both X-ray diffraction and nuclear Overhauser effect studies to show that the fused ring system in this compound adopts the same detailed conformation both in the solid state and in solution. The fused ring system in the penicillin sulfoxide molecule is very similar to that of the penicillins and of the 3- and 2-cephem derivatives. Thus, most likely these latter ring systems

---

* Brief portions of this section are reprinted by permission from Sweet and Dahl (1970).

are also sufficiently rigid to dictate the same conformation both in the solid state and in solution.

III. Structure–Activity Relationships

A. Introduction*

Having examined the detailed structures of various cephalosporin and penicillin derivatives and analogs, we are prepared to discuss the implications molecular structure has on the chemistry and biology of these compounds. As was mentioned earlier in the chapter, various workers have established that the penicillins and cephalosporins inhibit the terminal step in bacterial cell wall synthesis which is a peptide cross-linking of peptidoglycan strands catalyzed by the enzyme peptidoglycan transpeptidase. Tipper and Strominger (1965) suggested that the penicillins imitate a possible conformation of this enzyme's substrate, D-alanyl-D-alanine (Fig. 1). The enzyme mistakes the penicillin molecule for its proper substrate, cleaves the amide bond in the penicillin's β-lactam ring, is thus acylated, and is blocked irreversibly from further activity.

B. Substrate Recognition

These arguments require that the antibiotic have a molecular form which the enzyme to be inhibited recognizes as its substrate. Examination of molecular structures which are clearly acceptable, that is, active antibiotics which acylate the enzyme, is an obvious next step. The conformation of D-ala-D-ala which appears in Fig. 1 bears no part in this discussion. This is only one of many conformations this dipeptide can adopt, and it was designed solely to mimic penicillin. Clearly, examination of the static molecular forms of the antibiotics and their derivatives will tell more about the stereochemistry of the enzyme's preferred substrate than will speculation about a more flexible example of a substrate. Figure 2 shows the actual solid state conformation of the molecular nuclei of the penicillins (Pitt, 1952), the biologically active 3-cephem derivatives, and the biologically inactive 2-cephem derivatives (Sweet and Dahl, 1970). The drawings are arranged so that all of the β-lactams are in equivalent orientations. Presumably, the enzyme approaches the molecule roughly from the right. One might expect that the orientation of the carboxyl

* Brief portions of Sections III,A,B,C, and E are reprinted by permission from Sweet and Dahl (1970).

group, which is immediately adjacent to the β-lactam ring, is an important factor in the ability of the enzyme to recognize the antibiotic as its substrate. Although the penicillins and the 3-cephem derivatives are both recognized by the transpeptidase enzyme, the drawings clearly indicate that the conformations of carboxyl group relative to the lactam in these two molecular types are quite different. This suggests that the gross conformational requirements placed on the recognition by the enzyme of the antibiotic as its substrate are not very restrictive.

Consider now the stereochemistry of the 2-cephem nucleus shown in the same drawing (Fig. 2). The carboxyl group adopts a conformation relative to the β-lactam not unlike that of the penicillins. This stereochemistry in the 2-cephem certainly varies no more from that of either the penicillins or 3-cephems than they vary from each other. Thus, the enzyme may well recognize the 2-cephem ring system as well as the penicillin and 3-cephem moieties. Yet all 2-cephem derivatives are biologically inactive (Eardly et al., 1963). Earlier in this chapter the suggestion was made that in order to be an effective acylating agent for the enzyme, the antibiotic must have an amide bond which is more easily broken than a normal amide link. This could be possible in the antibiotics if the penicillin or cephalosporin β-lactam amide bond experiences less amide resonance than a free peptide bond does. We have already mentioned that the 2-cephem derivatives have considerably less biological activity than penicillins or 3-cephems. In addition, the well-known chemical stability of monocyclic β-lactams relative to the β-lactam antibiotics extends to the 2-cephems. These latter compounds are considerably more stable to such effects as basic hydrolysis than are the penicillins or 3-cephem derivatives (Van Heyningen and Ahern, 1968). Perhaps these differences in chemical and biological properties of the 2-cephem derivatives relative to the 3-cephems or penicillins are due to a difference in resonance properties of the β-lactam. Various physical evidence will tell if this difference exists.

C. Structural Chemistry of the β-Lactam

1. PLANARITY OF THE NITROGEN

To understand the effects which molecular structure can have on this sort of resonance, arguments made earlier by Woodward (1949) may be used to suggest that in a monocyclic β-lactam normal amide resonance (25) can occur

(25)

which tends to shorten the C–N and lengthen the C–O bonds. A principal requirement for maximization of this type of charge delocalization is that the three atoms connected to the nitrogen atom be coplanar with it so that the unshared electron pair of the nitrogen atom can be involved in π bonding with the adjacent carbonyl carbon atom. In the penicillins, however, the nitrogen atom cannot be planar for steric reasons. Data in Table III indicate the extent of this nonplanarity for several of these compounds. Infrared data (Bellamy, 1958) certainly indicate that the shift in C=O stretching frequency from unstrained β-lactams to the penicillins is toward less of this electron delocalization. This absorption band increases in frequency from about 1760 cm^{-1} for the free β-lactams to 1780 cm^{-1} for the penicillins as the planarity of the nitrogen atom decreases, which indicates an accompanying increase in double bond character between the carbon and oxygen atoms. A change in electron delocalization dramatic enough to be reflected in spectral changes as great as these certainly should be accompanied by detectable bond length changes. This is found to be the case, as is indicated in Tables III and IV. The weighted

Table IV

AVERAGED β-LACTAM PHYSICAL PARAMETERS

Compound	C=O stretching frequency (cm^{-1})	N–CO bond length (Å)	C=O bond length (Å)
Penicillins	1780–1770[a]	1.37(1)	1.20(1)
Cephalosporins	1776–1764[b]	1.38(1)	1.21(1)
Unstrained β-lactams	1760–1756[c]	1.347(7)	1.210(7)
Free amides	1680–1600[a]	1.32$_5$[d]	1.24[d]

[a] Bellamy (1958).

[b] Green et al. (1965).

[c] The C=O stretching frequency for the 2-cephem (Green et al., 1965) is in the same range as for most normal β-lactams (Bellamy, 1958).

[d] Marsh and Donohue (1967).

mean N–CO and C=O bond lengths respectively for the penicillins are 1.37(1) and 1.20(1) Å; for the 3-cephem derivatives, 1.38(1) and 1.21(1) Å; and for the 2-cephem, syn-pen, and syn-ceph β-lactams, 1.347(7) and 1.210(7) Å. Thus the decrease in amide resonance when the lactam nitrogen becomes less planar as one goes from unstrained β-lactams to the penicillins is followed by a significant increase of three standard deviations in N–CO bond length, and a systematic (though barely significant) decrease in C=O bond length which is paralleled by increased C=O stretching frequency.

2. ENAMINE RESONANCE

In the cephalosporins, however, another factor in addition to the lack of planarity of the amide nitrogen may add to the lability of the β-lactam amide bond. In these compounds, the possibility exists for normal enamine resonance, the delocalization of the nitrogen atom's unshared electron pair into the adjacent olefinic π-orbital system (26).

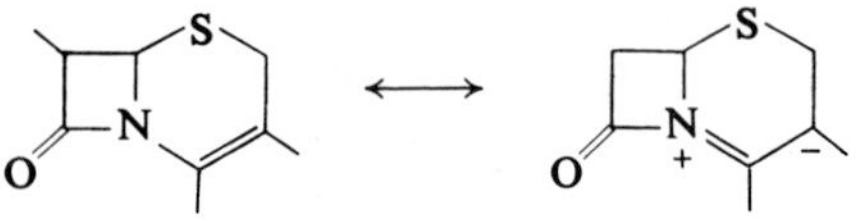

(26)

The weighted average values from cephaloridine and ceph C_c of the C(3)–C(4) (8) and C(4)–N(5) bond lengths are 1.355(8) and 1.400(8) Å, respectively. The first of these, a C=C double bond, is a bit longer while the second, the C–N single bond adjacent to it, is significantly shorter than the expected values (Pauling, 1960) of 1.33 Å for the double and 1.47 Å for the single bonds. This systematic shift in bond lengths from their expected values is certainly substantial evidence for the presence of enamine resonance. To the extent that this delocalization exists, the unshared electron pair of the nitrogen atom is involved in some π bonding even though the orbitals which contain it must possess s-orbital character because the atoms connected to the nitrogen atom are not coplanar with it. Thus, one might expect that in spite of the nonplanar nitrogen atom in the cephalosporin β-lactam, this atom's unshared electron pair could be involved to some degree in amide as well as enamine resonance. An increased contribution of one type of resonance will clearly decrease the contribution of the other type. Thus, one might suggest that enamine resonance plus the lack of planarity of the nitrogen atom combine to decrease the amide resonance in the lactam amide bond of the cephalosporins which otherwise occurs to a much larger extent in an unstrained β-lactam without the α,β unsaturation present in cephalosporins.

Morin and co-workers (1969) have provided additional evidence to illustrate the effect of the cephalosporin enamine on the β-lactam. These workers reported infrared data for the C=O stretch of the β-lactam in three types of compounds, i.e., penicillins (27), 3-cephems (28), and 2-cephems (29) where $R = -COCH_2OC_6H_5$. In each case the lactam absorption band was listed

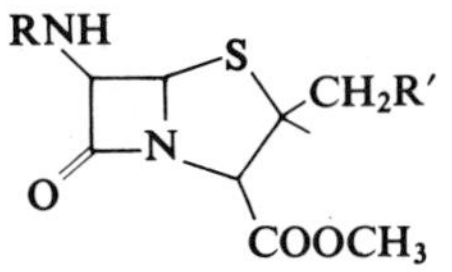

(27) 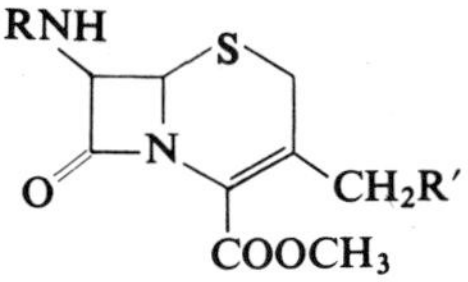   (28) 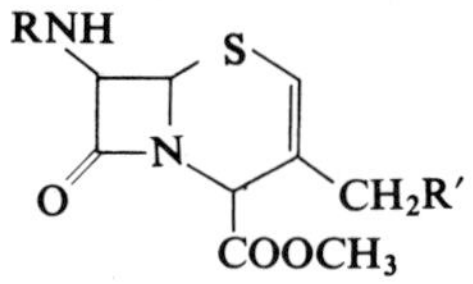   (29)

for the compounds where $R' = H$ and where $R' = OCOCH_3$. Rather clearly, the change of acetate for hydrogen at R' in (27) and (29) could have an effect on lactam amide resonance. Long-range electron withdrawal from the nitrogen atom by the more electronegative acetate group could decrease this electron delocalization. Apparently, this is the case since the shift in lactam absorption as one goes from $R' = H$ to $R' = OCOCH_3$ in (27) is $+5$ cm^{-1}, and in (29) it is $+4$ cm^{-1}. In the case of (28), however, the increase in electronegativity at R' as one goes from $R' = H$ to $R' = OCOCH_3$ helps to stabilize directly the proposed enamine delocalization (26). The shift in C=O absorption, hence the decrease in amide delocalization, is significantly larger, i.e., $+7$ cm^{-1}.

The structural chemistry of the β-lactam in Parthasarathy's compound (18) is substantially similar to that of the 3-cephems. The parachlorophenyl group bonded to the lactam nitrogen atom is very nearly coplanar with the lactam ring. This makes possible delocalization of the nitrogen atom's unshared electron pair into the phenyl ring (30). The lactam N–CO and C=O bond lengths of

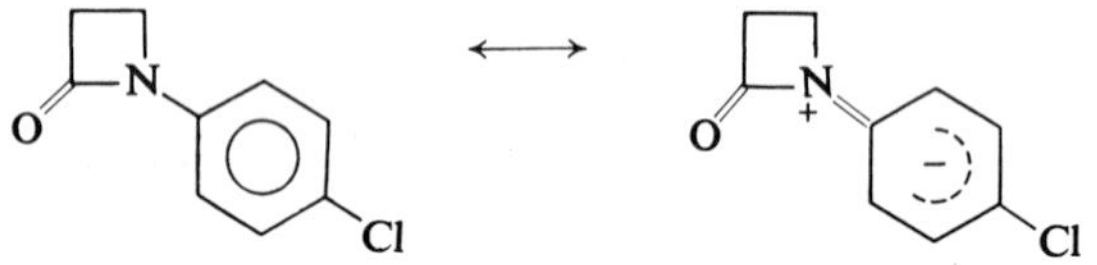

(30)

1.367(4) and 1.210(4) Å are sufficiently similar to those of the cephalosporins or penicillins (Table IV) to indicate that amide resonance in this lactam is being inhibited as in the antibiotics.

D. Conclusion

The evidence clearly shows that the amide bond in the β-lactam ring of the penicillin and cephalosporin antibiotics has electronic properties which are considerably different from those of β-lactams in an unstrained environment. The initial assertion was, however, that the antibiotic lactam amide bond must be more susceptible to cleavage than a normal amide. The physical data summarized in Table IV, namely, C=O stretching frequencies and mean C=O and N–CO bond lengths for normal amides, unstrained β-lactam amides, and antibiotic β-lactam amides, certainly indicate that the highly labile antibiotic β-lactams experience a minimum of amide resonance and unstrained β-lactams experience an intermediate amount. Loss by the antibiotic lactams of this amide resonance leaves the lactam carbonyl with electronic properties more like those of an aliphatic ketone than like a normal amide. That is, the unperturbed dipole moment of the carbonyl leaves the carbon atom with a slight positive charge relative to the oxygen atom. This situation certainly favors nucleo-philic attack at the carbonyl carbon atom of the sort which occurs during basic hydrolysis and which could occur on a hydrolytic enzyme.

E. An Anomaly

A crystal structure which has been very well determined but has been little discussed here is that of anhydro-α-phenoxymethylpenicillin (*14*) (Simon and Dahl, 1970). Because the nitrogen atom in the β-lactam must be nonplanar, equivalent to what is found in the penicillins, and because unsaturation exists α,β to the nitrogen atom, similar to that in the cephalosporins, one might expect even less amide resonance in the lactam ring. This hypothesis is supported by the following evidence. The infrared carbonyl band has shifted from 1775 cm^{-1} for penicillins to 1820 cm^{-1} for the anhydropenicillin (Wolfe *et al.*, 1968). The N–CO and C=O bonds have lengths 1.415(7) and 1.183(6) Å (Table II), respectively, compared to the mean values 1.37 and 1.20 Å for the penicillins. In spite of the apparent lack of amide resonance, however, significantly increased stability relative to that for the active penicillins is observed for this compound in that it is recovered unchanged after refluxing in various neutral solvents or from a melt (Wolfe *et al.*, 1968). This stability is completely in contrast with the known instability of the active cephalosporin systems and the penicillins. We shall await a further explanation of this unexpected difference in chemical activities.

IV. Summary*

In summary, structural comparisons have been made among the penicillins, the cephalosporins, and several other β-lactam-containing compounds by the use of detailed and accurate X-ray crystal structural results. The contrasting of the very different molecular forms of molecules known to inhibit the active site of the bacterial enzyme peptidoglycan transpeptidase indicates that the conformational requirements for substrate recognition by this enzyme may not be very restrictive. The penicillin and cephalosporin antibiotics are stereochemically similar, not in their detailed conformations or dimensions, but because each contains a N–CO bond in its β-lactam ring with less normal amide character than that in a free or unstrained β-lactam. This observed decrease in amide resonance character may well be the necessary activation of the lactam amide bond relative to normal amides which accounts for its rapid

---

* Brief portions of this section are reprinted by permission from Sweet and Dahl (1970).

cleavage on the enzyme or in basic solution. Naturally, the ability of a particular compound to acylate this transpeptidase in an *in vitro* preparation is not in itself a sufficient property for a successful antibiotic. Other considerations, such as permeability of the compound into an active site, can have a dramatic effect on its antibacterial activity. The ability of the compound to interact with the enzyme in the fashion discussed in this chapter is, however, clearly necessary for any sort of bactericidal action associated with inhibition of transpeptidation.

Note added in proof: As this book was being prepared to go to press, a letter by Dr. Byungkook Lee appeared in the *Journal of Molecular Biology* [*61*, 463 (1971)] which is pertinent to the subject matter of this chapter. In this letter, Dr. Lee published drawings similar to Fig. 1 and additionally made several. rather important suggestions about the conformational basis of biological activity in the β-lactam antibiotics.

Acknowledgments

The author gratefully acknowledges the gracious contribution of unpublished results for use in this chapter by Dorothy Hodgkin, J. Zanos Gougoutas, Mike James, V. Kalyani, Larry Dahl, and Gary Simon. The use of the facilities of the MRC Laboratory of Molecular Biology and· the support of the Damon Runyon Memorial Fund for Cancer Research is greatly appreciated.

References

Abrahamsson, S., Hodgkin, D. C., and Maslen, E. N. (1963). *Biochem. J.* **86**, 514.
Bellamy, L. J. (1958). "The Infrared Spectra of Complex Molecules," 2nd ed. Wiley, New York.
Cooper, R. D. G., DeMarco, P. V., Cheng, J. C., and Jones, N. D. (1969). *J. Amer. Chem. Soc.* **91**, 1408.
Crowfoot, D., Bunn, C. W., Rogers-Low, D. W., and Turner-Jones, A. (1949). *In* "The Chemistry of Penicillin" (H. T. Clarke, J. R. Johnson and R. Robinson, eds.), p. 310. Princeton Univ. Press, Princeton, New Jersey.
Diamond, R. D. (1963). A Crystallographic Study of the Structure of Some Antibiotics. D. Phil. Thesis, Univ. of Oxford.
Eardly, S., Gregory, G. I., Hall, M. E., and Long, A. G. (1963). Abstracts of 19th Int. Congr. of IUPAC, London, Sect. A8-6, p. 308.
Gougoutas, J. Z. (1970). Personal communication.
Green, G. F. H., Page, J. E., and Staniforth, S. E. (1965). *J. Chem. Soc.* 1595.
Hardcastle, G. A., Jr., Johnson, D. A., Panetta, C. A., Scott, A. I., and Sutherland, S. A. (1966). *J. Org. Chem.* **31**, 897.
Hodgkin, D. C., and Maslen, E. N. (1961). *Biochem. J.* **79**, 383.
Hunt, D. J., and Rogers, D. (1964). *Biochem. J.* **93**, 35C.
Izaki, K., Matsuhashi, M., and Strominger, J. L. (1966). *Proc. Nat. Acad. Sci.* **55**, 656.
Izaki, K., Matsuhashi, M., and Strominger, J. L. (1968). *J. Biol. Chem.* **243**, 3180.
James, M. N. G., Hall, D., and Hodgkin, D. C. (1968). *Nature* (London) **220**, 168.

Kalyani, V., and Hodgkin, D. C. (1970). Personal communication.

Marsh, R. E., and Donohue, J. (1967). *Advan. Prot. Chem.* **22**, 235.

Morin, R. B., Jackson, B. G., Mueller, R. A., Lavagnino, E. R., Scanlon, W. B., and Andrews, S. L. (1969). *J. Amer. Chem. Soc.* **91**, 1401.

Parthasarathy, R. (1970). *Acta Crystallogr.* **B26**, 1283.

Pauling, L. (1960). "The Nature of the Chemical Bond," 3rd ed., p. 224. Cornell Univ. Press, Ithaca, New York.

Pitt, G. J. (1952). *Acta Crystallogr.* **5**, 770.

Simon, G. L., and Dahl, L. F. (1970). Personal communication.

Strominger, J. L., Izaki, K., Matsuhashi, M., and Tipper, D. J. (1967). *Fed. Proc. Fed. Amer. Soc. Exp. Biol.* **26**, 9.

Sweet, R. M., and Dahl, L. F. (1969). *Biochem. Biophys. Res. Commun.* **34**, 14.

Sweet, R. M., and Dahl, L. F. (1970). *J. Amer. Chem. Soc.* **92**, 5489.

Tipper, D. J., and Strominger, J. L. (1965). *Proc. Nat. Acad. Sci.* **54**, 1133, and references cited therein.

Tipper, D. J., and Strominger, J. L. (1968). *J. Biol. Chem.* **243**, 3169.

Vaciago, A. (1960). *Atti. Accad. Nazion. Lincei, R. C., Cl. Sci. Fis. Mat. Nat.* **28**, 851.

Van Heyningen, E., and Ahern, L. K. (1968). *J. Med. Chem.* **11**, 933.

Wise, E. M., Jr., and Park, J. T. (1965). *Proc. Nat. Acad. Sci.* **54**, 75, and references cited therein.

Wolfe, S., Godfrey, J. C., Holdrege, C. T., and Perron, Y. G. (1968). *Can. J. Chem.* **46**, 2549.

Woodward, R. B. (1949). *In* "The Chemistry of Penicillin" (H. T. Clarke, J. R. Johnson, and R. Robinson, eds.), p. 440. Princeton Univ. Press, Princeton, New Jersey.

Chapter 8

PHYSICAL–CHEMICAL PROPERTIES OF CEPHALOSPORINS AND PENICILLINS

P. V. DEMARCO and R. NAGARAJAN

The organic chemist then must welcome the new physical
methods, as he has all their predecessors, as tools to
speed up structural work and give him the opportunity
of driving his subject further and deeper towards
our understanding of nature.

Lord Todd
Presidential Address, IUPAC Congress, 1963.

I. Introduction

Cephalosporins and penicillins constitute one of the most important classes of antibiotics used in antimicrobial chemotherapy. The problem of establishing the structure of various new products resulting from chemical conversions of these antibiotics is a complex one. In the past 20 years, the application of physical–chemical methods in organic chemistry has assumed immense importance. Problems in structure elucidation which took years of chemical work can now be solved within weeks by a judicious application of the correct physical–chemical methods. It requires a thorough knowledge of all the physical–chemical methods available today to be able to select the particular method that will solve a given problem in a minimum period. In this chapter some of the important physical–chemical methods used in cephalosporin and penicillin chemistry are discussed.

II. Dissociation Constants

Interpretation of the dissociation constants (pK_a) of penicillins played an important role in early penicillin chemistry, when a limited number of physical–chemical methods were available for structure elucidation of these antibiotics. An important argument used in favor of the β-lactam structure over the thiazolidine–oxazolone structure for penicillin was the fact that the pK_a measurements were consistent with the β-lactam structure (Woodward et al., 1949). As newer physical–chemical methods became available, the use of dissociation constants in structural studies of β-lactam antibiotics has diminished. To some extent this trend is inevitable, but not entirely warranted. The β-lactam antibiotics are amino acid derivatives, and amino acids are substituted bases and substituted acids at the same time. This confers on them the remarkable electrochemical property of being amphoteric electrolytes. Dissociation constant measurement provides a valuable tool to probe this unique property. Excellent review articles of the application of dissociation constants to elucidation of structure of natural products (King, 1963), amino acids (Greenstein and Winitz, 1961), and penicillins (Woodward et al., 1949) are available. Consequently, this section will deal only with the application of dissociation constants to cephalosporin chemistry.

An acid, as defined by Brönsted (1923), is a species which may lose a proton; a base is one which may add a proton. The dissociation constant of an acid or a base is a measure of this process. The dissociation constants discussed in this section are the apparent, and not the thermodynamic, dissociation constants. The former is just as useful and is easily measured.

A. Factors Affecting Dissociation Constants

The major external factor affecting the dissociation constant is the solvent. The pK_a values of cyclohexane carboxylic acid in the three commonly used solvents are different (Table I), and consequently, comparison of pK_a values in

Table I

DISSOCIATION CONSTANT OF CYCLOHEXANE CARBOXYLIC
ACID IN DIFFERENT SOLVENTS

Solvent	pK_a	Reference
Water	4.90	Dippy et al., 1954
H_2O:MCS[a] 12:88	7.43	Tichý et al., 1959
H_2O:DMF[b] 34:66	7.82	Stolow, 1959

[a] MCS = methyl cellosolve (2-methoxyethanol).
[b] DMF = dimethylformamide.

structural studies should be undertaken only when all measurements are conducted in the same solvent. The pK_a values reported in the literature are mostly for water solutions. For comparison, it would be ideal to determine the dissociation constants of cephalosporin derivatives in water. However, the solubility of these derivatives in water imposes restrictions. Consequently, the dissociation constants of the cephalosporin derivatives discussed in this section were measured in 66% DMF (by volume). The other minor external factor affecting the dissociation constants is temperature; this effect is small and can be conveniently neglected.

In the application of dissociation constants to structural organic chemistry, it is important to know the pK_a values of different functional groups and their variation with structural changes. The most important factors which govern variations in pK_a's are inductive, resonance, and electrostatic effects, steric inhibition of resonance, steric shielding of solvation, and intramolecular hydrogen bonding. For a detailed discussion of the above effects, the reader is referred to a number of excellent reviews (King, 1963; Greenstein and Winitz, 1961; Wheland, 1955). The effect of the variation of functional groups in the close vicinity of a carboxyl and amino group is shown in Table II. The examples chosen are particularly relevant to the discussion of dissociation constants of

Table II

VARIATION IN THE pK_a'S OF CARBOXYL AND AMINO
FUNCTIONS WITH STRUCTURAL CHANGES

	pK_a (in water)		pK_a (in 66% DMF)[a]		
Compound	Carboxyl	Amino	Carboxyl	Amino	Reference
$\overset{+}{N}H_3CH_2COO^-$	2.4	9.8	3.6	10.2	King, 1951
$\overset{+}{N}H_3$ | $CH(CH_2)_3COOH$ | COO^-	2.2 9.7 4.3		3.7 10.7 6.9		
$ClCH_2COOH$	2.9		5.0		Feates and Ives, 1956
$CH_3CONHCH_2COOH$	3.7				King and King, 1956
CH_3COOH	4.8		7.0		Harned and Ehlers, 1932
CH_3NH_2		10.6		10.3	Everett and Wynne-Jones, 1941
$C_6H_5CH_2NH_2$		9.4		9.1	Carothers et al., 1927
$NH_2COCH_2NH_2$		7.9			Zief and Edsall, 1937

[a] The pK_a in 66% DMF was determined by Mr. D. O. Woolf and his associates at the Lilly Research Laboratories.

cephalosporin derivatives. The effect of most α substitution in a carboxylic acid is an increase in acid strength of the carboxyl group. Amino acids can be considered as substituted fatty acids. There is compelling evidence to show that the α-amino acids exist in their dipolar ionic form, i.e., $\overset{+}{N}H_3CHRCOO^-$ (Greenstein and Winitz, 1961). Among the groups that increase the acidity of the carboxyl group, one of the most powerful is the charged $\overset{+}{N}H_3$ group. This group causes a pK_a change from 4.8 to 2.4 in aqueous solution, and from 7.0 to 3.6 in 66% DMF. In contrast, the effect of the charged COO^- group on the dissociation constant of the amino group is relatively small; the pK_a changes from 10.6 to 9.8 in aqueous solution, and from 10.3 to 10.2 in 66% DMF. This is largely due to the fact that at the pH where the amino group ionizes, the carboxyl group is in the COO^- form.

B. Dissociation Constants of Cephalosporins

It is desirable to examine the dissociation constants of a few representative cephalosporin derivatives. In cephalosporin C and deacetoxycephalosporin

C, the pK_a values of 3.9 and 4.0 for the side-chain carboxyl group, and 10.4 and 10.6 for the side-chain amino group, are consistent with the values observed for an α-amino acid (Tables II and III). Acetylation of the amino group of the α-aminoadipyl side chain decreases the acidity of the side-chain carboxyl group in the N-chloroacetyl derivatives (3) and (4), in accordance with the decrease observed in pK_a values when comparing glycine and N-acetyl glycine. However, the acidity of the carboxyl group in the N-chloroacetyl derivatives (3) and (4) is greater than that observed for a normal fatty acid. This is due to the acidifying effect of the amide bond adjacent to the carboxyl group, as observed in the pK_a values of acetic acid and N-acetyl glycine.

Except for the low value observed for cephaloridine, the dissociation constants of the 4-carboxyl groups range from 4.7 to 6.7 for the cephalosporin derivatives (Table III). The 4-carboxyl group is more acidic than a normal aliphatic acid due to the close proximity of the electronegative sulfur, β-lactam amide, side-chain amide, and the acetoxy group (Woodward et al., 1949). Thus, the pK_a values of the 4-carboxyl group of 3-methyleneacetoxy cephalosporin derivatives range from 4.7 to 6.2; the corresponding range for 3-methyl cephalosporins is 5.3–6.7. The difference in these two values is certainly due to the acidifying effect of an acetoxy group at close proximity. The low pK_a value of cephaloridine is similar to the values observed for glycine, and the carboxyl group of the α-aminoadipyl side chain in cephalosporin C. Undoubtedly, this high acidity of the 4-carboxyl group has its origin in the close vicinity of the positively charged pyridinium ion at the 3 position, and it indicates that the carboxyl group exists in solution in the ionized COO^- form.

In cephaloglycin (7) and cephalexin (8), the pK_a values of the side-chain amino group are 7.3 and 7.4, respectively. Consequently, the side-chain amino group is less basic than a normal aliphatic amine. This decrease in basicity is due to the fact that the carbon that carries this amino group is flanked by electron-withdrawing phenyl and amide groups. As can be seen in Table II, both glycine amide and benzylamine are weaker bases than methylamine.

III. Infrared Spectroscopy

Characteristic stretching frequencies recorded in earlier studies for the different carbonyl groups in penams and cephems are summarized in Table IV. Most diagnostic, structure-wise, of the three carbonyl stretching frequencies in the spectra of penicillins and cephalosporins is that originating from the β-lactam carbonyl since the frequency of this group can give important information regarding the structural integrity of both the β-lactam and thiazolidine (or thiazine) rings, the state of oxidation at sulfur, and the relative configuration of β-lactam protons. Thus, for example, in normal penams the

Table III

DISSOCIATION CONSTANTS OF CEPHALOSPORINS[a]

Cephalosporin[b]	pK_a (in 66% DMF)	
	Carboxyl	Amino
Cephalosporin C (*1*)	3.9, 5.0	10.4
Deacetoxycephalosporin C (*2*)	4.0, 5.8	10.6
N-Chloroacetyl ceph C (*3*)	4.8, 6.2	
N-Chloroacetyl deacetoxy ceph C (*4*)	5.4, 6.7	
Cephalothin (*5*)	5.0	
Cephaloridine (*6*)	3.4	
Cephaloglycin (*7*)	4.7	7.4
Cephalexin (*8*)	5.3	7.3

[a] These values were determined by Mr. D. O. Woolf and his associates at the Lilly Research Laboratories.

[b] Key to numbers:

$$(1)\ R_1 = NHCO(CH_2)_3\overset{\overset{+}{N}H_3}{\underset{|}{C}}HCOO^-,\ R_2 = COOH,\ R_3 = OCOCH_3$$

$$(2)\ R_1 = NHCO(CH_2)_3\overset{\overset{+}{N}H_3}{\underset{|}{C}}HCOO^-,\ R_2 = COOH,\ R_3 = H$$

$$(3)\ R_1 = NHCO(CH_2)_3\overset{NHCOCH_2Cl}{\underset{|}{C}}HCOOH,\ R_2 = COOH,\ R_3 = OCOCH_3$$

$$(4)\ R_1 = NHCO(CH_2)_3\overset{NHCOCH_2Cl}{\underset{|}{C}}HCOOH,\ R_2 = COOH,\ R_3 = H$$

(*5*) $R_1 = Th^*$, $R_2 = COOH$, $R_3 = OCOCH_3$

(*6*) $R_1 = Th$, $R_2 = COO^-$, $R_3 = $ pyridinium

$$(7)\ R_1 = NHCO\overset{NH_2}{\underset{|}{C}}HC_6H_5,\ R_2 = COOH,\ R_3 = OCOCH_3$$

$$(8)\ R_1 = NHCO\overset{NH_2}{\underset{|}{C}}HC_6H_5,\ R_2 = COOH,\ R_3 = H$$

carbonyl stretching frequency for the β-lactam carbonyl occurs in the 1790- to 1770-cm^{-1} range while in unfused β-lactam compounds of the type depicted by structure (9) and desthiopenicillin (10) the absorption peaks for corresponding carbonyls shift to considerably lower frequencies, i.e., 1680 cm^{-1} and 1739 cm^{-1}, respectively.

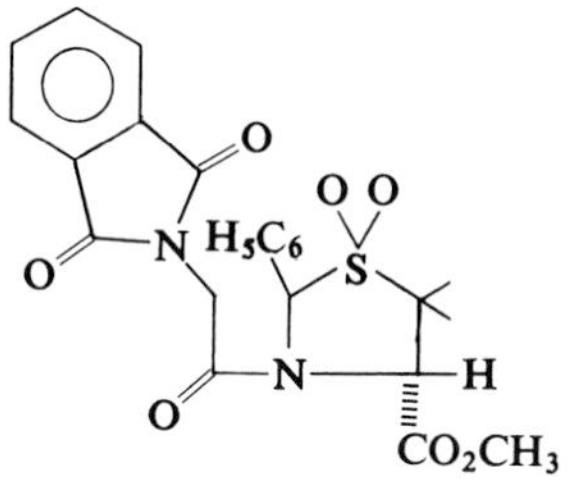

(9) 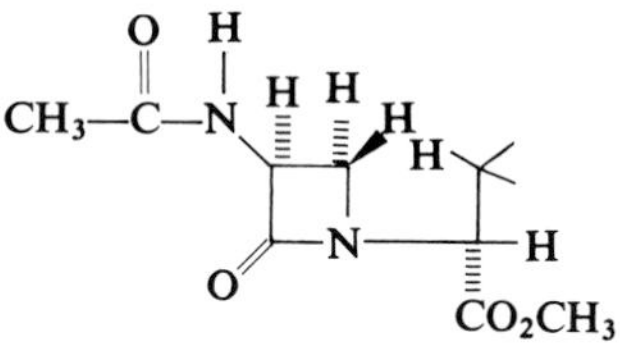   (10)

The state of oxidation at sulfur in penicillins and cephalosporins is also a factor affecting the frequency position of the β-lactam carbonyl. This was first illustrated by Thompson et al. (1949) and Sheehan et al. (1951) who recorded a shift of 45 cm^{-1} to higher frequency for the β-lactam absorption band of phthalimidopenicillin (11) upon oxidation to the corresponding sulfone (12). Shifts to shorter wavelength (into the 1800-cm^{-1} range) for the β-lactam carbonyl band in both penams and cephams have also been recorded following oxidation of the sulfur to a sulfoxide. Morin and co-workers (1969) have shown that β-lactam carbonyl absorption appears at a frequency approximately 15 cm^{-1} higher in the spectrum of phenoxymethylpenicillin sulfoxide

---

* Throughout this chapter, we have used the following abbreviations:

A = NHCOCH$_3$

Het = 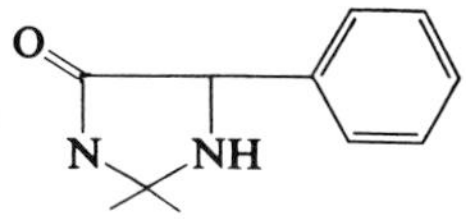   (6[D(−)-2,2-dimethyl-5-oxo-4-phenyl-1-imidazolidinyl])

Pht = N   (phthalimido)

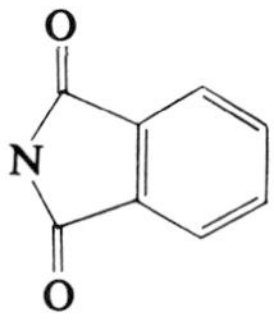

Th = NHCOCH$_2$ 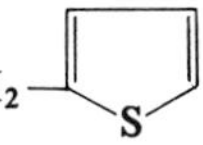   (thiopheneacetamido)

V = NHCOCH$_2$OC$_6$H$_5$ (phenoxyacetamido).

Table IV

CARBONYL ABSORPTION FREQUENCIES IN
PENICILLINS AND CEPHALOSPORINS

	β-Lactam carbonyl (cm^{-1})	Secondary amide carbonyl (cm^{-1})	Ester carbonyl (cm^{-1})
Penams[a,b]	1790–1770	1690–1680 1515–1510	1750
Penam sulfoxide[b]	1805	1695	1755
Penam sulfones[a,c]	1815–1805		1750
3-Cephems[d,e]	1792–1782	1680–1678 1505–1504	1736–1720
3-Cephem sulfoxides[e]	>1800	1695–1690	1740
2-Cephems[d,e]	1784–1772	1678–1676 1505–1504	1744–1740
Cephams[b]	1784–1780		
Unfused β-lactams[a]	1760–1730		
Desthiopenicillin[a]	1739		

[a] Bellamy (1958) and references cited therein.
[b] Morin et al. (1969).
[c] Sheehan et al. (1951).
[d] Green et al. (1965).
[e] Wright et al. (1971).

(*20a*) (1795 cm^{-1}) than in the parent sulfide (*20*) (1780 cm^{-1}). Similarly, conversion of cephalosporins (*13*) and (*14*) to their corresponding sulfoxides

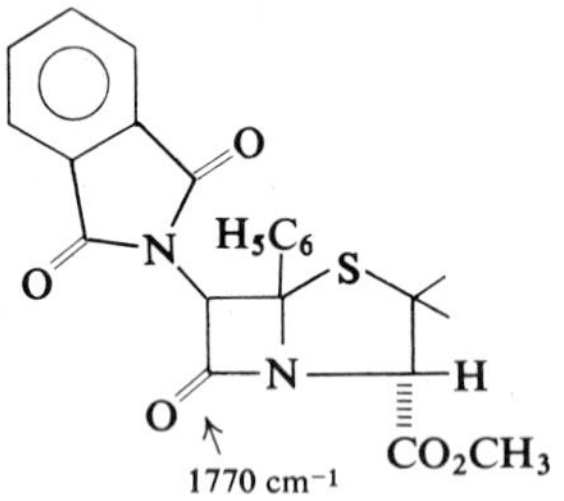

(*11*)

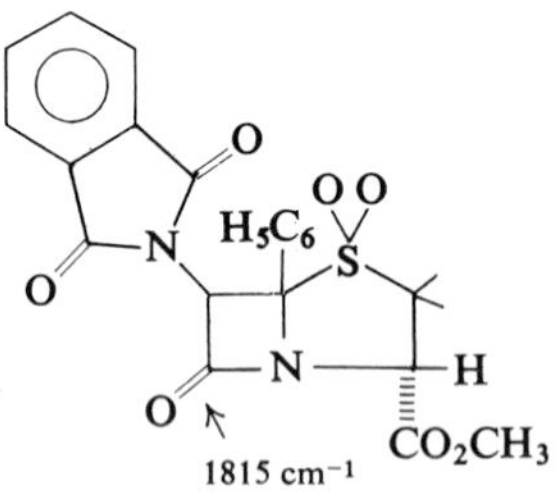

(*12*)

(*13a* and *14a*) results in shifts of the lactam carbonyl absorptions from the 1792- to 1782-cm^{-1} region into the 1800-cm^{-1} region (Wright et al., 1971). It is of interest to note from Table IV that the secondary amide carbonyl band is also shifted to higher frequency in the process of oxidation. One possible explanation for this shift is the formation of an intramolecular hydrogen bond, previously shown to exist from NMR studies (Cooper *et al.*, 1969a; Archer and Demarco, 1969), between the amido proton and sulfoxide or sulfone oxygen.

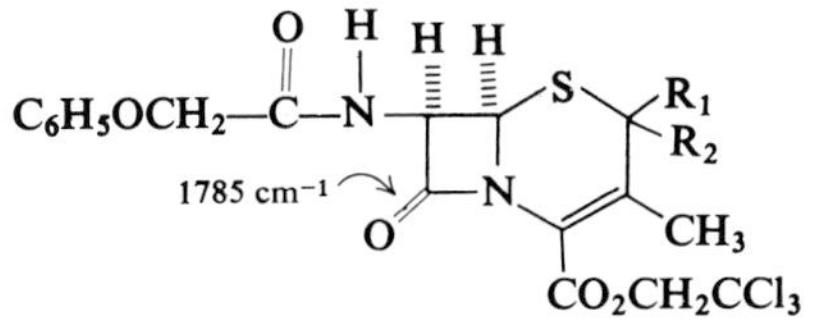

(*13*) $R_1 = H$, $R_2 = CH_3$ (*13a*) $R_1 = H$, $R_2 = CH_3$

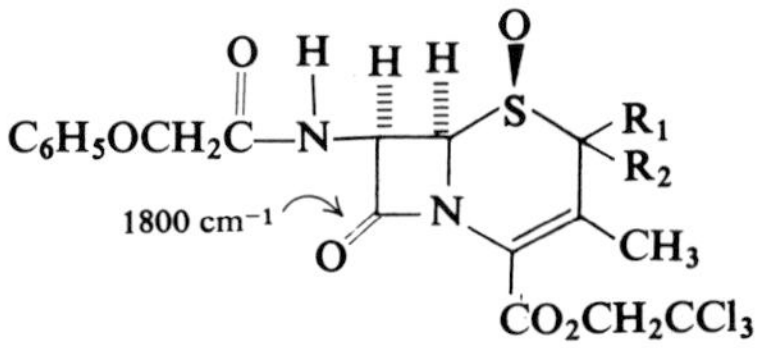

(*14*) R_1, $R_2 = CH_2$ (*14a*) R_1, $R_2 = CH_2$

According to the recent findings of Johnson *et al.* (1968), the relative configuration of β-lactam ring protons is also a factor affecting β-lactam carbonyl stretching frequency. Thus, hetacillin (*15*) and epihetacillin (*16*), which contain

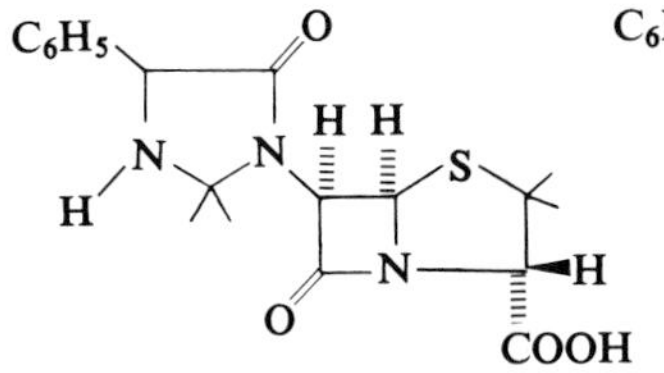

(*15*) 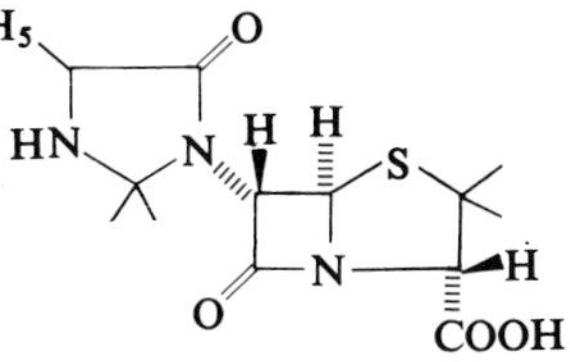   (*16*)

cis- and *trans*-substituted β-lactam moieties respectively, give rise to β-lactam carbonyl frequencies which are substantially different, the lactam carbonyl in the *cis* system (*15*) absorbing in the expected region (1775 cm^{-1}) while in the *trans* system (*16*) at much higher frequency (1800 cm^{-1}).

One further point of interest regarding the β-lactam carbonyl group is the relationship between its infrared stretching frequency and biological activity. Morin and co-workers (1969) have shown that, provided a direct correlation exists between β-lactam C=O stretching frequency and acylation ability* (i.e., the higher the frequency, the higher the acylation ability), a rough but positive relationship between acylation ability and biological activity can be inferred from their IR data, recorded from studies with a variety of penicillins and cephalosporins. This rationale has been projected further by Sweet and Dahl (1970) who, on the basis of X-ray structure data on various penicillins and cephalosporins, have suggested that, as the biological activity increases, the

---

* That is the ability to act antibacterially by acylating irreversibly the transpeptidase enzyme which is necessary for cross-linking in bacterial cell wall formation.

lactam C=O stretching frequency increases, the lactam nitrogen planarity decreases, and the ease of basic hydrolysis of the lactam amide bond increases. Further discussion of planarity and other X-ray structure correlations may be found in Chapter 7.

The carbonyl stretching band for the secondary amide group of penicillins appears at slightly higher values (1690–1680 cm^{-1} and 1515–1510 cm^{-1}) than that of the 3-cephems (1680–1678 cm^{-1} and 1505–1504 cm^{-1}) and 2-cephems (1678–1676 cm^{-1} and 1505–1504 cm^{-1}). Similarly, the ester carbonyl band of penicillins appears at higher frequency range (1755–1750 cm^{-1}) than that of 2-cephems (1744–1740 cm^{-1}) which in turn appears at a higher range than that of 3-cephems (1736–1720 cm^{-1}).

IV. Mass Spectrometry

Mass spectrometry was introduced as a tool to solve structural problems about a decade ago, and since then it has made enormous strides. One particular advantage of this physical method is that it requires small quantities of the compound whose mass spectrum is to be determined. There is a large amount of literature available in this field today. However, published information concerned with the mass spectra of penicillins (Richter and Biemann, 1964; Bochkarev et al., 1967; Moll and Hannig, 1970a, b) and cephalosporins (Richter and Biemann, 1965) is scant.

Penicillin and cephalosporin derivatives have several polar groups. In order to obtain useful information from the mass spectra of these compounds, it is necessary to derivatize the carboxyl and amino groups and convert them to neutral compounds with higher volatility. Analysis of the high-resolution mass spectra of these compounds affords a wealth of structural information, and this powerful tool is bound to become popular in penicillin and cephalosporin chemistry.

A. β-Lactams

A structural feature common to both penicillin and cephalosporin is the β-lactam moiety, and a discussion of the fragmentation pattern of a simple β-lactam on electron impact in the mass spectrometer is appropriate. The mass spectrum of desthio-6-aminopenicillanic acid (*17a*) has been reported (Moll and Hannig, 1970b). These data, along with the mass spectral analysis of the readily available desthiopenicillin G methyl ester (*17*) (Kaczka and Folkers, 1949; see appendix), give a clue to the fragmentation pattern of the β-lactam

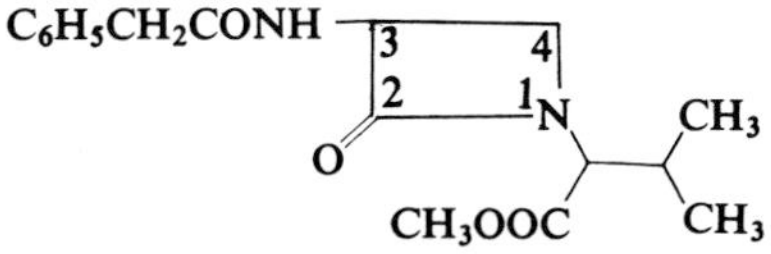

$C_6H_5CH_2CONH$ [ring, positions 3, 4, 2, 1, N]
with O, N, CH₃ substituents:

$C_6H_5CH_2CONH$—[β-lactam ring with C-3, C-4, C-2, C-1, N]—N—CH(CH₃)—CH₃ ; CH_3OOC

(17)

antibiotics. There are four modes of cleavage involving fission of the four-membered β-lactam ring, and one at the C-3 amido group on the β-lactam ring, to give the 3-amino β-lactam fragment (Nagarajan, 1971).

The probable structure of the fragments is shown below.

1. FISSION OF β-LACTAM RING

a. CLEAVAGE ACROSS C-1–C-2 AND C-3–C-4 BONDS:

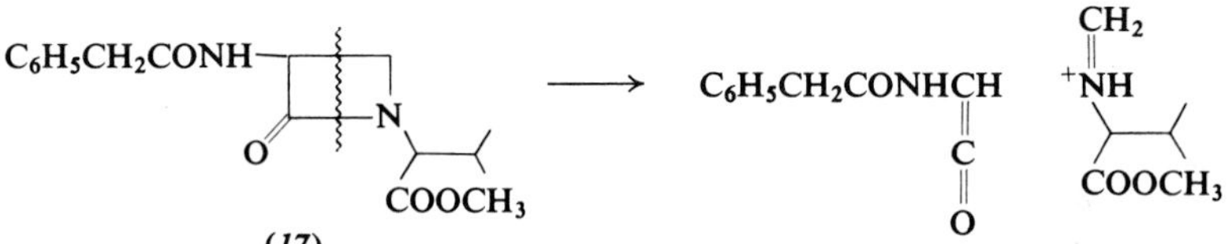

$C_6H_5CH_2CONH$—[ring, O, N, COOCH₃]

(17)

$\longrightarrow$

$C_6H_5CH_2CONHCH$ (with C=O below, =CH₂ above)

(17b) m/e 175

$CH_2{=}{}^+NH$ with COOCH₃ and isopropyl

(17c) m/e 144

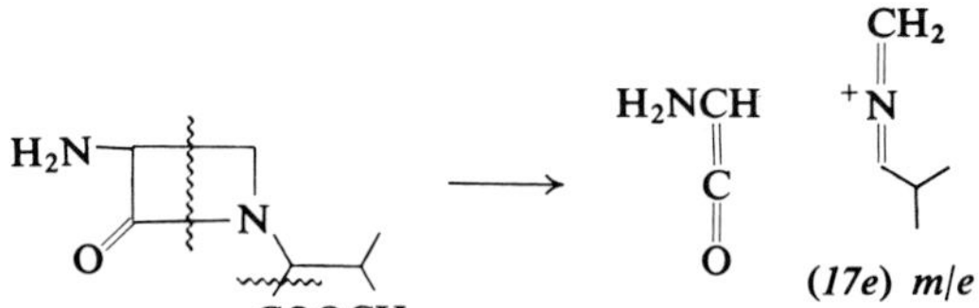

H_2N—[ring, O, N, COOCH]

(17a)

$\longrightarrow$

H_2NCH (with C=O below)

(17d)

$CH_2{=}{}^+N$ with isopropyl

(17e) m/e 84

b. CLEAVAGE ACROSS C-1–C-4 AND C-2–C-3 BONDS:

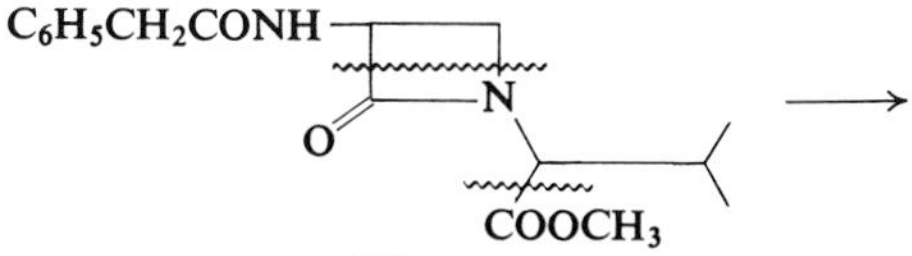

$C_6H_5CH_2CONH$—[ring, O, N, COOCH₃]

(17)

$\longrightarrow$

$C_6H_5CH_2CONHCH{=}CH_2$
(17f) m/e 161

$O{=}C{=}\overset{+}{N}{=}CHCH(CH_3)_3$
(17g) m/e 98

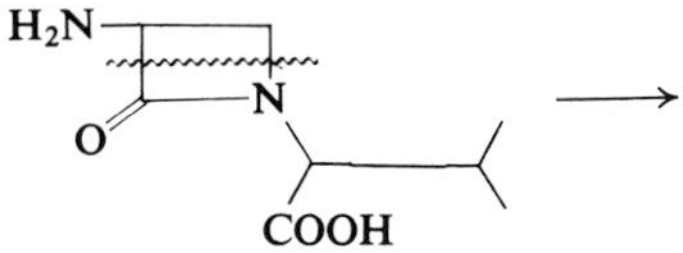

H_2N—[ring, O, N, COOH]

(17a)

$\longrightarrow$

$\overset{+}{H_3}NCH{=}CH_2$
(17h) m/e 44

$O{=}C{=}NCHCH(CH_3)_2$ with COOH
(17i)

c. Cleavage at C-1–C-2 and C-2–C-3 Bonds:

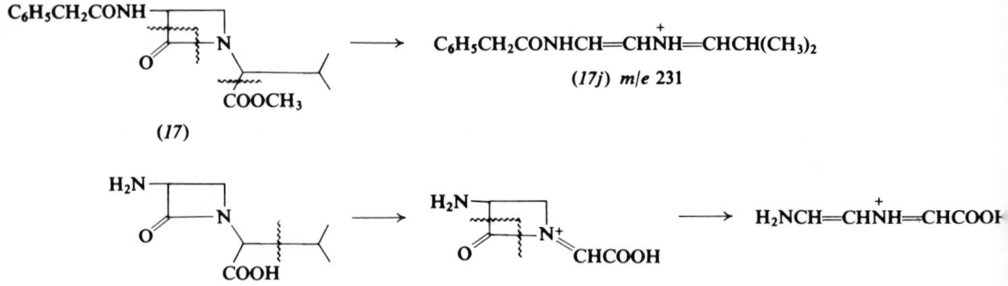
C6H5CH2CONH
N
O
COOCH3
C6H5CH2CONHCH=CHNH=CHCH(CH3)2
H2N
N
O
COOH
H2N
N+
O
CHCOOH
H2NCH=CHNH=CHCOOH

(17) (17j) m/e 231

(17a) (17k) (17l)

d. Cleavage at C-1–C-2 and C-1–C-4 Bonds:

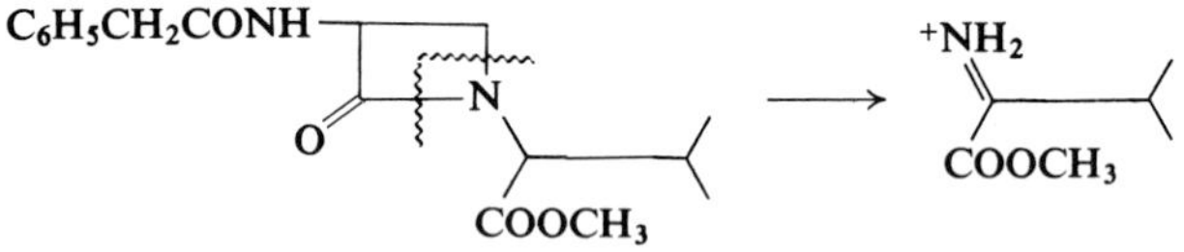
C6H5CH2CONH
N
O
COOCH3
+NH2
COOCH3

(17) (17m) m/e 130

2. Fragmentation of Substituents

a. Cleavage at 3-Amido Group:

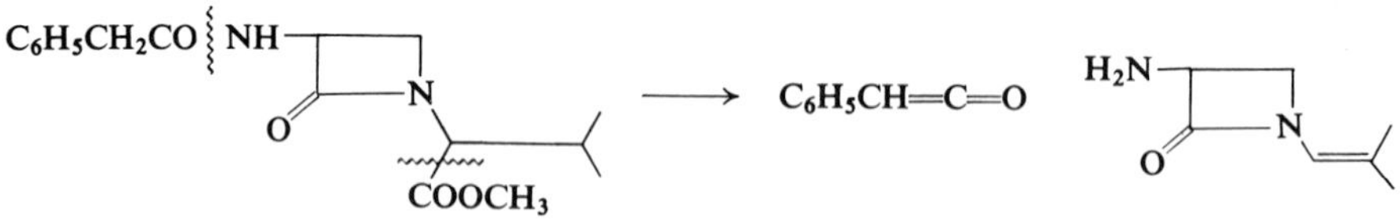
C6H5CH2CO NH
N
O
COOCH3
C6H5CH=C=O
H2N
N
O

(17) (17n) m/e 118 (17p) m/e 140

b. Cleavage of the Carbomethoxy Group:

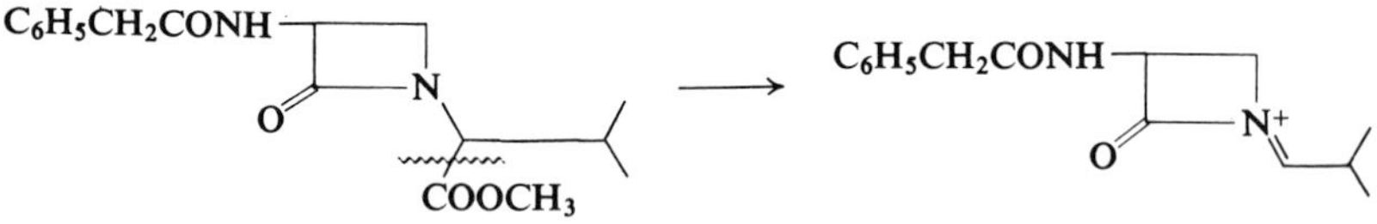
C6H5CH2CONH
N
O
COOCH3
C6H5CH2CONH
N+
O

(17) (17q) m/e 259

Based on knowledge of the modes of fragmentation of the above β-lactams, one would expect that fragmentations analogous to the cleavage across C-1–C-2 and C-3–C-4 bonds, cleavage at C-1–C-2 and C-2–C-3 bonds and at the C-3 amido group in β-lactam (*17*) would also occur in penicillin and cephalosporin. As we will see later, this is indeed so. The two other cleavages observed in (*17*), i.e., fission across C-1–C-4 and C-2–C-3 bonds, and at C-1–C-2 and C-1–C-4 bonds, would involve the thiazolidine and dihydrothiazine rings in penicillin and cephalosporin respectively, and these are not the major mode of fragmentation.

B. Penicillins

Penicillins undergo a number of fragmentations on electron impact in the mass spectrometer (Richter and Biemann, 1964; Bochkarev *et al.*, 1967; Moll and Hannig, 1970a). There are seven modes of fragmentation which are useful in structure determination which are discussed below.

1. FRAGMENTATION ACROSS THE β-LACTAM RING

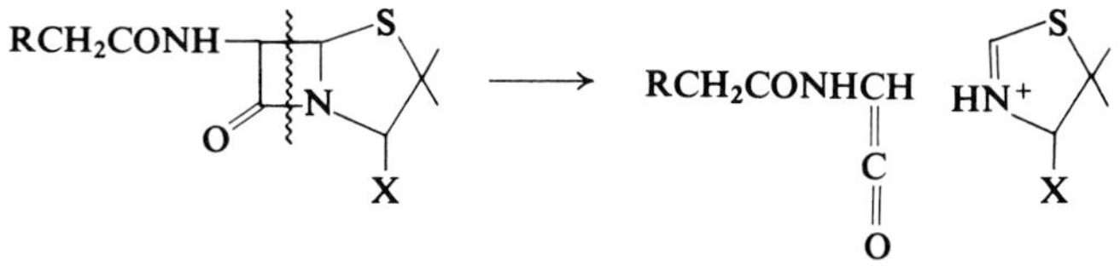

RCH₂CONH ⟶ RCH₂CONHCH ... HN⁺

(18)   (18a)   (18b)

This mode of fragmentation is general for penicillin, and highly diagnostic. The well-stabilized thiazolidine ion (*18b*) usually dominates the mass spectrum.

Fragment (18a) and (18b) can undergo further fragmentation as shown below.

$$RCH_2CONHCH=C=O \longrightarrow \overset{+}{R}CH_2$$

(18a)   (18c)

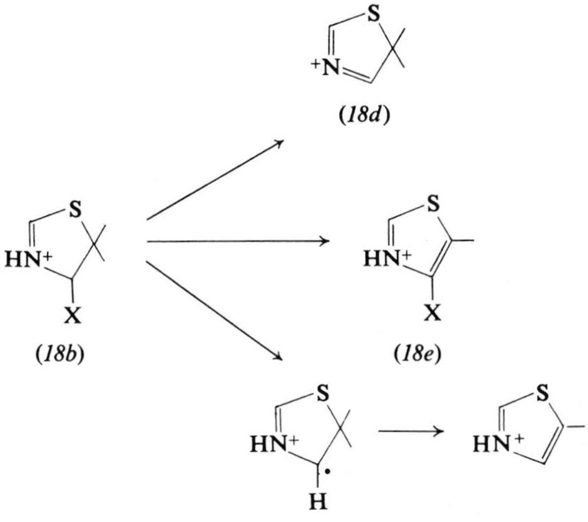

(18d)

(18b)   (18e)

(18f) ⟶ (18g)

When X $=$ COOCH$_3$ in ion (*18b*), the loss of CH$_3$OH occurs.

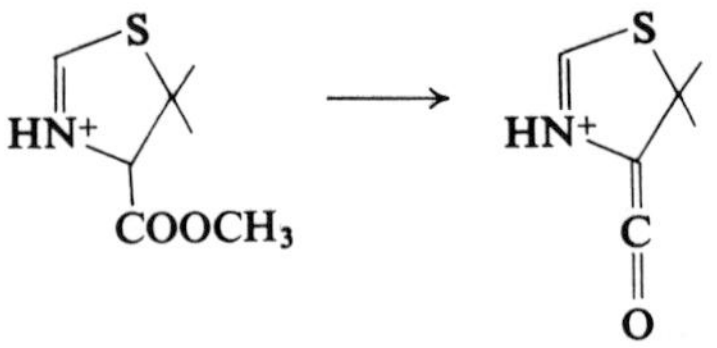

(*18b*)   (*18h*)

When X $=$ CH$_2$CONHC$_6$H$_5$ in (*18b*), further fragmentation takes place.

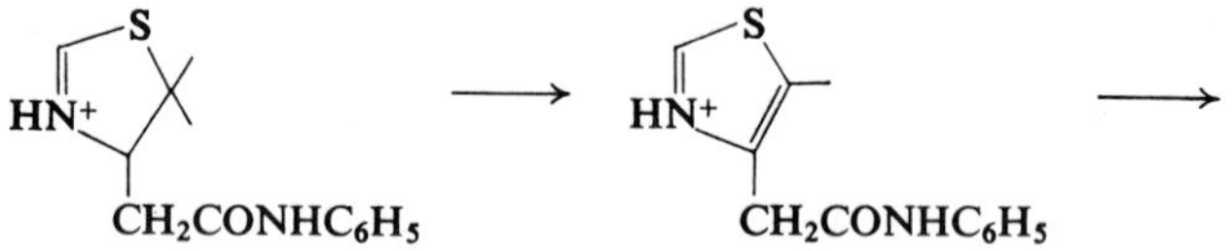

(*18b*)   (*18i*)

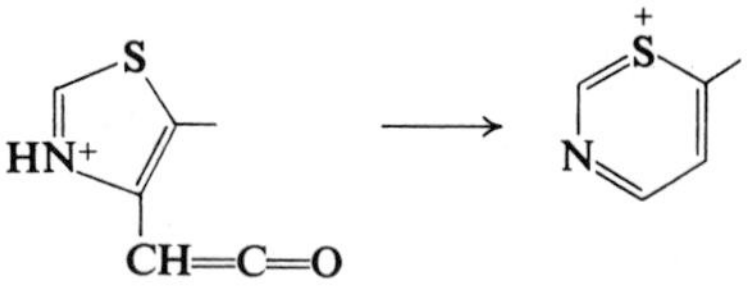

(*18j*)   (*18k*)

2. FRAGMENTATION OF THIAZOLIDINE RING

The two modes of fragmentation of the thiazolidine ring afford fragments (*18l*) and (*18m*). Fragment (*18m*) affords information on the nature of the substituent X at the C-4 position.

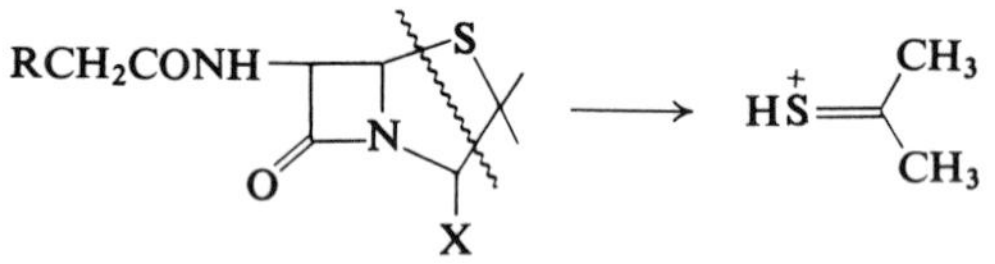

(*18*)   (*18l*)

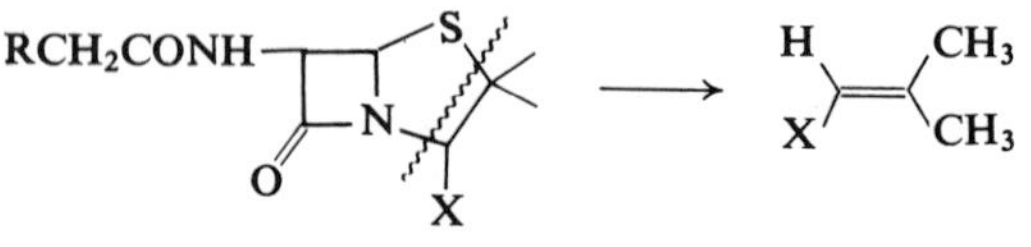

(*18*)   (*18m*)

3. FRAGMENTATION ACROSS THE THIAZOLIDINE AND β-LACTAM RINGS

There are two modes of fragmentation across both the thiazolidine and β-lactam rings, and the fragments afford information on the C-6 side chain.

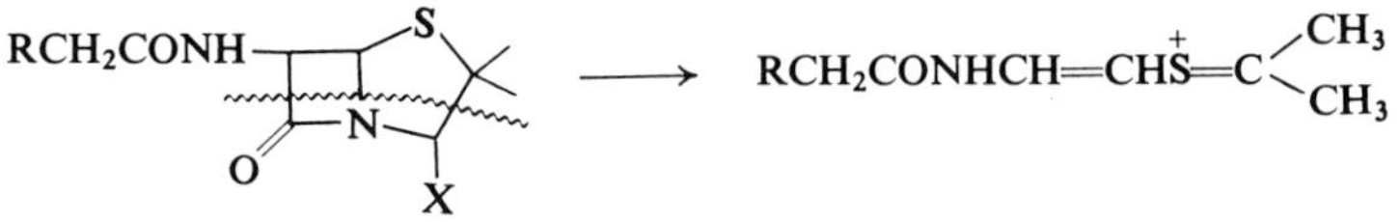

RCH₂CONH—[...] (18) ⟶ RCH₂CONHCH=CHS=C(CH₃)(CH₃) (18n)

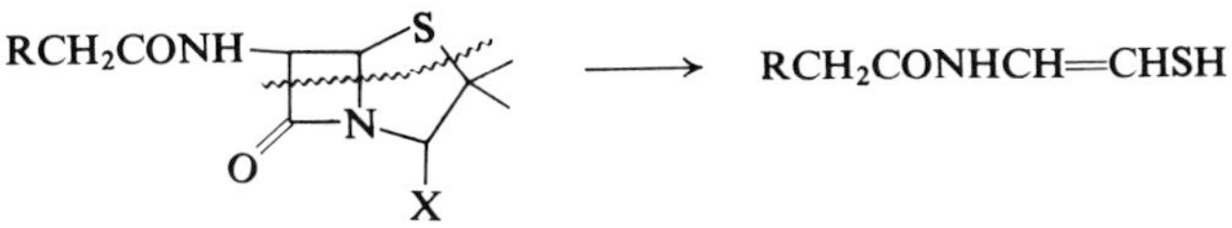

RCH₂CONH—[...] (18) ⟶ RCH₂CONHCH=CHSH (18p)

4. FRAGMENTATION OF SUBSTITUENTS ON THE PENAM SKELETON

Fragmentation of the C-6 amido group affords the 6-aminopenicillanic acid fragment, and cleavage of the C-4 substituent yields the fragment devoid of that substituent. These two fragmentations afford information on the nature of the C-4 and C-6 substituents of the penicillin under investigation.

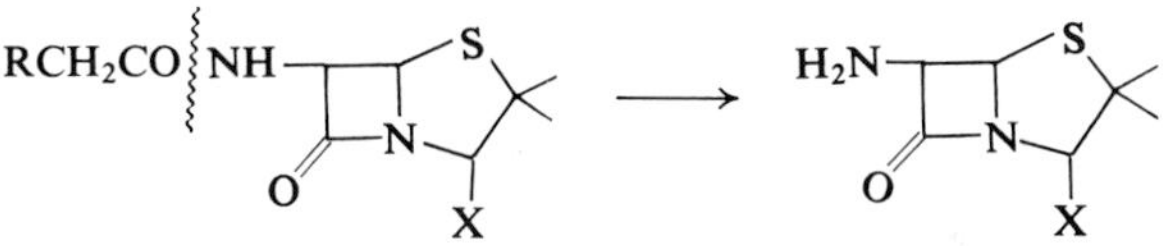

RCH₂CO⫶NH—[...] (18) ⟶ H₂N—[...] (18q)

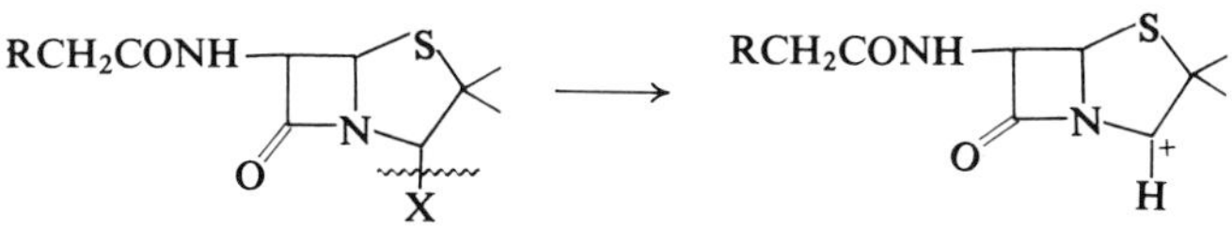

RCH₂CONH—[...] (18) ⟶ RCH₂CONH—[...] (18r)

C. Cephalosporins

Cephalosporin (19) undergoes a number of fragmentations (Richter and Biemann, 1965). The major fragmentation of diagnostic value is discussed below.

1. FRAGMENTATION ACROSS β-LACTAM RING

As in the case of penicillins, this fragmentation is observed in all cephalosporins. The dihydrothiazine ions (*19a* and *19f*) are usually the most intense ions in the spectrum and are extremely useful for diagnostic purposes.

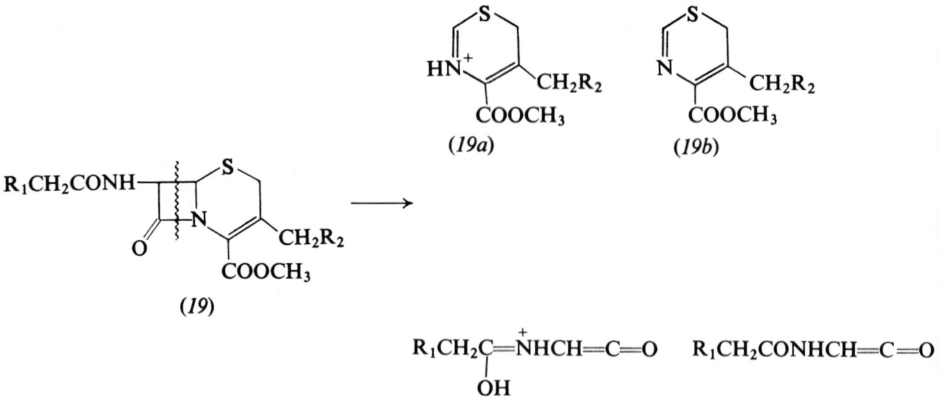

(*19a*)

(*19b*)

(*19*)

$$R_1CH_2\overset{+}{C}{=}NHCH{=}C{=}O$$
$$\underset{OH}{|}$$

$$R_1CH_2CONHCH{=}C{=}O$$

(*19c*)   (*19d*)

The ion (*19a*) undergoes further fragmentation.

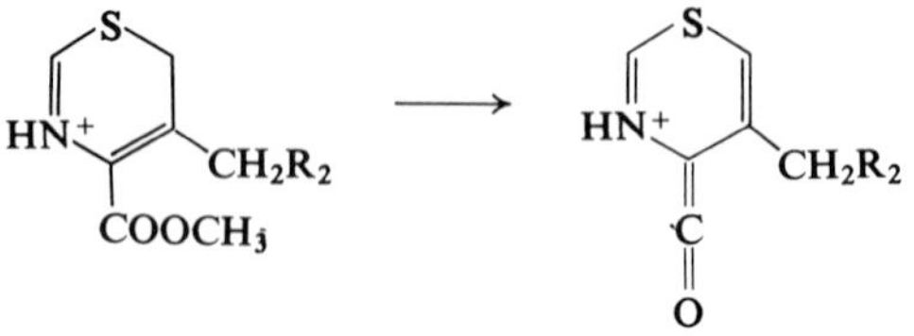

(*19a*)   (*19e*)

When $R_2 = OCOCH_3$ in (*19*), *19b* undergoes fragmentation to the stable allyl cation (*19f*).

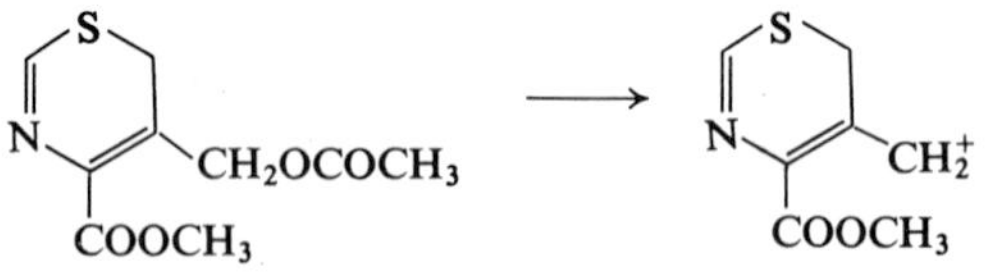

(*19b*)   (*19f*)

When $R_2 = H$ in (*19*), the ion (*19a*) fragments further as shown below (Nagarajan, 1971; see appendix).

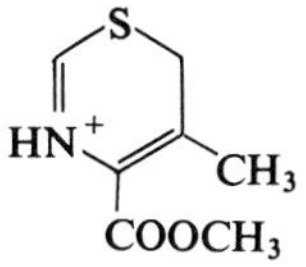

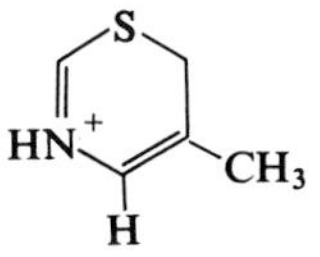

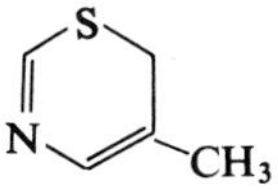

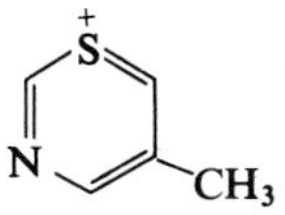

(19a)   (19g) m/e 114   (19h) m/e 113   (19i) m/e 112

In the lower mass region, the resonance stabilized thiazonium ion (19i) is one of the most intense ions and could be used effectively for diagnostic purposes.

2. FRAGMENTATION OF SUBSTITUENTS ON THE 3-CEPHEM MOIETY

When $R_2 = OCOCH_3$ in (19), two modes of cleavage of the 3 substituent occur.

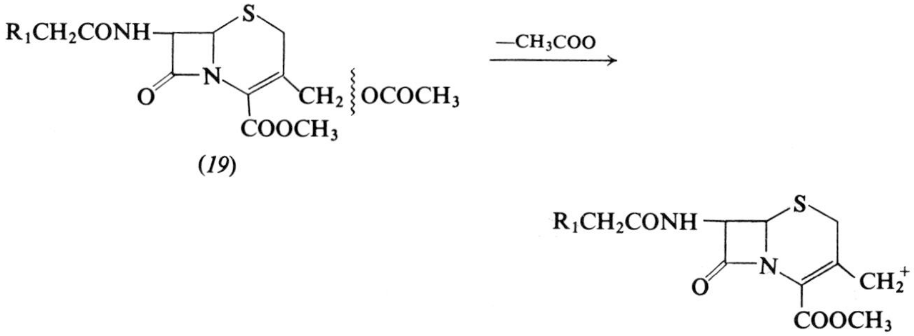

(19) $-CH_3COO \longrightarrow$

(19j)

(19) $-\overset{+}{C}H_2OCOCH_3 \longrightarrow$

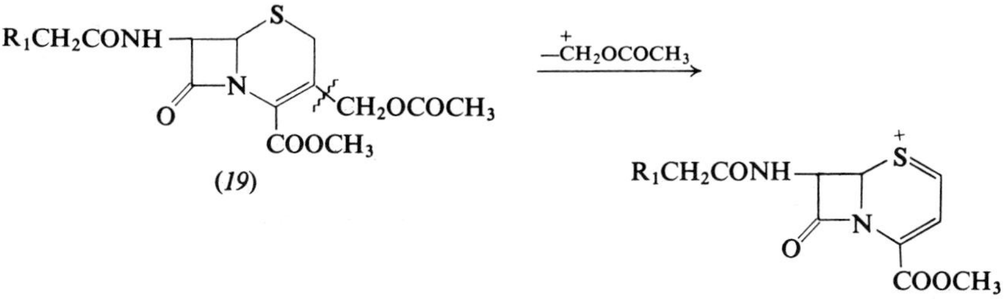

(19k)

When $R_2 = H$ in (19), the 4 substituent can be expelled (Nagarajan, 1971).

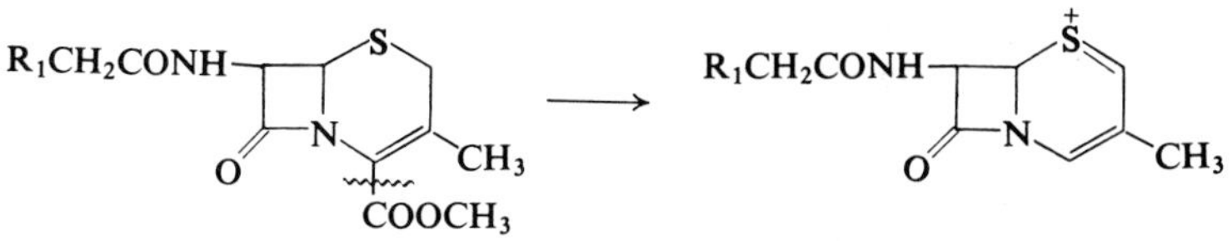

(19) $\longrightarrow$ (19l)

In cephalosporins with an easily expellable group at the 3 position, the molecular ion is of low intensity, and in the higher mass region the resonance stabilized, high-intensity allyl cation (19j) is important.

Cleavage at the C-7 amido side chain affords the 7-aminocephalosporanic acid fragment. This type of cleavage is observed in penicillin, and is analogous to one of the main pathways of peptide fragmentation, and used in peptide sequencing. However, because of the low intensity of the ions (18q) and (19m) in penicillin and cephalosporin, respectively, they are not very useful.

(19)   (19m)   (19n)

D. High-Resolution Mass Spectrometry

Penicillins and cephalosporins contain the heteroatoms oxygen, nitrogen, and sulfur. Derivatives of 6-aminopenicillanic acid and 7-aminocephalo-sporanic acid contain at least O_3N_2S and O_5N_2S, respectively. In the mass spectra of penicillin and cephalosporin derivatives, one or more heteroatoms are usually present in the fragments. The presence or absence of the heteroatom in the fragment results in small, but measurable, mass differences. High-resolution mass spectrometry is useful in the determination of exact mass of a fragment, and these data can be used effectively in structure elucidation of unknown penicillin and cephalosporin derivatives. The modes of fragmentation discussed in this section for the model β-lactam, (17), and the penicillin and cephalosporin derivatives have been confirmed by high-resolution mass spectral data (see appendix). Richter and Biemann (1964) have shown the effectiveness of high-resolution mass spectrometry in the unambiguous interpretation of the modes of fragmentation of the penicillin derivatives (18s) and (18t). The fragment with mass 114 occurs in the mass spectra of both compounds and, consequently, could not arise from a fragment containing the R group.

Examination of (18s) and (18t) by high-resolution mass spectrometry reveals that the mass 114 is a doublet with values of 114.0373 and 114.0664 for (18s) and 114.0380 and 114.0690 for (18t), respectively. The intensities of the two lines are in the ratio 9:1. The elemental composition of the fragments (18u), (18v), and (18w) are $C_4H_4NO_3$, C_5H_8NS, and $C_6H_{10}O_2$, respectively. The exact masses of the corresponding three fragments are 114.0191, 114.0377, and 114.0680. Consequently, of these three fragmentations, (a) is insignificant, (c) plays a minor role, and (b) affords most of the mass 114.

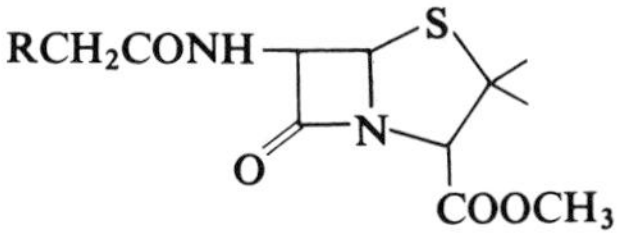

(a) $O{=}C{=}\overset{+}{N}CHCOOCH_3$

(18u)

RCH₂CONH — [β-lactam structure with S]

O

N

COOCH₃

(18s) R = C₆H₅
(18t) R = C₆H₅O

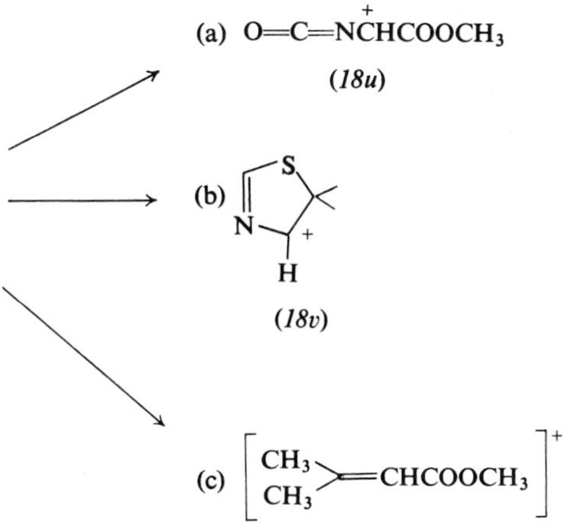

(b) [thiazolidine cation structure]

N

H

(18v)

(c) $\left[\begin{array}{c}CH_3\\CH_3\end{array}\right]{=}CHCOOCH_3\Bigg]^{+}$

(18w)

E. Use of Natural Isotopes

The presence in a penicillin or a cephalosporin derivative of an element with two abundant natural isotopes could be used in solving structural problems. The mass spectrum of 6-chloropenicillanic acid (Richter and Biemann, 1964) yields the molecular ion as a doublet of mass 249 and 251, and $M^+{-}COOCH_3$ ions at m/e 190 and 192. The relative intensities of the doublet are 3:1, in agreement with the natural abundance ratio for $^{35}Cl:^{37}Cl$ of 75.5:24.5. The corresponding thiazolidine fragments derived from M^+ and $M^+{-}COOCH_3$ occur at m/e 174 and 114, respectively, and are singlets. Consequently, the chlorine is at the 6 position.

The natural abundance ratio of $^{32}S:^{34}S$ is 95.0:4.2. In the mass spectrum of (19p), the measurement of ions m/e 172 and 174 by high-resolution technique reveals them as singlets with exact masses of 172.04274 and 174.04233, respectively (Nagarajan, 1971; see appendix). The calculated values for the ^{32}S and

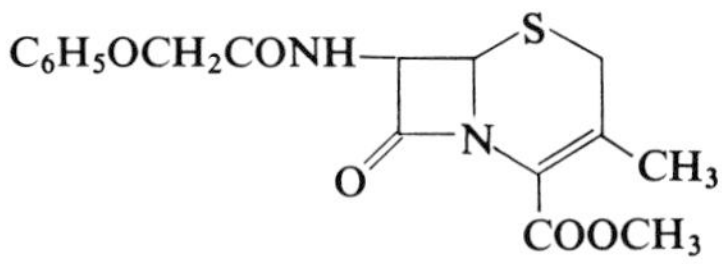

C₆H₅OCH₂CONH — [cephalosporin structure with S]

O

N

CH₃

COOCH₃

(19p)

^{32}S [structure]

HN⁺

CH₃

COOCH₃

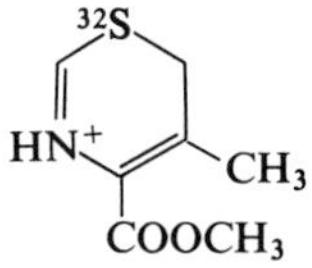

(19q)

$C_7H_{10}O_2N^{32}S$

172.04323

(−0.5 mmU)

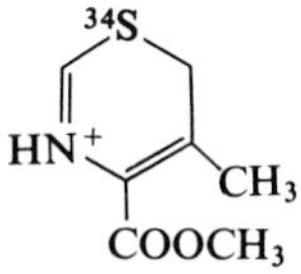

^{34}S [structure]

HN⁺

CH₃

COOCH₃

(19r)

$C_7H_{10}O_2N^{34}S$

174.04261

(−0.4 mmU)

[34]S dihydrothiazine ions (*19q*) and (*19r*) are 172.04323 and 174.04261, respectively, in excellent agreement with the observed values. Since the high-intensity thiazolidine and dihydrothiazine ions are the most important fragments for diagnostic purposes in penicillin and cephalosporin, and they both contain sulfur, the determination of the [32]S and [34]S fragments provides additional evidence and puts the assignments on a firm basis.

V. Nuclear Magnetic Resonance

Nuclear magnetic resonance spectroscopy has evolved into one of the more important physical methods used in the characterization and identification of penicillin and cephalosporin compounds. In this section, the various NMR techniques shown to be of use in penicillin–cephalosporin structure studies are discussed and their application illustrated with respect to appropriate examples from the field.

A. General NMR Spectral Characteristics

Tables V and VI summarize recorded NMR data for a variety of penicillin and cephalosporin derivatives, respectively, while Figs. 1–4 (shown in appendix) illustrate typical spectra obtained on some of the more common penicillin and cephalosporin antibiotics, namely, phenoxymethylpenicillin (penicillin V), cephalothin, cephalexin, and cephalosporin C.

1. β-LACTAM RESONANCES

Most characteristic of the NMR spectra of pencillins and cephalosporins are the single proton doublet and quartet signals originating from the two β-lactam ring protons, H_A and H_B, common to both systems (see schematic below). H_A, which corresponds to H-5 in penicillins and H-6 in cephalosporins,

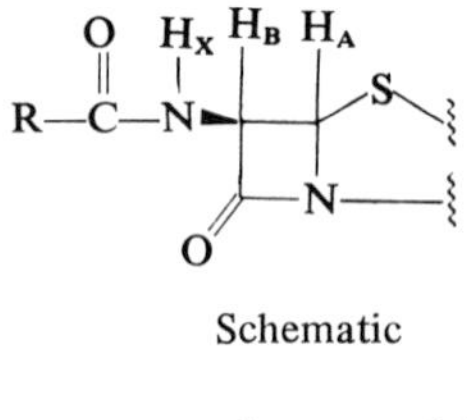

Schematic

is situated adjacent to one proton only, namely, H_B, and gives rise to the β-lactam doublet [$J_{AB}(cis) = 4$–5 Hz, $J_{AB}(trans) = 1.5$–2 Hz] (Barrow and Spotswood, 1965; Luche *et al.*, 1968; Johnson *et al.*, 1968; Gutowski, 1970), while

Table V

¹H NMR Data[a] for Some Penicillins[b] and Some Corresponding Sulfoxides

Compound[c]	2α-CH₃	2β-CH₃	H-3	H-5	H-6	CH₂OAc
				Resonance		
(20)[d]	1.49[1.13], s	1.60[1.20], s	4.47[4.39], s	5.58[5.11], d, $J = 4.5$	5.74[5.54], q, $J = 4.5, 9$	
(20a)[d]	1.23[0.51], s	1.73[1.25], s	4.69[4.65], s	5.03[3.77], d, $J = 4.5$	6.10[5.93], 1, $J = 4.5, 10$	
(20b)[e]	1.32[1.18], s	1.68[1.37], s	4.41[4.42], s	4.78[4.38], d, $J = 4.5$	5.55[4.60], q, $J = 4.5, 8$	
(20c)[d]	1.32, s	1.50, s	4.38, s	4.66	6.10	
(21)[e]	1.51[1.19], s	1.67[1.34], s	4.44[4.41], s	4.54[5.11], d, $J = 4.5$	5.72[5.50], q, $J = 4.5, 10.5$	
(21a)[e]	1.24[0.54], s	1.73[1.29], s	4.67[4.67], s	5.03[3.82], d, $J = 4.5$	6.08[5.91], q, $J = 4.5, 9$	
(21b)[e]	1.25[1.32], s	1.68[1.70], s	4.38[4.40], s	4.72[4.25], d, $J = 4.5$	5.51[4.46], q, $J = 4.5, 10$	
(21c)[e]	1.42[0.94], s	1.61[1.16], s	4.51[4.42], s	4.77[3.85], d, $J = 4.5$	6.15[5.88], q, $J = 4.5, 8$	
(22)[f]	1.51[1.25], s	1.82[1.67], s	4.68[4.72], s	5.60[5.29], d, $J = 4.5$	5.68[5.30], q, $J = 4.5, 10$	
(22b)[f]	1.33[1.17], s	1.83[1.46], s	4.61[4.57], s	4.86[4.36], d, $J = 4.5$	5.89[5.29], q, $J = 4.5, 9$	
(23)[e]	1.24[0.54], s	1.75[1.29], s	4.67[4.67], s	5.03[3.82], d, $J = 4.5$	6.08[5.91], q, $J = 4.5, 9$	
(24)[g]	s	s	s		5.42, q, $J = 4.5, 10$; q, $J = 1.5, 8$	

Table V —continued

Compound[c]	Resonance					
	2α-CH$_3$	2β-CH$_3$	H-3	H-5	H-6	CH$_2$OAc
(25)[h]	1.41[1.04] s	1.61[1.10] s	4.55[4.32] s	5.35[5.14] d, $J = 1.5$	4.75[4.24] q, $J = 1.5, 9$	
(25a)[h]	1.24[0.59] s	1.70[1.19] s	4.55[4.42] s			
(26)[f]	1.49[1.21] s	1.66[1.14] s	4.63[4.50] s	5.57[5.54] d, $J = 1.5$	5.39[5.48] d, $J = 1.5$	
(26a)[f]	1.29[0.73] s	1.73[1.35] s	4.58[4.58] s	5.35[4.66] d, $J = 1.5$	5.79[6.13] d, $J = 1.5$	
(22b)[f]	1.46[0.77] s	1.51[1.15] s	4.60[4.27] s	5.16[5.23] d, $J = 1.5$	5.65[5.60] d, $J = 1.5$	
(27)[i]	1.47	1.62 s	4.56 s	5.49 d, $J = 1.5$	4.67 d, $J = 1.5$	
(28)[j]	1.32 s		4.88 s	4.87 d, $J = 4$	5.89 d, $J = 4$	4.41, 4.68 AB, $J = 12$
(29)[j]		1.84 s	4.61 s	5.04 d, $J = 4$	5.88 d, $J = 4$	4.35, 4.48 AB, $J = 13$
(30)[j]	1.38 s		4.67 s	4.89 d, $J = 4$	5.63 q, $J = 4, 8$	4.50, 4.41 AB, $J = 13$
(31)[j]		1.75 s	4.52 s	5.00 d, $J = 4$	5.45 q, $J = 4, 8$	4.40, 4.50 AB, $J = 13$
(32)[j]	1.51 s		4.67 s	5.64 d, $J = 4$	5.78 q, $J = 4, 10$	3.80, 4.55 AB, $J = 12$
(32a)[j]	1.25 s		4.68 s	5.06 d, $J = 4$	6.13 q, $J = 4, 10$	4.57, 4.71 AB, $J = 12$

[a] In parts per million relative to TMS as internal reference. Unbracketed and bracketed shift values are for CDCl$_3$ and C$_6$D$_6$ solutions, respectively. J values are reported in hertz; s = singlet, d = doublet, q = quartet, b = broad.
[b] For a definition of symbols indicating penicillin C-6 side-chain substituents, refer to asterisk footnote of Footnote b, Table III.
[c] Key to numbers:

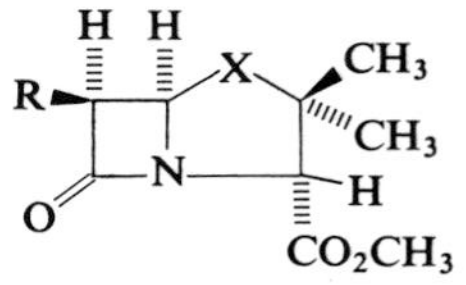

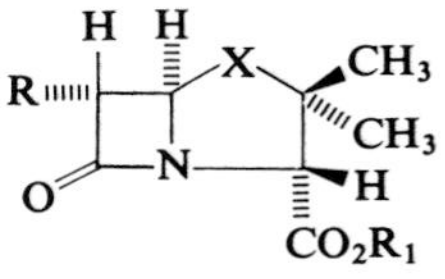

	X	R	R₁
(24)	S→O	V	CH_2CCl_3
(25)	S	Cl	CH_3
(25a)	S→O	Cl	CH_3
(26)	S	Pht	CH_3
(26a)	S→O	Pht	CH_3
(26b)	S⋯O	Pht	CH_3
(27)	S	Het	CH_3

	X	R
(20)	S	V
(20a)	S→O	V
(20b)	S⋯O	V
(20c)	SO_2	V
(21)	S	A
(21a)	S→O	A
(21b)	SO_2	A
(21c)	S	A
(22)	S⋯O	Pht
(22b)	S⋯O	Pht
(23)	S→O	A

Table V—continued

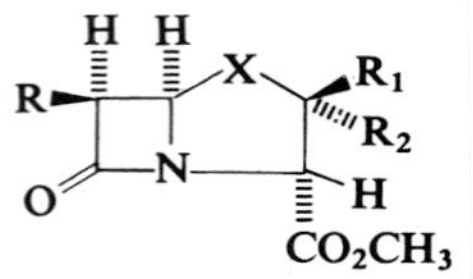

	X	R	R_1	R_2
(28)	S···O	Pht	CH_2OAc	CH_3
(29)	S···O	Pht	CH_3	CH_2OAc
(30)	S···O	A	CH_2OAc	CH_3
(31)	S···O	A	CH_3	CH_2OAc
(32)	S	A	CH_2OAc	CH_3
(32a)	S→O	A	CH_2OAc	CH_3

[d] Cooper et al. (1969a).
[e] Archer and Demarco (1969).
[f] Cooper et al. (1969b).
[g] Gutowski (1970).
[h] Cooper (1969).
[i] Johnson et al. (1968).
[j] Spry (1970).

¹H NMR DATA[a] FOR DIFFERENT CEPHALOSPORINS AND SOME CORRESPONDING SULFOXIDES[b]

Compound[c]	Resonance (ppm)							
	H-2α	H-2β	2-CH₃	3-CH₃	H-4	H-6	H-7	C=$<^H_H$
(33)[d]	3.56[2.55] d, J = 19	3.23[2.23] d, J = 19		2.21[1.67] s		5.05[4.20] d, J = 4.5	5.88[5.72] q, J = 4.5, 9	
(33a)[d]	3.27[1.77] dd, J = 1.9, 19.0	3.70[2.53] d, J = 19.0		2.24[1.63] s		4.56[3.14] dd, J = 1.9, 4.5	6.15[6.04] q, J = 4.5, 10.5	
(33b)[d]	3.52[2.78] d, J = 16.5	4.11[3.54] d, J = 16.5		2.36[1.79] s		4.63[3.99] d, J = 4.5	5.50[4.53] q, J = 4.5, 8.0	
(34)[e]	3.66 dd J = 7.5, <1.0		1.45 d J = 7.5	2.09 bs J = 1.0		5.16 d J = 5.0	5.80 q J = 5.0, 9.0	
(34a)[e]	3.27 dq J = 1.5, 8.0		1.78 d J = 8.0	2.16 s		4.71 dd J = 1.5, 5.0	6.17 q J = 5.0, 10.0	
(35)[e]		3.46 q J = 7.5	1.57 d J = 7.5	2.50 s		5.13 d J = 5.0	5.95 q J = 5.0, 9.0	
(35a)[e]		3.60 q J = 7.5	1.32 d J = 7.5	2.26 s		4.55 d J = 5.0	6.21 q J = 5.0, 11.0	
(36)[e]				2.30 s		5.17 d J = 5.0	5.92 q J = 5.0, 9.0	5.68, 5.91 AB, J = 1.0
(36a)[e]				2.31 s		4.71 d J = 5.0	6.16 q J = 5.0, 10.0	6.12, 6.26 AB, J = 1.0
(37)[e]				2.20 s		5.10 d J = 5.0	5.87 q J = 5.0, 8.0	5.57, 5.80 bs
(37a)[e]				2.20 s		4.60 d J = 5.0	6.08 q J = 5.0, 10.0	5.98, 6.10 bs
(38)[f]	3.45 d J = 14.0	2.51 dd J = 1.0, 14.0		1.30 s	4.81 d J = 1.0	5.31 d J = 4.5	5.54 q J = 4.5, 9.0	
(38a)[f]	2.85 d J = 14.5	3.35 dd J = <1.0, 14.5		1.35 bs	4.92 d J < 1.0	5.08 d J = 4.5	6.15 q J = 4.5, 10.5	
(39)[g]	3.75 d J = 14	3.20 d J = 14		1.54 s	4.40 s	5.30 d J = 4.5	5.58 q J = 4.5, 9	

Table VI—continued

Compound[c]	H-2α	H-2β	2-CH₃	3-CH₃	H-4	H-6	H-7	C=$\langle$H/H
(39a)[g]	3.35 d, J=15	4.33 d, J=15		1.58 s	4.60 s	4.97 d, J=4.5	6.00 q, J=4.5, 10	
(39b)[g]	3.30 d, J=14	3.80 d, J=14		1.65 s	4.90 s	4.24 d, J=4.5	5.27 q, J=4.5, 8	
(39c)[g]	4.07 d, J=14	3.90 d, J=14		1.57 s	4.44 s	5.14 d, J=4.5	5.99 q, J=4.5, 10	
(40)[h]	3.52 d, J=14	2.54 dd, J=14, <1.0		1.36 s	4.61 bs	5.46 d, J=4.5	5.61 q, J=4.5, 9	
(40b)[h]	3.30 d, J=14	3.61 bd, J=<1.0, 14		1.40 s	4.54 s, J=<1.0	5.09 d, J=4.5	5.92 q, J=4.5, 10	
(41)[i]	3.52 dd, J=6.5, 14.0	3.28 dd, J=4.5, 14.0		1.15 d, J=6.5	4.50 dd, J=1.0, 4.0	5.04 d, J=4.5	5.63 qd, J=1.0, 4.5, 9.0	
(42)[i]	3.40 dd, J=13.0, 14.5	2.91 dd, J=3.0, 14.5, <1.0		1.08 d, J=6.5	4.61 bd, J=5.5, <1.0	5.09 d, J=4.5	6.04 q, J=4.5, 11.0	
(43)[j]								
(44)[j]	5.90 m, J=1.3, 2.0			1.90 d, J=1.3	4.66 bs, J≃0.4, 2.0	5.32 bs, J=4.5	5.74 q, J=4.5, 9.0	
(44a)[j]	6.71 m, J=1.3, 2.1			2.06 d, J=1.3	4.95 bs, J≃0.4, 2.1	4.75 d, J=4.5	6.13 q, J=4.5, 11.0	
(44b)[j]	6.22 m, J=1.3, 2.0			2.01 d, J=1.3	4.57 bs, J≃0.4, 2.0	4.82 d, J=4.5	5.71 q, J=4.5, 9.0	
(45)[e]		1.90 s		1.90 s	4.93 s	5.39 d, J=4.0	5.72 q, J=4.0, 9.0	
(46)[i]			2.25 q, J=1.3	1.86 q, J=1.3		4.80 d, J=4.5	5.99 q, J=4.5, 11.0	
(47)[k]	3.62 d, J=18	3.28 d, J=18				4.96 d, J=5	5.82 d, J=5.0, 9	

$(47a)^e$	3.24 dd, $J=1.0, 18.0$	3.73 d, $J=18.0$		4.49 dd, $J=1.0, 5.0$	6.00 q, $J=5.0, 10.0$
$(48)^l$			7.12	4.81 d, $J=5$	5.23 q, $J=5, 8.5$
$(49)^d$	1.72 bs	3.42 bd, $J=17.5, 2.1, <1.0$	2.92 bd, $J=17.5, 0.4$	6.45 bs	4.92 d, $J=5.0$	5.75 q, $J=5.0, 9.0$
$(50)^l$				7.12	4.90 d, $J=2.5$	4.85 q, $J=2.5, 8.5$
$(51)^m$	2.16 s	3.50 d, $J=18.0$	3.21 d, $J=18.0$		4.75 d, $J=1.8$	5.08 q, $J=1.8, 8.0$
$(52)^n$	2.08 d, $J=1.0$	3.62 dd, $J=1.0, 18.0$			4.98, $J=1.8$	5.18 d, $J=1.8$

[a] See Footnote a in Table V.
[b] For a definition of symbols indicating cephalosporin C-7 side-chain substituents, refer to asterisk footnote to Footnote b in Table III.
[c] Key to numbers:

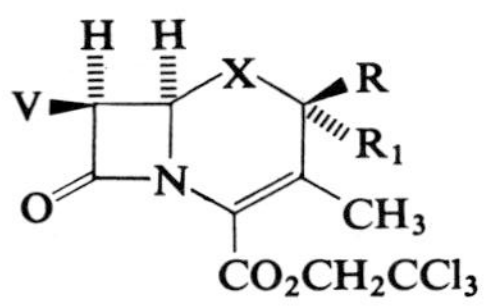

	X	R	R₁
(33)	S	H	H
(33a)	S→O	H	H
(33b)	S···O	H	H
(34)	S	CH₃	H
(34a)	S→O	CH₃	H
(35)	S	H	CH₃
(35a)	S→O	H	CH₃

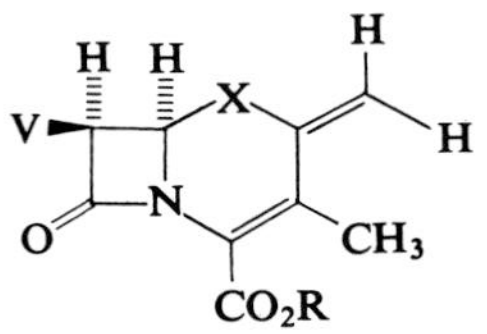

	X	R
(36)	S	CH₂CCl₃
(36a)	S→O	CH₂CCl₃
(37)	S	C(CH₃)₃
(37a)	S→O	C(CH₃)₃

Table VI—continued

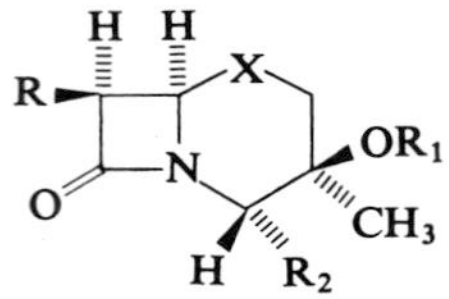

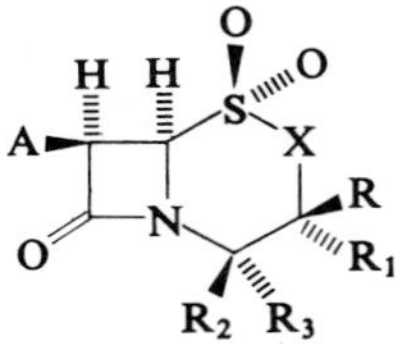

	X	R	R₁	R₂	R₃
(41)	CH₂	CH₃	H	CO₂CH₃	H
(42)	CH₂	H	CH₃	H	CO₂CH₃
(43)	O	H	CH₃	CH₃C=CH₂	H

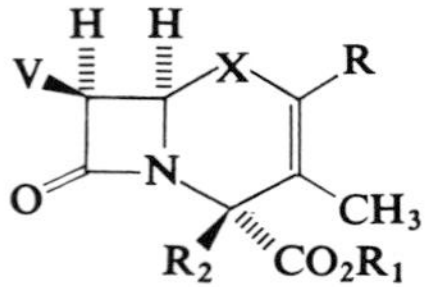

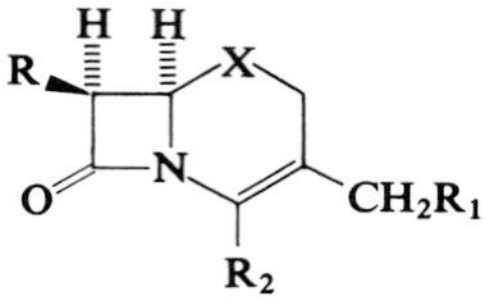

	X	R	R₂	R₁
(47)	S	Th	CO₂CH₃	OAc
(47a)	S→O	Th	CO₂C(CH₃)₃	OAc

	X	R	R₁	R₂
(38)	S	V	H	CO₂CH₂CCl₃
(38a)	S→O	V	H	CO₂CH₂CCl₃
(39)	S	V	COCH₃	CONHC(CH₃)₃
(39a)	S→O	V	COCH₃	CONHC(CH₃)₃
(39b)	S···O	V	COCH₃	CONHC(CH₃)₃
(39c)	SO₂	V	COCH₃	CONHC(CH₃)₃
(40)	S	Pht	H	CO₂CH₃
(40b)	S···O	Pht	H	CO₂CH₃

	X	R	R₁	R₂
(44)	S	H	C(CH₃)₃	H
(44a)	S→O	H	C(CH₃)₃	H

	X	R	R_1	R_2
(44b)	$S\cdots O$	H	$C(CH_3)_3$	H
(45)	S	CH_3	CH_2CCl_3	H
(46)	$S{\rightarrow}O$	CH_3	CH_2CCl_3	CH_3
(48)	$S{\rightarrow}O$	Th	H	OAc
(49)	S	V	H	H

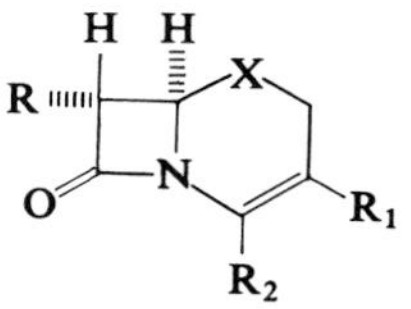

	X	R	R_1	R_2
(50)	$S{\rightarrow}O$	Th	CH_2OAc	H
(51)	S	V	CH_3	$CO_2CH_2CCl_3$
(52)	S	OH	CH_3	$CO_2CH_2C_6H_4NO_2(p)$

[d] Cooper et al. (1970a).
[e] Wright et al. (1971).
[f] Gutowski et al. (1971).
[g] Barton et al. (1970).
[h] Cooper et al. (1970b).
[i] Spry (1971).
[j] Cooper et al. (1970b).
[k] Green et al. (1965).
[l] Sassiver and Shepherd (1969).
[m] Gutowski (1970).
[n] Lunn (1970).

H_B, which corresponds to H-6 in penicillins and H-7 in cephalosporins, is located vicinal to both H_A and the amido proton H_X, and gives rise to the quartet (J_{AB} = same as above, J_{AX} = 8–11 Hz). Confirmation of these relative assignments can be obtained by simple deuterium exchange of the amido proton (accomplished by the addition of a drop of D_2O to a solution of a given penicillin or cephalosporin in an organic solvent, followed by shaking) and observing the collapse of the H_B quartet to a doublet. The following shift ranges summarized in Table VII for *cis*-β-lactam protons are evident from the

Table VII

RANGE OF SHIFTS[a] FOR *cis*-β-LACTAM PROTONS

	H-5	H-6	H-7
Penicillins	4.66–5.60	5.42–6.15	
Cephalosporins		4.24–5.46	5.23–6.21

[a] In parts per million.

data recorded in Tables V and VI. It is clear from these results that the ring junction β-lactam proton, H_A, generally resonates at higher field than its neighbor, H_B, located on the adjacent β-lactam carbon to which the side chain is attached. This observation can be of use in the relative assignment of β-lactam protons in systems where, because of the absence of an amido side-chain proton [e.g., compounds (22), (26), (28), and others], both β-lactam protons give rise to doublet signals and are rendered indistinguishable on the basis of their coupling patterns. Of further interest is the earlier observation that epimerization at C-6 in penicillins or C-7 in cephalosporins, giving the *trans*-β-lactam system, results in a large upfield shift (≈ 0.7–0.8 ppm) for the protons at these positions (Gutowski, 1970; Sassiver and Shepherd, 1969).

2. THIAZOLIDINE AND DIHYDROTHIAZINE RESONANCES

In addition to the β-lactam resonances, the NMR spectra of penicillin derivatives are further characterized by the presence of two methyl singlets corresponding to 2α-(δ1.23–1.66) and 2β-(δ1.49–1.84) geminal methyl groups and a one-proton singlet (δ4.38–4.92), corresponding to H-3. This is in striking contrast to the spectra of cephalosporins (compare Fig. 1 with Figs. 2–4 in appendix), which, in place of *gem*-dimethyl singlets, give rise to a two-proton AB quartet (δ3.23–3.70) in 3-cephems [see compounds (33), (33a), (33b), and (38–40b), Table VI] and a one-proton vinyl multiplet (δ5.90–6.71) in 2-cephems [see compounds (44–45), Table VI]. A three-proton vinyl methyl singlet originating from 3-CH_3 is also common to the spectra of 3-(δ2.20–2.36) and 2-(1.90–2.06) cephems. 2-Cephem spectra are further characterized by a broadened singlet resonance (δ4.57–4.95) originating from H-4.

3. Side-Chain Methylene Resonances

Not recorded in Tables V and VI are chemical shift positions for the methylene protons in some of the more common penicillin and cephalosporin side chains. These are summarized here. Methylene protons of phenylacetamido ($C_6H_5CH_2CONH-$), phenoxyacetamido ($C_6H_5OCH_2CONH-$), and thienylacetamido ($C_4H_3SCH_2CONH-$) all give rise to sharp two-proton singlets ranging from δ4.25–4.24, δ4.54–4.62, and δ3.75–3.86, respectively.

B. Nuclear Overhauser Effects

The nuclear Overhauser effect (NOE) (Anet and Bourn, 1965) is a well-substantiated method for probing three-dimensional identities of molecular entities as well as for establishing signal assignment for protons indistinguishable on the basis of their signal multiplicity. In its simplest terms, the nuclear Overhauser effect can be defined as follows. If two protons in a molecule are spatially proximal, i.e., R (the vector distance between them) $\leqslant \approx 3$ Å, saturation of one of these nuclei with an intense rf field will cause an increase in the integrated intensity of the other, the magnitude of which will be proportional to $1/R^6$. It is therefore possible to estimate from experimentally determined NOE values not only which nuclei in a molecule are responsible for the relaxation of a particular nucleus but also the relative distances between the interacting nuclei.*

Until recently, NMR investigations of penicillins and cephalosporins were mainly concerned with spectral analysis as a means of structural elucidation with little emphasis directed to the use of this technique for defining conformation and configuration. The first application of NOE to *conformational problems* in the penicillin field was carried out by Cooper et al. (1969a) on phenoxymethylpenicillin (*20*) and its corresponding sulfoxide (*20a*). The purpose of the study was (a) to establish whether thiazolidine ring conformation in (*20*) and (*20a*) was the same in solution as that previously reported to exist in crystal from X-ray investigations (Crowfoot et al., 1949; Cooper et al., 1969a), i.e., as conformation A in the sulfide (*20*) and conformation B in the sulfoxide

---

* Nuclear Overhauser effects are designated in structural formulas in this section by inserting the group undergoing saturation in square brackets, placing an asterisk beside the group showing the integrated intensity increase, and connecting the two with a double-headed arrow.

(20a) (see Fig. 1) and (b) to determine relative assignments for the two *gem*-dimethyl singlets in the spectra of (20) and (20a). It was shown that irradiation at the low ($\delta 1.54$) and high ($\delta 1.45$) field methyl singlets in (20) resulted in integrated intensity increases* of 21 and 7% respectively for H-3 with no detectable increases (NOE's) recorded for H-5 upon saturation of either singlet. Similar experiments on (20a) resulted in a 26% NOE for H-3, only when the low field methyl singlet ($\delta 1.70$) was saturated and a 14% NOE for H-5, only when the high field methyl singlet ($\delta 1.18$) was saturated. These results necessitate that H-3, and not H-5, be spatially proximal to both 2α- and 2β-CH$_3$ in (20), as shown in Fig. 1A, while in (20a) H-3 be spatially proximal to the low field

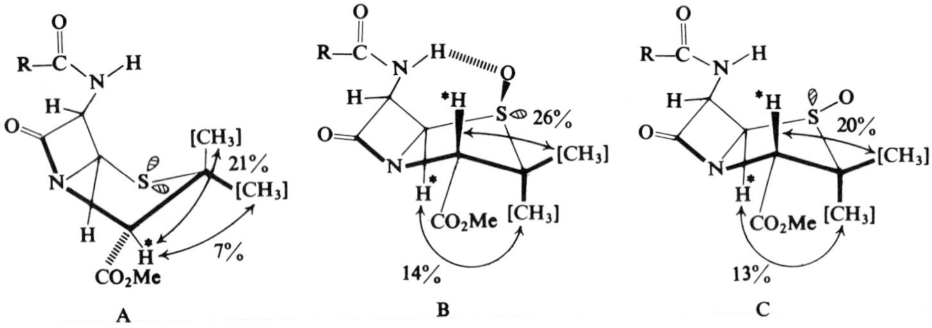

Fig. 1. Thiazolidine ring conformations and NOE's in penicillin and related sulfoxides.

methyl (which is accordingly assigned to 2β-CH$_3$) and H-5 be spatially proximal to the high field methyl (which is accordingly assigned to 2α-CH$_3$) (see Fig. 1B). Relative assignment of the two methyl singlets in (20) is based on the fact that the low field methyl group, which gives the larger NOE of the two for H-3, must correspond to 2β-CH$_3$ since this group, irrespective of the conformation adopted by the thiazolidine ring, is always spatially more proximal to H-3 than 2α-CH$_3$.

Similar studies by Archer and Demarco (1969) on methylpenicillin-*R*-sulfoxide (21b) have shown that inversion of sulfoxide configuration is of little consequence to thiazolidine conformation in penicillins, i.e., thiazolidine conformation is the same in (20a) and (20b) (see Fig. 1C) but different from that in (20).

NOE studies on phthalimidopenicillin sulfoxides (Cooper *et al.*, 1969b) have also been useful in making spectral assignments for H-5 and H-6, which give rise to identical doublet signals in these systems due to the absence of a

---

* NOE values reported in this section are expected to be accurate to ±10% of the reported values.

C-6 side-chain amido proton. Thus, assignments for 2α-CH_3 ($\delta1.33$) and H-5 ($\delta4.86$) in methyl phthalimidopenicillin-R-sulfoxide (*22b*) were confirmed by observation of a 9% NOE between these protons. An additional NOE (18%) noted between 2β-CH_3 ($\delta1.83$) and H-3 ($\delta4.61$) confirmed not only assignments for the remaining protons in the system but also demonstrated striking similarity in thiazolidine conformation in penicillin sulfoxides with different C-6 side chains, e.g., acetamido, phenoxyacetamido, phthalimido, etc.

A small but nevertheless significant NOE of 5–8% observed between 3-CH_3 and H-4 in cephalosporin derivatives (*38*)–(*39c*), shown in Fig. 2 (Barton *et al.*, 1970; Gutowski *et al.*, 1971), gives some evidence for tetrahydrothiazine conformation. Molecular models show that the tetrahydrothiazine ring can adopt

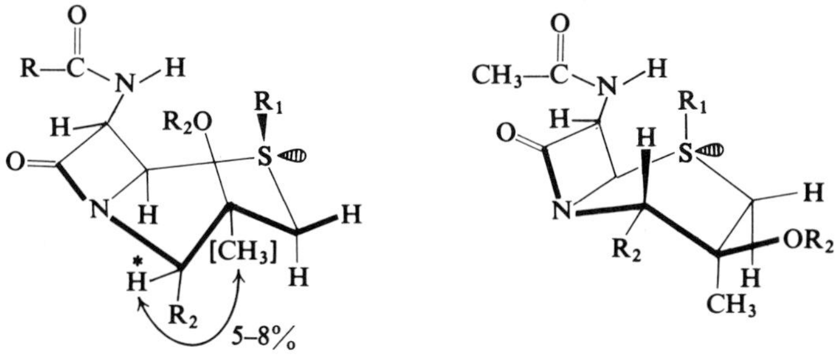

Fig. 2. Possible tetrahydrothiazine ring conformations for saturated cephalosporins (*36*)–(*41*).

either conformation A, a flattened chair in which 3-CH_3 and H-4 are oriented *trans*-diequatorial to each other, or conformation B, a boat in which 3-CH_3 and H-4 are oriented vicinal *trans*-diaxial to each other (see Figs. 2A and B). Of the two possible conformations, only A can reasonably account for the occurrence of an NOE between 3-CH_3 and H-4 since in this conformation these protons meet the requirement of spatial proximity (i.e., $R \leqslant 3$ Å). This conclusion is further supported by the absence of an NOE between 3-CH_3 and H-5, which would be expected if conformation B were adopted, and from hydrogen-bonding studies described later in this chapter.

Two applications of NOE to *configurational analysis* in penicillins and cephalosporins have recently been reported. In the conversion of penicillin to cephalosporin via double sulfoxide rearrangement, two isomeric 2-methylene substituted penicillins of the type shown in Figs. 3A and B were isolated by Spry (1970). Determination of the relative configuration at C-2 in the two epimers was shown to be a simple matter by NOE analysis. Thus, saturation of the C-2 methyl singlet in (*28*) and (*30*) gave an approximate 6–10% NOE for H-5 and no NOE for H-3 (see Fig. 3A) while, in (*29*) and (*31*), saturation of this same methyl resulted in a negligible NOE for H-5 but an approximate 12% NOE for H-3 (see Fig. 3B). These results can only be satisfied by assigning C-2 configurations as shown in Figs. 3A and B.

Kaiser *et al.* (1971) have utilized NOE studies to establish the configuration about the *exo* double bond in 2-thiomethylene cephalosporins of the type shown in Fig. 3C. It was reasoned that, if the *exo*-vinyl proton were oriented *syn* to 3-CH$_3$, a sizable NOE would be expected between this proton and 3-CH$_3$,

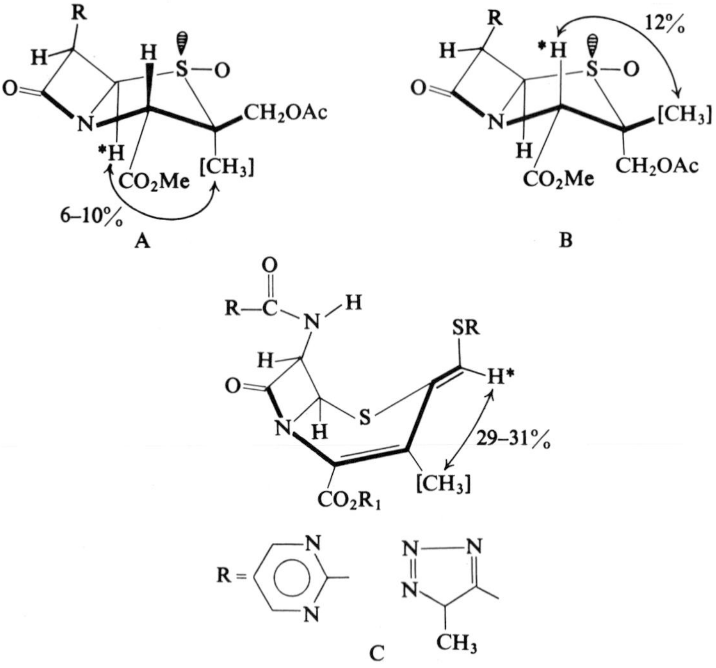

Fig. 3. NOE's recorded in epimeric C-2 methylene penicillin sulfoxides (A and B) and in a C-2 *exo*-vinyl cephalosporin (C).

while if the reverse configuration were the case, no intramolecular relaxation effect would be expected between these protons. As shown in Fig. 3C, irradiation at 3-CH$_3$ results in a 29–31% NOE for the vinyl proton, thus confirming its *syn* relationship to 3-CH$_3$.

C. Proton Spin–Spin Coupling

1. GEMINAL

Since the magnitude of geminal H–H coupling (J_{gem}) for methylene protons depends upon the number and conformation of adjacent π bonds as well as on the configuration of p orbitals on adjacent heteroatoms (Cookson et al., 1966; Allingham et al., 1968; and Bhacca and Williams, 1964), measurement of J_{gem} for the C-2 methylene protons in cephalosporins can provide important information regarding their structure.

For example, Cooper et al. (1970a) have recently shown that the relative magnitudes of J_{gem} for the C-2 methylene protons in 3-cephem-S- and -R-sulfoxides [(33a) and (33b) respectively in Table VI] are important in deciding between two possible conformations, A and B (see Fig. 4), for the dihydrothiazine ring in these systems. Since an axial lone pair of electrons on a heteroatom is more effective in transferring its electrons into the antisymmetric molecular orbitals of an adjacent methylene group (producing a positive change in J_{gem}) (Pople and Bothner-By, 1965) than is an equatorial lone pair, the observed

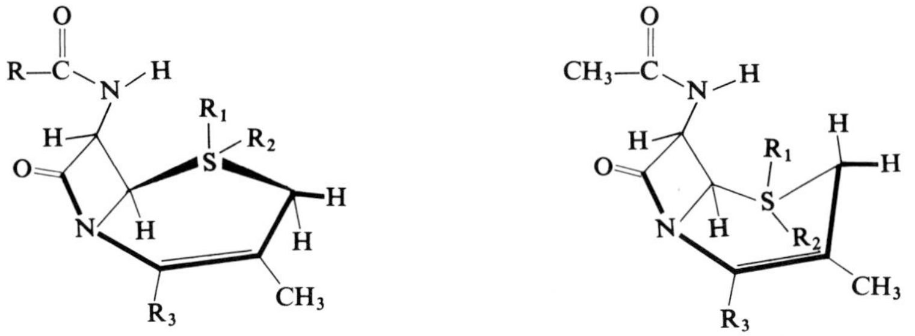

Fig. 4. Possible dihydrothiazine ring conformations in 3-cephems.

greater negative geminal coupling in (33a) ($J_{gem} = -19$ Hz) relative to (33b) ($J_{gem} = -17$ Hz) is only compatible with conformation A in which a sulfur lone pair is axial in (33b) (R-sulfoxide) and equatorial in (33a) (S-sulfoxide). Alternatively, in light of having established a preferred conformation for the dihydrothiazine ring in 3-cephem derivatives, measurement of J_{gem} can provide a simple method for ascertaining sulfoxide stereochemistry in such systems, i.e., the *S-sulfoxide gives rise to a smaller* (*more negative*) J_{gem} *than the R-sulfoxide*. This conclusion appears to be further supported by an example from the tetrahydrothiazine series of compounds shown in Table VI. Thus, compound (39a), which has an S-sulfoxide, gives a J_{gem} of -15.0 Hz, while compound (39b), which has an R-sulfoxide, gives a J_{gem} of -14.0 Hz.

The magnitude of J_{gem} also reflects the state of hybridization at C-3 in cephalosporins (Nagarajan et al., 1971). When a methylene group forms part of a cyclic system with an adjacent π system, as in 3-cephems, the π contribution (J^{π}) to J_{gem} will vary with the angle ϕ between the methylene group and the adjacent π bond (Bhacca and Williams, 1964). In the case of 3-cephems, $\phi = 30$–35 for a J^{π} contribution to J_{gem} of about 4 Hz (see Fig. 5). J_{gem} *values for 3-cephems are consequently smaller (more negative) than corresponding values in fully saturated cephalosporins having a tetrahydrothiazine ring.* This is borne out by data in Table VI. Thus, J_{gem} for 3-cephem compounds (*33*), (*33a*), (*33b*), and (*47–52*) ranges from -16.5 to -19.0 Hz while J_{gem} for the saturated tetrahydrothiazine cephalosporins (*38–40b*) ranges from -13.0 to -15.0 Hz.

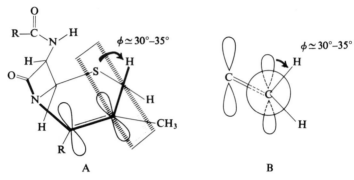

A   B

Fig. 5. Angular relationship of the C-2 methylene protons in 3-cephems with the adjacent π bond.

2. VICINAL

Most diagnostic of the relative configuration of β-lactam protons in penicillins and cephalosporins is the magnitude of their vicinal coupling (J_{gem}) since previous investigations have shown that $J_{cis} > J_{trans}$. Coupling between *cis*-β-lactam protons has been shown in the range 4–6 Hz (Barrow and Spotswood, 1965; Luche *et al.*, 1968; Allingham *et al.*, 1968) while coupling between *trans*-β-lactam protons in 6-epipenicillins and 7-epicephalosporins has been shown in the range 1.5–3 Hz (Barrow and Spotswood, 1965; Gutowski, 1970; Johnson *et al.*, 1968; Sassiver and Shepherd, 1969; Wolfe and Lee, 1968).

3. FOUR BOND COUPLING, ^4J

A number of four bond couplings have been observed in cephalosporin derivatives, the most common of which are the following: (a) ^4J coupling through four σ bonds oriented in a "W" or "zigzag" all *s-trans* conformation (see Fig. 6A) (Wiberg *et al.*, 1962; Rassat *et al.*, 1964) and (b) ^4J coupling through the agency of a π system, i.e., allylic coupling (Karplus, 1960, and Fraser, 1960). Typical ^4J values usually lie in the range 0–3 Hz. Long-range W coupling, between H-2 and H-4, has been observed in cephalosporin derivatives of the type shown in Fig. 6B [e.g., compounds (*38*), (*38a*), and (*42*) in Table VI] and range from 0 to 1 Hz in magnitude. The significance of such coupling is manifest in making relative assignments for H-2β and H-2α, which give rise to otherwise identical doublet signals and are readily distinguished on the basis of a long-range ^4J coupling between H-2β and H-4. Accordingly, *H-2β and H-2α are assigned to the high and low field doublets respectively in the spectra of cephalosporin sulfides [e.g., (38), (39), and (40)] while in the corresponding sulfoxides [e.g., (38a), (39a), and (40b)], reverse assignment is shown to be the case (see Table VI).*

Of further interest is a rather unique ^4J W coupling (<1 Hz) observed to exist between the C-3 OH and the C-3 methyl protons in (38a) (see Fig. 6C). This, presumably, is a consequence of the formation of intramolecular hydrogen bond between 3β-OH and the S-sulfoxide oxygen (evidence for this is presented later in this section), locking the O–H bond into a W conformation with

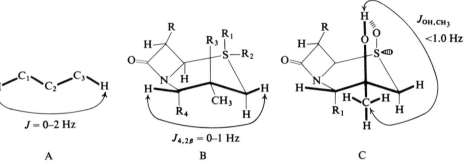

Fig. 6. (A) W or zigzag requirement for long-range four bond coupling. (B and C) W couplings in cephalosporins.

C-3 methyl protons (see Fig. 6C). Verification of this coupling comes from the fact that deuterium exchange of the hydroxyl proton results in the disappearance of this coupling in the 3-CH$_3$ signal.

^4J allylic couplings (Karplus, 1960; Bothner-By *et al.*, 1962) have been reported by Cooper *et al.* (1970a) in 2-cephems. Important to emphasize, once again, is their use in making C-2 proton assignments. Since the magnitude of $^4J_{al}$ is dependent upon the angle (ϕ) between the plane of the double bond and an adjacent C–H bond (Garbisch, 1964) (see Fig. 7A), allylic coupling involving H-2 and H-4 in 2-cephems will be stereospecific. The allylic couplings shown in Fig. 7B have been observed in 2-cephems (44–45). Thus, the observed large J_{al} coupling between H-2 and H-4 (1.9–2.2 Hz) not only supports the proposed conformation for the dihydrothiazine ring in compounds (44)–(45) (Cooper *et al.*, 1970a) but also confirms the previously assigned β configuration for H-4 (Van Heyningen and Ahern, 1968) in these systems.

An observed allylic coupling of 2.1 Hz between H-4 and the low field H-2 proton in the spectrum of (49) (see Fig. 7C) establishes the assignment of H-2α

and H-2β to the low and high field doublets. An additional coupling of approximately 0–1.0 Hz between the C-3 methyl and C-2 protons has also been observed in the spectra of 3-cephems (see Fig. 7D). As with allylic coupling, the largest coupling to the C-3 methyl group originates from the C-2 proton most orthogonal to the plane of the adjacent C-3–C-4 double bond. Thus, in

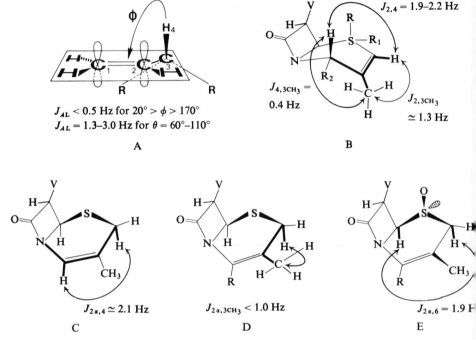

$$J_{AL} < 0.5 \text{ Hz for } 20° > \phi > 170°$$
$$J_{AL} = 1.3\text{–}3.0 \text{ Hz for } \theta = 60°\text{–}110°$$

A

$$J_{2,4} = 1.9\text{–}2.2 \text{ Hz}$$
$$J_{4,3CH_3} = 0.4 \text{ Hz}$$
$$J_{2,3CH_3} \simeq 1.3 \text{ Hz}$$

B

$$J_{2\alpha,4} \simeq 2.1 \text{ Hz}$$

C

$$J_{2\alpha,3CH_3} < 1.0 \text{ Hz}$$

D

$$J_{2\alpha,6} = 1.9 \text{ H}$$

E

Fig. 7. (A) Illustration of angular dependency of allylic coupling. (B–E) Allylic and other four bond couplings in cephalosporins.

the spectrum of (*49*), the low field C-2 geminal doublet exhibits the larger coupling to 3-CH$_3$ ($\simeq$1.0 Hz) and is attributed to H-2α, while the high field doublet exhibits the smaller coupling to 3-CH$_3$ (0.4 Hz) and is attributed to H-2β.

A unique long-range coupling of 1.9 Hz has been previously reported to exist between H-2α and H-6 in 3-cephem-*S*-sulfoxides (see Fig. 7E) (Cooper *et al.*, 1970a) which is absent in the spectra of corresponding sulfides, *R*-sulfoxides, and related tetrahydro derivatives (*38–39b*). Although the origin of this coupling is not apparent, it is believed that the *S*-sulfoxide bond is in some way responsible for the transfer of spin coupling information from C-2 to C-6.

4. FIVE BOND COUPLING, ^5J

Long-range ^5J couplings, hitherto unobserved in the spectra of cephalosporins, have been observed for compounds (*41*), (*43*), and (*46*) (see Figs. 8A and B) whose syntheses have recently been reported (Spry, 1971; Cooper et al., 1970b). Mutual coupling between the vinyl methyl protons ($J_{CH_3, CH_3} = 1.3$ Hz) in the spectrum of (*46*) presumably originate from a homoallylic rather than a through space coupling mechanism. The observed coupling between H-4α and H-7 ($J_{4\alpha,7} \simeq 1.0$ Hz) in (*41*) and (*43*) is stereospecific as it requires

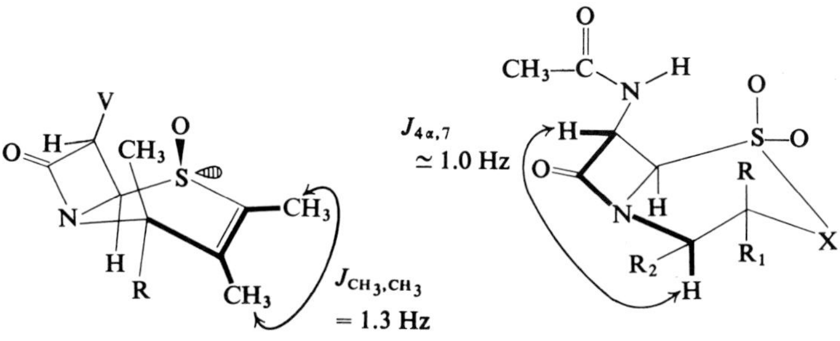

Fig. 8. Five bond couplings (J) observed in cephalosporins.

the C-4 proton be in the α-axial configuration. Thus, reversal of the configuration at C-4 as in (*42*) (see Table VI) results in the disappearance of coupling between the two protons in question. Investigation of H-4 and H-7 multiplicity in cephalosporins can therefore be of use in establishing the configuration at C-4.

D. Sulfoxide Bond Screening Effects

Investigation of proton chemical shift changes induced in penicillin and cephalosporin derivatives as a result of oxidation at sulfur (i.e., the introduction of either an *R*- or *S*-sulfoxide into the ring system) can furnish considerable information concerning configuration of the sulfoxide bond and conformation of both thiazolidine and thiazine ring systems (Morin et al., 1969; Cooper et al., 1969a, b, 1970a; Archer and Demarco, 1969; Barton et al., 1969).

On the assumption that the sulfoxide bond possesses axial symmetry and therefore has acetylenic-like* anisotropy, the screening environment around an S → O can be described by Eq. (1), the McConnell point dipole approximation (McConnell, 1957), which relates the magnitude of nuclear screening at a given proton to

$$\sigma = \varDelta\chi[(1 - 3\cos^2\theta)/R^3] \tag{1}$$

its position in space relative to the symmetry axis of an anisotropic function. In Eq. (1), R is the vector distance between a given proton and the electrical center of gravity of the anisotropic bond, θ is the angle between R and the symmetry axis of the bond, and $\varDelta\chi$ is a constant characteristic of the magnetic

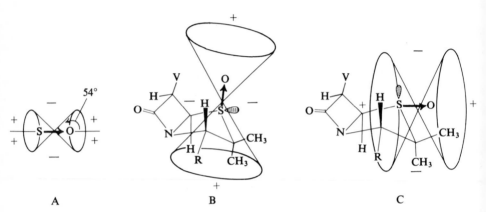

Fig. 9. (A) Pictorial representation of screening environment around a sulfoxide bond. (B and C) Screening effect of sulfoxide bond on protons in S- and R-sulfoxides.

anisotropy of the bond under consideration. For the S → O bond* $\varDelta\chi$ is assumed to be negative, in accord with previously reported negative $\varDelta\chi$ values for the acetylenic bond (Castellano and Lorenc, 1965; Pople, 1962). Thus, calculation from Eq. (1) of the sign of σ for varying increment values of θ ($0° < \theta < 360°$) gives a qualitative description of the screening environment around the S → O bond which is illustrated in Fig. 9A. Negative and positive values indicate deshielding and shielding regions respectively.

Using this model for the screening environment around an S → O bond, different groups have investigated sulfoxide bond stereochemistry in the major oxidation product of penicillin (Morin et al., 1969; Cooper et al., 1969a; Barton et al., 1969). It was reasoned that in the S configuration, shown in Fig. 9B, the S → O bond would exert deshielding effects on H-3, H-6, and 2β-CH₃

---

* It appears to be firmly established that the sulfur–oxygen bond in sulfoxides is a p^2–pd hybrid double bond. However, because of d, p–π overlap, the S → O bond is considered to be "electronically a triple bond" (Burg, 1961).

and shielding effects on H-5 and 2α-CH₃ while, in the R configuration shown in Fig. 9C, all protons were expected to be deshielded except H-3, which was expected to be shielded. As observed, shifts for the different protons in the process, sulfide → sulfoxide, were shown to correspond most closely to the former case. The S → O bond of the major oxidation product was accordingly assigned the S configuration.

Application of these calculations to the photochemically inverted epimer of (20a) [i.e., the R-sulfoxide (20b)] gave, in general, similar agreement between observed and calculated shifts (Archer and Demarco, 1969) with one notable exception, namely, H-5. The observed shift of 0.80 ppm to higher field for this proton when compared with this same proton in the parent sulfide was unexpected in light of its position in the deshielding region of the R-sulfoxide

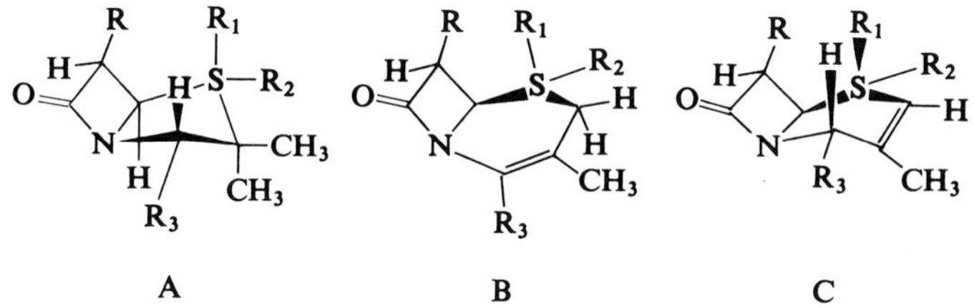

Fig. 10. Conformations proposed for thiazolidine ring in penicillin sulfoxides (A) and for the dihydrothiazine ring in 3- and 2-cephem sulfoxides (B and C).

bond (see Fig. 9C). One explanation offered (Archer and Demarco, 1969; Barton et al., 1969) for this unexpectedly large upfield shift was the shielding caused by the *trans*-oriented sulfur lone-pair electrons since similar effects have been observed in thione-1-oxide (Lambert and Keske, 1966a, b). Presumably this phenomenon, along with that for the effect of axial lone-pair electrons on the magnitude of geminal coupling constants (Cookson et al., 1966; Pople and Bothner-By, 1965) have a common origin, i.e., the ability of an axial lone pair on a heteroatom to transfer electron density into adjacent antisymmetric methylene or methine orbitals.

Sulfoxide bond chemical shift perturbations have also been useful in assigning configuration and conformation in both 3- and 2-cephem derivatives (Cooper et al., 1970a). It was inferred from observed parallel shift trends for corresponding protons in penicillin and cephalosporin (see Table VIII) that conformational similarities exist between 3- and 2-cephems and analogous penicillin derivatives, i.e., H-5, H-6, and H-3 in penicillins are situated, relative to the sulfoxide bond, at approximately the same spatial positions as H-7, H-6, and H-4, respectively, in cephalosporin derivatives. Cephalosporin conformations most consistent with these data are shown in Fig. 10.

Table VIII

PROTON RESONANCE SHIFTS INDUCED BY THE SULFOXIDE BOND $(\Delta_{SO})^{a}$ IN PENICILLINS AND CEPHALOSPORINS

In penicillins (ppm)

	Example	$2\alpha\mathrm{CH}_3$	$2\beta\mathrm{CH}_3$	H-3	H-5	H-6
S → S=O	$(20) \to (20a)$	+0.26	−0.13	−0.22	+0.55	−0.36
	$(21) \to (21a)$	+0.27	−0.06	−0.23	+0.51	−0.36
	$(25) \to (25a)$	+0.17	−0.09	0.00		
	$(26) \to (26a)$	+0.20	−0.07	+0.05	+0.22	−0.40
	$(32) \to (32a)$	+0.26		−0.01	+0.58	−0.35
S → S···O	$(20) \to (20b)$	+0.17	−0.08	+0.06	+0.80	+0.19
	$(21) \to (21b)$	+0.26	−0.01	+0.06	+0.72	+0.21
	$(22) \to (22b)$	+0.18	−0.01	+0.07	+0.74	−0.21
	$(26) \to (26b)$	+0.20	−0.02	+0.03	+0.41	−0.26

In cephalosporins (ppm)

	Example	$\text{H-}2\alpha$	$\text{H-}2\beta$	$2\alpha\mathrm{CH}_3$	$2\beta\mathrm{CH}_3$	H-4	H-6	H-7
S → S=O	$(33) \to (33a)$	+0.29	−0.47				−0.49	−0.27
	$(34) \to (34a)$	+0.39					−0.45	−0.37
	$(35) \to (35a)$		−0.14	+0.25	−0.33		−0.58	−0.26
	$(36) \to (36a)$						−0.46	−0.24
	$(37) \to (37a)$						−0.50	−0.21
	$(38) \to (38a)$	+0.60	−0.84			−0.11	−0.23	−0.61
	$(39) \to (39a)$	+0.40	−1.13			−0.20	−0.33	−0.42
	$(44) \to (44a)$	+0.38	−0.45			−0.29	−0.57	−0.39
	$(47) \to (47a)$						−0.47	−0.18
S → S···O	$(33) \to (33b)$	+0.04	−0.41				+0.42	+0.38
	$(39) \to (39b)$	+0.35	−0.60				+1.06	+0.31
	$(40) \to (40b)$	+0.22	−1.07			+0.07	+0.37	−0.31
	$(44) \to (44b)$					+0.09	+0.50	+0.03

^{a} $\Delta_{SO} = \delta_{\text{sulfoxide}} - \delta_{\text{sulfide}}$. Positive and negative signs indicate upfield and downfield shifts respectively resulting from the process, sulfide → sulfoxide.

Table VIII, which is derived from data in Tables V and VI, summarizes the observed sulfoxide perturbation shifts (Δ_{SO}) for pertinent protons in the different penicillins and cephalosporins. The recorded data clearly show that, without exception, *protons and/or methyl groups located vicinal and trans diaxial to either a sulfoxide bond or a sulfur lone pair are shielded in the process sulfide → sulfoxide.* Note, for example, upfield shifts recorded for 2α-CH$_3$ and H-5 in penicillins and 2α-CH$_3$, H-2α, and H-6 in cephalosporins.

Most indicative of differences between R- and S-sulfoxides are resonances arising from H-3, H-5, and H-6 in penicillins and H-4, H-6, and H-7 in cephalosporins. Thus, in penicillin- and cephalosporin-S-sulfoxides, H-3 and H-4 respectively are deshielded relative to their parent sulfides, while in the corresponding R-sulfoxides these same protons are shielded. The downfield shifts experienced by H-3 and H-4 in the former case are a consequence of *syn*-1,3- and *syn*-1,4-diaxial deshielding effects respectively (Buck *et al.*, 1966; Foster *et al.*, 1968; Sollman *et al.*, 1967).

Additionally, H-5 and H-6 in penicillins and H-6 and H-7 in cephalosporins experience screening effects of opposite sign in the process sulfide → R-sulfoxide [see, e.g., (*22* → *22b*), (*26* → *26b*), and (*40* → *40b*) in Table VIII].

E. Inter- and Intramolecular Solvent and Hydrogen-Bonding Effects

Investigation of aromatic-solvent-induced shifts (ASIS) (Laszlo, 1967) and hydrogen-bonding behavior in penicillin and cephalosporin sulfoxides has furnished considerable information regarding the chirality at sulfur in these systems (Cooper *et al.*, 1969a, b, 1970a; Barton *et al.*, 1969). The phenomenon of ASIS (ASIS $= \delta_{CDCl_3} - \delta_{C_6D_6}$) originates from the fact that (a) aromatic solvents, such as benzene, display a strong tendency to coordinate at electron-deficient sites within a solute molecule (Bhacca and Williams, 1964), i.e., at the positive end of a solute dipole* and (b) the anisotropy in the magnetic susceptibility of the associated aromatic nucleus results in large screening effects for solute protons situated in the vicinity of, and on the same side of, the solute as the site of association. Since the magnitude and sign of shifts induced for different protons in penicillin and cephalosporin sulfoxides in benzene, relative to chloroform, will be characteristic of the geometry of the associated complex, which in turn will depend upon sulfoxide configuration, benzene association with S- and R-sulfoxides should take place from the α and β sides of these systems respectively.

---

* Ledaal (1968) has recently proposed a model for benzene–polar solute associations which is common for all polar solutes. The model presumes that the dipole axis of a polar function in a solute is located along the sixfold axis of symmetry of the benzene system with the positive end of the polar function nearest and the negative end farthest away from it.

Accordingly, the large ASIS values recorded for α-face protons in the major oxidation products of penicillins (i.e., 2α-CH$_3$ and H-5), 3-cephems (i.e., H-2α and H-6), and 2-cephems (i.e., H-2 and H-6) (see Figs. 11A–C for recorded ASIS values*) were presented as strong evidence in support of the S configuration for the S → O bond in these systems (Cooper *et al.*, 1969a, 1970a; Barton *et al.*, 1969). Although ASIS have been recorded for similar protons in related epimeric cephalosporin-*R*-sulfoxides (Cooper *et al.*, 1970a) and in phthalimidopenicillin-*R*-sulfoxides (Cooper *et al.*, 1969b), the observed shifts for such systems do not correspond to ASIS values expected, *a priori*, on

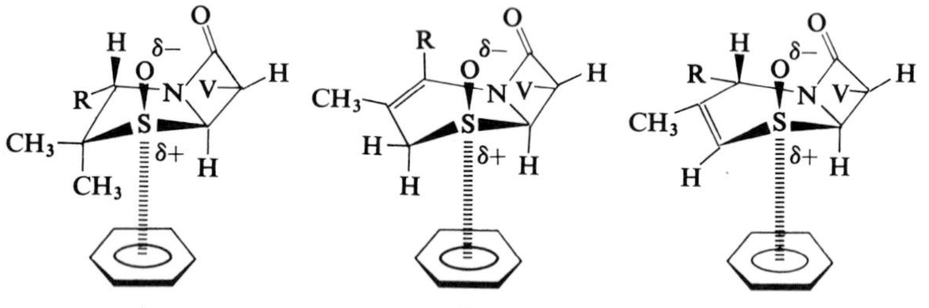

Fig. 11. Proposed geometries of benzene–solute collision complexes for penicillin (A) and cephalosporin (B and C) *S*-sulfoxides.

the basis of benzene solvation from the positive end of the *R*-sulfoxide dipole, i.e., from the β face of the molecule. These discrepancies were rationalized in terms of steric prevention of benzene association from the β face by the bulky C-6 phenoxyacetamido side chain. Indeed, investigation of ASIS in systems where the bulky C-6 substituent can no longer prevent steric interference from the β face, such as, for example, in 6-epiphthalimidopenicillin-*R*-sulfoxides (Cooper *et al.*, 1969b) gives the expected upfield shifts for β-face protons H-3 and 2β-CH$_3$ (see Fig. 12), which is consistent with a mode of association taking place from the β face.

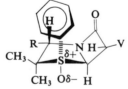

Fig. 12. Proposed geometry of benzene–solute collision complex for 6-epipenicillin-*R*-sulfoxides.

* ASIS values discussed here are net values resulting from subtraction of ASIS for a sulfoxide from its corresponding sulfide (i.e., ASIS$_{sulfoxide}$ − ASIS$_{sulfide}$). The resulting ASIS values are thus a reflection of benzene–solute association at the S → O bond only.

Recorded ASIS, listed in Table IX, show that epimeric sulfoxides of both penicillins and cephalosporins can be readily distinguished on the basis of their empirical shift differences alone. Thus, a large positive ASIS value for H-6 in a penicillin or H-7 in a cephalosporin is strongly indicative of R-sulfoxide stereochemistry while large positive ASIS values for 2α-CH$_3$ and H-5 in penicillins and H-2α and H-6 in cephalosporins are characteristic of S-sulfoxide configuration.

Table IX

Recorded Net ASIS[a] for Isomeric Sulfoxides

	Penicillins				
	2α-CH$_3$	2β-CH$_3$	H-3	H-5	H-6
S-sulfoxide	+0.27–0.35	+0.04–0.11	−0.03–0.14	+0.50–0.79	−0.03–0.06
R-sulfoxide	−0.22	−0.09	−0.09	−0.07	+0.75
	Cephalosporins				
	H-2α	H-2β	H-4	H-6	H-7
Δ^3-S-sulfoxide	+0.49	+0.17		+0.57	−0.05
Δ^3-R-sulfoxide	+0.27	+0.43		−0.21	+0.80
Δ^2-S-sulfoxide			+0.21	+0.52	−0.17
Δ^2-R-sulfoxide			+0.21	−0.03	+0.57

[a] Net ASIS = ASIS (sulfide)-ASIS (sulfoxide); in parts per million.

The intra- and intermolecular hydrogen-bonding behavior of the C-6 side-chain amido proton has also been shown to be a useful probe for investigating sulfoxide stereochemistry. Since the internuclear distance* R (i.e., the distance of closest approach) between the side-chain amido proton and the oxygen of an S- and R-sulfoxide is approximately 1.6 and 3.2 Å respectively in both penicillins and cephalosporins (see Fig. 13), it is clear that an intramolecular N–H$\cdots$O–S hydrogen bond can be formed only in the former case. As hydrogen bonding results in a shift to lower field for the proton in question (Pimentel and McClellan, 1960), the amido proton of an S-sulfoxide should resonate at lower field than this same proton in an epimeric R-sulfoxide or corresponding sulfide.

That this is indeed the case was illustrated by Cooper et al. (1969a) and Archer and Demarco (1969) in both phenoxymethyl- and methylpenicillin

* As measured from Dreiding molecular models.

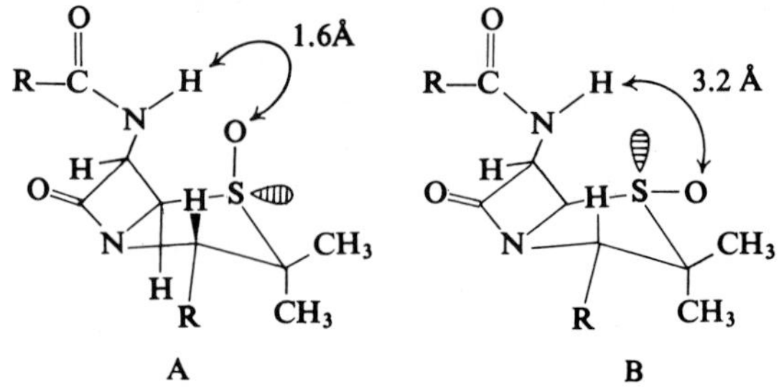

Fig. 13. Internuclear distances between the amido proton and sulfoxide oxygen in penicillin S- and R-sulfoxides (A and B respectively).

systems. Hydrogen-bonding data for the amido proton is recorded in Table X and shows that in compounds (*20a*) and (*21a*) the major oxidation products of penicillins (*20*) and (*21*) respectively, the amido proton resonates at considerably lower field than in the corresponding sulfides (*20* and *21*) or photochemically inverted sulfoxides (*20b* and *21b*). Sulfoxide configuration was accordingly assigned as S in (*20a*) and (*21a*) and R in (*20b*) and (*21b*).

Table X

NH PROTON SHIFTS[a]

Compound	δCDCl$_3$	δDMSO-d$_6$	Δ[b]
Phenoxymethylpenicillin (*20*)	7.83	8.64	1.26
Phenoxymethylpenicillin-*S*-sulfoxide (*20a*)	8.27	8.27	0.00
Phenoxymethylpenicillin-*R*-sulfoxide (*20b*)	7.34	9.21	1.87
Methylpenicillin (*21*)	6.35	8.64	2.29
Methylpenicillin-*S*-sulfoxide (*21a*)	7.03	7.81	0.78
Methylpenicillin-*R*-sulfoxide (*21b*)	6.65	9.00	2.35

[a] In parts per million relative to TMS as internal standard.
[b] $\Delta = \delta_{CDCl_3} - \delta_{DMSO-d_6}$.

Further support for these configurational assignments evolves from the *intermolecular* hydrogen-bonding behavior of their N–H protons in DMSO-d$_6$. Thus, in penicillin-S-sulfoxides where an *intramolecular* N–H $\cdots$ O–S hydrogen bond has already been indicated to exist, the amido proton displays little tendency to hydrogen bond to the oxygen of DMSO solvent, as evidenced by the absence of shift (on going from CDCl$_3$ to DMSO-d$_6$) for this proton in (*20a*) ($\Delta = 0.0$ ppm) and the relatively small shift for this proton in (*21a*) ($\Delta = 0.78$ ppm). This is in contrast to sulfides (*20*) and (*21*) and R-sulfoxides (*20b*) and (*21b*) where large solvent Δ values (see Table X) for N–H protons confirm that extensive solute–solvent *intermolecular* N–H $\cdots$ O–S hydrogen bonding is occurring in DMSO-d_6.

Similar hydrogen-bonding behavior has been noted for the N–H proton in cephalosporins and has been used, in addition to other evidence, to confirm sulfoxide configuration in cephalosporins (Cooper et al., 1970a).

A rather dramatic illustration of the use of hydrogen-bonding information as an aid in both conformational and configurational analysis is exemplified by saturated cephalosporin systems (Gutowski et al., 1971) shown in Fig. 14. Hydrogen-bonding NMR information for both the OH and NH protons in (38) and (38a) is shown in Table XI.

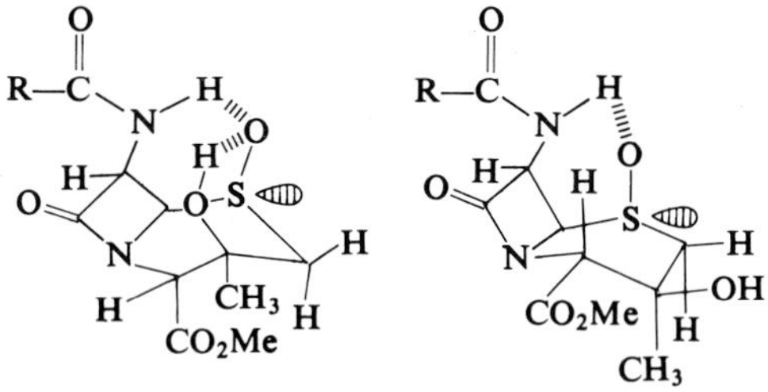

Fig. 14. Possible conformations for tetrahydrothiazine ring in saturated cephalosporins.

Molecular models indicate that the tetrahydrothiazine ring in (38) and (38a) could adopt either conformation A, in which the 3β-hydroxyl function is oriented 1,3-diaxial to either the sulfur lone pair (38) or the sulfoxide bond (38a), or conformation B, in which the 3β-hydroxyl function is oriented pseudo-equatorial and distant from the sphere of the sulfur atom. A strong intra-molecular hydrogen bond between the amide proton and the sulfoxide

Table XI

NH^a PROTON SHIFTS

Compound	Resonance	Solvent		Δ^b
		CDCl$_3$	DMSO-d_6	
(38)	NH	8.55	10.02	−1.47
(X = S)	OH	4.00	5.51	−1.51
(38a)	NH	8.09	8.27	−0.18
(X = S ◄ O)	OH	6.47	6.64	−0.17

^{a} In parts per million relative to TMS as internal standard.

^{b} $\Delta = \delta_{CDCl_3} - \delta_{DMSO-d_6}$.

oxygen in (*38a*) is inferred from the fact that the amide proton of (*38a*) suffers no appreciable shift to lower field ($\Delta = -0.18$ ppm) in DMSO-d_6 relative to CDCl$_3$. This is in contrast to the analogous proton in sulfide (*38*) which is extensively shifted to lower field ($\Delta = -1.47$ ppm) (see Table XI) and thus confirms the *S*-sulfoxide configuration.

Empirical hydrogen-bonding data recorded in Table XI shows that the C-3 hydroxyl proton is also involved in intramolecular hydrogen bonding. This is inferred from the fact that (a) the OH proton of the S-sulfoxide derivative resonates at considerably lower field ($\delta 6.47$) than the corresponding proton in the parent sulfide ($\delta 4.00$) and that (b) the OH proton of the *S*-sulfoxide suffers a negligible shift to lower field in DMSO-d_6 relative to CDCl$_3$ ($\Delta = -0.17$ ppm). This is in contrast to a large shift for this proton in the parent sulfide ($\Delta = -1.51$ ppm). Since, from molecular models, it can be seen that an intramolecular hydrogen bond can be formed between C-3 OH and the *S*-sulfoxide oxygen in conformation A only, conformation A is strongly favored over conformation B from hydrogen-bonding data.

The above data supporting conformation A (Fig. 13) is in accord with previously reported W couplings (see section on long-range couplings) between H-4 and H-2β and between the OH proton and the C-3 methyl protons.

F. Carbon-13 Nuclear Magnetic Resonance

Carbon-13 NMR promises to be equally as important as ^{1}H NMR in structural studies of penicillin and cephalosporin antibiotics since ^{13}C shifts are sensitive to steric, conformational, and electronic changes in a molecule. The first application of ^{13}C NMR to the study of phenoxymethyl- and methylpenicillins [(*20*), (*20a*), and (*21a–21c*)] was reported by Archer *et al.* (1970) who have demonstrated considerable correspondence of ^{13}C chemical shift trends with known steric and conformation changes in the process sulfide → sulfoxide. Carbon-13 chemical shift assignments recorded for penicillin derivatives (*20*), (*20a*), and (*21a–21c*) by these investigators are listed in Table XII and a typical ^{13}C NMR spectrum of a penicillin derivative is shown in Fig. 15.

It is clear from this study that from an analysis of ^{13}C shifts it is possible to recognize not only incipient changes in thiazolidine ring conformation but also sulfoxide bond configuration. Thus, large upfield shifts for the 2α-CH$_3$ signals in the process sulfide → sulfoxide is indicative of a conformationally induced 1,3-diaxial juxtaposition of a 2β-CH$_3$ to H-5 in this process. Alternatively, upfield shifts recorded for 2β-CH$_3$ [13]C signals are satisfactorily explained on the basis of their steric proximity to the sulfoxide oxygen which in turn is dependent upon sulfoxide configuration.

With the advent of fourier transform methods, ^{13}C NMR will undoubtedly

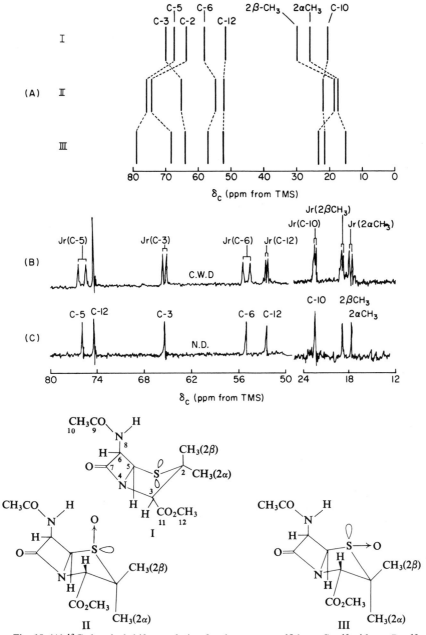

Fig. 15. (A) ^{13}C chemical shift correlation for the process sulfide → S-sulfoxide → R-sulfoxide. (B) C.W.D. spectrum of *(21a)* (0.2 gm) in DMSO. (C) N.D. spectrum of *(21a)*. Spectra shown in B and C were run at 25.2 MHz and are the result of time averaging 100 scans each at 50 seconds of scan time.

Table XII

^{13}C Chemical Shift Assignments^a for Penicillin
Derivatives (20), (20a), and (21–21b)

	(20)	(20a)	(21)	(21a)	(21b)
C-2	64.0	74.9	63.6	74.1	68.1
C-3	70.0	65.8	69.7	65.1	63.9
C-5	67.4	76.0	67.1	75.5	78.7
C-6	58.4	54.8	58.3	55.5	57.0
2β-CH₃	31.0	19.0	30.0	18.7	23.4
2α-CH₃	26.6	18.0	26.1	17.6	15.3
–CO₂CH₃	52.1	52.8	51.7	52.2	52.2
R-CH₂CO–	65.6	67.0	20.8	22.1	21.6
C-7^b	167.6	167.3	—	168.1	167.3
C-9	167.6	167.7	—	169.2	169.5
CO₂CH₃	172.6	173.8	—	173.8	170.2

^{a} In parts per million from ^{13}C resonance of Me₄Si chemical shifts were measured relative to external Me₂SO and corrected to Me₄Si as internal reference by the relationship $\delta_C(Me_4Si)$ = 40.4 − $\delta_C(Me_2SO)$.

^{b} The bracket indicates that the relative assignment of C-7 and C-9 have not been established. Reverse assignment is also possible.

become even more applicable to the study of penicillin and cephalosporin antibiotics since it will be possible to readily obtain ^{13}C natural abundance spectra on sample concentrations as small as 15 mg/ml in times as short as 30–90 minutes.

VI. Ultraviolet Spectroscopy

The penam moiety of penicillins is devoid of characteristic absorption spectra, and the compounds show only end absorption. However, ultraviolet spectroscopy has been valuable in elucidation of the structure of some degradation products of penicillin, and an excellent review article is available (Woodward et al., 1949). In contrast, the ultraviolet spectrum of the 3-cephem chromophore, the basic skeleton of the cephalosporins, has evoked considerable comment. Abraham and Newton (1961) pointed out that the absorption maxima of cephalosporins at ~260 nm occur at longer wavelength than expected for a normal N-acyl-α,β-unsaturated amino acid (Table XIII). The model compound α-acetamido-ββ-dimethyl acrylic acid showed absorption maximum at 223 nm. They suggested that the unexpected red shift in the ultra-violet spectrum of cephalosporin may be another consequence of the suppression of the normal amide resonance in a fused β-lactam, a postulate first put forth by Woodward (1949) to explain the anomalous infrared absorption of β-lactam carbonyl in penicillin.

Two groups synthesized and studied the ultraviolet spectra of 3-hydroxy and 3-aminofuran-2(5H)-ones (Table XIV), (Barrett *et al.*, 1964b; Long and Turner, 1963; Green *et al.*, 1964) and partially supported the hypothesis of the

Table XIII

Ultraviolet Spectral Data of Cephalosporin C Derivatives

Compound	Solvent	λ_{max} (nm)	ϵ	Reference
Cephalosporin C	W	260	8900	Abraham and Newton, 1961
Deacetyl cephalosporin C[a]	W	260	7100	Nagarajan, 1971
Deacetyl cephalosporin C lactone (cephalosporin C_c)	W	257	7900	Abraham and Newton, 1961
Deacetoxy cephalosporin C[a]	W	260	6000	Nagarajan, 1971

[a] These compounds may not be absolutely pure; consequently, the pure compounds could have higher extinction coefficients. W = water; E = ethanol; M = methanol.

Oxford group (Abraham and Newton, 1961), that the suppression of the amide resonance allowed the lone-pair electrons of the nitrogen of the β-lactam to become part of the double bond chromophore in cephalosporin.

Both of these groups (Barrett *et al.*, 1964a; Green *et al.*, 1964) reported the first synthesis and ultraviolet spectra of 3,6-dihydro-2(H)-1,3-thiazine ring systems, present in deacetoxy cephalosporin C (Table XV).

A comparison of the absorption spectra of dialkyl sulfides and β,γ-unsaturated sulfides reveals that even though the sulfur and the double bond are insulated by a methylene group, a bathochromic shift occurs, suggesting some sort of an interaction between the two chromophores (Fehnel and Carmack, 1949a; Koch, 1949a; Price and Oae, 1962a). In view of such an effect in β,γ-unsaturated sulfides, the Glaxo group (Green *et al.*, 1964) suggested that the *d*-orbital of the sulfur may be involved in the electronic excited state to give rise to structures (*53a*) and (*53b*), and that the sulfur, ring

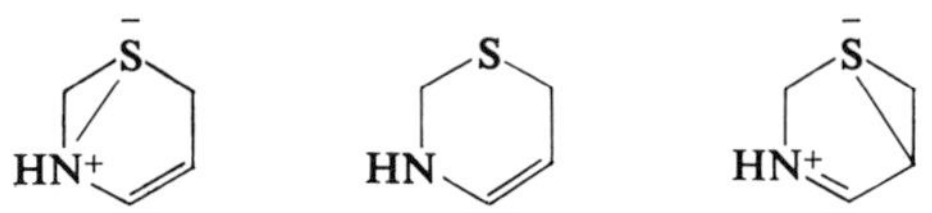

(53a)   *(53)*   *(53b)*

Table XIV

ULTRAVIOLET SPECTRAL DATA OF FURAN-2(5H)-ONES

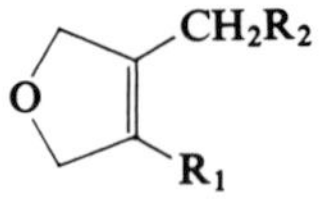

(8)

Compound	Solvent	λ_{max} (nm)	ϵ	Reference
(58a) $R_1 = OH, R_2 = H$	W	232	6,310	Abraham and Newton, 1961
	E	232	11,900	Green et al., 1964
(58b) $R_1 = OH, R_2 =$ 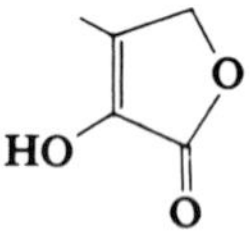	W	238	17,600	Green et al., 1964
	E	237	11,700	Long and Turner, 1963
(58c) $R_1 = OH, R_2 =$ 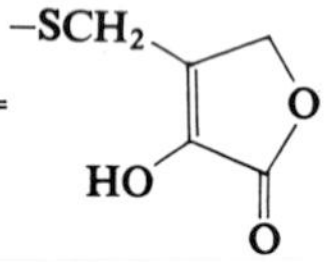	W	235	15,000	Abraham and Newton, 1961
	E	236	14,800	Long and Turner, 1963
(58d) $R_1 = OH, R_2 = SCH_2C_6H_5$	E	232	19,800	Long and Turner, 1963
(58e) $R_1 = NH_2, R_2 = H$	W	248	8,700	Barrett et al., 1964b
	E	255	8,400	Barrett et al., 1964b
(58f) $R_1 = N$, $R_2 = H$ 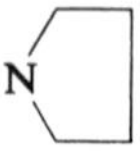	E	290	4,660	Galantay et al., 1964
(58g) $R_1 = NH_2, R_2 =$ 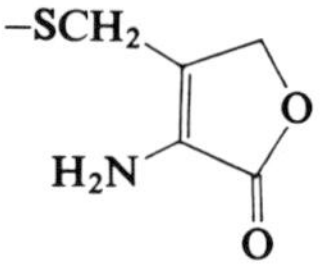	E	268	7,800	Galantay et al., 1964
(58h) $R_1 = NH_2,$ $R_2 = SCH_2C_6H_5$	E	266	10,600	Long and Turner, 1963

nitrogen, and the double bond of the 3-cephem skeleton may be essential for the absorption.

Synthesis of the 3,6-dihydro-2[H]-1,3-thiazine lactone system present in cephalosporin C_c was subsequently reported by two groups of workers (Stork and Cheung, 1965; Dolfini et al., 1969). The absorption spectra of these compounds are similar to cephalosporins. There are two points of interest in the spectra of the dihydrothiazines. There is a considerable red shift between the monocyclic and bicyclic dihydrothiazines (Table XV). Further, in the bicyclic dihydrothiazines there is negligible difference between the enamine and enamide dihydrothiazine derivatives.

Table XV

ULTRAVIOLET SPECTRAL DATA OF DIHYDROTHIAZINES

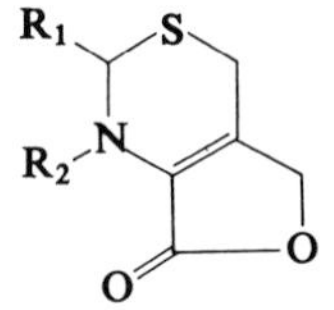

(59)

(59a) $R_1 = C_6H_5$, $R_2 = H$
(59b) $R_1 = C_6H_5$, $R_2 = COCH_3$
(59c) $R_1 = PhtCH_2$, $R_2 = H$
(59d) $R_1 = PhtCHCOOC(CH_3)_3$, $R_2 = H$

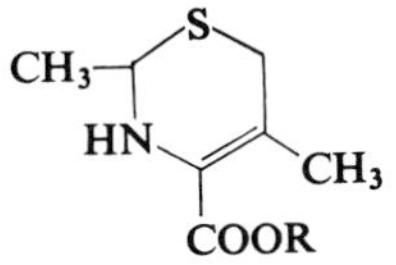

(59e) $R = C_2H_5$
(59f) $R = CH_2C_6H_5$

Compound	Solvent	λ_{max} (nm)	ϵ	Reference
(59a)	E	269	4220	Dolfini et al., 1969
(59b)	M	268	4500	Stork and Cheung, 1965
				Dolfini et al., 1969
(59c)	E	272	4490	Dolfini et al., 1969
(59d)	E	268	4700	Dolfini et al., 1969
(59e)	E	285	3100	Green et al., 1964
(59f)	E	285	3300	Barrett et al., 1964a

The ultraviolet and circular dichroism spectra of the 3-methyl-3-cephem derivative (60n) (Morin et al., 1969), and its carboxy derivatives (60b) and (60c), show that the 4-carboxy function contributes a red shift of about 10 nm (Nagarajan and Spry, 1971a). (For a complete discussion of the circular dichroism curves of cephalosporins see Chapter 15, Section VII.) Extension of the enamide chromophore by substituting a group containing a π-electron system at the 3-position produces the expected large bathochromic shift (Chamberlin and Campbell, 1967). Table XVI shows the absorption spectra of representative 3-cephem derivatives. Substitution of the acetoxy function on the 3-methylene group of the cephalosporin by an oxygen of a lactone (*60k*), a methoxy (*60l*), or ethylene ketal oxygens (*60m*) (Table IV) produces negligible change in the absorption spectra. A nitrogen function on the 3-methylene would be expected to produce no large change (Leonard and Locke, 1955), and a sulfur produces a red shift of about 5 nm (*60h* and *60i*). If we assume a bathochromic shift of similar magnitude for the ring sulfur of the 3-cephem nucleus, then the ring sulfur *d*-orbital involvement in the electronic excited state accounts for a red shift of about 5 nm. Reduction of the double bond in cephalosporin results in loss of absorption at 260 nm. It might be of interest to point out here that computing for the known differences in the absorption maxima of *cis* disubstituted and trisubstituted olefins, the absorption maximum of the simple 3-cephem chromophore (*54*) would be expected to be about 245 nm.

(*54*)

There are two structural features of the 3-cephem chromophore which have not been pointed out previously, and which should be taken into consideration in making comparisons with model compounds. In the 3-cephem moiety, the nitrogen is tertiary, and the double bond and nitrogen atom are part of a ring system. An examination of the absorption spectra of amines reveals that tertiary amines absorb at longer wavelength (Vencov, 1943; Pickett *et al.*, 1953; Tannenbaum *et al.*, 1953). It would be reasonable to expect a similar red shift in the absorption maximum of tertiary enamine, and the spectra of 3-aminofuran-2(5H)-ones (*58e*) and (*58f*) confirm it. A bathochromic shift is observed in absorption spectra of enamines, when both the nitrogen and double bond are part of a ring system. A second red shift occurs on reducing the size of the ring (Leonard and Locke, 1955).

The X-ray structural analysis of cephalosporin C reveals that the six-membered dihydrothiazine ring is rather flat, that the C-2, C-3, C-4, and N-5 atoms lie in a plane with the C-6 atom 0.6 Å below, and the sulfur atom 0.6 Å above, this plane (Hodgkin and Maslen, 1961) (see Chapter 7). Recently, the X-ray analysis of two synthetic cephalosporins have been reported, and the bond lengths suggest that, in the 3-cephem moiety, the lone-pair electrons of the nonplanar nitrogen are involved to some degree in amide (*55*) as well as enamine (*56*) resonance (Sweet and Dahl, 1970).

Table XVI

ULTRAVIOLET SPECTRAL DATA OF SYNTHETIC CEPHALOSPORINS

Compound[a]	Solvent	λ_{max} (nm)	ϵ	Reference
(60a)	W	262	8000	Nagarajan and Spry, 1971b
(60b)	M	262	8000	Nagarajan and Spry, 1971a
(60c)	E	261	7900	Nagarajan and Spry, 1971a
(60d)	E	263	9000	Nagarajan and Spry, 1971a
(60e)	W	262	7000	Nagarajan and Spry, 1971b
(60f)	W	261	8400	Nagarajan and Spry, 1971b
(60g)	M	264	8600	Nagarajan and Spry, 1971b
(60h)	E	266	8500	Nagarajan and Spry, 1971b
(60i)	E	267	2100	Nagarajan and Spry, 1971a
(60j)	E	260	7180	Chamberlin and Campbell, 1967
(60k)	E	260	7020	Chamberlin and Campbell, 1967
(60l)	W	260	8600	Webber et al., 1971
(60m)	E	260	7370	Chamberlin and Campbell, 1967
(60n)	E	256	9150	Morin et al., 1969

[a] Key to numbers:

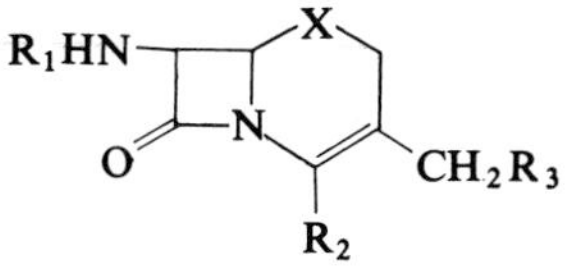

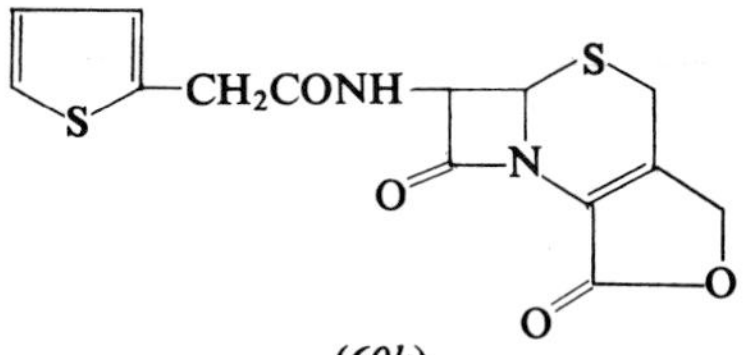

(60k)

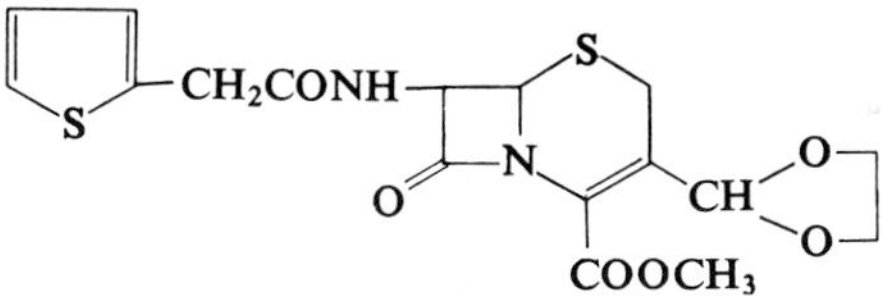

(60m)

(60a) $R_1 = H$, $R_2 = COOH$, $R_3 = OCOCH_3$, $X = S$
(60b) $R_1 = COCH_3$, $R_2 = COOH$, $R_3 = OCOCH_3$, $X = S$
(60c) $R_1 = COCH_3$, $R_2 = COOCH_3$, $R_3 = OCOCH_3$, $X = S$
(60d) $R_1 = COCH_3$, $R_2 = COOCH_3$, $R_3 = OCOCH_3$, $X = SO_2$
(60e) $R_1 = H$, $R_2 = COOH$, $R_3 = H$, $X = S$
(60f) $R_1 = COCH_3$, $R_2 = COOH$, $R_3 = H$, $X = S$
(60g) $R_1 = COCH_3$, $R_2 = COOCH_3$, $R_3 = H$, $X = S{\rightarrow}O$
(60h) $R_1 = COCH_3$, $R_2 = COOH$, $R_3 = SCH_3$, $X = S$
(60i) $R_1 = COCH_3$, $R_2 = COOCH_3$, $R_3 = SCH_3$, $X = S$
(60j) $R_1 = Pht$, $R_2 = COOCH_3$, $R_3 = OH$, $X = S$
(60l) $R_1 = Pht$, $R_2 = COOH$, $R_3 = OCH_3$, $X = S$
(60n) $R_1 = COCH_2OC_6H_5$, $R_2 = H$, $R_3 = H$, $X = S$

(55)   (56)

The absorption spectra of sulfones are transparent in the ultraviolet region, at least above 200 nm (Fehnel and Carmack, 1949b; Koch, 1949b; Szmant and McIntosh, 1951; Price and Oae, 1962b), due to the fact that the sulfur atom has no lone-pair electrons and the oxygen electrons are bound tightly. Unlike the red shift observed for β,γ-unsaturated sulfides, no similar effect is observed in β,γ-unstaurated sulfones (Fehnel and Carmack, 1949a). Consequently, it would be expected that the absorption maximum of a sulfone (60d) would be at lower wavelengths than would the sulfide (60c). Though the ultraviolet spectra of (60c) and (60d) do not substantiate this prediction, the circular dichroism curves reveal a blue shift of about 5 nm (Nagarajan and Spry, 1971a). It would be of interest to compare the absorption spectrum of the 3-cephem

(57)

chromophore with that of the as yet unknown, non-sulfur-containing analog (57). The latter compound would be expected to show an absorption maximum at about 240 nm.

References

Abraham, E. P., and Newton, G. G. F. (1961). *Biochem. J.* **79**, 377.
Allingham, Y., Cookson, R. C., and Crabb, T. A. (1968). *Tetrahedron* **24**, 1989.
Anet, F. A. L., and Bourn, A. J. R. (1965). *J. Amer. Chem. Soc.* **87**, 5250.
Archer, R. A., and Demarco, P. V. (1969). *J. Amer. Chem. Soc.* **91**, 1530.
Archer, R. A., Cooper, R. D. G., Demarco, P. V., and Johnson, L. F. (1970). *Chem. Commun.* 1291.
Barrett, G. C., Eggers, S. H., Emerson, T. R., and Lowe, G. (1964a). *J. Chem. Soc.* **788**.
Barrett, G. C., Kane, V. V., and Lowe, G. (1964b). *J. Chem. Soc.* 783.
Barrow, K. D., and Spotswood, T. M. (1965). *Tetrahedron Lett.* 3325.
Barton, D. H. R., Comer, F., and Sammes, P. G. (1969). *J. Amer. Chem. Soc.* **91**, 1529.
Barton, D. H. R., Comer, F., Greig, D. G. T., Lucente, G., Sammes, P. G., and Underwood, W. G. E. (1970). *Chem. Commun.* 1059.
Bellamy, L. J. (1958). *In* "The Infra-Red Spectra of Complex Molecules." Wiley, New York.
Bhacca, N. S., and Williams, D. H. (1964). *In* "Applications of NMR Spectroscopy in Organic Chemistry." Holden-Day, San Francisco, California.
Bochkarev, V. N., Ovchinnikova, N. S., Vul'fson, N. S., Kleiner, E. M., and Khokhlov, A. S. (1967). *Dokl. Akad. Nauk SSSR* **172**, 1079.
Bothner-By, A. A., Naar-Colin, C., and Günther, H. (1962). *J. Amer. Chem. Soc.* **84**, 2748.
Brönsted, J. N. (1923). *Rec. Trav. Chim. Pays-Bas* **42**, 718.

Buck, K. W., Foster, A. B., Pardoe, W. D., Qadir, M. H., and Webber, J. M. (1966). *Chem. Commun.* 759.

Burg, A. B. (1961). *In* "Organic Sulfur Compounds" (N. Kharasch, ed.), Vol. I, p. 36. Pergamon Press, New York.

Carothers, W. H., Bickford, C. F., and Hurwitz, G. J. (1927). *J. Amer. Chem. Soc.* **49**, 2908.

Castellano, S., and Lorenc, J. (1965). *J. Phys. Chem.* **69**, 3552.

Chamberlin, J. W., and Campbell, J. B. (1967). *J. Med. Chem.* **10**, 966.

Cookson, R. C., Crabb, T. A., Frankel, J. J., and Hudec, J. (1966). *Tetrahedron Suppl.* **22**, 355.

Cooper, R. D. G. (1969). Unpublished results.

Cooper, R. D. G., Demarco, P. V., Cheng, J. C., and Jones, N. D. (1969a). *J. Amer. Chem. Soc.* **91**, 1408.

Cooper, R. D. G., Demarco, P. V., and Spry, D. O. (1969b). *J. Amer. Chem. Soc.* **91**, 1528.

Cooper, R. D. G., Demarco, P. V., Murphy, C. F., and Spangle, L. A. (1970a). *J. Chem. Soc. C* 340.

Cooper, R. D. G., Hatfield, L. D., José, F., and Spry, D. O. (1970b). Unpublished results.

Crowfoot, D., Bunn, C. W., Rogers-Low, B. W., and Turner-Jones, A. (1949). *In* "The Chemistry of Penicillin" (H. T. Clarke, J. R. Johnson, and R. Robinson, eds.), p. 310. Princeton Univ. Press, Princeton, New Jersey.

Dippy, J. F. J., Hughes, S. R. C., and Laxton, J. W. (1954). *J. Chem. Soc.* 4102.

Dolfini, J. E., Schwartz, J., and Weisenborn, F. (1969). *J. Org. Chem.* **34**, 1582.

Everett, D. H., and Wynne-Jones, W. F. K. (1941). *Proc. Roy. Soc. (London)* **A177**, 499.

Feates, F. S., and Ives, D. J. G. (1956). *J. Chem. Soc.* 2798.

Fehnel, E. A., and Carmack, M. (1949a). *J. Amer. Chem. Soc.* **71**, 84.

Fehnel, E. A., and Carmack, M. (1949b). *J. Amer. Chem. Soc.* **61**, 231.

Foster, A. B., Inch, T. D., Qadir, M. H., and Webber, J. M. (1968). *Chem. Commun.* 1086.

Fraser, R. R. (1960). *Can. J. Chem.* **38**, 549.

Galantay, E., Engel, H., Szabo, A., and Fried, J. (1964). *J. Org. Chem.* **29**, 3560.

Garbisch, Jr., E. W. (1964). *J. Amer. Chem. Soc.* **86**, 5561.

Green, D. M., Long, A. G., May, P. J., and Turner, A. F. (1964). *J. Chem. Soc.* 766.

Green, G. F. H., Page, J. E., and Staniforth, S. E. (1965). *J. Chem. Soc.* 1595.

Greenstein, J. P., and Winitz, M. (1961). *In* "Chemistry of the Amino Acids," Vol. I, p. 435. Wiley, New York.

Gutowski, G. E. (1970). *Tetrahedron Lett.* 1779.

Gutowski, G. E., Daniels, C. J., and Cooper, R. D. G. (1971). *Tetrahedron Lett.* 3429.

Harned, H. S., and Ehlers, R. W. (1932). *J. Amer. Chem. Soc.* **54**, 1350.

Hodgkin, D. C., and Maslen, E. N. (1961). *Biochem. J.* **79**, 393.

Johnson, D. A., Mania, D., Panetta, C. A., and Silvestri, H. H. (1968). *Tetrahedron Lett.* 1903.

Kaczka, E., and Folkers, K. (1949). *In* "The Chemistry of Penicillin" (H. T. Clarke, J. R. Johnson, and R. Robinson, eds.), p. 243. Princeton Univ. Press, Princeton, New Jersey.

Kaiser, G. V., Ashbrook, C. W., Goodson, T., Wright, I. G., and Van Heyningen, E. M. (1971). *J. Med. Chem.* **14**, 426.

Karplus, M. (1960). *J. Chem. Phys.* **33**, 1842.

King, E. J. (1951). *J. Amer. Chem. Soc.* **73**, 155.

King, E. J., and King, G. W. (1956). *J. Amer. Chem. Soc.* **78**, 1089.

King, J. F. (1963). *In* "Technique of Organic Chemistry" (A. Weissberger, ed.), "Elucidation of Structures by Physical and Chemical Methods" (K. W. Bentley, ed.), Vol. XI, Part 1, p. 317. Wiley (Interscience), New York.

Koch, H. P. (1949a). *J. Chem. Soc.* 387.

Koch, H. P. (1949b). *J. Chem. Soc.* 408.

Lambert, J. R., and Keske, R. G. (1969a). *J. Amer. Chem. Soc.* **88**, 620.
Lambert, J. R., and Keske, R. G. (1969b). *J. Org. Chem.* **31**, 3429.
Laszlo, P. (1967). *In* "Progress in Nuclear Magnetic Resonance Spectroscopy," Vol. III, p. 348. Pergamon Press, Oxford.
Ledaal, T. (1968). *Tetrahedron Lett.* 1683.
Leonard, N. J., and Locke, D. M. (1955). *J. Amer. Chem. Soc.* **77**, 437.
Long, A. G., and Turner, A. F. (1963). *Tetrahedron Lett.* 421.
Luche, J. L., Kagan, H. B., Parthasarathy, R., Tsoucaris, G., deRango, C., and Zelwer, C. (1968). *Tetrahedron* **24**, 1275.
Lunn, W. H. W. (1970). Unpublished results.
McConnell, H. M. (1957). *J. Chem. Phys.* **27**, 226.
Moll, F., and Hannig, M. (1970a). *Arch. Pharm.* **303**, 321.
Moll, F., and Hannig, M. (1970b). *Arch. Pharm.* **303**, 831.
Morin, R. B., Jackson, B. G., Mueller, R. A., Lavagnino, E. R., Scanlon, W. B., and Andrews, S. L. (1969). *J. Amer. Chem. Soc.* **91**, 1401.
Nagarajan, R. (1971). Unpublished results.
Nagarajan, R., and Spry, D. O. (1971a). *J. Amer. Chem. Soc.* **93**.
Nagarajan, R., and Spry, D. O. (1971b). Unpublished results.
Nagarajan, R., Boeck, L. D., Gorman, M., Hamill, R. L., Higgens, C. E., Hoehn, M. M., Stark, W. M., and Whitney, J. G. (1971). *J. Amer. Chem. Soc.* **93**.
Pickett, L. W., Corning, M. E., Wieder, G. M., Semenow, D. A., and Buckley, J. M. (1953). *J. Amer. Chem. Soc.* **75**, 1618.
Pimentel, G. C., and McClellan, A. L. (1960). *In* "The Hydrogen Bond," Chapter 4. Freeman, San Francisco, California.
Pople, J. A. (1962). *J. Chem. Phys.* **37**, 53.
Pople, J. A., and Bothner-By, A. A. (1965). *J. Chem. Phys.* **42**, 1339.
Price, C. C., and Oae, S. (1962a). *In* "Sulfur Bonding," p. 30. Ronald Press, New York.
Price, C. C., and Oae, S. (1962b). *In* "Sulfur Bonding," p. 94. Ronald Press, New York.
Rassat, A., Jefford, C. W., Lehn, J. M., and Waegell, B. (1964). *Tetrahedron Lett.* 233.
Richter, W., and Biemann, K. (1964). *Monatsh. Chem.* **95**, 766.
Richter, W., and Biemann, K. (1965). *Monatsh. Chem.* **96**, 484.
Sassiver, M. L., and Shepherd, R. G. (1969). *Tetrahedron Lett.* 3993.
Sheehan, J. C., Hill, W. H., Jr., and Buhle, E. L. (1951). *J. Amer. Chem. Soc.* **73**, 4373.
Sollman, P. B., Nagarajan, R., and Dodson, R. M. (1967). *Chem. Commun.* 552.
Spry, D. O. (1970). *J. Amer. Chem. Soc.* **92**, 5006.
Spry, D. O. (1971). Unpublished results.
Stolow, R. D. (1959). *J. Amer. Chem. Soc.* **81**, 5806.
Stork, G., and Cheung, H. T. (1965). *J. Amer. Chem. Soc.* **87**, 3783.
Sweet, R. M., and Dahl, L. F. (1970). *J. Amer. Chem. Soc.* **92**, 5489.
Szmant, H. H., and McIntosh, J. J. (1951). *J. Amer. Chem. Soc.* **73**, 4356.
Tannenbaum, E., Coffin, E. M., and Harrison, A. J. (1953). *J. Chem. Phys.* **21**, 311.
Thompson, H. W., Brattain, R. R., Randall, H. M., and Rasmussen, R. S. (1949). *In* "The Chemistry of Penicillin" (H. T. Clarke, J. R. Johnson, and R. Robinson, eds.), p. 409. Princeton Univ. Press, Princeton, New Jersey.
Tichý, M., Jonás, J., and Sicher, J. (1959). *Collect. Czech. Chem. Commun.* **24**, 3434.
Van Heyningen, E. M., and Ahern, L. K. (1968). *J. Med. Chem.* **11**, 933.
Vencov, S. (1943). *Bull. Sect. Sci. Acad. Roumaine* **26**, 89.
Webber, J. A., Huffman, G. W., Koehler, R. E., Murphy, C. F., Ryan, C. W., Van Heyningen, E. M., and Vasileff, R. T. (1971). *J. Med. Chem.* **14**, 113.
Wheland, G. W. (1955). *In* "Resonance in Organic Chemistry," p. 354. Wiley, New York.

Wiberg, K. B., Lowry, B. R., and Nist, B. J. (1962). *J. Amer. Chem. Soc.* **84**, 1594.

Wolfe, S., and Lee, W. S. (1968). *Chem. Commun.* 242.

Woodward, R. B. (1949). *In* "The Chemistry of Penicillin" (H. T. Clarke, J. R. Johnson, and R. Robinson, eds.), p. 443. Princeton Univ. Press, Princeton, New Jersey.

Woodward, R. B., Neuberger, A., and Tenner, N. R. (1949). *In* "The Chemistry of Penicillin" (H. T. Clarke, J. R. Johnson, and R. Robinson, eds.), p. 415. Princeton Univ. Press, Princeton, New Jersey.

Wright, I. G., Ashbrook, C. W., Goodson, T., Kaiser, G. V., and Van Heyningen, E. M. (1971). *J. Med. Chem.* **14**, 420.

Zief, M., and Edsall, J. T. (1937). *J. Amer. Chem. Soc.* **59**, 2245.

Chapter 9

MICROBIAL SYNTHESIS OF CEPHALOSPORIN AND PENICILLIN COMPOUNDS

PAUL A. LEMKE and DONALD R. BRANNON

I. Introduction

The β-lactam antibiotics are made available for use in human medicine by virtue of microbial synthesis. Biogenesis of these compounds has intrigued scientists for decades, ever since Sir Alexander Fleming (1929) observed antibiosis between a *Penicillium* mold and neighboring bacterial cultures. The antibacterial substance of Fleming's experiments proved to be penicillin (Florey *et al.*, 1949), the oldest recognized antibiotic and the progenitor of the most significant chemotherapeutic agents developed during the past 30 years.

The introduction of penicillin to medicine was brought about by a cooperative Anglo-American effort during the second world war. The success of this enterprise was due largely to the rapid development of a fermentation process for large-scale production of antibiotic (Moyer and Coghill, 1946a, b, 1947) and to the selection of *Penicillium* strains superior for antibiotic synthesis (Raper *et al.*, 1944; Raper and Alexander, 1945).

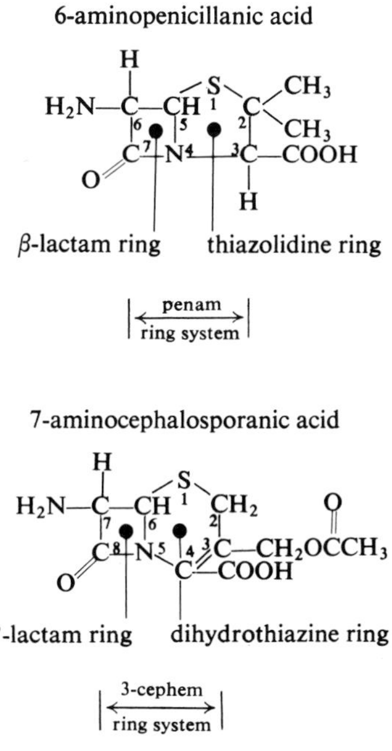

Fig. 1. β-Lactam ring systems.

In time, penicillin proved not to be a single compound or even a unique series of compounds. The cephalosporin antibiotics were subsequently discovered, and these proved to be structurally related to penicillin (Abraham and Newton, 1961, 1965; Nagarajan *et al.*, 1971). Penicillins and cephalosporins are unusual molecules owing to a four-membered β-lactam ring common to their respective heterocyclic ring systems (Fig. 1).

The β-lactam ring is biologically quite rare and chemically difficult to construct. Enzymatic reactions leading to formation of this ring have not been resolved. Nevertheless, the β-lactam compounds are preeminently natural products, and industrial production of all β-lactam antibiotics depends on microbial fermentation. Total chemical syntheses of penicillin and cephalosporin have been successful (Sheehan and Henery-Logan, 1959; Woodward et al., 1966; Woodward, 1966; Heusler, 1968), but these efforts have not been competitive with microbial synthesis.

A. Distribution of β-Lactam Antibiotics

The β-lactam antibiotics are synthesized, for no apparent reason, by only a few microorganisms. All of the organisms recognized to produce β-lactam antibiotics are filamentous microorganisms, but not all of these microorganisms are taxonomically related. Some are true fungi (eukaryotes), whereas others are streptomycetes. The streptomycetes are indisputably gram-positive filamentous bacteria (prokaryotes) (Waksman, 1967).

The fungal contaminant of Fleming's original experiment was *Penicillium notatum*. Subsequently, several other species of *Penicillium* were demonstrated to produce penicillin (Sanders, 1949). The fungus selected for the commercial production of penicillin was *P. chrysogenum* (Raper *et al.*, 1944). Penicillins have been reported from species of fungi other than *Penicillia* (Sanders, 1949). These include *Aspergillus* species (Dulaney, 1947); two dermatophytes, *Trichophyton mentagrophytes* and *Epidermophyton floccosum* (Cole, 1966a; Uri *et al.*, 1965; Sanders, 1949); *Cephalosporium* species (Brotzu, 1948; Gottshall *et al.*, 1951; Roberts, 1952; Newton and Abraham, 1953; Abraham *et al.*, 1954; Sukapure and Thirumalachar, 1963); *Emericellopsis* species (Grosklags and Swift, 1957; Bhuyan and Johnson, 1958; Kavanagh *et al.*, 1958a; Elander *et al.*, 1961; Cole and Rolinson (1961); *Paecilomyces persicinus* (Pisano *et al.*, 1961); and a thermophilic fungus, *Malbranchea pulchella* (Rode *et al.*, 1947). The last-named organism, according to Dodge (1935), may be an actinomycete (prokaryote). A penicillin has also been reported from streptomycetes (Miller *et al.*, 1962; Nagarajan *et al.*, 1971).

Cephalosporin compounds have been identified from a single *Cephalosporium* species (Abraham and Newton, 1961) and from two species of *Streptomyces* (Nagarajan *et al.*, 1971), *S. lipmanii* and *S. clavuligerus* (Higgens and Kastner, 1971). Details may be found in Chapter 15.

The β-lactam antibiotics, recognized for their antimicrobial activity, represent a biased sample of β-lactam compounds. Synthesis of β-lactam compounds among diverse organisms now appears to be more common than previously expected. Two compounds with a four-membered β-lactam ring have been reported from a higher plant *Pachysandra terminalis* (Kikuchi and Uyeo, 1967). These compounds are not antibiotics but are steroidal alkaloids. A β-lactam compound has also been identified from a bacterium, *Pseudomonas tabaci*, and is associated with "wildfire" disease of tobacco (Stewart, 1971).

B. Classification of β-Lactam Antibiotics

All β-lactam antibiotics are derivatives of a bicyclic ring system. All, with the exception of 6-aminopenicillanic acid (6-APA) and 7-aminocephalosporanic acid (7-ACA), have an acyl group attached as a side chain to the amino group of a heterocyclic nucleus. The penicillin ring system (penam) contains a four-membered β-lactam ring fused with a five-membered thiazolidine ring. The cephalosporin ring system (3-cephem) differs insofar as the four-membered β-lactam ring is fused with an unsaturated six-membered dihydrothiazine ring (Fig. 1). The penicillins and cephalosporins are thus distinguished chemically on the basis of ring system.

Classification of β-lactam antibiotics with regard to biosynthesis rests upon certain other criteria. There are two recognizable biogenetic patterns for β-lactam antibiotics. These patterns are herein designated as the *Penicillium*-type and the *Cephalosporium*-type.

The *Penicillium*-type is characterized by the microbial synthesis of an extensive series of penicillin compounds. These penicillins are variable with regard to N-acyl side chain. The N-acyl side chains include L-α-aminoadipic acid or any of several other carboxylic acid derivatives. The synthesis of specific penicillins is generally in direct response to the addition of specific side-chain precursors to the culture medium. The *Penicillium*-type fermentation accumulates 6-aminopenicillanic acid, especially in the absence of side-chain precursors. All organisms in this category are eukaryotic. These *Penicillium*-type organisms are not known to synthesize cephalosporin compounds. *Penicillium chrysogenum* typifies organisms of the *Penicillium*-type.

By contrast, the *Cephalosporium*-type is characterized by the synthesis of a single penicillin with a D-α-aminoadipyl side chain. This fermentation is insensitive to the addition of side-chain precursors and little or no 6-aminopenicillanic acid is formed. The *Cephalosporium*-type includes prokaryotic as well as eukaryotic organisms. Certain of these organisms can elaborate cephalosporin compounds. All cephalosporin compounds known to be formed biosynthetically possess the D-α-aminoadipyl side chain. No 7-aminocephalosporanic acid is formed. The pattern of antibiotic synthesis by *C. acremonium* typifies the *Cephalosporium*-type.

The principal β-lactam compounds formed by microbial synthesis are indicated in Table I.

Table I

MAJOR β-LACTAM ANTIBIOTICS PRODUCED BY DIRECT FERMENTATION

Penicillium-type penicillins

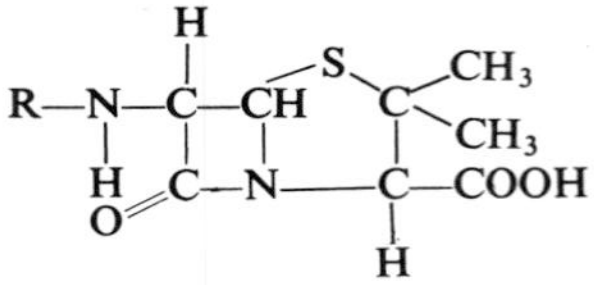

$$R-N-C-CH \underset{\underset{O}{\overset{\|}{C}}-N}{\overset{S}{\diagdown}} C \overset{CH_3}{\underset{CH_3}{\diagup}} C-COOH$$

R (*N*-Acyl side chain)	Common name(s)	References
H–	Penicin	Kato (1953a, b)
	Penicillin nucleus (6-Aminopenicillanic acid)	Batchelor *et al.* (1959)
HO₂C–CH(NH₂)(CH₂)₃–CO– (L-α-Aminoadipic acid)	Isopenicillin N	Flynn *et al.* (1962)
	Penicillin M	Cole and Batchelor (1963)
CH₃CH₂CH=CHCH₂CO– (β,γ-Hexenoic acid)	Penicillin F (2-Pentenylpenicillin)	Florey *et al.* (1949)
CH₃(CH₂)₄–CO– (Caproic acid)	Penicillin dihydro F (Amylpenicillin)	Florey *et al.* (1949)
CH₃(CH₂)₆–CO– (Octanoic acid)	Penicillin K (Heptylpenicillin)	Florey *et al.* (1949)
C₆H₅–CH₂–CO– (Phenylacetic acid)	Penicillin G (Benzylpenicillin)	Moyer and Coghill (1946a, b, 1947)
p-OH–C₆H₅–CH₂–CO– (p-Hydroxyphenylacetic acid)	Penicillin X (p-Hydroxybenzylpenicillin)	Raper and Fennel (1946)
C₆H₅–O–CH₂–CO– (Phenoxyacetic acid)	Penicillin V (Phenoxymethylpenicillin)	Behrens (1949)

Cephalosporium-type penicillins

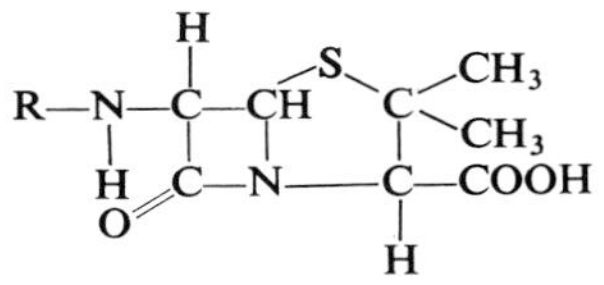

R (*N*-Acyl side chain)	Common name(s)	References
H–	Penicillin nucleus (6-Aminopenicillanic acid)	Cole and Rolinson (1961)
HO₂C–CH(NH₂)(CH₂)₃–CO– (D-α-Aminoadipic acid)	Penicillin N, Synnematin B, Cephalosporin N	Florey (1955), Olson et al. (1953), Crawford et al. (1952)

Cephalosporium-type cephalosporins

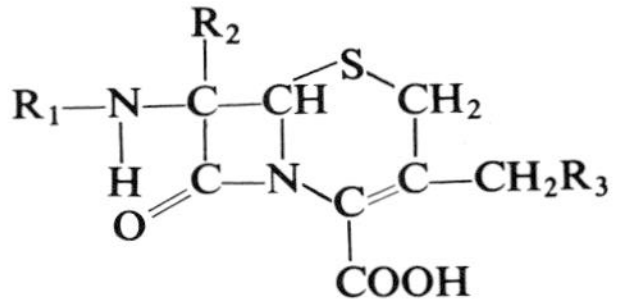

R₁	R₂	R₃	Common name	References
HO₂C–CH(NH₂)(CH₂)₃–CO– (D-α-Aminoadipic acid)	H	–OCOCH₃	Cephalosporin C	Abraham and Newton (1961)
HO₂C–CH(NH₂)(CH₂)₃–CO– (D-α-Aminoadipic acid)	H	–OH	Deacetylcephalosporin C	Jeffery et al. (1961)
HO₂C–CH(NH₂)(CH₂)₃–CO– (D-α-Aminoadipic acid)	OCH₃	–OCOCH₃	7-Methoxycephalosporin C	Nagarajan et al. (1971)
HO₂C–CH(NH₂)(CH₂)₃–CO– (D-α-Aminoadipic acid)	H	–OCONH₂	Deacetyl-3-O-carbamoylcephalosporin C	Nagarajan et al. (1971)
HO₂C–CH(NH₂)(CH₂)₃–CO– (D-α-Aminoadipic acid)	OCH₃	–OCONH₂	Deacetyl-3-O-carbamoyl-7-methoxycephalosporin C	Nagarajan et al. (1971)

1. THE *Penicillium*-TYPE

Until crystalline forms of an American and a British penicillin were available for analysis, it was not realized that the two were chemically different. They differed with regard to side chain (Florey *et al.*, 1949). The British penicillin (2-pentenylpenicillin) was named penicillin F, whereas the American penicillin (benzylpenicillin) was named penicillin G. Penicillin synthesized by *P. chryso-genum* eventually proved to be a heterogeneous assemblage of penicillin compounds and to be influenced qualitatively as well as quantitatively by ingredients added to the fermentation medium.

Benzylpenicillin was fermented inadvertently at Peoria, Illinois by the addition of corn steep liquor to the fermentation medium. Only later was it realized that the phenylacetic acid content of corn steep liquor served as a precursor for the side chain of penicillin G (Moyer and Coghill, 1946a, b). The addition of this side-chain precursor not only enhanced the specific formation of benzylpenicillin at the expense of other penicillins but greatly increased the overall titer of penicillin (Higuchi *et al.*, 1946; Moyer and Coghill, 1947; Wolff and Arnstein, 1960). Thus, one of the major rate-limiting factors for the synthesis of penicillin appeared to be the availability of side-chain precursor. Addition of a large variety of potential side-chain precursors to fermentation medium has yielded a correspondingly large variety of penicillins. Over 100 penicillins can be produced by the method of precursor supplementa-tion (Behrens *et al.*, 1948a, b; Behrens, 1949; Cole, 1966b). All potential side-chain precursors have proven to be aliphatic or arylaliphatic carboxylic acids or derivatives of these acids.

In the absence of specific precursor additions, or even in a chemically defined growth medium, several penicillins can be formed by *P. chrysogenum*. These include an indefinite number of penicillins with side chains derived from natural carboxylic acids, e.g., penicillins K, F, dihydro F, etc. (Cole, 1966b). Two unusual penicillin compounds accumulate during fermentation, especially if the availability of side-chain precursors in the medium is limited. These compounds are isopenicillin N (Flynn *et al.*, 1962; Cole and Batchelor, 1963) and 6-aminopenicillanic acid (Kato, 1953a, b; Batchelor *et al.*, 1959, 1961a). Isopenicillin N is an unusual penicillin since it has a hydrophilic, amino acid side chain, L-α-aminoadipic acid, and is not extractable into solvent at low pH. 6-Aminopenicillanic acid also has a free amino group and is not solvent extractable. 6-Aminopenicillanic acid is essentially devoid of antibacterial activity.

Several compounds which form in the *Penicillium* fermentation are regarded as artifacts rather than significant compounds in penicillin biosynthesis. These are derivatives or degraded forms of 6-aminopenicillanic acid. 6-Aminopenicillanic acid in aqueous solution can dimerize to form biologically more active molecules (Dennen, 1967). It can also react nonenzymatically with respiratory carbon dioxide to form 8-hydroxypenicillic acid (Batchelor et al., 1961c; Ballio et al., 1961; Johnson and Hardcastle, 1961). Several species of bound 6-aminopenicillanic acid, such as N-glucosyl derivatives, can be detected in fermentation broths (Moss and Cole, 1964). 6-Aminopenicillanic acid bound to carbohydrate is recoverable by mild acid hydrolysis.

Several other penicillin-producing species synthesize a spectrum of penicillins comparable to that of P. chrysogenum (Cole, 1966b). These include certain other Penicillia, species of Aspergillus, and two species of dermatophytes, Trichophyton and Epidermophyton. These fungi produce 6-aminopenicillanic acid and respond to the addition of specific carboxylic acid precursors for penicillin synthesis.

Only two of the many penicillin antibiotics produced by direct fermentation have proven to be clinically useful, benzylpenicillin and phenoxymethylpenicillin. The latter penicillin, penicillin V, is obtained by addition of phenoxyacetic acid to fermentation medium. This penicillin is acid stable and an effective oral antibiotic (Brandl et al., 1953). 6-Aminopenicillanic acid can be N-acylated by chemical methods (Batchelor et al., 1959) and is an important intermediate for the preparation of semisynthetic penicillins (Jones, 1970; Hoover and Stedman, 1970; Cole, 1969c).

2. THE Cephalosporium-TYPE

Discovery of the cephalosporin compounds developed from interest in a new penicillin. Penicillin N, D-α-aminoadipylpenicillin, was isolated and identified from a Cephalosporium sp. CMI 49,137 (Crawford et al., 1952; Abraham et al., 1953, 1954; Newton and Abraham, 1953). This antibiotic-producing culture was collected from seawater near the effluent of a Sardinian sewer and was identified as a species of Cephalosporium related to C. acremonium (Brotzu, 1948). The name C. acremonium was taken up but has apparently been misapplied to this culture. The Brotzu isolate has been reclassified and transferred to another fungal species, Acremonium chrysogenum (Gams, 1971; Lemke and Nash, 1972).

Interest in the Brotzu culture was immediate since penicillin N had superior activity to that of benzylpenicillin against certain gram-negative bacteria. An antibiotic with properties similar to penicillin N had been independently discovered in Cephalosporium (Tilachlidium) salmosynnematum (Gottshall et al., 1951; Roberts, 1952). This antibiotic, called synnematin B (Olson et al., 1953), was characterized further and shown to be chemically identical with penicillin N (Abraham et al., 1955; Fusari and Machamer, 1958). When the perfect or sexual stage of C. salmosynnematum was discovered, the fungus was renamed *Emericellopsis salmosynnemata* (Grosklags and Swift, 1957). Other species were subsequently recognized to produce penicillin N (Kavanagh *et al.*, 1958a; Bhuyan and Johnson, 1958; Cole and Rolinson, 1961; Elander *et al.*, 1961; Pisano *et al.*, 1961; Miller *et al.*, 1962; Higgens and Kastner, 1971).

Species that produce penicillin N produce no other major penicillin compound and are insensitive to incorporation of extraneous side-chain precursors into antibiotic (Arnstein, 1958). Mere traces of 6-aminopenicillanic acid have been detected in the fermentation broth of *Emericellopsis minima*, *E. salmosynnemata*, and *Cephalosporium acremonium* (Cole and Rolinson, 1961; Lemke and Nash, 1972). The amount of 6-aminopenicillanic acid detectable is negligible compared to that amount observed from strains of *P. chrysogenum*, especially industrial strains of *Penicillium* developed for high penicillin production. Indeed, no penicillin of consequence other than penicillin N is formed by microbes of the *Cephalosporium*-type. However, certain of these organisms do produce nonpenicillin antibiotics.

Cephalosporin C, D-α-aminoadipylcephalosporin, was first recognized as a chemical contaminant of partially purified penicillin N from *C. acremonium* (Abraham and Newton, 1954; Newton and Abraham, 1955, 1956, see Chapter 1). This cephalosporin compound possessed good activity against gram-negative bacteria and had only about $\frac{1}{10}$% the activity of benzylpenicillin against gram-positive bacteria. The chemical structure of cephalosporin C was determined (Abraham and Newton, 1961; Hodgkin and Maslen, 1961) and differs from penicillin N by substitution of a dihydrothiazine ring for a thiazolidine ring and by the presence of an acetoxy group attached to the carbon of the methyl group at C-3 of the cephalosporin ring system (Table I).

7-Aminocephalosporanic acid has not been found in fermentation nor has the production of other cephalosporins been induced by addition of carboxylic acid derivatives to fermentation medium (Ott *et al.*, 1962). All known natural cephalosporins as well as penicillin N possess the D-α-aminoadipyl side chain.

Deacetylcephalosporin C is present in fermentation broth of *C. acremonium* (Abraham, 1962; Jeffery *et al.*, 1961) and may be a degradation product of cephalosporin C following attack by acetylesterase. A nonenzymatic derivative of cephalosporin C was observed following addition of sodium thiosulfate to fermentation medium (Demain *et al.*, 1963b). This compound is apparently the thiosulfate derivative of deacetylated cephalosporin C (Cocker *et al.*, 1965).

A non-β-lactam antibiotic activity is produced by *C. acremonium* and is solvent extractable (Burton and Abraham, 1951). This activity, designated cephalosporin P, is represented among a series of closely related steroid compounds. The principal compound, cephalosporin P_1, is an acidic steroid (Chou *et al.*, 1967) chemically related to helvolic acid (Iwasaki *et al.*, 1970). The biosynthesis of cephalosporin P compounds is related to general steroid biosynthesis. The label from [2-^{14}C]mevalonic acid, an established intermediate for steroid metabolism (Wagner and Folkers, 1961), was efficiently incorporated into antibiotic (Baird *et al.*, 1961).

Cephalosporin antibiotics, all containing the D-α-aminoadipyl side chain, are produced by two streptomycetes (Higgens and Kastner, 1971; Nagarajan *et al.*, 1971). Both streptomycetes produce penicillin N as well as cephalosporin compounds. The cephalosporin compounds formed by these species are chemically quite closely related to cephalosporin C. *Streptomyces lipmanii* can synthesize 7-methoxycephalosporin C; *S. clavuligerus* can synthesize deacetyl-3-*O*-carbamoylcephalosporin C and deacetyl-3-*O*-carbamoyl-7-methoxycephalosporin C (Table I).

The fact that all β-lactam antibiotics of the *Cephalosporium*-type are invariable with regard to *N*-acyl side chain is in marked contrast to the extended series of *N*-acyl penicillin compounds produced by direct fermentation of the *Penicillium*-type.

II. Tripeptide Theory

The formal molecular units that comprise β-lactam antibiotics are well known. Those β-lactam antibiotics containing the α-aminoadipyl side chain are essentially heterocyclic tripeptides composed of modified α-aminoadipic acid, cysteine, and valine (Fig. 2). All other biosynthetic penicillins are dipeptides possessing an *N*-acyl side chain derived from a carboxylic acid and a heterocyclic nucleus composed of cysteinyl and valinyl residues.

Biosynthesis of β-lactam peptides may be considered in the broader context of the synthesis of microbial peptides. The β-lactam compounds possess many features in common with other peptide antibiotics. Certain structural criteria have been recognized as diagnostic for peptide antibiotics (Abraham, 1957; Abraham *et al.*, 1965; Bodanszky and Perlman, 1969, 1971). These criteria include formation of atypical cyclic structures, frequent occurrence of amino acid residues with a D configuration, presence of amino acids or substituted amino acids not normally found in cellular protein, and limitation in molecular size. Biosynthesis of peptide antibiotics is often temporally dissociated from rapid growth or from those conditions optimal for net synthesis of cellular protein (Abraham *et al.*, 1965). The biosynthesis of many peptide antibiotics, including penicillins and cephalosporins, is maximal when exponential growth is arrested (Jarvis and Johnson, 1947; Hockenhull, 1959; Smith *et al.*, 1967).

The synthesis of peptide antibiotics may be mechanistically uncoupled from protein synthesis. The enzymatic synthesis of gramicidin S by *Bacillus brevis* has become a model for understanding synthesis of a peptide antibiotic (Saito *et al.*, 1970). Synthesis of gramicidin is not ribosomal dependent nor mediated by transfer ribonucleic acids (*t*-RNA). The component amino acids

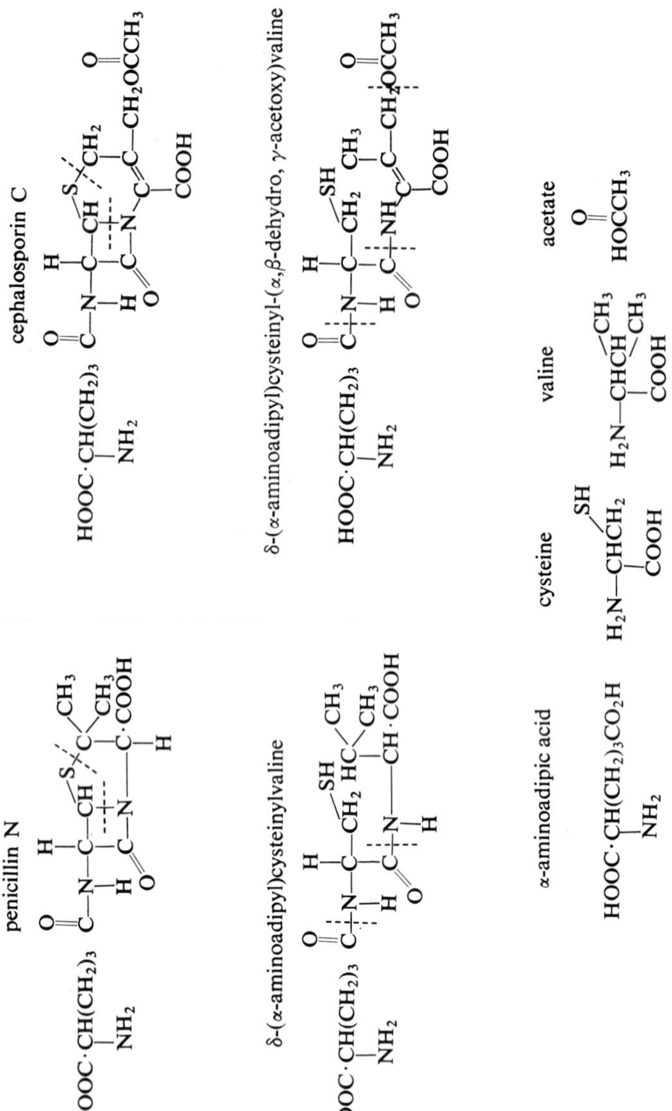

Fig. 2. Tripeptide antibiotics and related compounds.

of gramicidin are activated by specific amino-acid-activating enzymes. The free, activated amino acids are able to recognize an enzyme template and are assembled directly on this enzyme. Accordingly, the pentapeptide subunit of gramicidin S can be constructed in the absence of ribosomes. Total synthesis of gramicidin S, a cyclic decapeptide containing two residues of D-phenyl-alanine and two residues of L-ornithine, can be accomplished by a cell-free, soluble enzyme system.

It is not known if the biosynthesis of β-lactam antibiotics occurs in a manner similar to that of gramicidin S. General guidelines for study of the biosynthesis of peptide antibiotics have been presented (Bodanszky and Perlman, 1968, 1969, 1971), whereby consideration should be given to each of the following: (a) the mechanism by which component amino acids are combined, (b) the formation and incorporation of D-amino acids into peptide, and (c) the formation of the cyclic or hypercyclic ring systems. Each of these considerations has been largely a matter of speculation for biosynthesis of β-lactam antibiotics.

A. Isolation and Characterization of Tripeptide

The isolation of a noncyclic peptide corresponding empirically with penicillin N was reported by Arnstein et al. (1959, 1960) and by Arnstein and Morris (1960c). These reports initiated the tripeptide theory for penicillin synthesis. The tripeptide theory has dominated the subject of β-lactam biosynthesis for a decade.

1. THE ARNSTEIN TRIPEPTIDE (Penicillium)

The Arnstein tripeptide was obtained from mycelia of P. chrysogenum. The peptide was oxidized with performic acid during isolation and, upon hydrolysis, yielded residues of α-aminoadipic acid, cysteic acid, and valine (Arnstein et al., 1959, 1960). Arnstein and Morris (1960c) established the structure of the tripeptide to be δ-(α-aminoadipyl)cysteinylvaline (Fig. 2).

Since no other small peptides containing both cysteine and valine were recovered from mycelial extracts, Arnstein and co-workers (1960) suggested that α-aminoadipic acid might play a central role in penicillin biosynthesis. Analogy of the tripeptide with penicillin N was recognized, and the suggestion was made that all other penicillins might be obtained from penicillin N by enzymatic reactions involving a side-chain transferase (Arnstein and Morris, 1960c; Wolff and Arnstein, 1960). Penicillin N, however, was not a recognized penicillin of Penicillium. Only later was an α-aminoadipyl-containing penicillin detected in culture filtrates of P. chrysogenum (Flynn et al., 1962).

The configuration of the N-terminal α-aminoadipyl group of the tripeptide was not determined although free α-aminoadipic acid found in P. chrysogenum was of the L configuration (Arnstein and Morris, 1960c). The α-aminoadipyl side chain of penicillin N from *Cephalosporium* was earlier determined to be of the D configuration (Newton and Abraham, 1953).

The tripeptide theory is simple and, therefore, attractive. It implies that three amino acids from the cellular pool of amino acids simply combine to initiate penicillin biosynthesis. A sequence for peptide bond formation in the synthesis of tripeptide has been implied from data concerning the incorporation of label from a radioisotopic precursor into penicillin. The disulfide form of the dipeptide, L-cysteinyl-L-[1-^{14}C]valine, can be directly utilized for penicillin synthesis by *P. chrysogenum* (Arnstein and Morris, 1960a, b). These data have been interpreted to indicate that cysteinylvaline is an intermediate for synthesis of tripeptide and that the N-terminal α-aminoadipic acid is the last amino acid to be incorporated into tripeptide (Cole, 1966b; Sermonti, 1969), but clearly this interpretation was not favored by Arnstein and Morris (1960a, b).

The Arnstein tripeptide has been formed from component amino acids by cell-free extracts of *P. chrysogenum* (Bauer, 1970). The sequence for incorporation of amino acids into tripeptide was not determined. Tripeptide can be synthesized by chemical methods (Bauer, 1970).

2. THE OXFORD PEPTIDES (*Cephalosporium*)

A peptide with the same electrophoretic mobility as the sulfonic acid of δ-(α-aminoadipyl)cysteinylvaline was detected after oxidation of a crude mixture of peptides from cells of *C. acremonium* (Abraham *et al.*, 1964). This peptide was labeled readily with carbon-14 from either L-α-aminoadipic acid, L-cysteine, or L-valine and proved to be rapidly metabolized without being excreted (Smith *et al.*, 1967). The amount of this peptide found in *Cephalosporium* appeared to be considerably less than the amount of tripeptide isolated from *Penicillium*.

The intracellular, sulfur-containing peptides from *Cephalosporium* have been resolved further (Loder and Abraham, 1971a, b). Small, sulfur-containing peptides can be selectively extracted from *Cephalosporium* according to a procedure developed for isolation of glutathione from animal tissue (Waelsch and Rittenberg, 1941). Represented among peptides isolated from *Cephalosporium* is the Arnstein tripeptide (Loder and Abraham, 1971a). Mass spectrographic analysis demonstrated this peptide to be δ-(α-aminoadipyl)cysteinylvaline. Optical configurations of the component amino acids were determined by circular dichroism, which showed the tripeptide from *Cephalosporium* to be δ-(L-α-aminoadipyl)-L-cysteinyl-D-valine.

The principal sulfur-containing peptide found in *Cephalosporium* is glutathione, γ-(glutamyl)cysteinylglycine (Abraham *et al.*, 1964). In biosynthesis of glutathione, glycine is incorporated as the final amino acid (Snoke,

1955; Loder and Abraham, 1971a, b). The synthesis of δ-(α-aminoadipyl)-cysteinylvaline by *Cephalosporium* proceeds in a similar manner. Mycelial extracts of *Cephalosporium* synthesized tripeptide in the presence of a dipeptide precursor, δ-(L-α-aminoadipyl)-L-cysteine (Loder and Abraham, 1971b). Synthesis of the tripeptide was not observed in the presence of δ-(D-α-amino-adipyl)-L-cysteine (Loder *et al.*, 1969; Loder and Abraham, 1971b) or of either L-cysteinyl-L-valine or L-cysteinyl-D-valine (Loder and Abraham, 1971b). Dipeptides of cysteinylvaline were neither hydrolyzed nor taken up by intact cells of *Cephalosporium*.

In addition to Arnstein's tripeptide, related peptides have been isolated from *C. acremonium*. These contain glycine as well as α-aminoadipic acid and cysteine. They are tetrapeptides which have been designated P_1 and P_2 and are electrophoretically distinct. The former contains a residue of β-hydroxyvaline, whereas the latter contains valine.

3. OXIDATION OF THE VALINYL MOIETY

The entire carbon skeleton of L-valine is an established precursor of penicillin and cephalosporin (Arnstein and Clubb, 1957; Stevens and DeLong, 1958; Warren *et al.*, 1967b). Derivation of the thiazolidine ring of penicillin and the dihydrothiazine ring of cephalosporin requires that this valinyl moiety at some time undergo oxidation. A different oxidation may be appropriate for each ring system.

Hockenhull and co-workers (1949) have suggested that β-hydroxyvaline, by analogy with the formation of cystathionine from homoserine (Horowitz, 1947), might condense with cysteine to form dimethyllanthionine (*I*) and that this compound might be an intermediate for the penicillin ring system.

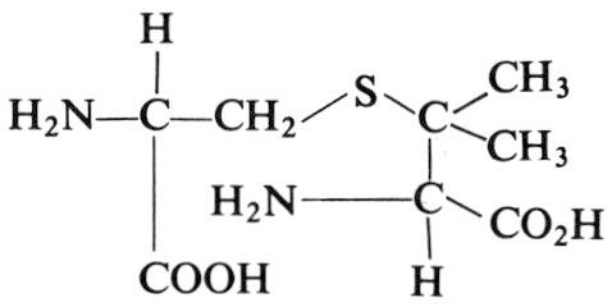

(*I*)

This proposal was shown to be untenable when dimethyllanthionine failed to depress incorporation of label from L-cysteine into penicillin (Stevens *et al.*, 1954a). Subsequent results (Arnstein and Clubb, 1958) indicated that various *N*-cysteinyl derivatives of dimethyllanthionine were also noncompetitive with cysteine in penicillin biosynthesis. These studies did not present evidence to indicate that dimethyllanthionine or its derivatives penetrated cells of *Penicillium*. Thus, the competitive nature of these compounds at the site of antibiotic synthesis has not been adequately investigated.

Arnstein and Clubb (1957) observed that label from DL-[1-^{14}C]-β-hydroxy-valine was not incorporated in the valinyl moiety of penicillin but at the C-7 position. This indicated that β-hydroxyvaline was converted to glycine. Label from glycine might then be transferred to the cysteinyl moiety of penicillin. Free β-hydroxyvaline has not been detected in cells of P. chrysogenum (Stevens and Halpern, 1949).

Trown and co-workers (1963a) have shown that in C. acremonium the α,β-dehydro-γ-hydroxyvaline moiety of deacetylcephalosporin C is derived from valine. However, γ-hydroxyvaline is a less efficient precursor than L-valine for antibiotic synthesis (Warren et al., 1967b). Addition of DL-γ-hydroxyvaline to resting cells of Cephalosporium depressed synthesis of penicillin N. Free γ-hydroxyvaline could not be found in C. acremonium (Abraham et al., 1964) nor was it detected after addition of D- or L-[1-^{14}C]-valine.

From the foregoing data, oxidized forms of free valine do not appear to be the precursors of the valinyl portion of β-lactam antibiotics. The oxidation required for cyclization must occur after formation of peptide(s). This is also evident from the observation by Loder and Abraham (1971a) that a peptide present in Cephalosporium, presumably related to antibiotic synthesis, contains β-hydroxyvaline.

B. Cyclization of the Tripeptide

Arnstein's tripeptide is the only noncyclic compound that has been formally implicated as an intermediate for β-lactam biosynthesis (Arnstein and Morris, 1960c). The discovery of this tripeptide led to several proposals for its cyclization to form the penam and 3-cephem bicyclic ring systems (Abraham and Newton, 1961, 1965; Demain 1963a, 1966a). These hypotheses have had to account for the following: (a) the occurrence of the D configuration of the valinyl moiety of penicillin (Arnstein, 1958; Arnstein and Clubb, 1957), (b) the sequence of formation for the β-lactam and thiazolidine or dihydrothiazine rings, (c) the point of divergence from the tripeptide toward the synthesis of 3-cephem as well as penam antibiotics, and (d) the origin of numerous penicillins as well as 6-aminopenicillanic acid (i.e., Penicillium-type antibiotics) from a common tripeptide.

Experimental evidence for direct utilization of α-aminoadipylcysteinylvaline or any derivative of the tripeptide in the synthesis of β-lactam antibiotics has not been obtained. This has not discouraged hypotheses regarding the pathway of β-lactam biosynthesis from specific peptides (Abraham, 1962; Abraham and Newton, 1965, 1967; Abraham et al., 1964; Arnstein, 1958; Arnstein and Morris, 1960c; Demain, 1963a, 1966a). These hypotheses consider iso-penicillin N to be a major biosynthetic penicillin.

1. Isopenicillin N

The tripeptide theory gained considerable support with the discovery of isopenicillin N, L-α-aminoadipylpenicillin, in *P. chrysogenum* (Flynn *et al.*, 1962; Cole and Batchelor, 1963). This penicillin represents an isomer of penicillin N. A small amount of isopenicillin N along with 6-aminopenicillanic acid were produced in the culture filtrates of *Penicillium*, when the mold was grown in medium to which side-chain precursors had not been added (Flynn *et al.*, 1962). Isopenicillin N (= penicillin M) as well as 6-aminopenicillanic acid were also detected in mycelia of *P. chrysogenum*, and the intracellular concentrations of both compounds were reported to be relatively high as compared to other penicillins (Cole and Batchelor, 1963).

Isopenicillin N has been regarded not only as the initial biosynthetic penicillin but also as a common intermediate for the synthesis of 6-aminopenicillanic acid and all other *N*-acyl penicillins (Demain, 1963a, 1966a). Enzymatic conversion of isopenicillin N to form 6-aminopenicillanic acid or other penicillins has not been demonstrated in studies involving penicillin acylase (Vanderhaeghe *et al.*, 1968). However, isopenicillin N does appear to be a substrate for an acyltransferase system in *Penicillium* (P. B. Loder and E. P. Abraham, personal communication).

2. Origin of the β-Lactam–Thiazolidine Ring System

Virtually nothing is known concerning the biological formation of the β-lactam ring of penicillin and cephalosporin. It is assumed that this ring is the first to be formed in β-lactam biosynthesis, and a plausible mechanism for its formation has been presented (Arnstein, 1958; Arnstein and Crawhall, 1957; Birch and Smith, 1958). This mechanism is based on evidence for the incorporation of tritium from DL-[2,2'-³H]cystine and DL-[3,3'-³H]cystine into benzylpenicillin. It was determined that tritium from these cysteine precursors was retained in the C-5 and C-6 positions of antibiotic. These results precluded the possibility of ring closure involving either a carbonyl at the C-5 or a double bond between the C-5 and C-6 of the cysteinyl residue of antibiotic. A noncyclic intermediate (2) was therefore proposed (Arnstein and Crawhall, 1957) as a precursor for a possible monocyclic form of penicillin (3).

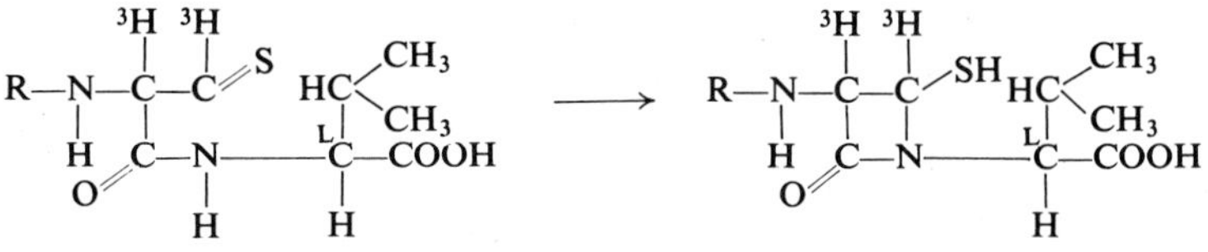

(2)   (3)

It has been implied that formation of the β-lactam ring might be followed by dehydrogenation of the valinyl residue to yield a monocyclic α,β-dehydrovaline intermediate (4) (Arnstein, 1958; Demain, 1959). This hypothetical α,β-dehydrovaline derivative could be subsequently converted to penicillin (5) by addition of the thiol group to the double bond. Cyclization could concomitantly invert the valinyl residue of penicillin to a D configuration at the C-3 position if the reaction was stereospecific. However, such inversion of the valinyl moiety

```
    H   SH                           H   S
    |   |    CH3                      |  / \   CH3
R—N—C—CH C<                 R—N—C—CH C<
    |   |  | ‖  CH3                   |   |  | D|  CH3
    H   C—N—C—COOH                    H   C—N—C—COOH
      O                                 O         |
                                                  H
     (4)                              (5)
```

during cyclization now seems improbable in view of the determination of a D configuration for the valine residue of tripeptide from *Cephalosporium* (Loder and Abraham, 1971a, b).

It has been proposed that formation of isopenicillin N by *Penicillium* occurs via cyclization of the Arnstein tripeptide and involves monocyclic and unsaturated intermediates similar to compounds (3) and (4) (Demain, 1963a, 1966a; Abraham and Newton, 1965, 1967). It has also been suggested that isopenicillin N is an immediate precursor of penicillin N in *Cephalosporium* (Demain, 1963a), but neither isopenicillin N nor the racemase required to convert isopenicillin N to penicillin N has been demonstrated in this fungus.

3. ORIGIN OF THE DIHYDROTHIAZINE RING

The biosynthesis of cephalosporin C has been related to the biosynthesis of penicillin and to the tripeptide theory (Demain, 1963a, 1966a; Abraham and Newton, 1965, 1967). The detection of peptides in *Cephalosporium* (Abraham *et al.*, 1964) similar to the tripeptide of *Penicillium* (Arnstein *et al.*, 1959) has fostered speculation concerned with biosynthesis of the 3-cephem structure of cephalosporin C in accordance with tripeptide theory.

Demain (1963a, 1966a) proposed that 3-cephem as well as penam antibiotics could be derived from a common α,β-dehydrovaline derivative of tripeptide (4). The dihydrothiazine ring of cephalosporin could result from dehydrogenation of the thiol group and one of the methyl carbons of the dehydrovalinyl moiety (Abraham and Newton, 1961). The resultant compound would be a deacetoxycephalosporin (6). The specific cephalosporin predicted to be formed from the Arnstein tripeptide was L-α-aminoadipyldeacetoxycephalosporin or the hypothetical isodeacetoxycephalosporin C (Demain, 1966a). This cephalosporin compound would be further oxidized and acetylated to yield isocephalosporin C. Finally, isocephalosporin C would be inverted at the α-amino group by a racemase to give cephalosporin C. However, deacetoxycephalosporin C

H   SH
| /
R—N—C—CH   CH$_3$ −2H   H H
| C—N   C—CH$_3$ ⟶   R—N—C—C^{S}CH$_2$
H   ‖   C | C—N   C—CH$_3$
O | H   ‖   C
        COOH   O |
        (4)   COOH
                                              (6)

has not been found in *C. acremonium* (Jeffery *et al.*, 1961). Furthermore, neither isocephalosporin C nor a cephalosporin racemase have been identified from *Cephalosporium*.

Alternative hypotheses have been proposed for the oxidation of the valine moiety prior to formation of the 3-cephem ring system. Abraham and Newton (1965) have outlined several possible pathways for cephalosporin biosynthesis. One such hypothesis is that penicillin N and cephalosporin C are synthesized from separate tripeptides and thus diverge early in their biosynthesis. Another hypothetical pathway involves a monocyclic, β-lactam intermediate with both methyl groups of the valinyl moiety oxidized (7). Cyclization of this intermediate would yield deacetylcephalosporin C (8). This cephalosporin would be acetylated by acetate to form cephalosporin C. The acetyl group of cephalosporin C has been shown to arise from an acetate precursor (Trown *et al.*, 1962).

H H   H H
R—N—C—C^{S}CH$_2$OH   ⟶   R—N—C—C^{S}CH$_2$
| C—N   C—CH$_2$OH | C—N   C—CH$_2$OH
H   ‖   C   H   ‖   C
O | O |
        COOH   COOH
        (7)   (8)

Another hypothetical mechanism for the biosynthesis of a 3-cephem compound is via ring expansion of a preformed penam compound (Abraham and Newton, 1965, 1967). Specifically, cephalosporin C could be synthesized from penicillin N. Conversion of the thiazolidine ring to the dihydrothiazine ring has proven to be chemically feasible (Morin *et al.*, 1963; Wolfe *et al.*, 1963), as diagrammed below. Morin and co-workers found that refluxing the methyl ester of phenoxymethylpenicillin sulfoxide (9) in xylene with a trace of *p*-toluenesulfonic acid gave the corresponding methyl ester of the deacetoxy-cephalosporin (11) via a hypothetical intermediate (10).

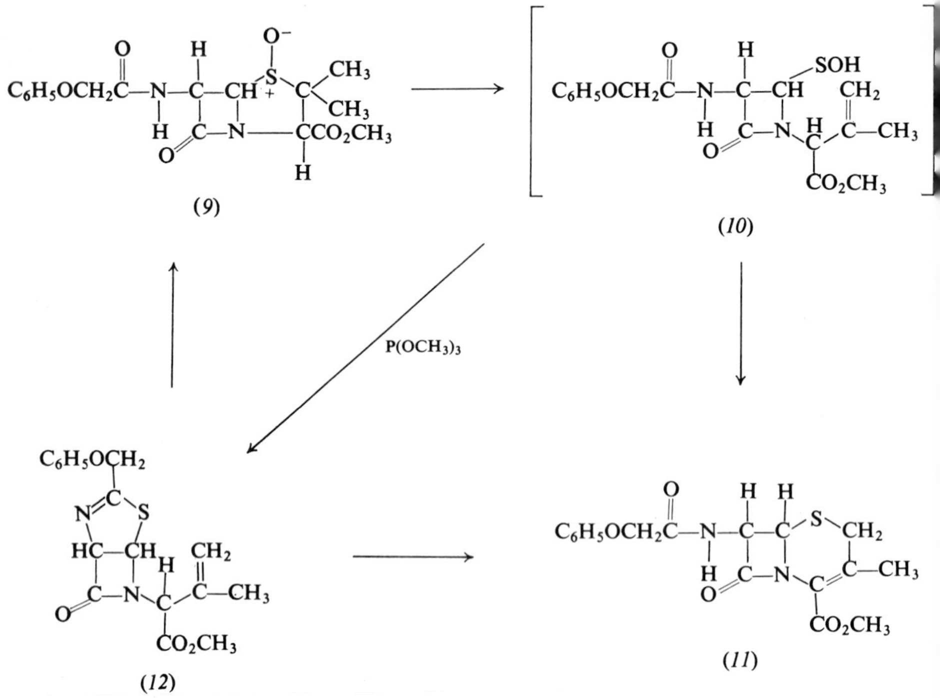

388

This sulfenic acid intermediate (*10*) in the presence of alkyl phosphite forms a thiazolidine compound (*12*) which, according to Cooper and José (1972); can be converted to compounds with penam (*9*) or 3-cephem (*11*) ring systems. The valinyl moiety of compound (*12*) resembles that of hypothetical intermediates of β-lactam biosynthesis (Demain, 1963a, 1966a; Abraham and Newton, 1965, 1967).

Wolfe and co-workers (1963) reported that the penam ring system of anhydropenicillin (*13*) could be expanded to the 3-cephem ring system. The anhydropenicillin was converted via allylic bromination with *N*-bromosuccinimide to give an intermediate (*14*) that, either upon treatment with base or by microbial hydroxylation, yielded a cephalosporin (*15*).

The ring expansion theory, which calls for rearrangement of the thiazolidine component of a penam to form the dihydrothiazine portion of a 3-cephem, is appealing as an explanation of the origin of cephalosporins. The idea has not been tested directly under biological conditions. However, a starting material which would support such a theory is available to cephalosporin-producing microorganisms since all of them produce penicillin N. Indeed, many organisms of the *Cephalosporium*-type seem to produce only penicillin N, and mutants of *C. acremonium* have been isolated which are unable to synthesize cephalosporin

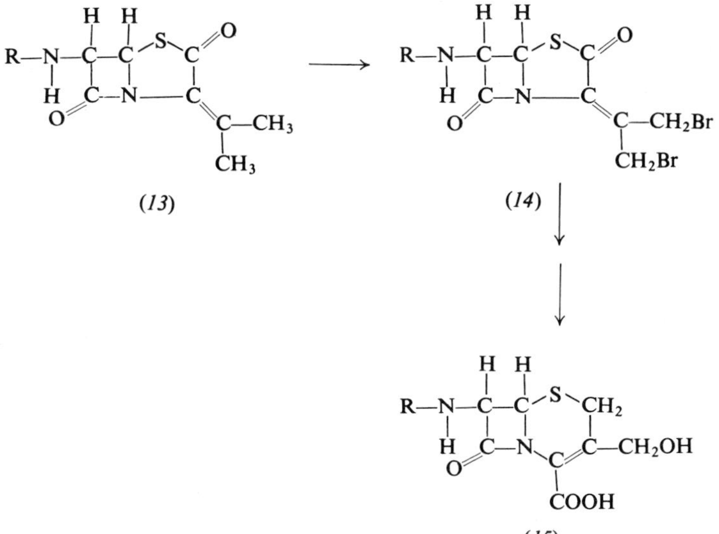

C but still retain the potential to synthesize penicillin N (Lemke and Nash, 1972).

An attempt to demonstrate microbial conversion of penicillin N to cephalosporin C was aborted since the label from exogenous [^{14}C]penicillin N did not enter mycelia of *Cephalosporium* (Smith *et al.*, 1967). The conversion of penicillin N to cephalosporin C by *Cephalosporium* is difficult to reconcile with the evidence that synthesis of penicillin N can be selectively depressed by D-valine (Abraham *et al.*, 1964; Warren *et al.*, 1967b).

It is generally agreed that the essential difference in biosynthesis of penicillins and cephalosporins involves oxidation of the valinyl moiety. It is not known whether this differential oxidation occurs early, at the level of tripeptide, or later, at the level of cyclic intermediates.

One of the main unresolved aspects of β-lactam biosynthesis is the origin of the cephalosporin ring system. Another major unresolved aspect of β-lactam biosynthesis is the origin of 6-aminopenicillanic acid.

C. Origin of 6-Aminopenicillanic Acid

Prior to 1953, all recognized penicillins from *Penicillium* were potent antimicrobial compounds against gram-positive bacteria, and virtually all known penicillins were extractable into solvent at low pH. In 1953, Kato reported an unusual penicillin formed by *P. chrysogenum* in the absence of side-chain precursor. This imperfect penicillin, called penicin (Kato, 1953a, b), was a poor antibiotic and was not extractable into butyl acetate at pH 2. The compound was regarded as a possible precursor of penicillin since it could be detected by the iodometric assay for penicillin and could induce formation of penicillinase in *Bacillus cereus*.

Kato's compound proved to be 6-aminopenicillanic acid (Batchelor *et al.*, 1959). The compound was detected by a discrepancy between chemical and biological assays for penicillin produced in a nonprecursed *Penicillium* fermentation. It was isolated and characterized as the free amino form of penicillin, a compound that could be converted to antibiotic by direct chemical acylation. 6-Aminopenicillanic acid reacted *in vitro* with phenylacetyl chloride to yield benzylpenicillin (Batchelor *et al.*, 1959; Wolff and Arnstein, 1960). The advent of 6-aminopenicillanic acid through fermentation profoundly influenced the design of new penicillin compounds by chemical acylation. The formation of semisynthetic penicillins by chemical acylation of 6-aminopenicillanic has sustained interest in penicillin chemotherapy (Hoover and Stedman, 1970).

Several factors influence the biosynthesis of 6-aminopenicillanic acid by *Penicillium* (Batchelor *et al.*, 1961a; Cole, 1966c). A deficiency of side-chain precursors in the fermentation medium enhances synthesis of 6-aminopenicillanic acid relative to most other penicillins. Overall penicillin synthesis is inhibited by a limitation of side-chain precursor. If cellular respiration is limited to 60% of maximum, then 6-aminopenicillanic acid is synthesized at a maximal rate. Overall penicillin synthesis is maximal in the presence of side-chain precursors and at a maximal rate of respiration. Superior penicillin-producing strains of *Penicillium*, obtained by genetic mutation, generally have an increased potential to synthesize 6-aminopenicillanic acid. However, a direct relationship between increased production of penicillin and the formation of 6-aminopenicillanic acid has not been observed in all mutants of *Penicillium* (Fuska and Welwardová, 1969).

The heterocyclic ring system of 6-aminopenicillanic acid can be envisioned as a bicyclic fusion product of L-cysteine and D-valine (Hockenhull, 1959; Arnstein and Morris, 1960b). Arnstein and Morris proposed that 6-aminopenicillanic acid could arise by cyclization of cysteinylvaline. This dipeptide theory for the synthesis of penicillin has been seriously considered by several investigators.

Derivatives of cyclic cysteinylvaline (*16*) labeled with carbon-14 at the C-6 position were tested as precursors for penicillin synthesis (Sjöberg *et al.*, 1965). Label from these compounds was not incorporated into antibiotic and no evidence was presented to indicate uptake of cyclic cysteinylvaline by *Penicillium* cells.

It has been claimed that 6-aminopenicillanic acid can be synthesized directly by mycelial mats of *P. chrysogenum* as a condensation product of cysteine,

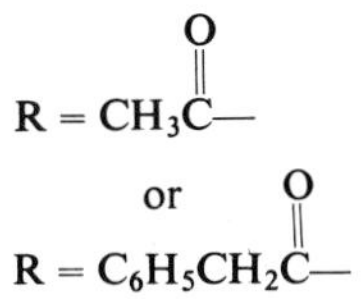

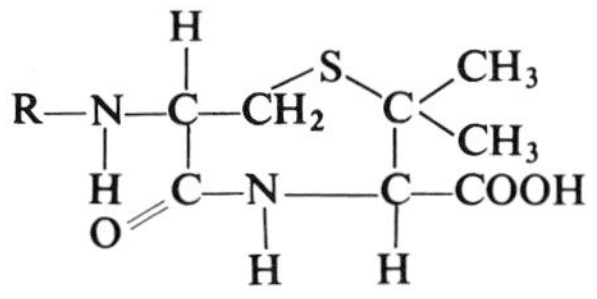

R = CH$_3$C—

or

R = C$_6$H$_5$CH$_2$C—

(16)

acetone, and glycine (Shimi and Imam, 1968). The reaction is reversible and influenced by coenzyme A. The amino acid L-valine is involved, but it is degraded to form acetone and glycine. This acetone and glycine are then reassembled to form the D-valinyl moiety of penicillin upon condensation with cysteine (Fig. 3).

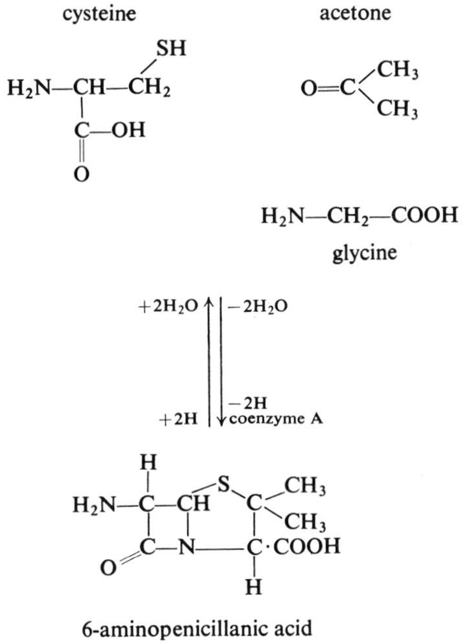

cysteine   acetone

H$_2$N—CH—CH$_2$ (SH)

C—OH

O=C (CH$_3$ CH$_3$)

H$_2$N—CH$_2$—COOH

glycine

+2H$_2$O ↑ | −2H$_2$O

+2H | −2H coenzyme A

6-aminopenicillanic acid

Fig. 3. Synthesis of the valinyl moiety of 6-aminopenicillanic acid by degraded valine.

The isolation of tripeptide (Arnstein et al., 1959) and the discovery of iso-penicillin N (Flynn et al., 1962; Cole and Batchelor, 1963) in Penicillium prompted speculation that 6-aminopenicillanic acid could be derived from isopenicillin N and was not an intermediate for penicillin biosynthesis (Arnstein and Morris, 1960c; Demain, 1963a). 6-Aminopenicillanic acid would thus arise by enzymatic deacylation of isopenicillin N. An enzyme, penicillin acylase, is recognized in Penicillium (Sakaguchi and Murao, 1950), but to date, this enzyme has not been shown to remove the L-α-aminoadipyl side chain from isopenicillin N (Vanderhaeghe et al., 1968).

Only trace amounts of 6-aminopenicillanic acid have been observed in fermentations of *C. acremonium* and *Emericellopsis minima* (Cole and Rolinson, 1961), and 7-aminocephalosporanic acid is not formed biologically (Ott et al., 1962). Mutant strains of *Cephalosporium* with increased antibiotic productivity do not accumulate 6-aminopenicillanic acid (Lemke and Nash, 1972). The negligible amount of 6-aminopenicillanic acid present in culture filtrates of *Cephalosporium* may arise by chemical rather than biological hydrolysis of penicillin N. Penicillin N is not a substrate for penicillin acylase (Claridge et al., 1963; Hamilton-Miller, 1966).

It is still not known if 6-aminopenicillanic acid is a precursor in penicillin synthesis or a product from preformed penicillin. The evidence that 6-amino-penicillanic acid may be synthesized by *Penicillium* from nonpeptide precursors (Shimi and Imam, 1968) suggests that its synthesis may be an ancillary aspect of β-lactam biosynthesis, divorced or unrelated to the biosynthesis of the tripeptide antibiotics. The diversity of the *Penicillium*-type penicillins with regard to side chain remains difficult to reconcile with tripeptide theory unless it can be specifically determined that isopenicillin N is an efficient substrate for penicillin acyltransferase. Numerous *N*-acyl penicillins can be formed from 6-aminopenicillanic acid and derivatives of carboxylic acids in the presence of penicillin acylase (Hamilton-Miller, 1966). 6-Aminopenicillanic acid is thus an attractive intermediate for synthesis of these penicillins.

The Arnstein tripeptide may be an intermediate only for the synthesis of tripeptide antibiotics, e.g., isopenicillin N, penicillin N, and cephalosporin C. 6-Aminopenicillanic acid might be synthesized via a separate biosynthetic pathway and serve as an intermediate for synthesis of all other penicillin compounds. This pathway would be unique to those organisms producing *Penicillium*-type antibiotics. Such a distinct pathway for the synthesis of 6-aminopenicillanic acid and the *N*-acyl penicillins seems unlikely since α-aminoadipic acid not only stimulates but is apparently required for synthesis of all penicillin compounds (Somerson et al., 1961; Cole and Batchelor, 1963; Goulden and Chattaway, 1968).

The data from primary metabolism generally support tripeptide theory.

III. Biosynthesis of β-Lactam Antibiotics and Primary Metabolism

The β-lactam antibiotics are secondary metabolites derived principally from compounds of primary metabolism. As pointed out in previous discussion, isopenicillin N, penicillin N, and cephalosporin C can each be formally divided into three amino acid residues—amino acids that are normal constituents of cellular metabolism (Fig. 2). Confirmative evidence that β-lactam compounds can be synthesized from specific amino acids has been based on experiments designed to test the incorporation of isotopic label from precursors into antibiotic. These biochemical data indicate that the component amino acids of tripeptide can be individually incorporated into antibiotic in a manner consistent with the tripeptide theory (Abraham et al., 1964; Demain, 1966a). Thus, α-aminoadipic acid is a direct precursor for the side chain of penicillin N and cephalosporin C. Cysteine provides the carbon of the β-lactam ring and the sulfur of antibiotic. Valine contributes to the thiazolidine portion of penicillin and to the dihydrothiazine portion of cephalosporin.

The β-lactam compounds are, therefore, what they seem to be, i.e., peptide antibiotics. The consensus is that tripeptide theory is attractive but not unequivocally established. The mechanisms by which the units of tripeptide are assembled and converted into heterocyclic antibiotics still have to be resolved. This is the hard core of β-lactam biosynthesis and the subject of considerable speculation in the absence of direct experimental evidence.

Experiments designed to trace incorporation of radioisotopic label from suspected precursors into antibiotic have characterized the study of β-lactam biosynthesis during the past 25 years. Such experiments have not and may not resolve the pathway of β-lactam biosynthesis. Although simple amino acid precursors have been taken up effectively by cells and incorporated into antibiotic, uptake of more complex compounds has proven to be inefficient. The distribution of label from large compounds often reflects turnover and is thus more difficult to interpret. There is no indication that intact β-lactam compounds are able to enter cells, which makes improbable the success of experiments for antibiotic conversion. The need for a cell-free system to further the study of β-lactam biosynthesis has been indicated (Demain, 1963a, b), but an adequate cell-free enzyme system has not yet been devised. There is no assurance that even a cell-free system will be suitable for the task.

In addition to an analysis of the biochemical pathway for β-lactam formation, other aspects of β-lactam biogenesis are worthy of consideration. The interrelationship of primary metabolism and antibiotic formation has not been clarified. Virtually nothing is known regarding the genetic basis for antibiotic synthesis. These aspects of biosynthesis go beyond pathway analysis.

Genetic mutations that enhance antibiotic productivity in Penicillium and Cephalosporium have been obtained by mutation induction and random selection (Backus and Stauffer, 1955; Stauffer et al., 1966). Such mutations have contributed substantially to the success of the antibiotic industry. The nature of mutations responsible for increases in antibiotic yield has for some time been difficult to comprehend. Data is slowly evolving to indicate that many, if not all, of the mutations toward greater antibiotic productivity are mutations that affect regulatory mechanisms in cells.

Demain (1966b) has reviewed several examples of regulatory mechanism from primary metabolism that are known to influence antibiotic synthesis. Three general types of enzyme regulation are recognized in metabolism: (1) repression or derepression of enzyme formation (regulation of protein synthesis), (2) noncompetitive or feedback inhibition (the end product of a pathway binds to an enzyme in the pathway and inhibits enzymatic activity by changing the structural conformation of the active site of the enzyme), and (3) competitive inhibition (substrate and molecules which mimic substrate compete for the active site of the enzyme). These regulatory mechanisms are subject to mutation.

With knowledge of antibiotic structure, an understanding of the physiological requirements for antibiotic synthesis and an insight into the regulation of primary metabolism it has been possible to design selective methods to obtain desirable mutations. Specific examples of genetic changes that have enhanced β-lactam productivity by altering primary metabolism are available (Segel and Johnson, 1961, 1963; Tardrew and Johnson, 1958, 1959; Goulden and Chattaway, 1969; Nüesch et al., 1970). It is apparent from such studies that antibiotic synthesis can be profoundly stimulated by mutational changes in the regulation of primary metabolism.

The potential for antibiotic production may afford a cell metabolic plasticity in the event that regulatory processes are altered. Secondary metabolism in general might be regarded as a consequence of disruption in the regulation of basic cellular metabolism. Antibiotics and other nonessential compounds could represent compensatory metabolites—compounds formed in response to deregulation of the cell's essential metabolism.

Three metabolic pathways and their regulation are known to influence directly the synthesis of β-lactam antibiotics.

A. The α-Aminoadipyl Moiety and Lysine Metabolism

α-Aminoadipic acid is not a universal metabolite among life forms (Vogel, 1960). It is considered to be absent from prokaryotic organisms such as bacteria and streptomycetes (Waksman, 1967) but is a common intermediate for the synthesis of lysine in higher fungi (Mitchell and Houlahan, 1948; Yura and Vogel, 1957; Strassman et al., 1964; Sinha and Bhattacharjee, 1970). Prokaryotic cells synthesize lysine by decarboxylation of another intermediate, 2,6-diaminopimelic acid.

The presence of α-aminoadipic acid in the β-lactam antibiotics elaborated by streptomycetes is anomalous from the standpoint of comparative biochemistry. The origin of the α-aminoadipic acid for these antibiotics is of further interest since the cell wall of the antibiotic-producing *Streptomyces*

Fig. 4. Biosynthesis of lysine in higher fungi: CoASH = reduced coenzyme A; NADP = oxidized nicotinamide adenine dinucleotide phosphate; NADPH = reduced nicotinamide adenine dinucleotide phosphate; PP_i = inorganic pyrophosphate; AMP = adenosine monophosphate; ATP = adenosine triphosphate.

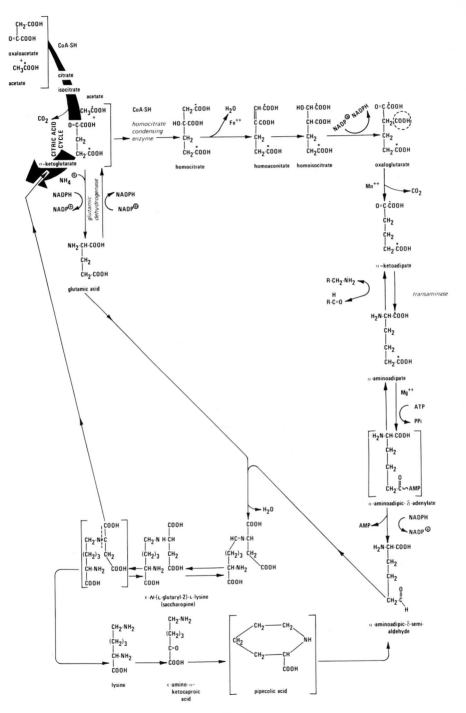

Fig. 4.

contains diaminopimelic acid (Higgens and Kastner, 1971), a characteristic component of the *Streptomyces* cell wall (Lechevalier and Lechevalier, 1967) and a normal intermediate for lysine metabolism in streptomycetes. It is not known if the α-aminoadipic acid used for the synthesis of β-lactam antibiotics in the *Streptomyces* is an intermediate for lysine or is obtained from lysine. Apparently, a few prokaryotic systems can catabolize lysine to α-aminoadipic-δ-semialdehyde (Calvert and Rodwell, 1966; Soda *et al.*, 1968; Ichihara and Ichihara, 1960). Higher fungi may well have reversed a catabolic sequence of prokaryotic origin in order to synthesize lysine.

The discontinuity between prokaryotic and eukaryotic organisms with regard to lysine metabolism is certainly not complete (Cohen, 1970). Lower fungi, algae, and higher plants possess diaminopimelic acid (Vogel, 1960, 1964). Certain mammalian cells, although unable to synthesize lysine, contain mitochondria with α-aminoadipate aminotransferase (Nakatani *et al.*, 1970). The presence of this enzyme in mitochondria of animals could be indicative of a vestigial lysine pathway in a "prokaryotic" organelle. Several of the early enzymes in the lysine pathway of yeast are apparently also localized in mitochondria (Betterton *et al.*, 1968). If mitochondria are considered to be subcellular prokaryotes, then there are precedents to indicate synthesis of α-aminoadipic acid in prokaryotic forms.

Data from studies with *Penicillium* and *Cephalosporium* indicate that the α-aminoadipic acid of antibiotic is obtained as an intermediate of lysine biosynthesis. Lysine metabolism in these fungi appears, thus far, to be consistent with the general pathway of lysine biosynthesis in higher fungi (Fig. 4) (Kuo *et al.*, 1962, 1964; Aspen and Meister, 1962; Strassman and Ceci, 1964; Strassman *et al.*, 1964; Mitchell and Houlahan, 1948; Yura and Vogel, 1957). α-Aminoadipic-δ-adenylate, an activated form of α-aminoadipic acid, has been recognized in yeast to be an intermediate in the conversions of α-aminoadipic acid to α-aminoadipic-δ-semialdehyde (Sinha and Bhattacharjee, 1970). α-Aminoadipic-δ-adenylate may be the specific compound required to initiate the biosynthesis of β-lactam antibiotics in *Penicillium* and *Cephalosporium*.

1. THE *Penicillium*-TYPE AND LYSINE METABOLISM

Lysine was observed by Demain (1957a) to inhibit benzylpenicillin synthesis in *P. chrysogenum* even before the tripeptide theory was formulated. Support for the tripeptide theory followed with the observation that lysine inhibition of penicillin synthesis could be reversed by addition of α-aminoadipic acid to the *Penicillium* fermentation (Somerson *et al.*, 1961). The implication was that an α-aminoadipyl-containing penicillin might be an intermediate in the synthesis of all other penicillins. Lysine inhibited general penicillin synthesis by feedback regulation of the lysine pathway, thereby limiting the endogenous supply of α-aminoadipic acid. Cole and Batchelor (1963) specifically demonstrated that α-aminoadipic acid stimulated and lysine inhibited synthesis of isopenicillin N.

Goulden and Chattaway (1968) have reported convincing genetic evidence that α-aminoadipic acid is an obligatory intermediate for synthesis of all penicillins by *Penicillium*. Mutations that specifically block the lysine pathway fall into two phenotypic classes. One class is blocked prior to synthesis of α-aminoadipic acid. Mutants of this class are unable to synthesize any penicillin although they do grow well when supplemented with lysine. Mutants of a second class are blocked after synthesis of α-aminoadipic acid and synthesize antibiotic if grown in the presence of lysine supplementation. Mutants of the first class grown in the presence of lysine are able to synthesize antibiotic, but only if exogenous α-aminoadipic acid is supplied to the culture.

Bonner (1947) had earlier surveyed biochemically deficient mutants of *Penicillium* for potential to produce antibiotic. He observed that one-fourth of the lysine-requiring mutants were deficient for penicillin synthesis. These early data suggested that lysine and penicillin might have a common precursor. The common precursor has proven to be L-α-aminoadipic acid (Mitchell and Houlahan, 1948; Yura and Vogel, 1957; Arnstein and Morris, 1960c; Somerson *et al.*, 1961; Goulden and Chattaway, 1968).

2. THE *Cephalosporium*-TYPE AND LYSINE METABOLISM

Penicillin N and cephalosporin C differ from isopenicillin N in possessing the D configuration of the α-aminoadipyl side chain. Nevertheless, the L isomer of [6-^{14}C]-α-aminoadipic acid can be incorporated into the side chain of *Cephalosporium* antibiotics more efficiently than the corresponding D isomer (Abraham *et al.*, 1964; Warren *et al.*, 1967a).

Lysine does not inhibit, and α-aminoadipic acid does not stimulate, antibiotic synthesis of the *Cephalosporium*-type (Bhuyan and Johnson, 1958; Demain *et al.*, 1963a; Ott *et al.*, 1962; Trown *et al.*, 1963b; Abraham and Newton, 1965). Fungi of the *Cephalosporium*-type may synthesize an excess of α-aminoadipic acid (Demain, 1966a).

Lysine has been reported to stimulate penicillin N synthesis in an *Emericellopsis* species (Nara and Johnson, 1959) and certain analogs of lysine, ε-amino-*n*-caproic acid and ε-*N*-acetyllysine, have been reported to stimulate cephalosporin C synthesis in *C. acremonium* (Demain *et al.*, 1963a). Addition of [1-^{14}C]lysine to cells of *Cephalosporium* resulted in a small amount of label in saccharopine and glutamic acid, but no label was detected in free α-aminoadipic acid or in antibiotic (Abraham *et al.*, 1964).

The evidence that L-α-aminoadipic acid is an intermediate for lysine metabolism in *Cephalosporium* as well as a precursor to the D-α-aminoadipyl side chain of antibiotic is based on a series of experiments using radioisotopic label

(Trown *et al.*, 1962, 1963a, b; Abraham *et al.*, 1964; Warren *et al.*, 1967a; Neuss *et al.*, 1971). *Cephalosporium* grown in the presence of [1-^{14}C]acetate synthesized cephalosporin C labeled in the acetoxy group as well as in the C-1 and C-6 positions of the D-α-aminoadipyl side chain (Trown *et al.*, 1962). Cephalosporin C produced by cells grown in the presence of [5-^{14}C]-α-keto-glutarate was labeled almost exclusively in the C-6 of side chain (Trown *et al.*, 1963a). Label from DL-[1-^{14}C]-α-aminoadipic acid can be incorporated effectively into antibiotic and also appears in saccharopine, lysine, and protein (Abraham *et al.*, 1964). Virtually all endogenous α-aminoadipate detectable in *Cephalosporium* is of the L isomer (Warren *et al.*, 1967a).

Confirmation of results obtained by Trown *et al.* (1962) has come from studies designed to test incorporation of [^{13}C]acetate into cephalosporin C (Neuss *et al.*, 1971). Incorporation of carbon-13 can be measured directly by nuclear magnetic resonance spectroscopy (Tanabe *et al.*, 1970). The [1-^{13}C]-acetate was incorporated into cephalosporin C in the carboxyl carbon of the acetoxy group and in the C-1 and C-6 positions of the side chain. The corres-ponding [2-^{13}C]acetate was incorporated, as anticipated, in the methyl carbon of the acetoxy group and in the C-2, C-3, C-4, and C-5 positions of side chain. Dispersion of label from [2-^{13}C]acetate in the side chain would be explained readily through cyclization of acetate via the citric acid cycle. These data as well as earlier data involving carbon-14 labeling of cephalosporin C (Trown *et al.*, 1962) demonstrate that the carbon skeleton of the α-aminoadipyl side chain is derived via condensation of α-ketoglutarate and acetyl coenzyme A (Fig. 4).

A lysine-requiring mutant of *C. acremonium* has been obtained (Lemke and Nash, 1972). The strain is deficient for synthesis of antibiotic when grown in basal medium supplemented with lysine. This mutant appears to be blocked for lysine metabolism after synthesis of α-aminoadipic acid, since it will not grow on α-aminoadipic acid. The mutant strictly requires lysine for growth. Antibiotic is produced by this culture only when grown in the presence of both lysine and α-aminoadipic acid. Apparently, lysine is a potent inhibitor of α-aminoadipic acid synthesis in the mutant since exogenous α-aminoadipic acid is required for antibiotic synthesis by this culture.

B. The Cysteinyl Moiety and Sulfur Metabolism

In microorganisms, the sulfur in cysteine can be derived via the reduction of sulfate and can be transferred to methionine. This transfer in bacteria is efficient and mediated by nonreversible β- and γ-cystathionases (Delavier-Klutchko and Flavin, 1965). In fungi (Fig. 5) reverse transsulfuration occurs from methionine to cysteine and is mediated by a reversible β-cystathionase and a γ-cystathionase (Flavin and Slaughter, 1967; Kerr and Flavin, 1970).

While bacteria are compelled to take up inorganic sulfur for synthesis of cysteine, the fungi exercise their option and are prone to assimilate methionine (Stevens *et al.*, 1953; Segel and Johnson, 1961, 1963; Wiebers and Garner, 1960; Caltrider and Niss, 1966; Benko *et al.*, 1967). In some fungi modest uptake of sulfate is a major limitation for synthesis of cysteine via the sulfate reduction pathway (Marzluf, 1970a, b; Caltrider and Niss, 1966).

Methionine can repress reverse transsulfuration by inhibiting β- as well as γ-cystathionase (Flavin and Slaughter, 1967). A derivative of methionine, *S*-adenosylmethionine, specifically inhibits cystathionine-γ-synthase in the

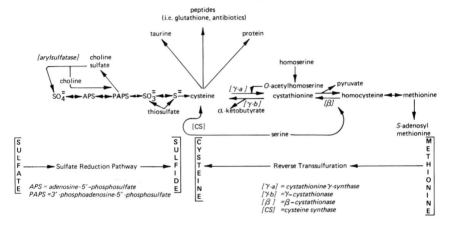

Fig. 5. Sulfur metabolism in fungi.

direction of methionine biosynthesis (Kerr and Flavin, 1970). Inhibition of cystathionine-γ-synthase, by repressing cystathione synthesis from cysteine, indirectly prevents dissimilation of cysteine carbon to pyruvate. The desulfhydration of cysteine to form pyruvate involves β-cystathionase (Flavin and Slaughter, 1964).

Sulfate can be stored by fungal cells in the form of choline sulfate, and the enzyme that catalyzes the release of stored sulfate is arylsulfatase (Fig. 5) (Harada and Spencer, 1962; Siddiqi *et al.*, 1966). Sulfate and compounds of the sulfate reduction pathway are recognized repressors of arylsulfatase activity (Scott and Spencer, 1968). Even cysteine, the terminal compound of sulfate reduction, inhibits arylsulfatase in many fungi. Methionine derepresses arylsulfatase in *Cephalosporium* (Dennen and Carver, 1969) although methionine is not recognized to derepress arylsulfatase in other fungi (Harada and Spencer, 1962; Siddiqi *et al.*, 1966; Metzenberg and Parson, 1966).

The carbon skeleton for cysteine comes from serine (Abelson and Vogel, 1955) and can be donated via either of two pathways (Fig. 5). The first involves condensation of serine and homocysteine and is mediated by β-cystathionase to form cystathionine, the precursor of cysteine via reverse transsulfuration. Alternatively, serine can complex with reduced sulfur to form cysteine, a condensation catalyzed by cysteine synthase (Leinweber and Monte, 1965). Cysteine synthase is inhibited by methionine in some fungi (Wiebers and Garner, 1967).

The β-lactam antibiotics possess a single sulfur atom derived from cysteine. Cysteine is truly at the crossroads of sulfur metabolism in fungi since it can be formed via either the sulfate reduction pathway or the reverse transsulfuration pathway. These two pathways are under coordinate controls that are not now fully elucidated. Accordingly, sulfate and methionine are alternative sulfur sources for cysteine and potential sulfur sources for antibiotic.

In *Penicillium*, the sulfur for penicillin is derived efficiently via the sulfate reduction pathway from sulfate but can also be derived via reverse transsulfuration from methionine (Stevens *et al.*, 1953; Segel and Johnson, 1963). In *Cephalosporium*, the sulfur for antibiotic is derived expeditiously from methionine via reverse transulfuration (Caltrider and Niss, 1966; Nüesch *et al.*, 1970).

1. THE *Penicillium*-TYPE AND SULFUR METABOLISM

Early labeling experiments established that cysteine and its metabolic precursors could be incorporated into the cysteinyl moiety of penicillin. Carbon-14 from cystine, serine, and glycine (Arnstein and Grant, 1954a, b) as well as from acetate and formate (Martin *et al.*, 1953; Tome *et al.*, 1953) served as precursors.

Triply labeled DL-[3-^{14}C, ^{15}N, ^{35}S]cystine, upon reduction to cysteine, proved to be a direct precursor of penicillin. The ratio of three labels found in benzylpenicillin was similar to that of initial precursor, but some turnover was observed (Arnstein and Grant, 1954a, b). Singly labeled L-cystine proved to be a more efficient precursor of penicillin than the corresponding D isomer.

Sulfur-35 from sodium sulfate enters penicillin (Howell *et al.*, 1948; Stevens *et al.*, 1953). This incorporation was significantly inhibited by L-cysteine. Several organic sulfur compounds were utilized preferentially over sulfate as a source for penicillin sulfur (Stevens *et al.*, 1953, 1954a). Sulfur from methionine, homocysteine, and cystathionine was incorporated into penicillin, which indicated a role for reverse transsulfuration in penicillin synthesis.

The role of the reverse transsulfuration pathway in formation of penicillin by industrial strains of *Penicillium* has been a relatively minor one. High penicillin-producing strains are efficient for sulfate anabolism (Segel and Johnson, 1961, 1963). Such mutant strains have an increased ability to concentrate intermediates of the sulfate reduction pathway and have apparently relaxed control for mechanisms regulating inorganic sulfur uptake and transfer to cysteine.

Addition of cysteine to *P. chrysogenum* fermentation medium containing inorganic sulfate does not stimulate penicillin productivity (Hockenhull, 1948). Stimulation with cysteine has been observed only with starved mycelial suspensions (Demain, 1956).

Sulfur-35 from methionine can be incorporated into penicillin (Stevens *et al.*, 1953), but methionine does not stimulate *Penicillium*-type antibiotic synthesis.

2. THE *Cephalosporium*-TYPE AND SULFUR METABOLISM

Methionine has a marked stimulatory effect on the synthesis of penicillin N (Gr. Brit. Patent 759,624) and cephalosporin C (Ott *et al.*, 1962; Demain and Newkirk, 1962) by *C. acremonium*. Stimulation of antibiotic synthesis by methionine is consistent in several media and occurs even if inorganic sulfate is supplied (Caltrider and Niss, 1966; Nüesch *et al.*, 1970).

Synthesis of penicillin N by several other *Cephalosporium*-type fungi is also enhanced by methionine, particularly the D isomer of methionine (Kavanagh *et al.*, 1958b). Kavanagh and co-workers suggested that D-methionine could serve as a precursor for the D-α-aminoadipyl side chain of penicillin N. This postulated mode of action for methionine is now questionable since carbon-14 from DL-[1-^{14}C]methionine did not label the α-aminoadipyl side chain of *Cephalosporium* antibiotics (Abraham *et al.*, 1964).

Methionine has multiple effects upon the *Cephalosporium* fermentation (Demain and Newkirk, 1962; Demain *et al.*, 1963a; Caltrider *et al.*, 1968; Dennen and Carver, 1969), but its principal role is that of a sulfur source for antibiotic (Caltrider and Niss, 1966; Nüesch *et al.*, 1970). Caltrider and Niss (1966) demonstrated that virtually all of the sulfur for cephalosporin C synthesis in complex medium was derived from methionine since sulfur-35 of the antibiotic was incorporated from [^{35}S]methionine without dilution. Studies in a synthetic medium, using specific biochemical mutants of *Cephalosporium*, confirm that methionine uptake and reverse transsulfuration of methionine to cysteine are necessary for efficient synthesis of cephalosporin C (Nüesch *et al.*, 1970). The role of methionine as a sulfur donor for antibiotic has been unequivocally established by these studies.

Methionine has other effects of a regulatory nature upon the metabolism of *Cephalosporium*. Cells of *C. acremonium* when grown in the presence of methionine as opposed to sulfate have a different morphology, an increased rate of respiration and a reduced rate of growth (Caltrider *et al.*, 1968). Moreover, methionine derepresses arylsulfatase in *Cephalosporium* (Dennen and Carver, 1969), especially in superior cephalosporin-producing mutants.

Demain and Newkirk (1962) postulated that methionine could enhance antibiotic synthesis in *C. acremonium* by preventing depletion of cysteine. It was suggested that methionine might specifically inhibit activity of a cysteine-degrading enzyme, cysteine desulfhydrase. This enzyme may be identical with β-cystathionase (Mondovi *et al.*, 1963), an enzyme which is able to convert cysteinyl carbon to pyruvate (Flavin and Slaughter, 1964). Since β-cystathionase activity is required for reverse transsulfuration of methionine, there is an apparent conflict between the hypothesis of Demain and Newkirk (1962) and the data of Caltrider and Niss (1966). The conflict is resolvable with the assumption that in *Cephalosporium* methionine prevents depletion of cysteine by inhibiting cystathionine-γ-synthase rather than β-cystathionase. Methionine, or more specifically *S*-adenosylmethionine, is an inhibitor of cystathionine-γ-synthase in other fungi (Kerr and Flavin, 1970).

Methionine derepresses arylsulfatase in *C. acremonium* (Dennen and Carver, 1969). In other fungi methionine can repress activity of cysteine synthase, the enzyme that condenses sulfide with serine to form cysteine (Leinweber and Monte, 1965; Wiebers and Garner, 1967). Concurrent derepression of arylsulfatase and repression of cysteine synthase by methionine should result in accumulation of sulfide.

Endogenous sulfide restricts methionine uptake by *Cephalosporium* (Nüesch *et al.*, 1970). These investigators obtained a mutant of *C. acremonium* blocked in the sulfate reduction pathway prior to sulfide formation. This biochemical mutant was able to assimilate more exogenous methionine and had the potential to synthesize fourfold more antibiotic than its sulfide proficient parent.

Cysteine, not methionine, is the direct precursor for β-lactam antibiotics of *Cephalosporium*. Carbon-14-labeled cysteine was incorporated into cephalosporin C (Trown *et al.*, 1962, 1963b) but was not taken up by cells readily (Abraham *et al.*, 1964). Methionine exogenously supplied, is simply a more expedient source of sulfur for antibiotic than inorganic sulfate or cysteine.

Mutants of *Cephalosporium* have now been obtained that utilize sulfate well to make antibiotic. This feature of these mutants resembles the facility for sulfate transfer in synthesis of penicillin by *P. chrysogenum*. Mutants were obtained by selection for resistance to specific toxicants. One such mutant possessed increased permeability for sulfate and was relatively insensitive for derepression of arylsulfatase by methionine (H. F. Niss and C. H. Nash, personal communication). This strain was competent to synthesize antibiotic from sulfate (U.S. Pat. 3,539,694). The native inability of *C. acremonium* to utilize sulfate well for antibiotic synthesis may be explained by assuming that sulfate assimilation by that organism is under strict negative control. Such control can be altered by mutation in the case of certain mutants resistant to specific toxicants.

Cysteine and methionine are subject to oxidative deamination by enzymes from *Cephalosporium* (Nüesch *et al.*, 1970). Amino acid oxidases and transaminases are recognized as common enzymes in fungi and prokaryotic microorganisms (Aurich, 1966; Burton, 1951; Chen and Duerre, 1970; Inove, 1960; Meister *et al.*, 1960; Sentheshanmuganathan and Nickerson, 1962; Thayer and Horowitz, 1951; Belg. Patent 736,934). In *C. acremonium* a constitutive, intracellular D-amino acid oxidase has been isolated (Benz *et al.*, 1971). This enzyme exhibits specificity for D-monoamino acids and is especially reactive with D-methionine and other D-amino acids related to methionine. Deamination proceeds at pH 8.5 with a K_m of 3.2×10^{-3} M for D-methionine and 7.6×10^{-3} M for D-cysteine. The deamination of D-methionine yields 2-keto-4-methylthiobutyric acid, and this reaction is competitively inhibited by several D-amino acids—particularly D-norleucine, D-norvaline, and D-leucine.

An L-amino acid transaminase has also been isolated from *C. acremonium* (M. Liersch, personal communication). This enzyme catalyzes a reversible reaction between α-ketoglutaric acid and any one of numerous L-amino acids. The 2-keto-4-methylthiobutyric acid, a compound formed by enzymatic deamination of D-methionine, is apparently also a substrate for this L-amino acid transaminase. Accordingly, 2-keto-4-methylbutyric acid can be enzymatically converted to L-methionine, which is then available for reverse transsulfuration. Therefore, successive activities of two enzymes, D-amino acid oxidase and L-amino acid transaminase can explain the ability of *Cephalosporium* to utilize the sulfur of D-methionine for synthesis of antibiotic.

The β-lactam antibiotics formed by *Streptomyces* will certainly derive their sulfur from sulfate if these antibiotic-producing cultures are consistent in their sulfur metabolism with other prokaryotic organisms.

C. The Valinyl Moiety and Valine Metabolism

Biosynthesis of valine is related to that of two other branched-chain amino acids, leucine and isoleucine (Umbarger and Davis, 1962). Formation of valine is initiated by enzymatic conversion of pyruvate to acetolactate by acetohydroxyacid synthetase (Fig. 6). This enzyme is subject to feedback inhibition by L-valine (Magee and deRobichon-Szulmajster, 1968; Goulden and Chattaway, 1969).

The pathway of valine metabolism in fungi (Strassman *et al.*, 1960; Radhakrishnan *et al.*, 1960) is comparable to that of bacteria (Umbarger and Davis, 1962), although considerably more is known from bacterial studies regarding the genetic regulation of enzymes involved in the biosynthesis (Umbarger, 1970). In fungi as well as in bacteria the later steps in the synthesis of isoleucine and valine are catalyzed by a single sequence of enzymes.

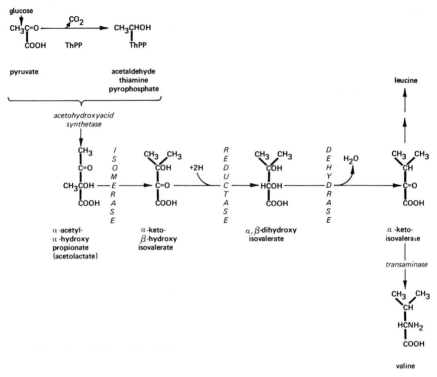

Fig. 6. Biosynthesis of valine: ThPP = thiamine pyrophosphate.

Leucine and valine are synthesized from a common intermediate, α-ketoiso-valeric acid, but in yeast only valine is an effective feedback inhibitor of aceto-hydroxy acid synthetase (Magee and deRobichon-Szulmajster, 1968).

1. THE *Penicillium*-TYPE AND VALINE METABOLISM

The valinyl moiety of penicillin exists in the D configuration since degrada-tion of penicillin yields the D isomer of penicillamine (Arnstein and Clubb, 1957). The actual precursor for the valinyl portion of antibiotic is apparently L-valine, which might undergo change in configuration either during formation of tripeptide (Loder and Abraham, 1971) or as a consequence of cyclization during formation of the thiazolidine ring (Arnstein, 1958). The L isomer of valine appears to be a better precursor for penicillin than the D isomer (Arnstein and Clubb, 1957; Stevens *et al.*, 1956). D-Valine is a poor precursor even if correction is made for its slow uptake into mycelia (Arnstein and Margreiter, 1958). However, conversion of D-valine to L-valine by *P. chrysogenum* has been demonstrated (Stevens and DeLong, 1958), and the mold contains a valine oxidase (Emerson *et al.*, 1950) that may be specific for the D isomer.

Valine can be incorporated directly into antibiotic. The label from DL-[γ,γ'-^{14}C]valine was introduced into the penicillamine fragment of benzylpenicillin, but localization of this label in specific carbons of antibiotic was not determined (Arnstein and Grant, 1954a). In another study, uniformly labeled [^{14}C]valine was incorporated intact into penicillin (Arnstein and Clubb, 1957). Furthermore, doubly labeled L-[1-^{14}C,^{15}N]valine was incorporated into the thiazolidine portion of penicillin without loss of the ^{15}N or the ^{14}C (Stevens and DeLong, 1958).

Label from an oxidized form of valine, L-[1-^{14}C]-β-hydroxyvaline, did not precurse the valinyl moiety of penicillin (Arnstein and Clubb, 1957) but was incorporated into that portion of antibiotic attributable to the cysteinyl moiety. The isotopic carbon from β-hydroxyvaline was apparently exchanged by the transfer of label to glycine, then to serine, and eventually to cysteine (Fig. 5).

The addition of [1-^{14}C]acetate to growing cells of *Penicillium* can also label the valine portion of penicillin, presumably by the conversion of carbon from acetate to acetaldehyde and ultimately to valine (Tome *et al.*, 1953).

Evidence has been presented that the valine portion of penicillin can be constructed biologically from acetone and glycine (Shimi and Imam, 1968). These authors had previously observed that mycelial mats of *P. chrysogenum* could degrade the valine portion of benzylpenicillin to acetone and glycine (Shimi and Imam, 1966). A mixture of acetone, glycine, and cysteine stimulated formation of a 6-aminopenicillanic acid, and this synthesis was enhanced further by addition of coenzyme A to resting mycelia. Shimi and Imam (1968) suggest that inversion of the L-valine of metabolism into the D-valine of antibiotic could involve transitory breakdown of L-valine to form glycine and acetone, with subsequent reassemblage of the degraded valine to form the D isomer present in penicillin (Fig. 3).

Demain (1966a) has presented evidence that benzylpenicillin synthesis can be stimulated by L-valine and inhibited by D-valine, provided the amino acid is added to cells starved for carbohydrate. However, stimulation of penicillin synthesis by exogenously supplied valine was not observed for cultures grown in complex media (Behrens, 1949).

The accumulation of endogenous valine can apparently influence production of penicillin by *Penicillium*. The enzyme acetohydroxyacid synthetase was compared in a high penicillin-producing mutant and in a low penicillin-producing strain of *Penicillium* (Goulden and Chattaway, 1969). The enzyme in both cultures was sensitive to feedback inhibition by L-valine, but the mutant superior for antibiotic productivity was less sensitive. Enzyme from the mutant strain was altered insofar as it retained only one of two binding sites for valine.

This valine-deregulated mutant was not subject to the same degree of feedback inhibition for valine synthesis present in the low penicillin-yielding strain.

2. The *Cephalosporium*-Type and Valine Metabolism

The valinyl moiety of penicillin N is also in the D configuration and the valinyl fragment of cephalosporin C is α,β-unsaturated and substituted with an acetoxy group at the γ-carbon position. Neither D-valine nor oxidized forms of free valine can be incorporated into these antibiotics as efficiently as L-valine (Abraham *et al.*, 1964; Warren *et al.*, 1967b).

D-[1-^{14}C]valine is taken into cells of *C. acremonium* more slowly than its L isomer and can be converted to L-valine readily (Warren *et al.*, 1967b). This situation in *Cephalosporium* is comparable to that in *Penicillium*. Addition of D-valine to resting cells of *C. acremonium* inhibited penicillin N synthesis without affecting synthesis of cephalosporin C. This might suggest that the D isomer of valine is a better precursor for cephalosporin C than it is for penicillin N. However, neither antibiotic incorporated label from D-[1-^{14}C]-valine readily (Abraham *et al.*, 1964).

Free γ-hydroxyvaline has not been found in cells of *Cephalosporium*, but if added to resting cells, it will decrease the yield of cephalosporin C without affecting penicillin N synthesis (Abraham *et al.*, 1964; Warren *et al.*, 1967b). It is, therefore, unlikely that free γ-hydroxyvaline is a precursor for cephalosporin C. Oxidation of the methyl group of the valine portion of cephalosporin must take place at some later stage in biosynthesis (Abraham and Newton, 1965).

The label from L-[1-^{14}C]valine, when added to *Cephalosporium*, is labile (Abraham and Newton, 1965). Over 65% of this carboxyl label could not be recovered after 15 minutes. Forty percent of the added label appeared as $^{14}CO_2$ via rapid decarboxylation of valine. The remainder of the label did get into antibiotics and into α-ketoisovaleric acid, peptides, and protein. With reference to the antibiotics, a pattern of labeling was evident. Label was detected in penicillin N prior to its appearance in cephalosporin C. The ratio of label detectable in the cephalosporins was initially higher in deacetylcephalosporin C than in cephalosporin C. This apparent sequence of labeling by valine might suggest conversion of penicillin N to deacetylcephalosporin C and, subsequently, conversion of deacetylcephalosporin C to cephalosporin C. A second interpretation of these data is that incorporation of L-valine into cephalosporin C might somehow be selectively inhibited (Abraham *et al.*, 1964).

IV. The Biology of *Penicillium* and *Cephalosporium*

The microorganisms that produce β-lactam antibiotics are in themselves interesting biological systems representing widely divergent taxonomic species.

The scattered appearance of β-lactam compounds among unrelated taxa, prokaryotes as well as eukaryotes, suggests that these compounds are of no fundamental evolutionary significance.

Each of three basic biological phenomena—growth, cellular organization, and genetic structure—influence the synthesis of β-lactam antibiotics.

A. Major Strains and Growth Media

The efficiency for microbial synthesis of β-lactam antibiotics is variable. The amount of antibiotic formed is dependent upon the genetic endowment of a specific strain and upon rather specialized conditions for growth. These attributes for efficient synthesis of antibiotic were recognized early in the development of a process for large-scale production of penicillin.

1. THE PEORIA ISOLATE AND DESCENDANTS (*Penicillium*)

A specific strain of *P. chrysogenum* proved to respond well under conditions of submerged fermentation (Raper, 1946; Moyer and Coghill, 1946a, b, 1947). This strain, designated NRRL 1951, was isolated from a cantaloupe in Peoria, Illinois. All major industrial strains employed for penicillin production are descendants of NRRL 1951 (Elander, 1967; Sermonti, 1969).

Substantial yield improvements for penicillin have been obtained by random screening of variant strains following mutation induction (Backus and Stauffer, 1955). Various mutagens—nitrogen mustard, ultraviolet light, X irradiation—have been used to obtain superior antibiotic-producing strains of *P. chrysogenum*. Specialized media have been developed for production of penicillin by submerged fermentation (Arnstein and Grant, 1956). In all media a high rate of aeration is required for efficient yield of antibiotic (Jarvis and Johnson, 1947), and the rate of antibiotic synthesis reaches a maximum after a phase of exponential growth (Koffler *et al.*, 1945). The development of complex media for penicillin production has been largely empirical (Moyer and Coghill, 1947; Olson *et al.*, 1954; Moss and Cole, 1964). Fermentation media for penicillin production are generally supplemented with specific carboxylic acid precursors in order to condition formation of specific penicillin compounds. The average fermentation proceeds at 25°C and lasts 5–7 days.

The *Penicillium* fermentation has been categorically divided into three phases (Koffler *et al.*, 1945; Hockenhull, 1959): (1) an initial phase of exponential growth with accumulation of biomass, (2) a phase of maturation with a maximal rate of penicillin production, and (3) a final phase of senescence with cellular autolysis. Glucose is readily metabolized by *P. chrysogenum* and the level of glucose during fermentation is critical for penicillin formation (Stefaniak *et al.*, 1946). Glucose, if continuously provided to a culture in critical amounts, can sustain the phase of penicillin production (Davey and Johnson, 1953). Although substantial accretion of penicillin follows a phase of rapid growth, experiments with continuous cultures of *P. chrysogenum* have indicated that penicillin synthesis is dependent upon continued growth (Pirt and Righelato, 1967). Cytological changes during autolysis of *Penicillium* have been characterized (Trinci and Righelato, 1970).

Systematic approaches to the development of synthetic fermentation media have been outlined (Perlman, 1966), and chemically defined media for penicillin synthesis have been proposed (Hockenhull, 1959; Verkhovtseva *et al.*, 1970; Lemke and Ness, 1970). Media for surface growth and sporulation of *P. chrysogenum* have been developed and are useful for genetic investigations (Macdonald *et al.*, 1963).

2. THE SARDINIAN ISOLATE AND DESCENDANTS (*Cephalosporium*)

At about the time penicillin was introduced for clinical use, an antibiotic-producing fungus was isolated from the Gulf of Cagliari, Sardinia (Brotzu, 1948). The fungus was transmitted to England for further study, whereupon it was designated CMI 49,137 (Abraham, 1962; Van Heyningen, 1967; see Chapter 1). A significant strain, culture 8650, was obtained from CMI 49,137 following mutagenesis with ultraviolet light. It was from culture filtrates of 8650 that cephalosporin C was isolated (Abraham and Newton, 1961). Mutant 8650 possessed increased potential for synthesis of cephalosporin C but not for synthesis of penicillin N. The 8650 culture has been a parent for obtaining several mutant cultures superior for cephalosporin C synthesis (Stauffer *et al.*, 1966; Dennen and Carver, 1969; Nüesch *et al.*, 1970).

Industrial production of cephalosporin C occurs by submerged fermentation in complex media and requires a high efficiency of aeration (Jones, 1970; Cole, 1969c; Caltrider and Niss, 1966; Caltrider *et al.*, 1968; Auden *et al.*, 1969; Feren and Squires, 1969). Poor aeration increases penicillin N production relative to that of cephalosporin C. Antibiotic production by *Cephalosporium* resembles penicillin formation by *Penicillium* insofar as the maximal rate of antibiotic formation occurs after rapid cellular growth (Smith *et al.*, 1967).

Two synthetic media have been formulated for fermentation of cephalo-sporin C. The medium of Demain and co-workers (1963a) has been modified by Dennen and Carver (1969), and the medium of Ott and co-workers (1962) has been modified by Benz and associates (1971). Sporulation medium for *Cephalosporium* has also been developed (Lemke and Nash, 1972).

A chemically defined medium for production of penicillin N by *Emericel-lopsis* has been proposed (Harvey and Olson, 1958).

Cells of *C. acremonium* actively engaged in antibiotic synthesis can be removed from fermentation medium, whereupon antibiotic synthesis does not immediately cease (Ott *et al.*, 1962; Demain, 1963b). Washed cell suspensions of *Cephalosporium* have been used successfully to evaluate incorporation of labeled precursors into antibiotic (Abraham *et al.*, 1964; Nash and Huber, 1971). Disrupted cell preparations of *Cephalosporium* have proven to be inefficient for antibiotic synthesis, and to date, cell-free synthesis of β-lactam antibiotics has not been adequately demonstrated (Demain, 1966a).

B. Cellular Organization

The greatest evolutionary discontinuity in the biological world is indicated by the degree of cellular organization that distinguishes eukaryotic organisms from prokaryotic organisms (Stanier *et al.*, 1963; Charles and Knight, 1970; Margulis, 1968). *Penicillium chrysogenum* and *Cephalosporium acremonium* are eukaryotic organisms and are related insofar as they belong to the same taxonomic family of higher fungi, the Family *Moniliaceae* of the Class *Fungi Imperfecti*.

As eukaryotic organisms, *Penicillium* and *Cephalosporium* possess membrane-bound nuclei with chromosomal organization and a cytoplasm with relatively complex membranous structures (e.g., mitochondria, endoplasmic reticulum). As higher fungi, the basic cellular form of *Penicillium* and *Cephalosporium* is the septate hypha, a vegetative filament of indeterminant length bound by a cell wall (Ainsworth and Sussman, 1965). As imperfect fungi, *Penicillium* and *Cephalosporium* reproduce asexually by mitosis and cellular elongation. The asexual spore form for both *Penicillium* and *Cephalosporium* is a unicellular, uninucleate conidium, a type of cell produced upon the hypha (Fig. 7A).

The streptomycetes are filamentous microorganisms with relatively simple prokaryotic organization (Waksman, 1967). The nuclei of streptomycetes are not membrane bound. The cell wall of streptomyces resembles that of gram-positive bacteria and not that of higher fungi.

1. CELL WALL BIOCHEMISTRY OF *Penicillium*

Intracellular antibiotic titer in *P. chrysogenum* (Demain, 1957b) and *C. acremonium* (Smith *et al.*, 1967) is low compared to extracellular accumulation of antibiotic. The β-lactam antibiotics are apparently excreted across a concentration gradient, and such active transport seemingly occurs at or near the cell surface. The site of antibiotic synthesis in *Penicillium* and *Cephalosporium* is unknown. Neither cell wall nor cell membrane has been formally implicated in β-lactam biosynthesis.

The cell walls of fungi are formidable structures. The cell walls of the imperfect fungi are composed substantially of chitin and β-glucan (Bartnicki-Garcia, 1969). Biochemical studies indicate that β-lactam antibiotics are not

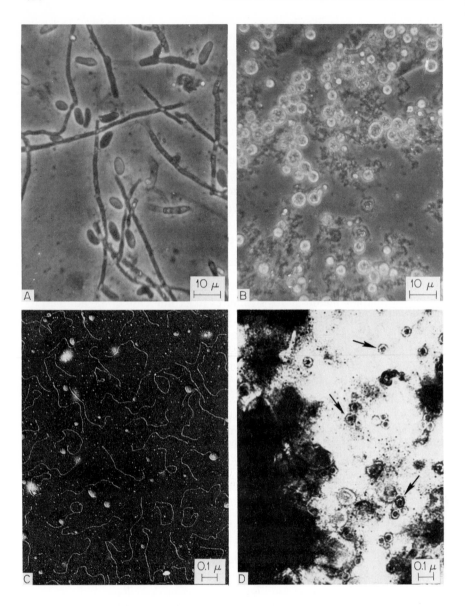

Fig. 7. Biological aspects of *Penicillium* and *Cephalosporium*: (A) hyphae and conidia of *C. acremonium*, (B) arthrospores of *C. acremonium* formed during submerged fermentation, (C) molecules of double-stranded ribonucleic acid (2×10^6 daltons) extracted from *P. chrysogenum*, and (D) virus particles present in mycelia of *C. acremonium*.

involved in cell wall structure (Applegarth, 1967; Troy and Koffler, 1969; Rizza and Kornfeld, 1969). The amino acids detected in the cell wall of *Penicillium* are those normally associated with cellular protein. Moreover, the conidial cell wall contains typical amino acids (Rizza and Kornfeld, 1969). The bound or *N*-glucosyl derivative of 6-aminopenicillanic acid detected in *P. chrysogenum* (Moss and Cole, 1964) is doubtfully related to cell wall structure.

Mucopeptides containing unusual amino acids are characteristic of the cell walls of streptomycetes and bacteria (Lechavalier and Lechavalier, 1967; Strominger *et al.*, 1968). The β-lactam antibiotics are generally antagonistic to cell wall synthesis of these prokaryotic organisms. The mode of antimicrobial action by penicillin is recognized (Strominger *et al.*, 1968). Two enzymatic reactions involved in bacterial cell wall synthesis, peptidoglycan transpeptidase and D-alanine carboxypeptidase, are sensitive to penicillin. Actinomycetes are generally sensitive to β-lactam antibiotics (Waksman, 1967; Lemke, 1969). Accordingly, species of *Streptomyces* that produce β-lactam antibiotics are anomalous for their insensitivity to these antibiotics.

2. MORPHOGENESIS IN *Cephalosporium*

Cells of *C. acremonium* are morphologically heterogeneous in submerged culture (Smith *et al.*, 1967). The maximal rate of antibiotic synthesis during fermentation is temporally associated with morphogenesis—differentiation of hyphal filaments (Fig. 7A) into swollen, highly septate fragments (arthrospores, Fig. 7B).

Four cell types of *C. acremonium* are recognized: hyphae, arthrospores, conidia, and germinated conidia (Nash and Huber, 1971). These cell types were separated by sucrose density-gradient centrifugation. Gradient fractions were then evaluated for potential to synthesize antibiotic. Fractions containing arthrospores were 40% more efficient for antibiotic synthesis than fractions containing other cell types. The arthrospore has been implicated as the cell type of *C. acremonium* most actively engaged in antibiotic synthesis (Smith *et al.*, 1967; Nash and Huber, 1971). However, mutants of *Cephalosporium* which are unable to synthesize antibiotic do form arthrospores normally (Lemke and Nash, 1972).

3. MYCOPHAGES OF *Penicillium* AND *Cephalosporium*

Viruses were unknown in fungi until rather recently (Hollings and Stone, 1969). The first demonstration of mycophage in the *Fungi Imperfecti* developed from the study of statolon, a fermentation product of *Penicillium stoloniferum* (Ellis and Kleinschmidt, 1967). Statolon induces interferon in laboratory animals (Kleinschmidt and Murphy, 1967), and the active antiviral component of statolon is now recognized to be double-stranded ribonucleic acid of viral origin (Kleinschmidt *et al.*, 1968).

Viruses containing double-stranded RNA are also present in *P. chrysogenum* (Banks *et al.*, 1969; Lemke and Ness, 1970; Fig. 7C) and *C. acremonium* (Day and Ellis, 1971; Fig. 7D). The significance of such viruses in these fungi is unknown at present. The mycophages of *Penicillium* and *Cephalosporium* appear to be avirulent since host cultures are not lysed in a general or predictable manner. Nevertheless, double-stranded RNA is not a normal constituent of the eukaryotic cell, and its presence would constitute extrachromosomal genetic material. Mycophages may influence profoundly the biology of *Penicillium* and *Cephalosporium*.

Strains of *P. chrysogenum* have been recognized as unstable (Foster and Karow, 1945; Backus and Stauffer, 1955). Strains sector for growth rate, sporulation efficiency, and antibiotic productivity. The frequency of this sectoring is too high to be explained either by spontaneous genetic mutation or normal mitotic segregation. Future studies will surely determine if viral nucleic acid in *Penicillium* undermines cultural stability. Ribonucleic acid can act as a template for synthesis of deoxyribonucleic acid by certain RNA viruses (Temin, 1964; Spiegelman *et al.*, 1970). Such RNA-dependent DNA synthesis by these tumor viruses demonstrates the potential of viral RNA to influence the genetics of a eukaryotic cell. Polymerase activity, basically RNA polymerase activity, has been reported recently in association with purified mycophages (Lemke and Nash, 1971; Lapierre *et al.*, 1971), but no DNA-copy for these viruses is now known. Nevertheless, genetic determination in *P. chrysogenum* may prove to be a highly complicated affair involving viral genes as well as host cell genome. In any event, *P. chrysogenum* is a model experimental system for study of RNA virus in a eukaryotic microorganism.

The genetic basis for antibiotic synthesis by *Penicillium* and *Cephalosporium* remains fair game for critical genetic investigation.

C. Genetic Studies

Although imperfect fungi lack sexual reproduction, the genetics of many of these fungi can be studied by parasexual methods (Pontecorvo *et al.*, 1953). Parasexuality is based on mitotic recombination of genetic material during somatic reproduction. The essential features of the parasexual process are: (a) formation of a heterokaryon via introduction of genetically dissimilar nuclei into a common cytoplasm, (b) recovery of a heterozygous diploid strain from a resident heterokaryon, and (c) detection of recombinants, diploid as well as haploid, formed by genetic crossover or chromosomal loss (nondisjunction) during mitotic reproduction of a heterozygous diploid strain.

The overall results of the parasexual cycle are similar to those accomplished by meiosis and sexuality, but the parasexual events—heterokaryosis, diploidization, mitotic recombination, and haploidization—are irregular and occur at relatively low frequencies. Selective genetic techniques are required to demonstrate parasexual phenomena. Both *P. chrysogenum* (Pontecorvo and Sermonti, 1954) and *C. acremonium* (Nüesch *et al.*, 1970) exhibit parasexuality. In some fungi, as in *Aspergillus nidulans*, the parasexual cycle may be accompanied by a bona fide sexual cycle. Moreover, a third phenomenon for genetic recombination occurs in *A. nidulans* and has been termed mitotic nonconformity (Azevedo and Roper, 1970; Roper, 1971). According to this phenomenon, parental and daughter nuclei do not necessarily conform in genotype due to some intrinsic infidelity in the mitotic process. Loss and gain of genetic material through mitotic nonconformity could explain a high incidence of instability for a culture. Mitotic infidelity in *A. nidulans* is related to crossover events within inversion loops of chromosomes. Extensive segments of chromosomes apparently invert in *A. nidulans* at a high frequency, and crossover within an inversion loop during mitosis could generate deletion as well as tandem duplication of genetic material. Tandem duplication of an inverted chromosomal segment would invoke even further instability during subsequent mitoses. Thus, mitotic nonconformity would lead to successive and transposable genetic heterogeneity within a culture. A high frequency of chromosomal imbalance (aneuploidy) would result. Loss of genetic material via a crossover mechanism is analogous to the release of a bacteriophage in an integrated state.

Mitotic nonconformity may also exist in *P. chrysogenum* (Ball, 1969, 1971), and this phenomenon may explain the intrinsic instability of that culture (Pathak and Elander, 1971). Elander (1967) and Elander and co-workers (1970) have observed considerable variability among strains of *P. chrysogenum* with respect to content of deoxyribonucleic acid within conidia. This is indicative evidence for rampant aneuploidy in *Penicillium*. It is unlikely that such aneuploidy is an incidental effect. The evidence for virus in *P. chrysogenum* warrants consideration for a possible cause–effect relationship between mycophage and mitotic non-conformity.

1. PARASEXUAL GENETICS OF *Penicillium* AND *Cephalosporium*

The genetics of antibiotic-producing microorganisms has been reviewed by Sermonti (1969). More recent contributions to this subject were included in a symposium devoted to the genetics of industrial microorganisms (Elander *et al.*, 1970; Ball, 1970).

The genetics of *P. chrysogenum* can be studied formally by parasexual methods (Pontecorvo and Sermonti, 1954; Sermonti, 1957). Penicillin productivity by *P. chrysogenum* has also been studied through parasexual methods (Sermonti, 1956, 1959a; Macdonald, 1966; Macdonald *et al.*, 1963, 1965; Elander, 1967; Elander *et al.*, 1970; Ball, 1971). Heterokaryons, heterozygous diploids, and recombinants from diploids have all been evaluated for potential to synthesize antibiotic. Interpretation of data from these studies has been exceedingly difficult, and there is no agreement among investigators regarding the merit of parasexual genetics for industrial strain improvement.

Genetic experiments concerned with penicillin production by *P. chrysogenum* have been handicapped in two ways. First, these experiments constitute inbreeding since all strains involved in crosses have been descendants of a single strain, NRRL 1951. It is unlikely that such crosses would demonstrate hybrid vigor (heterosis) or yield superior recombinants often generated through hybridization. Secondly, parasexual experiments have been conducted against a background of intrinsic genetic instability. The general instability of *P. chrysogenum* has been discussed previously.

There exists considerable variation for penicillin synthesis among diploids, even diploids synthesized from the same parents (Macdonald *et al.*, 1965; Elander, 1967). Determination of penicillin productivity appears generally to reside in nuclear genes (Sermonti, 1959a, b; Macdonald *et al.*, 1963) although cytoplasmic genes for "dwarfism" have been shown to influence the growth of *Penicillium* (Sermonti, 1959b). Cytoplasmic genes that undermine stability for growth rate in *P. chrysogenum* would indirectly affect penicillin synthesis. A genetic program for *P. chrysogenum* has only recently been designed whereby parental strains are selected for stability prior to parasexual analysis (Ball, 1971).

A series of diploid cultures has been extensively characterized by Pathak and Elander (1971), Diploids were compared to haploids with respect to antibiotic synthesis, growth rate, conidiation, sugar utilization, oxygen uptake, and the levels of three enzymes—glucose oxidase, alkaline protease, and β-galactosidase. Diploids were clearly superior to haploids on all accounts save penicillin biosynthesis. Certain relatively stable diploid cultures were merely comparable to their haploid parents in ability to synthesize antibiotic. No strain of *P. chrysogenum* developed through parasexual methods has, thus far, been adopted for industrial production of penicillin.

Cephalosporium acremonium has been adapted for genetic investigation via parasexual techniques (Nüesch *et al.*, 1970). As a genetic system, *C. acremonium* differs from *P. chrysogenum* in several respects. Heterokaryons and diploids are relatively difficult to obtain with *C. acremonium*. Cells of the fungus are characteristically uninucleate, a condition that physically restricts heterokaryosis (Fig. 8a, b). Only a small percentage of cells possess more than one nucleus (Fig. 8c, d). Accordingly, heterokaryons are structurally delimited,

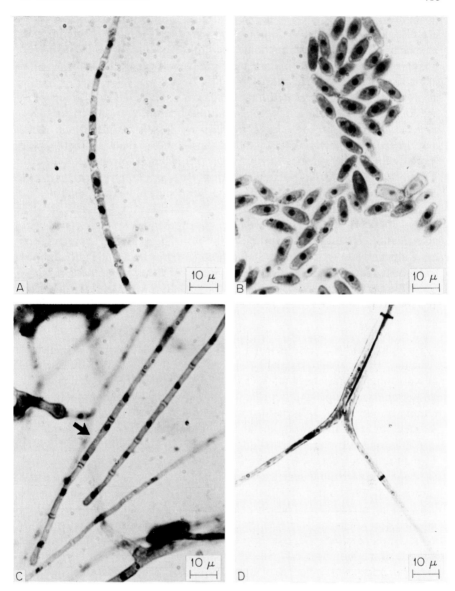

Fig. 8. Cytological aspects of *Cephalosporium*: (A) haploid hypha composed of uninucleate cells, (B) uninucleate conidia, (C) rare binucleate cell (arrow), and (D) cytological
evidence for hyphal anastomosis and heterokaryosis. (Courtesy of H. J. Treichler, CIBA–
Geigy Ltd.)

grow slowly, and are metabolically unbalanced. Diploids of *C. acremonium* are also atypical. Cells of *C. acremonium* are analogous to bacterial cells insofar as they do not accommodate the diploid condition well. Diploid cell lines grow poorly, do not conidiate, but exhibit mitotic segregation for parental as well as recombinant cell lines.

Most species of *Emericellopsis* are similar to *C. acremonium* with regard to the uninucleate condition of vegetative cells (Benson and Grosklags, 1969). *Emericellopsis* differs from *Cephalosporium* by possession of a sexual cycle, and the species of *Emericellopsis* studied thus far are sexually self-compatible (homothallic). The genetics of antibiotic (penicillin N) production by two *Emericellopsis* species has been investigated (Fantini, 1962). Heterokaryosis in *Emericellopsis* was found to be limited in frequency and extent, and meiotic recombination (sexuality) was found to occur rarely.

The β-lactam producing *Streptomyces* are potential systems for genetic investigation of antibiotic synthesis. Streptomycetes are in some respects more amenable to genetic investigation than are imperfect fungi although the techniques required to investigate the genetics of either group have much in common. Sermonti (1969) has reviewed the general genetics of streptomycetes and imperfect fungi.

2. Mutations that Impair the Synthesis of β-Lactam Antibiotics

Penicillin synthesis is at the mercy of the general genetics of *P. chrysogenum* (Bonner, 1946, 1947; Macdonald *et al.*, 1963; Ball, 1971). Biochemical (auxotrophic) mutations, mutations that delete synthesis of essential metabolites, often decrease penicillin synthesis. This is especially true of mutants that require amino acids. In general, mutants that require vitamins or mutants selected for resistance to antimetabolites are not significantly impaired for synthesis of antibiotic (Macdonald *et al.*, 1963; Lemke, 1969; Ball, 1971). Two mutants of *C. acremonium* should be mentioned in this context. A *Cephalosporium* mutant specifically blocked for the formation of sulfide was shown to possess superior potential for synthesis of cephalosporin C in the presence of methionine (Nüesch *et al.*, 1970). A second mutant, a mutant selected for resistance to a specific toxicant, proved to be deregulated for assimilation of sulfate and could synthesize cephalosporin C efficiently in the absence of methionine (H. F. Niss and C. H. Nash, personal communication; U.S. Pat. 3,539,694). Influence of antibiotic synthesis through mutations which affect primary metabolism is well established. In addition, antibiotic synthesis per se is subject to mutation.

Nine mutants of *P. chrysogenum* which were inactive for antibiotic synthesis were studied by Caglioli and Sermonti (1956). All mutants were apparently blocked for penicillin synthesis at the same genetic locus. This was indicated through complementation analysis. Complementation analysis involves the introduction of mutant genotypes into a common cytoplasm (heterokaryon or diploid) in order to test for mutual correction of a lost function by separate genetic deficiencies. Lack of complementation is indicative of common genetic deficiencies. Antibiotic synthesis was not reinstated in diploids formed by pairing the nine penicillin-negative mutants. Sermonti (1956) demonstrated further, again through complementation analysis, that intermediates of penicillin synthesis are intracellular and not diffusible between cell lines. Two mutants, one inactive and one semiactive, were obtained from a parental strain of *Penicillium* fully active for penicillin synthesis. The two mutants, when copropagated as individual cell lines in one medium, remained deficient for antibiotic synthesis. However, complementation, active synthesis of penicillin, occurred in a heterokaryon and a diploid formed from the two mutant cell lines.

Mutants of *C. acremonium* fall into four phenotypic classes based on potential to synthesize antibiotic (Lemke and Nash, 1972). Strains of each class were obtained as products of an extensive industrial strain improvement program and represent mutant survivors of treatment with either ultraviolet light (Stauffer *et al.*, 1966) or *N*-methyl-*N'*-nitro-*N*-nitrosoguanidine (Lemke, 1969). The four mutant classes include: (1) strains with increased potential to synthesize cephalosporin C, (2) strains unable to synthesize antibiotic, (3) strains able to synthesize only penicillin N, and (4) strains able to synthesize a large amount of penicillin N and a trace of 6-aminopenicillanic acid.

Seven mutants of the second class, negative for β-lactam synthesis, have been characterized further. Only one mutant was biochemically deficient (auxotrophic). This mutant required lysine and could synthesize a small amount of antibiotic if grown in the presence of α-aminoadipic acid. The remaining six were prototrophic and were consistently negative for antibiotic synthesis.

Mutants were examined for potential to incorporate either [^{14}C]valine or [^{14}C]-α-aminoadipic acid into sulfur-containing peptides—the peptides implicated as intermediates in the synthesis of β-lactam antibiotics (Abraham *et al.*, 1964). Peptides were isolated according to a procedure developed to extract glutathione from animal cells (Waelsch and Rittenberg, 1941). Two of the six prototrophic mutants did not form intermediate peptides as indicated by an inability to incorporate labeled valine or α-aminoadipic acid into sulfur-containing peptides. Four of the six β-lactam negative strains did accumulate the sulfur-containing peptides. These data indicate that genetic mutations present among the six mutants represent at least two mutations, one that blocks synthesis of intermediate peptides and one that blocks the conversion of peptides into antibiotic. Formation of the intermediate peptides by the lysine auxotroph of *Cephalosporium* proved to be conditional. Intermediate peptides were not formed if this strain was grown in media supplemented by lysine alone. Antibiotic as well as intermediate peptides were formed if the strain was grown in media supplemented with lysine and α-aminoadipic acid. These data provide confirmative evidence that specific peptides are related to the synthesis of antibiotics by *Cephalosporium.*

A thorough biochemical characterization of peptides formed by mutants blocked for the biosynthesis of β-lactam antibiotics is needed. These mutants should also be examined through complementation analysis to test for the conversion of suspected intermediates into antibiotic. Such approaches to biosynthesis, the use of specific mutations and complementation analysis, have been applied extensively and successfully to analyze biosynthetic pathways in other fungi (Yanofsky, 1960; Beadle, 1945; Esser and Kuenen, 1967). These techniques have contributed significantly to our understanding of primary metabolism and will ultimately be brought to bear on problems of secondary metabolism as well.

V. Modification of β-Lactam Antibiotics by Enzymes from *Penicillium* and *Cephalosporium*

The β-lactam compounds are not biologically stable. Several enzymes degrade or modify penicillin and cephalosporin antibiotics. Certain of these enzymes are produced by *Penicillium* and *Cephalosporium*, while others are foreign.

The most destructive of enzymes are bacterial β-lactamases (Abraham and Sabath, 1965; Abraham, 1968), enzymes that hydrolyze the β-lactam ring to yield biologically inactive derivatives of penicillin and cephalosporin (Newton *et al.*, 1968; Hamilton-Miller *et al.*, 1970). The β-lactamases vary in their specificity for penicillin and cephalosporin as substrates (Newton and Abraham, 1956; Crompton *et al.*, 1962; Abraham, 1968). Recently, a fungal "β-lactamase" called arylamidase was isolated from *Cephalosporium* and partially purified (Dennen *et al.*, 1971). Penicillin N as well as a variety of other *N*-acylpenicillins proved to be inert substrates for arylamidase. The enzyme hydrolyzes specifically the β-lactam ring of cephalosporins and could adversely affect the accumulation of cephalosporin C during fermentation.

An enzyme that modifies the D-α-aminoadipyl side chain of cephalosporin C and, presumably also, penicillin N has been reported in a Belgium patent (Belg. Patent 736,934). The enzyme is an unusual D-amino acid oxidase isolated from *Aspergillus flavus*. This enzyme oxidizes the α-amino group of side chain to form an unstable α-iminoadipyl-containing cephalosporin. This intermediate can be readily hydrolyzed to yield cephalosporin with an α-ketoadipyl side chain. This specific enzyme has not been reported from *P. chrysogenum* or *C. acremonium*. However, D-amino acid oxidases from fungi are common, intracellular enzymes which act preferentially on D-monoamino acids.

The acetoxy group of cephalosporin C can be attacked by an acetylesterase from citrus rind (Jeffery *et al.*, 1961). The reaction forms deacetylcephalosporin C. Deacetylcephalosporin C is also present in culture filtrates of *Cephalosporium* and could be derived enzymatically from cephalosporin C. General esterase activity has been detected in numerous species of *Cephalosporium* (Pisano and Capone, 1967) as well as in bacteria and actinomycetes (Demain *et al.*, 1963c).

The cleavage as well as the formation of an amide bond between β-lactam nucleus and various acyl side chains can be brought about enzymatically. The enzymes that catalyze such reactions have been studied extensively and bear several names—"amidase," "acylase," "acyltransferase," etc. (Claridge *et al.*, 1963; Hamilton-Miller, 1966). Recent information concerning these enzymes has made their nomenclatural differentiation obscure, if not meaningless.

A. Acylase and Acyltransferase

For the purpose of the present discussion, it seems useful to group acylating enzymes into two general classes (Fig. 9), acylases and acyltransferases, based upon substrate differences of specific reactions rather than upon classification of the proteins involved. Spencer and Maung (1970) have implied that one protein in *P. chrysogenum* has multiple activities and may catalyze most of the reactions indicated in Fig. 9.

The enzymes reported to cleave penicillins were initially referred to as "amidases" (Murao, 1955). Enzyme preparations were subsequently found that could synthesize penicillins from side-chain precursors and 6-aminopenicillanic acid (Rolinson *et al.*, 1960), and such enzymes were called "acylases." Certain enzymes proved to be reversible (Erickson and Dean, 1966), e.g., to possess "amidase" as well as "acylase" activity. It now appears probable that all penicillin amidases, under certain conditions and with appropriate substrates, are penicillin acylases. To distinguish these enzymes by name would be superfluous. The term "penicillin acylase" is now preferred although it should be emphasized that the hydrolytic potential of these enzymes has thus far proven to be far greater than their synthetic potential.

The term "penicillin acylase" is too restrictive in yet another sense. Enzymes which transfer an acyl side chain from an activated intermediate (e.g., phenylacetyl-CoA) to penicillin nucleus or from one penicillin (phenoxymethylpenicillin) to another penicillin (benzylpenicillin) have been reported (Brunner *et al.*, 1968). These enzymes have been referred to as acyltransferases. It seems plausible that all such enzymatic transacylation would involve activation of the side-chain precursor prior to transfer of the acyl moiety to the amino group of

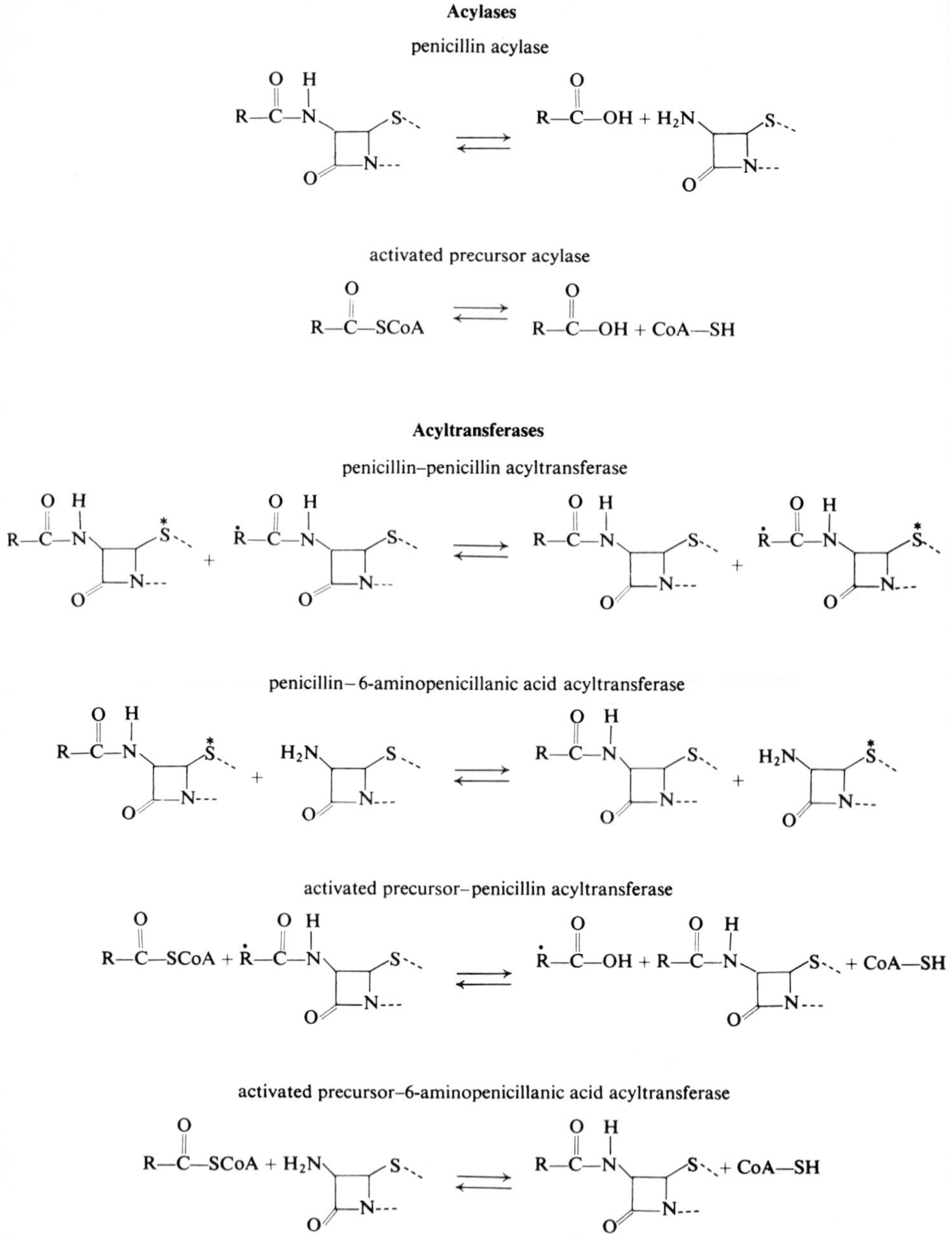

PAUL A. LEMKE AND DONALD R. BRANNON

Acylases

penicillin acylase

activated precursor acylase

$$R-C-SCoA \rightleftharpoons R-C-OH + CoA-SH$$

Acyltransferases

penicillin–penicillin acyltransferase

penicillin–6-aminopenicillanic acid acyltransferase

activated precursor–penicillin acyltransferase

activated precursor–6-aminopenicillanic acid acyltransferase

Fig. 9. Enzymatic activities, real and hypothetical, encompassed by the terms acylase and acyltransferase.

the β-lactam nucleus. Enzymatic hydrolysis of activated precursor, phenyl-acetyl-CoA, has recently been reported (Spencer and Maung, 1970) as an additional activity of an enzyme from *P. chrysogenum*. This enzyme has been termed "activated side chain acylase" (Fig. 9).

1. DISTRIBUTION OF PENICILLIN ACYLASES

All penicillin-producing fungi investigated possess penicillin acylase activity (Cole, 1966a). The first report of penicillin acylase in *P. chrysogenum* (Saka-guchi and Murao, 1950) has been repeatedly confirmed (Erickson and Bennett, 1961, 1965; Murao and Kishida, 1961; Claridge *et al.*, 1963; Erickson and Dean, 1966; Vanderhaeghe *et al.*, 1968). A mutant strain of *Penicillium*, which was unable to produce penicillin, retained the penicillin acylase (Erickson and Bennett, 1965).

Penicillin acylases from microbial sources appear to be of two types (Huang *et al.*, 1963). Type I, also known as phenoxymethylpenicillin acylase, occurs in molds, yeast, and *Streptomyces* and deacylates phenoxymethylpenicillin more efficiently than benzylpenicillin (Batchelor *et al.*, 1961b). Type II, or benzyl-penicillin acylase, occurs in bacteria and in *Nocardia* (Rolinson *et al.*, 1960) and cleaves benzylpenicillin efficiently. This bacterial-type acylase seems to recognize the phenylacetyl moiety readily, as numerous phenylacetyl derivatives other than benzylpenicillin are hydrolyzed by type II enzyme (Rolinson *et al.*, 1960; Cole, 1964, 1966a, c, 1969a, b). *Penicillium* and *Cephalosporium* possess the fungal-type of type I acylase (Hamilton-Miller, 1966). This penicillin acylase appears to be predominantly extracellular (Batchelor *et al.*, 1961b; Cole, 1966a, c).

A difference between penicillin acylase and acyltransferase may be that the latter is primarily an intracellular or cellular dependent form of the former. If true, this would imply that acyltransferase activity is biologically significant only insofar as it may have ability to modify intracellular penicillins. It should be recalled that the principal intracellular penicillins of *Penicillium* are iso-penicillin N and 6-aminopenicillanic acid. Isopenicillin N has not been identified from *Cephalosporium*, and the amount of 6-aminopenicillanic acid produced by this fungus is negligible.

2. SUBSTRATE SPECIFICITY

The significance of the hydrolysis of benzylpenicillin by mycelial extracts of *Penicillium* (Sakaguchi and Murao, 1950) was not fully appreciated until 6-aminopenicillanic acid was identified in fermentation broths of *P. chryso-genum* (Batchelor *et al.*, 1959). The biogenesis of this penicillin compound, once recognized, stimulated the search for other penicillin acylases. These studies were further encouraged by the fact that 6-aminopenicillanic acid proved to be a valuable intermediate for preparation of new penicillins by chemical acylation.

The substrate specificity of penicillin acylases was soon determined. All naturally occurring penicillins, with the exception of isopenicillin N and penicillin N, are now confirmed substrates for penicillin acylase (Hamilton-Miller, 1966).

Soon after the structure of cephalosporin C was determined (Abraham and Newton, 1961), this compound was tested as a substrate for penicillin acylase (Claridge et al., 1963). The results were discouragingly negative but consistent with the observed absence of 7-aminocephalosporanic acid from the *Cephalosporium* fermentation (Ott et al., 1962). Evidence that penicillin acylase was unable to remove the D-α-aminoadipyl moiety from penicillin N had been reported previously (Cole and Rolinson, 1961). These data indicated that penicillin acylases were ineffective where polar acyl side chains were involved. The specificity of penicillin acylases does in fact reside with the *N*-acyl side chain rather than with the β-lactam ring system (Cole, 1964; Kaufmann and Bauer, 1964). Cephalosporin compounds possessing *N*-acyl side chains other than D-α-aminoadipic acid can be chemically prepared, and these are hydrolyzed by acylases as are their corresponding penicillin analogs (Huang et al., 1963).

The substrate specificity of penicillin acylase from *P. chrysogenum* has been given particular attention. Phenoxymethylpenicillin is a better substrate for this acylase than is benzylpenicillin, and enzyme activity favors nonpolar side chains of moderate length (Claridge et al., 1963).

Several laboratories have searched for an acylase to cleave the native D-α-aminoadipyl side chain from penicillin N and cephalosporin C (Demain et al., 1963c; Nüesch et al., 1967). Only one laboratory has claimed to be successful. Walton (1964) developed an enrichment technique to screen for microorganisms able to hydrolyze *N*-adipyl-*p*-nitroaniline. An *Achromobacterium* sp. was found that could apparently deacylate both penicillin N and cephalosporin C. These antibiotics, when incubated in the presence of the *Achromobacterium* culture, were converted, respectively, into 6-aminopenicillanic acid and 7-aminodeacetylcephalosporanic acid. The *Achromobacterium* sp. appeared to possess an acetylesterase in addition to a unique penicillin acylase. The yield of β-lactam nucleus was not reported by Walton (1964), but his results were subsequently patented (U.S. Patent 3,239,394).

Penicillin acylase activity in *Cephalosporium*, comparable to acylase activity in *Penicillium*, has been reported (Cole and Rolinson, 1961; Cole, 1966a). The enzyme derived from *Cephalosporium* will not deacylate penicillin N or cephalosporin C, nor will it cleave the α-aminoadipyl moiety from a synthetic tripeptide, L-α-aminoadipyl-L-cysteinyl-L-valine (Loder et al., 1969). The enzyme did cleave two polar dipeptides, α-aminoadipylcysteine and glutamylcysteine, and exhibited greater specificity for the L-α-aminoadipyl and L-glutamyl isomers of the dipeptides.

According to Vanderhaeghe *et al.* (1968), penicillin acylase from *P. chrysogenum* did not deacylate a standard of isopenicillin N. This result is especially noteworthy since isopenicillin N has been implicated as the essential intermediate in the synthesis of all penicillins and 6-aminopenicillanic acid (Demain, 1963a, 1966a). Perhaps only intracellular isopenicillin N, either in an activated form or as some bound derivative, can be deacylated or transacylated by enzyme.

3. BIOSYNTHETIC POTENTIAL

The ability of a penicillin acylase to "synthesize" an *N*-acylpenicillin from 6-aminopenicillanic acid and a carboxylic acid was first demonstrated with enzyme preparations from *Escherichia coli* (Rolinson *et al.*, 1960; Kaufmann *et al.*, 1961; Szentrimai, 1966). This bacterial penicillin acylase, at pH 4.5, effectively reconstructed hydrolyzed benzylpenicillin. The synthetic potential of this enzyme for certain other penicillins, however, was relatively poor (Kaufmann *et al.*, 1961).

Penicillin acylase activity from *Streptomyces lavendulae* (Batchelor *et al.*, 1961b) and from *Alcaligenes faecalis* (Claridge *et al.*, 1960) subsequently proved to be reversible (Erickson and Dean, 1966). In general, the specificity of reverse reactions are identical with that of the hydrolytic reactions.

According to Kaufmann *et al.* (1961), enzymatic synthesis of benzylpenicillin and phenoxymethylpenicillin could be accelerated by the presence of "activated" side-chain precursors. Phenylacetylglycine and phenoxyacetylglutamate were more effective precursors, respectively, for benzylpenicillin and phenoxymethylpenicillin than were phenylacetic acid and phenoxyacetic acid. These data suggested that a transfer reaction involving energy-rich side-chain precursors might be responsible for the enzymatic acylation of 6-aminopenicillanic acid.

The reversibility of penicillin acylase in *P. chrysogenum* was postulated (Cole, 1966a) and confirmed (Erickson and Dean, 1966). Even a mutant *Penicillium*, a strain unable to synthesize penicillin, was able to acylate enzymatically a standard of 6-aminopenicillanic acid (Erickson and Dean, 1966). According to Cole (1966a), acylases from both *Penicillium* and *Cephalosporium* are largely extracellular and have limited biosynthetic potential.

Although certain of the natural penicillins have been prepared by the acylase activity of enzymes from *P. chrysogenum*, neither isopenicillin N nor penicillin N has been synthesized by enzymatic acylation of 6-aminopenicillanic acid with α-aminoadipic acid. Ballio *et al.* (1960) tested several dicarboxylic acids as side-chain precursors for acylase. Adipic acid in the presence of 6-aminopenicillanic acid and enzyme gave 4-carboxy-*n*-butylpenicillin.

424   PAUL A. LEMKE AND DONALD R. BRANNON

Brunner (1963) has suggested a requirement for activation of side-chain precursors by coenzyme A. In 1968, Brunner and co-workers reported an acyltransferase from *P. chrysogenum* that transferred phenylacetyl-CoA to 6-aminopenicillanic acid, e.g., activated precursor-6-aminopenicillanic acid acyltransferase (Fig. 9). These workers also found a coenzyme A ligase, an enzyme that could generate an acyl-coenzyme A derivative of free carboxylic acids. This is the enzyme termed "activated side-chain acylase" (Fig. 9).

Two additional reports appeared in 1968 concerning transacylation of activated precursors with 6-aminopenicillanic acid by an enzyme from *P. chrysogenum*. In one report (Gatenbeck and Brunsberg, 1968), the precursors were coenzyme A derivatives of phenylacetic acid, *p*-methoxyphenylacetic acid, phenoxyacetic acid, and octanoylacetic acid. All were substrates for acyl-transferase in the presence of 6-aminopenicillanic acid. The enzyme preparation used did not deacylate benzylpenicillin. In a second report (Spencer, 1968) phenylacetyl-CoA was enzymatically transacylated with [35S]-6-amino-penicillanic acid to form [35S]benzylpenicillin. The acyltransferase tested by Spencer (1968) was specific for the thiol-ester-activated coenzyme A derivative of precursor. Free phenylacetic acid, as well as conjugated phenylacetyl-phosphate, phenylacetyladenylate, and phenylacetylglycine, were all inert substrates for enzyme. Penicillamine, 7-aminocephalosporanic acid, 7-amino-deacetylcephalosporanic acid, and several peptides were all inactive as acyl acceptor substrates from a phenylacetyl-CoA donor.

An acyltransferase from *P. chrysogenum*, able to catalyze the exchange of *N*-acyl groups between benzylpenicillin and phenoxymethylpenicillin, was reported by Peterson and Wideburg (1960). Observation of this penicillin–penicillin acyltransferase (Fig. 9) was confirmed by Pruess and Johnson (1967). These authors demonstrated that an enzyme purified with calcium phosphate gel could catalyze acyltransfer not only between [35S]benzyl-penicillin and phenoxymethylpenicillin, but also between [35S]benzylpenicillin and 6-aminopenicillanic acid, e.g., penicillin-6-aminopenicillanic acid acyl-transferase (Fig. 9). Moreover, phenoxymethylpenicillin, heptylpenicillin, *p*-hydroxybenzylpenicillin, and amylpenicillin exchanged their respective side chains with [35S]-6-aminopenicillanic acid in the presence of enzyme. Penicillin N, methylpenicillin, and phenylpenicillin did not undergo acyltransfer with [35S]-6-aminopenicillanic acid. The enzyme did not deacylate penicillins to form 6-aminopenicillanic acid and side-chain acids.

Spencer (1968) further purified acyltransferase from *Penicillium* and demonstrated transfer of acyl groups from activated coenzyme A precursors to 6-aminopenicillanic acid, e.g., activated precursor-6-aminopenicillanic acid acyltransferase. Spencer did not observe penicillin acylase activity with purified acyltransferase in this instance.

Spencer and Maung (1970) subsequently reported that purified acyltransferase from *Penicillium* has multiple activities, that of penicillin–penicillin acyltransferase, activated precursor-6-aminopenicillanic acid acyltransferase, penicillin acylase, and activated precursor acylase, e.g., hydrolysis of phenyl-acetyl-coenzyme A.

Several critical experiments are now indicated regarding the role of acyl-transferase in the synthesis of β-lactam antibiotics. Does *Cephalosporium* possess an acyltransferase comparable to that of *Penicillium*? Are the terms "penicillin acylase" and "acyltransferase" synonyms for one protein in any system? Is isopenicillin N or isocephalosporin C a substrate for acyltransferase in either *Penicillium* or *Cephalosporium*? These compounds are hypothetical intermediates for synthesis of all other biosynthetic β-lactam compounds (Demain, 1966a; Abraham and Newton, 1967). There have been no reports to indicate efficient displacement of the L-α-aminoadipyl moiety of these anti-biotics in the presence of purified acyltransferase.

Loder and Abraham (personal communication) have tested standards of isopenicillin N and isocephalosporin C as substrates for an activated precursor-penicillin acyltransferase in *Penicillium*. Standards were combined with mycelial extracts in the presence of [^{14}C]phenylacetyl]-CoA. Isopenicillin N was apparently involved in an acyltransferase reaction since [^{14}C]benzyl-penicillin was formed in this complex reaction mixture. Isocephalosporin C did not react in this system.

B. Acetylesterase

Deacetylcephalosporin C is present in culture filtrates of *Cephalosporium* (Jeffery *et al.*, 1961). It is not known if this compound is an intermediate of cephalosporin C biosynthesis or merely a degraded form of cephalosporin C. Demain (1963a, 1966a) has suggested that deacetylcephalosporin C is an intermediate in cephalosporin C biosynthesis. Abraham (1962) earlier proposed that deacetylcephalosporin C might arise during fermentation from enzymatic deacetylation of cephalosporin C.

Addition of DL-[1-^{14}C]valine to *Cephalosporium* (Abraham *et al.*, 1965) resulted in radioactivity appearing in cephalosporin C prior to deacetyl-cephalosporin C. These results suggest that biosynthesis of cephalosporin C precedes that of a deacetyl derivative. Conceivably, the introduction of the acetyl of cephalosporin C would occur early, during cyclization, by transfer of an acetyl group from an S-acetyl precursor (Abraham *et al.*, 1965). Isotopic carbon from acetate does precurse cephalosporin C at the acetoxy position (Trown *et al.*, 1962; Neuss *et al.*, 1971), but the actual mechanism for this incorporation is unknown.

Label from DL-[1-^{14}C]valine was incorporated by resting cells of *C. acremonium* into both deacetylcephalosporin C and cephalosporin C (Abraham *et al.*, 1964), and the apparent ratio of label between deacetylcephalosporin C and cephalosporin C was higher initially than it was subsequently. This could indicate that deacetylcephalosporin C is converted to cephalosporin C.

Huber and co-workers (1968) examined the formation of deacetylcephalosporin C in *Cephalosporium* fermentation broth and concluded that it was formed by nonenzymatic hydrolysis of cephalosporin C. Rate constants for the deacetylation of cephalosporin C were identical in fermentation medium, either in the presence or absence of *Cephalosporium* cells.

An esterase which deacetylated *p*-nitrophenylacetate was detected in cellular extracts of *Cephalosporium* (Huber *et al.*, 1968). Deacetylation of cephalosporin C was not specifically measured with the intracellular extract. However, no inhibition of the hydrolysis of *p*-nitrophenylacetate was observed in the presence of cephalosporin C. Ethyl acetate decreased enzymatic hydrolysis of *p*-nitrophenylacetate as much as 61 %. The conclusion drawn was that cephalosporin C did not competitively inhibit the activity of this intracellular esterase and should not be regarded as a substrate.

Data to indicate the biosynthetic origin of deacetylcephalosporin C are ambivalent. The possibility remains that deacetylcephalosporin C is an intracellular precursor of cephalosporin C, rapidly acetylated without accumulation or release from the cell. The deacetylcephalosporin C present in broth might then be derived secondarily via chemical hydrolysis of preformed cephalosporin C. Enzymatic acetylation of deacetylcephalosporin C has not been reported.

Pisano and Capone (1967) found that mycelial extracts from 12 species of *Cephalosporium* possessed esterase activity with triacetin as substrate. Cephalosporin C was not tested as a substrate for this esterase activity. Esterases that will deacetylate cephalosporin C are ubiquitous and have been found in many nonfungal sources: citrus (Jeffery *et al.*, 1961), bacteria and actinomycetes (Demain *et al.*, 1963c), wheat germ (Belgian Patent 671,692), and animal tissue (O'Callaghan and Muggleton, 1963).

C. Arylamidase

An enzyme with cephalosporinase-like activity has been isolated from *Cephalosporium* (Dennen *et al.*, 1971). The enzyme arylamidase selectively destroys the antibacterial activity of cephalosporin compounds. Purification by DEAE-cellulose chromatography, gel filtration, and gel electrophoresis gave three aggregational forms of the enzyme. Hydrolysis of L-leucyl-β-naphthylamide by enzyme proceeded with a K_m of 4.2×10^{-4} M and was noncompetitively inhibited by cephalosporins. A variety of penicillins did not inhibit enzyme activity. The enzyme hydrolyzed the β-lactam ring of several cephalosporins, and the K_m for cephalosporin C was 9.09×10^{-4} M. Aryl-amidases may not severely affect the accretion of cephalosporin C during fermentation but could contribute to degradation of antibiotic in broth following fermentation.

It is a reflection upon the status of our knowledge concerning β-lactam biosynthesis that considerably more is known about enzymes that degrade these compounds than about biosynthetic enzymes.

VI. Conclusions

The pathway for biosynthesis of β-lactam antibiotics is a well-kept biological secret. Enzymatic formation of the four-membered β-lactam ring is without precedent. The suspected intermediates for *Penicillium*-type biosynthesis, tripeptide and isopenicillin N, have traditionally been inert substrates for penicillin acylase and acyltransferase, enzymes that would explain the origin of 6-aminopenicillanic acid and other penicillins from a common intermediate. Isopenicillin N in the presence of activated precursor has only recently proven to be a substrate for acyltransferase activity in *Penicillium*. This result is quite significant. It endorses isopenicillin N as a pivotal intermediate of penicillin biosynthesis and is consistent with the biochemical and genetic evidence that α-aminoadipic acid is required for biosynthesis of all β-lactam antibiotics.

The biosynthesis of *Cephalosporium*-type compounds is rather obscure. The origin and invariability of the D-α-aminoadipyl side chain of these antibiotics is unreconciled. A racemase able to convert isopenicillin N to penicillin N has been postulated, but neither this enzyme nor its substrate has been demonstrated in *Cephalosporium*. The synthesis of the cephalosporin ring system by ring-expansion of penicillin has been accomplished chemically. It would thus appear that the origin of cephalosporin C from preformed penicillin N is at least mechanistically feasible, although this conversion by enzyme is again without precedent.

There is convincing evidence that three primary amino acids, L-α-amino-adipic acid, L-cysteine, and L-valine, as well as an extended series of carboxylic acids can be incorporated more or less directly into penicillin formed by *Penicillium* (Fig. 10). There is correspondingly good evidence that the same three primary amino acids are ingredients for β-lactam antibiotics produced by *Cephalosporium* (Fig. 11). These data characterize the study of β-lactam biosynthesis during the past 25 years and, in essence, corroborate the tripeptide theory.

Tripeptide theory is attractive, but the evidence for it is still circumstantial. There is no direct evidence for conversion of tripeptide, substituted tripeptide, or any monocyclic derivatives of tripeptide into antibiotic. These compounds are

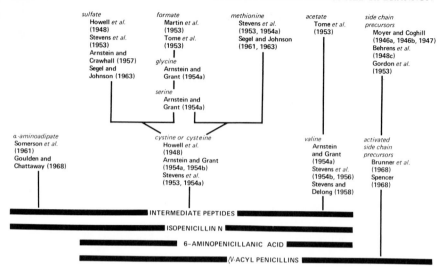

Fig. 10. Investigations on the biosynthesis of *Penicillium*-type antibiotics.

the suspected intermediates of β-lactam biosynthesis. Impermeability of cells to such intermediates has discouraged conversion testing. There is no indication that intact cells will take up an intermediate any more sophisticated than a polar dipeptide, and even these dipeptides are subject to substantial hydrolysis and turnover by cells. Studies involving incorporation of label into antibiotic by intact cells have apparently reached the point of diminishing return.

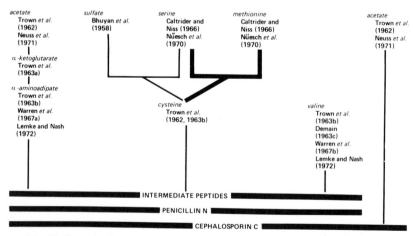

Fig. 11. Investigations on the biosynthesis of *Cephalosporium*-type antibiotics.

Cell-free synthesis of tripeptide δ(α-aminoadipyl)cysteinylvaline has been accomplished with mycelial extracts of *Penicillium* and *Cephalosporium*. However, cell-free enzyme preparations have not yet been devised that unequivocally demonstrate *de novo* synthesis of antibiotic. Initial attempts to obtain cell-free synthesis indicate a requirement for particulate or cellular substructure. Competence to produce antibiotic may even be dependent upon whole-cell machinery. Appropriate configuration of intermediates as well as the correct conformation of relevant enzymes may depend upon cellular integrity. There is no assurance that a cell-free system will reconstruct the pathway of β-lactam biosynthesis.

Biosynthesis can be studied critically in intact cells with the aid of genetic methods. It is regrettable that these genetic techniques have not been extensively applied to the task of elucidating biosynthesis of β-lactam antibiotics. Both *Penicillium* and *Cephalosporium* have been adapted for formal genetic studies, and mutations that impair the synthesis of antibiotics are obtainable in both systems. Such mutants should be extensively characterized for accumulation of suspected intermediates. Studies involving complementation analysis among impotent mutants should reveal if suspected intermediates of β-lactam biosynthesis are real.

Penicillin N and cephalosporin compounds are now recognized as products of prokaryotic organisms, *Streptomyces* species. These organisms have a simpler degree of cellular organization and may be more amenable for study of antibiotic biosynthesis. The presence of β-lactam antibiotics in streptomycetes is anomalous on two accounts. First, formation of these antibacterial compounds by filamentous bacteria is difficult to reconcile, especially since the general cell-wall chemistry of streptomycetes resembles that of gram-positive bacteria. Secondly, the presence of α-aminoadipic acid in products of a streptomycete is an enigma. This amino acid is not a recognized metabolite of prokaryotic cells.

Both *Penicillium* and *Cephalosporium* harbor mycophages, double-stranded ribonucleic acid viruses that may profoundly influence the synthesis of β-lactam antibiotics. Future studies concerning these organisms will surely decipher any relevance of mycophage to antibiotic synthesis.

Alteration of regulatory mechanisms has been shown to influence antibiotic synthesis by *Penicillium* and *Cephalosporium*. Perhaps it can be suggested that antibiotics are formed in response to deregulation of primary metabolism. Secondary metabolites, in general, may be compensatory metabolites, compounds invoked to accommodate deranged regulation. One thing is certain. We can truly claim to understand primary metabolism only when we understand secondary metabolism.

"We have not yet exhausted a consideration of the products of Brotzu's mould ... [Florey, 1955]."

430   PAUL A. LEMKE AND DONALD R. BRANNON

References

Abelson, P. H., and Vogel, H. J. (1955). *Biol. Chem.* **213**, 355.

Abraham, E. P. (1957). "Biochemistry of Some Peptide and Steroid Antibiotics," p. 33. Wiley, New York.

Abraham, E. P. (1962). *Pharmacol. Rev.* **14**, 473.

Abraham, E. P. (1968). *In* "Topics in Pharmaceutical Sciences" (D. Perlman, ed.), pp. 1–31. Wiley (Interscience), New York.

Abraham, E. P., and Newton, G. G. F. (1954). *Biochem. J.* **58**, 266.

Abraham, E. P., and Newton, G. G. F. (1961). *Biochem. J.* **79**, 377.

Abraham, E. P., and Newton, G. G. F. (1965). *Advan. Chemother.* **2**, 23.

Abraham, E. P., and Newton, G. G. F. (1967). *In* "Antibiotics" (D. Gottlieb and P. D. Shaw, eds.), Vol. 2, pp. 1–16. Springer-Verlag, New York.

Abraham, E. P., and Sabath, L. D. (1965). *Enzymologia* **29**, 221.

Abraham, E. P., Newton, G. G. F., Crawford, K., Burton, H. S., and Hale, C. W. (1953). *Nature* **71**, 343.

Abraham, E. P., Newton, G. G. F., and Hale, C. W. (1954). *Biochem. J.* **58**, 94.

Abraham, E. P., Olson, B. H., Newton, G. G. F., Schuurmans, D. M., Schenck, J. R., Fisher, M. W., Hargie, M. P., and Fusari, S. A. (1955). *Nature* **176**, 551.

Abraham, E. P., Newton, G. G. F., and Warren, S. C. (1964). *IAM Symp. Appl. Microbiol. Tokyo* **6**, 79.

Abraham, E. P., Newton, G. G. F., and Warren, S. C. (1965). *In* "Biogenesis of Antibiotic Substances" (Z. Vanek and Z. Hostalek, eds.), pp. 169–194. Academic Press, New York.

Ainsworth, G. C., and Sussman, A. S. (1965). "The Fungi." Academic Press, New York.

Applegarth, D. A. (1967). *Arch. Biochem. Biophys.* **120**, 471.

Arnstein, H. R. V. (1958). *Ann. Rep. Prog. Chem.* **54**, 339.

Arnstein, H. R. V., and Clubb, M. E. (1957). *Biochem. J.* **65**, 618.

Arnstein, H. R. V., and Clubb, M. E. (1958). *Biochem. J.* **68**, 528.

Arnstein, H. R. V., and Crawhall, J. C. (1957). *Biochem. J.* **67**, 180.

Arnstein, H. R. V., and Grant, P. T. (1954a). *Biochem. J.* **57**, 353.

Arnstein, H. R. V., and Grant, P. T. (1954b). *Biochem. J.* **57**, 360.

Arnstein, H. R. V., and Grant, P. T. (1956). *Bacteriol. Rev.* **20**, 133.

Arnstein, H. R. V., and Margreiter, H. (1958). *Biochem. J.* **68**, 339.

Arnstein, H. R. V., and Morris, D. (1960a). *Biochem. J.* **76**, 318.

Arnstein, H. R. V., and Morris, D. (1960b). *Biochem. J.* **76**, 323.

Arnstein, H. R. V., and Morris, D. (1960c). *Biochem. J.* **76**, 357.

Arnstein, H. R. V., Morris, D., and Toms, E. J. (1959). *Biochim. Biophys. Acta* **35**, 561.

Arnstein, H. R. V., Artman, N., Morris, D., and Toms, E. J. (1960). *Biochem. J.* **76**, 353.

Aspen, A. J., and Meister, A. (1962). *Biochemistry* **1**, 606.

Auden, J. A., Gruner, J., Liersch, M., and Nüesch, J. (1969). *Pathol. Microbiol.* **34**, 240.

Aurich, H. (1966). *Wiss. Z. Karl. Marz Univ. Leipzig. Math. Naturwiss. Reihe* **15**, 359.

Azevedo, J. L., and Roper, J. A. (1970). *Genet. Res.* **16**, 79.

Backus, M. P., and Stauffer, J. F. (1955). *Mycologia* **47**, 429.

Baird, B. M., Halsall, T. G., Jones, E. R. H., and Lowe, G. (1961). *Proc. Chem. Soc.* 257.

Ball, C. (1969). *Heredity* **24**, 691.

Ball, C. (1970). *Int. Symp. Genet. Ind. Microorgan., 1st, Abstr., Prague,* 1970, 178.

Ball, C. (1971). *J. Gen. Microbiol.* **66**, 63.

Ballio, A., Chain, E. B., Dentice Di Accadia, F., Mastropietro-Cancellieri, M. F., Morpurgo, G., Serlupi-Crescenzi, G., and Sermonti, G. (1960). *Nature* **185**, 97.

Ballio, A., Chain, E. B., Dentice Di Accadia, F., Mauri, M., Rauer, K., Schlesinger, M. J., and Schlesinger, S. (1961). *Nature* **191**, 909.

Banks, G. T., Buck, K. W., Chain, E. B., Dearbyshire, J. E., and Himmelweit, F. (1969). *Nature* **222**, 89.

Bartnicki-Garcia, S. (1969). *Phytopathology* **59**, 1065.

Batchelor, F. R., Doyle, F. P., Nayler, J. H. C., and Rolinson, G. N. (1959). *Nature* **183**, 257.

Batchelor, F. R., Chain, E. B., and Rolinson, G. N. (1961a). *Proc. Roy. Soc.* **B154**, 478.

Batchelor, F. R., Chain, E. B., Richards, M., and Rolinson, G. N. (1961b). *Proc. Roy. Soc.* **B154**, 522.

Batchelor, F. R., Gazzard, D., and Nayler, J. H. C. (1961c). *Nature* **191**, 910.

Bauer, K. (1970). *Z. Naturforsch.* **25**, 1125.

Beadle, G. W. (1945). *Chem. Rev.* **37**, 15.

Behrens, O. K. (1949). *In* "The Chemistry of Penicillin" (H. T. Clarke, J. R. Johnson, and R. Robinson, eds.), pp. 657–679. Princeton Univ. Press, Princeton, New Jersey.

Behrens, O. K., Corse, J., Jones, R. G., Mann, M. J., Soper, Q. F., Van Abeele, F. R., and Chiang, M. (1948a). *J. Biol. Chem.* **175**, 751.

Behrens, O. K., Corse, J., Edwards, J. P., Garrison, L., Jones, R. G., Soper, Q. F., Van Abeele, F. R., and Whitehead, C. W. (1948b). *J. Biol. Chem.* **175**, 793.

Behrens, O. K., Corse, J., Jones, R. G., Kleiderer, E. C., Soper, Q. F., Van Abeele, F. R. Larson, L. M., Sylvester, J. C., Haines, W. J., and Carter, H. E. (1948c). *J. Biol. Chem.* **175**, 765.

Belgium Patent 671,692.

Belgium Patent 736,934.

Benko, P. V., Wood, T. C., and Segel, I. H. (1967). *Arch. Biochem. Biophys.* **122**, 783.

Benson, B. W., and Grosklags, J. H. (1969). *Mycologia* **61**, 718.

Benz, F., Liersch, M., Nüesch, J., and Treichler, H. J. (1971). *Eur. J. Biochem.* **20**, 81.

Betterton, H., Fjellstedt, T., Matsuda, M., Ogur, M., and Tate, R. (1968). *Biochim. Biophys. Acta* **170**, 459.

Bhuyan, B. K., and Johnson, M. J. (1958). *J. Bacteriol.* **76**, 376.

Bhuyan, B. K., Mohberg, J., and Johnson, M. J. (1958). *J. Bacteriol.* **76**, 393.

Birch, A. J., and Smith, H. (1958). *In* "Amino Acids and Peptides with Antimetabolite Activity" (Ciba Foundation Symposium), p. 247. Churchill, London.

Bodanszky, M., and Perlman, D. (1968). *Antimicrob. Ag. Chemother.* **1967**, 464.

Bodanszky, M., and Perlman, D. (1969). *Science* **163**, 352.

Bodanszky, M., and Perlman, D. (1971). *Ann. Rev. Biochem.* **40**, 449.

Bonner, D. (1946). *Amer. J. Bot.* **33**, 788.

Bonner, D. (1947). *Arch. Biochem.* **13**, 1.

Brandl, E., Giovannini, M., and Margreiter, H. (1953). *Wien. Med. Wochschr.* **193**, 602.

Brotzu, G. (1948). *Lavori dell'istituto D'Igiene di Cagliari.*

Brunner, R. (1963). *Med. Welt.* 29.

Brunner, R., Rohr, M., and Zinner, M. (1968). *Z. Physiol. Chem.* **349**, 95.

Burton, H. S., and Abraham, E. P. (1951). *Biochem. J.* **50**, 168.

Burton, K. (1951). *Biochem. J.* **50**, 258.

Caglioli, M. T., and Sermonti, G. (1956). *J. Gen. Microbiol.* **14**, 38.

Caltrider, P. G., and Niss, H. F. (1966). *Appl. Microbiol.* **14**, 746.

Caltrider, P. G., Huber, F. M., and Day, L. E. (1968). *Appl. Microbiol.* **16**, 1913.

Calvert, A. F., and Rodwell, U. W. (1966). *J. Biol. Chem.* **241**, 409.

Charles, H. P., and Knight, B. C. J. G. (eds.). (1970). "Symp. Soc. Gen. Microbiol.," No. 20. Cambridge Univ. Press, London and New York.

Chen, S. S., and Duerre, J. A. (1970). *Bacteriol. Proc.* 142.

Chou, T. S., Eisenbraun, E. J., and Rapala, R. T. (1967). *Tetrahedron Lett.* 409.
Claridge, C. A., Gourevitch, A., and Lein, J. (1960). *Nature* 187, 237.
Claridge, C. A., Luttinger, J. R., and Lein, J. (1963). *Proc. Soc. Exp. Biol. Med.* 113, 1008.
Cocker, J. D., Cowley, B. R., Cox, J. S. G., Eardley, S., Gregory, G., Lazenby, J. K., Long, A. G., Sey, J. C. P., and Somerfield, G. A. (1965). *J. Chem. Soc.* 922, 5015.
Cohen, S. S. (1970). *Amer. Sci.* 58, 281.
Cole, M. (1964). *Nature* 203, 519.
Cole, M. (1966a). *Appl. Microbiol.* 14, 98.
Cole, M. (1966b). *Process Biochem.* 1, 334.
Cole, M. (1966c). *Process Biochem.* 1, 373.
Cole, M. (1969a). *Biochem. J.* 115, 733.
Cole, M. (1969b). *Biochem. J.* 115, 747.
Cole, M. (1969c). *Biochem. J.* 115, 757.
Cole, M., and Batchelor, F. R. (1963). *Nature* 198, 383.
Cole, M., and Rolinson, G. N. (1961). *Proc. Roy. Soc.* B154, 490.
Cooper, R. D. G., and José, F. L. (1972). *J. Amer. Chem. Soc.* 94, 1021.
Crawford, K., Heatley, N. G., Boyd, P. F., Hale, C. W., Kelley, B. K., Miller, G. A., and Smith, N. (1952). *J. Gen. Microbiol.* 6, 47.
Crompton, G., Jago, M., Crawford, K., Newton, G. G. F., and Abraham, E. P. (1962). *Biochem. J.* 83, 52.
Davey, V. F., and Johnson, M. J. (1953). *Appl. Microbiol.* 1, 208.
Day, L. E., and Ellis, L. F. (1971). *J. Appl. Microbiol.* 22, 919.
Delavier-Klutchko, C., and Flavin, M. (1965). *J. Biol. Chem.* 240, 2537.
Demain, A. L. (1956). *Arch. Biochem. Biophys.* 64, 74.
Demain, A. L. (1957a). *Arch. Biochem. Biophys.* 67, 244.
Demain, A. L. (1957b). *Antibiot. Chemother.* 7, 359.
Demain, A. L. (1959). *Advan. Appl. Microbiol.* 1, 23.
Demain, A. L. (1963a). *Trans. N.Y. Acad. Sci. II* 25, 731.
Demain, A. L. (1963b). *Clid. Med.* 70, 2045.
Demain, A. L. (1963c). *Biochem. Biophys. Res. Commun.* 10, 45.
Demain, A. L. (1966a). *In* "Biosynthesis of Antibiotics" (J. F. Snell, ed.), Vol. I, pp. 29–94. Academic Press, New York and London.
Demain, A. L. (1966b). *Advan. Appl. Microbiol.* 8, 1.
Demain, A. L., and Newkirk, J. F. (1962). *Appl. Microbiol.* 10, 321.
Demain, A. L., Newkirk, J. F., and Hendlin, D. (1963a). *J. Bacteriol.* 85, 339.
Demain, A. L., Newkirk, J. F., Davis, G. E., and Harman, R. E. (1963b). *Appl. Microbiol.* 11, 58.
Demain, A. L., Walton, R. B., Newkirk, J. F., and Miller, I. M. (1963c). *Nature* 199, 909.
Dennen, D. W. (1967). *J. Pharm. Sci.* 56, 1273.
Dennen, D. W., and Carver, D. D. (1969). *Can. J. Microbiol.* 15, 175.
Dennen, D. W., Allen, C. C., and Carver, D. D. (1971). *J. Appl. Microbiol.* 21, 907.
Dodge, C. W. (1935). "Medical Mycology," p. 705. Mosby, St. Louis, Missouri.
Dulaney, E. L. (1947). *Mycologia* 39, 570.
Elander, R. P. (1967). *In* "Induced Mutations and Their Utilizations" (H. Stubbe, ed.), pp. 403–423. Academic-Verlag, Berlin.
Elander, R. P., Stauffer, J. F., and Backus, M. P. (1961). *In* "Antimicrobial Agents Annual–1960" (P. Gray, B. Tabenkin, and S. G. Bradley, eds.), pp. 91–102. Plenum Press, New York.
Elander, R. P., Espenshade, M. A., Pathak, S. G., and Pan, C. H. (1970). *Int. Symp. Genet. Ind. Microorgan., 1st, Abstr., Prague, 1970*, 180.

Ellis, L. F., and Kleinschmidt, W. J. (1967). *Nature* **215**, 649.
Emerson, R. L., Puziss, M., and Knight, S. G. (1950). *Arch. Biochem. Biophys.* **25**, 299.
Erickson, R. C., and Bennett, R. E. (1961). *Bacteriol. Proc.* 65.
Erickson, R. C., and Bennett, R. E. (1965). *Appl. Microbiol.* **13**, 738.
Erickson, R. C., and Dean, L. D. (1966). *Appl. Microbiol.* **14**, 1047.
Esser, K., and Kuenen, R. (1967). "Genetics of Fungi." Springer-Verlag, Berlin.
Fantini, A. A. (1962). *Genetics* **47**, 161.
Feren, C. J., and Squires, R. W. (1969). *Biotech. Bioeng.* **11**, 583.
Flavin, M., and Slaughter, C. (1964). *J. Biol. Chem.* **239**, 2212.
Flavin, M., and Slaughter, C. (1967). *Biochim. Biophys. Acta* **132**, 406.
Fleming, A. (1929). *Brit. J. Exp. Pathol.* **10**, 226.
Florey, H. W. (1955). *Ann. Int. Med.* **43**, 480.
Florey, H. W., Chain, E. B., Heatley, N. G., Jennings, M. A., Sanders, A. G., Abraham, E. P., and Florey, M. E. (1949). "Antibiotics," Vol. 2. Oxford Univ. Press, London and New York.
Flynn, E. H., McCormick, M. H., Stamper, M. C., De Valeria, H., and Godzeski, C. W. (1962). *J. Amer. Chem. Soc.* **84**, 4594.
Foster, J. W., and Karow, E. O. (1945). *J. Bacteriol.* **49**, 19.
Fusari, S. A., and Machamer, H. E. (1958). In "Antibiotics Annual–1957–58" (H. Welch and F. Marti-Ibanez, eds.), pp. 529–537. Medical Encyclopedia, New York.
Fuska, J., and Welwardová, E. (1969). *Chem. Zvesti* **23**, 704.
Gams, W. (1971). "*Cephalosporium*—artige Schimmelpilze, Hyphomycetes." Fisher-Verlag, Stuttgart, Germany.
Gatenbeck, S., and Brunsberg, U. (1968). *Acta Chem. Scand.* **22**, 1059.
Gordon, M., Pan, S. C., Virgona, A., and Numerof, P. (1953). *Science* **118**, 43.
Gottshall, R. Y., Roberts, J. M., Portwood, L. M., and Jennings, J. C. (1951). *Proc. Soc. Exp. Biol. Med.* **76**, 307.
Goulden, S. A., and Chattaway, F. W. (1968). *Biochem. J.* **110**, 55P.
Goulden, S. A., and Chattaway, F. W. (1969). *J. Gen. Microbiol.* **59**, 111.
Great Britain Patent 759,624.
Grosklags, J. H., and Swift, M. E. (1957). *Mycologia* **49**, 305.
Hamilton-Miller, J. M. T. (1966). *Bacteriol. Rev.* **30**, 161.
Hamilton-Miller, J. M. T., Richards, E., and Abraham, E. P. (1970). *Biochem. J.* **116**, 385.
Harada, J., and Spencer, B. (1962). *Biochem. J.* **82**, 148.
Hardcastle, Jr., G. A., and Johnson, D.A. (1961). *J. Amer. Chem. Soc.* **83**, 3534.
Harvey, C. L., and Olson, B. H. (1958). *Appl. Microbiol.* **6**, 276.
Heusler, K. (1968). In "Topics in Pharmaceutical Sciences" (D. Perlman, ed.), Vol. I, pp. 33–53. Wiley (Interscience), New York.
Higgens, C. E., and Kastner, R. E. (1971). *Int. J. Syst. Bacteriol.* **21**, 326.
Higuchi, K., Jarvis, F. G., Peterson, W. H., and Johnson, M. J. (1946). *J. Amer. Chem. Soc.* **68**, 1669.
Hockenhull, D. J. D. (1948). *Biochem. J.* **43**, 498.
Hockenhull, D. J. D. (1959). *Prog. Ind. Microbiol.* **1**, 3.
Hockenhull, D. J. D., Ramachandran, K., and Walker, T. K. (1949). *Arch. Biochem.* **23**, 160.
Hodgkin, D. C., and Maslen, E. N. (1961). *Biochem. J.* **79**, 393.
Hollings, M., and Stone, O. M. (1969). *Sci. Progr. London* **57**, 371.
Hoover, J. R. E., and Stedman, R. J. (1970). In "Medicinal Chemistry" (A. Burger, ed.), pp. 371–408. Wiley (Interscience), New York.
Horowitz, N. H. (1947). *J. Biol. Chem.* **171**, 255.
Howell, S. F., Thayer, J. D., and Labaw, L. W. (1948). *Science* **107**, 299.

Huang, H. T., Seto, T. A., and Schull, G. M. (1963). *Appl. Microbiol.* **11**, 1.

Huber, F. M., Baltz, R. H., and Caltrider, P. G. (1968). *Appl. Microbiol.* **16**, 1011.

Ichihara, A., and Ichihara, E. A. (1960). *J. Biochem.* **49**, 154.

Inove, Y. (1960). *J. Antibiot. Tokyo, Ser. A* **14**, 221.

Iwasaki, S., Sair, M. I., Igaraski, H., and Okuda, S. (1970). *Chem. Commun.* 1119.

Jarvis, F. G., and Johnson, M. J. (1947). *J. Amer. Chem. Soc.* **9**, 3010.

Jeffery, J. D'A., Abraham, E. P., and Newton, G. G. F. (1961). *Biochem. J.* **81**, 591.

Jones, R. G. (1970). *Amer. Sci.* **58**, 404.

Kato, K. (1953a). *J. Antibiot. Tokyo Ser. A* **6**, 130.

Kato, K. (1953b). *J. Antibiot. Tokyo Ser. A* **6**, 184.

Kaufmann, W., and Bauer, K. (1964). *Nature* **203**, 520.

Kaufmann, W., Bauer, K., and Offe, H. A. (1961). *In* "Antimicrobial Agents Annual–1960" (P. Gray, B. Tabenkin, and S. G. Bradley, eds.), pp. 1–5. Plenum Press, New York.

Kavanagh, F., Tunin, D., and Wild, G. (1958a). *Mycologia* **50**, 370.

Kavanagh, F., Tunin, D., and Wild, G. (1958b). *Arch. Biochem. Biophys.* **77**, 268.

Kerr, D. S., and Flavin, M. (1970). *J. Biol. Chem.* **245**, 1842.

Kikuchi, T., and Uyeo, S. (1967). *Chem. Pharm. Bull.* **15**, 549.

Kleinschmidt, W. J., and Murphy, E. B. (1967). *Bacteriol. Rev.* **31**, 132.

Kleinschmidt, W. J., Ellis, L. F., Van Frank, R. M., and Murphy, E. B. (1968). *Nature* **220**, 167.

Koffler, H., Emerson, R. L., Perlman, D., and Burris, R. H. (1945). *J. Bacteriol.* **50**, 517.

Kuo, M. H., Saunders, P., and Broquist, H. P. (1962). *Biochem. Biophys. Res. Commun.* **8**, 227.

Kuo, M. H., Saunders, P. P., and Broquist, H. P. (1964). *J. Biol. Chem.* **239**, 508.

Lapierre, H., Astier-Manifacier, S., and Cornuet, P. (1971). *Compt. Rend. Acad. Sci., Paris, ser. D.* **273**, 992.

Lechevalier, H. A., and Lechevalier, M. P. (1967). *Ann. Rev. Microbiol.* **21**, 71.

Leinweber, F. J., and Monte, K. J. (1965). *J. Biol. Chem.* **240**, 782.

Lemke, P. A. (1969). *Mycopat. Mycol. Appl.* **38**, 49.

Lemke, P. A., and Nash, C. H. (1971). *Int. Mycol. Cong., 1st, Abstr., Exeter, 1971,* 56.

Lemke, P. A., and Nash, C. H. (1972). *Can. J. Microbiol.* **18**, 255.

Lemke, P. A., and Ness, F. M. (1970). *J. Virol.* **6**, 813.

Loder, P. B., and Abraham, E. P. (1971a). *Biochem. J.* **123**, 471.

Loder, P. B., and Abraham, E. P. (1971b). *Biochem. J.* **123**, 477.

Loder, P. B., Abraham, E. P., and Newton, G. G. F. (1969). *Biochem. J.* **112**, 389.

Macdonald, K. D. (1966). *Antonie van Leeuwenhoek J. Microbiol. Serol.* **32**, 431.

Macdonald, K. D., Hutchinson, J. M., and Gillet, W. A. (1963). *J. Gen. Microbiol.* **33**, 375.

Macdonald, K. D., Hutchinson, J. M., and Gillet, W. A. (1965). *Genetics* **36**, 378.

Magee, P. T., and deRobichon-Szulmajster, H. (1968). *Eur. J. Biochem.* **3**, 507.

Margulis, L. (1968). *Science* **161**, 1020.

Martin, E., Berky, J., Godzeski, C., Miller, P., Tome, J., and Stone, R. W. (1953). *J. Biol. Chem.* **203**, 239.

Marzluf, G. A. (1970a). *J. Bacteriol.* **102**, 716.

Marzluf, G. A. (1970b). *Arch. Biochem. Biophys.* **138**, 254.

Meister, A., Wellner, D., and Scott, S. J. (1960). *J. Nat. Cancer Inst.* **24**, 31.

Metzenberg, R. L., and Parson, J. W. (1966). *Proc. Nat. Acad. Sci.* **55**, 632.

Miller, I. M., Stapley, E. O., and Chaiet, L. (1962). *Bacteriol. Proc.* **39**,

Mitchell, H. K., and Houlahan, M. B. (1948). *J. Biol. Chem.* **174**, 883.

Mondovi, B., Scioscia-Santoro, A., and Cavallini, D. (1963). *Arch. Biochem. Biophys.* **101**, 363.

Morin, R. B., Jackson, B. G., Mueller, R. A., Lavagnino, E. R., Scanlon, W. B., and Andrews, S. L. (1963). *J. Amer. Chem. Soc.* **85**, 1896.
Moss, M. O., and Cole, M. (1964). *Biochem. J.* **92**, 643.
Moyer, A. J., and Coghill, R. D. (1946a). *J. Bacteriol.* **51**, 57.
Moyer, A. J., and Coghill, R. D. (1946b). *J. Bacteriol.* **51**, 79.
Moyer, A. J., and Coghill, R. D. (1947). *J. Bacteriol.* **53**, 329.
Murao, S. (1955). *Nippon Nogei Kagaku Kaishi* **29**, 400.
Murao, S., and Kishida, Y. (1961). *J. Agr. Chem. Soc. Japan* **35**, 607.
Nagarajan, R., Boeck, L. D., Gorman, M., Hamill, R. L., Higgens, C. E., Hoehn, M. M., Stark, W. M., and Whitney, J. G. (1971). *J. Amer. Chem. Soc.* **93**, 2308.
Nakatani, Y., Fujioka, M., and Higashino, K. (1970). *Biochem. Biophys. Acta* **198**, 219.
Nara, T., and Johnson, M. J. (1959). *J. Bacteriol.* **77**, 217.
Nash, C. H., and Huber, F. M. (1971). *J. Appl. Microbiol.* **22**, 6.
Neuss, N., Nash, C. H., Lemke, P. A., and Grutzner, J. B. (1971). *J. Amer. Chem. Soc.* **93**, 2337.
Newton, G. G. F., and Abraham, E. P. (1953). *Nature* **172**, 395.
Newton, G. G. F., and Abraham, E. P. (1955). *Nature* **175**, 548.
Newton, G. G. F., and Abraham, E. P. (1956). *Biochem. J.* **62**, 651.
Newton, G. G. F., Abraham, E. P., and Kuwabara, S. (1968). *Antimicrob. Ag. Chemother.* **1967**, 449.
Nüesch, J., Gruner, J., Knüsel, F., and Treichler, H. J. (1967). *Pathol. Microbiol.* **30**, 880.
Nüesch, J., Treichler, H. J., and Liersch, M. (1970). *Int. Symp. Genet. Ind. Microorgan., 1st, Abstr., Prague,* 1970, 160.
O'Callaghan, C. H., and Muggleton, P. W. (1963). *Biochem. J.* **89**, 304.
Olson, B. H., Jennings, J. C., and Junek, A. J. (1953). *Science* **117**, 76.
Olson, B. H., Jennings, J. C., Pisano, M. A., and Junek, A. J. (1954). *Antibiot. Chemother.* **4**, 1.
Ott, J. L., Godzeski, C. W., Pavey, D. E., Farran, J. D., and Horton, D. R. (1962). *Appl. Microbiol.* **10**, 515.
Pathak, S. G., and Elander, R. P. (1971). *Appl. Microbiol.* **22**, 366.
Perlman, D. (1966). *Ann. N.Y. Acad. Sci.* **139**, 258.
Peterson, W. H., and Wideburg, N. E. (1960). *Proc. Int. Congr. Biochem., 4th, Vienna,* 1958 136.
Pirt, S. J., and Righelato, R. C. (1967). *Appl. Microbiol.* **15**, 1284.
Pisano, M. A., and Capone, J. J. (1967). *Develop. Ind. Microbiol.* **8**, 417.
Pisano, M. A., Fleischman, A. I., Littman, M. L., Dutcher, J. D., and Pansy, F. E. (1961). *In* "Antimicrobial Agents Annual–1960" (P. Gray, B. Tabenkin, and S. G. Bradley, eds.), pp. 41–47. Plenum Press, New York.
Pontecorvo, G., and Sermonti, G. (1954). *J. Gen. Microbiol.* **11**, 94.
Pontecorvo, G., Roper, J. A., Hemmons, L. M., Macdonald, K. D., and Bufton, A. W. J. (1953). *Advan. Genet.* **5**, 141.
Pruess, D. L., and Johnson, M. J. (1967). *J. Bacteriol.* **94**, 1502.
Radhakrishnan, A. N., Wagner, R. P., and Snell, E. E. (1960). *J. Biol. Chem.* **235**, 2322.
Raper, K. B. (1946). *Ann. N.Y. Acad. Sci.* **48**, 41.
Raper, K. B., and Alexander, D. F. (1945). *J. Elisha Mithcell Sci. Soc.* **61**, 74.
Raper, K. B., and Fennel, D. I. (1946). *J. Bacteriol.* **52**, 761.
Raper, K. B., Alexander, D. F., and Coghill, R. D. (1944). *J. Bacteriol.* **48**, 639.
Rizza, V., and Kornfeld, J. M. (1969). *J. Gen. Microbiol.* **58**, 307.
Roberts, J. M. (1952). *Mycologia* **44**, 292.
Rode, L. J., Foster, J. W., and Schuhardt, V. T. (1947). *J. Bacteriol.* **53**, 565.
Rolinson, G. N., Batchelor, F. R., Butterworth, D., Cameron-Wood, J., Cole, M., Eustace, G. C., Hart, M. V., Richards, M., and Chain, E. B. (1960). *Nature* **187**, 236.

Roper, J. A. (1971). *Int. Symp. Genet. Ind. Microorgan., 1st, Abstr.*, Prague, 1970, 20.

Saito, Y., Otani, S., and Otani, S. (1970). *Advan. Enzymol.* 33, 337.

Sakaguchi, K., and Murao, S. (1950). *Nippon Nogei Kagaku Kaishi* 23, 411.

Sanders, A. G. (1949). In "Antibiotics" (H. W. Florey, E. B. Chain, N. G. Heatley, M. A. Jennings, A. G., Sanders, E. P. Abraham, and M. E. Florey, eds.), Vol. 2, pp. 672–685. Oxford Univ. Press, London and New York.

Scott, J. M., and Spencer, B. (1968). *Biochem. J.* 106, 471.

Segel, I. H., and Johnson, M. J. (1961). *J. Bacteriol.* 81, 91.

Segel, I. H., and Johnson, M. J. (1963). *Arch. Biochem. Biophys.* 103, 216.

Sentheshanmuganathan, S., and Nickerson, W. J. (1962). *J. Gen. Microbiol.* 27, 465.

Sermonti, G. (1956). *J. Gen. Microbiol.* 15, 599.

Sermonti, G. (1957). *Genetics* 42, 433.

Sermonti, G. (1959a). *Ann. N.Y. Acad. Sci.* 81, 950.

Sermonti, G. (1959b). *Selec. Sci. Pap. Ist. Super. Sanita* 2, 407.

Sermonti, G. (1969). "Genetics of Antibiotic-Producing Microorganisms." Wiley (Interscience), New York.

Sheehan, J. C., and Henery-Logan, K. R. (1959). *J. Amer. Chem. Soc.* 81, 5838.

Shimi, I. R., and Imam, G. M. (1966). *Biochem. J.* 101, 831.

Shimi, I. R., and Imam, G. M. (1968). *Arch. Microbiol.* 60, 275.

Siddiqi, O., Apte, B. N., and Pitale, M. P. (1966). *Cold Spring Harb. Symp. Quant. Biol.* 31, 381.

Sinha, A. K., and Bhattacharjee, J. K. (1970). *Biochem. Biophys. Res. Commun.* 39, 1205.

Sjöberg, B., Thelin, H., Nathorst-Westfelt, L., van Tamelen, E., and Wagner, E. R. (1965). *Tetrahedron Lett.* 281.

Smith, B., Warren, S. C., Newton, G. G. F., and Abraham, E. P. (1967). *Biochem. J.* 103, 877.

Snoke, J. E. (1955). *J. Biol. Chem.* 213, 813.

Soda, K., Misono, H., and Tamamoto, T. (1968). *Biochemistry* 7, 4102.

Somerson, N. L., Demain, A. L., and Nunheimer, T. D. (1961). *Arch. Biochem. Biophys.* 93, 238.

Spencer, B. (1968). *Biochem. Biophys. Res. Comm.* 31, 170.

Spencer, B., and Maung, C. (1970). *Biochem. J.* 188, 29.

Spiegelman, S., Burny, A., Das, M. R., Keydar, J., Schlon, J.,Trávníček, M., and Watson, K. (1970). *Nature* 228, 430.

Stanier, R. Y., Doudoroff, M., Adelberg, E. A. (1963). "The Microbial World." Prentice-Hall, Englewood Cliffs, New Jersey.

Stauffer, J. F., Schwartz, L. J., and Brady, C. W. (1966). *Develop. Ind. Microbiol.* 7, 104.

Stefaniak, J. J., Gailey, F. B., Jarvis, F. G., and Johnson, M. J. (1946). *J. Bacteriol.* 52, 119.

Stevens, C. M., and DeLong, C. W. (1958). *J. Biol. Chem.* 230, 991.

Stevens, C. M., and Halpern, P. E. (1949). *J. Biol. Chem.* 179, 389.

Stevens, C. M., Vohra, P., Inamine, E., and Roholt, O. A., Jr. (1953). *J. Biol. Chem.* 205, 1001.

Stevens, C. M., Vohra, P., Moore, J. E., and DeLong, C. W. (1954a). *J. Biol. Chem.* 210, 713.

Stevens, C. M., Vohra, P., and DeLong, C. W. (1954b). *J. Biol. Chem.* 211, 297.

Stevens, C. M., Inamine, E., and DeLong, C. W. (1956). *J. Biol. Chem.* 219, 405.

Stewart, W. W. (1971). *Nature* 229, 174.

Strassman, M., and Ceci, L. N. (1964). *Biochem. Biophys. Res. Commun.* 14, 262.

Strassman, M., Shalton, J. B., and Weinhouse, S. (1960). *J. Biol. Chem.* 235, 700.

Strassman, M., Ceci, L. N., and Silverman, B. E. (1964). *Biochem. Biophys. Res. Commun.* 14, 268.

Strominger, J., Izaki, K., Matsuhashi, M., and Tipper, D. J. (1968). In "Topics in Pharmaceutical Sciences" (D. Perlman, ed.), Vol. I pp. 53–84. Wiley (Interscience), New York.

Sukapure, R. S., and Thirumalachar, M. J. (1963). *Mycologia* **55**, 563.
Szentrimai, A. (1966). *Acta Microbiol. Acad. Sci. Hung.* **12**, 395.
Tanabe, M., Seto, H., and Johnson, L. (1970). *J. Amer. Chem. Soc.* **92**, 2157.
Tardrew, P. L., and Johnson, M. J. (1958). *J. Bacteriol.* **76**, 400.
Tardrew, P. L., and Johnson, M. J. (1959). *J. Biol. Chem.* **234**, 1850.
Temin, H. M. (1964). *Proc. U.S. Nat. Acad. Sci.* **52**, 323.
Thayer, P. S., and Horowitz, N. H. (1951). *J. Biol. Chem.* **192**, 755.
Tome, J., Zook, H. D., Wagner, R. B., and Stone, R. W. (1953). *J. Biol. Chem.* **203**, 251.
Trinci, A. P. J., and Righelato, R. C. (1970). *J. Gen. Microbiol.* **60**, 239.
Trown, P. W., Abraham, E. P., Newton, G. G. F., Hale, C. W., and Miller, G. A. (1962). *Biochem. J.* **84**, 157.
Trown, P. W., Sharp, M., and Abraham, E. P. (1963a). *Biochem. J.* **86**, 280.
Trown, P. W., Smith, B., and Abraham, E. P. (1963b). *Biochem. J.* **86**, 284.
Troy, F. A., and Koffler, H. (1969). *J. Biol. Chem.* **244**, 5563.
Umbarger, H. E. (1970). *Int. Symp. Genet. Ind. Microorgan., 1st, Abstr., Prague*, 1970, 86.
Umbarger, H. E., and Davis, B. D. (1962). In "The Bacteria" (J. C. Gunsalus and R. Y. Stanier, eds.), pp. 167–251. Academic Press, New York.
United States Patent 3,239,394.
United States Patent 3,539,694.
Uri, J., Juhasz, P., and Csoban, G. (1965). *Pharmazie* **10**, 709.
Vanderhaeghe, H., Claesen, M., Vlietinck, A., and Parmentier, G. (1968). *Appl. Microbiol.* **16**, 1557.
Van Heyningen, E. (1967). *Advan. Drug. Res.* **4**, 1.
Verkhovtseva, T. P., Lurie, L. M., and Levitov, M. M. (1960). *Antibiotiki.* **15**, 876.
Vogel, H. J. (1960). *Biochim. Biophys. Acta* **41**, 172.
Vogel, H. J. (1964). *Amer. Natur.* **98**, 435.
Waelsch, H., and Rittenberg, D. (1941). *J. Biol. Chem.* **139**, 761.
Wagner, A. F., and Folkers, K. (1961). *Endeavour* **20**, 177.
Waksman, S. (1967). "The Actinomycetes." Ronald Press, New York.
Walton, R. B. (1964). *Develop. Ind. Microbiol.* **5**, 349.
Warren, S. C., Newton, G. G. F., and Abraham, E. P. (1967a). *Biochem. J.* **103**, 891.
Warren, S. C., Newton, G. G. F., and Abraham, E. P. (1967b). *Biochem. J.* **103**, 902.
Wiebers, J. L., and Garner, H. R. (1960). *J. Bacteriol.* **80**, 51.
Wiebers, J. L., and Garner, H. R. (1967). *J. Biol. Chem.* **242**, 12.
Wolfe, S., Godfrey, J. C., Haldrege, C. T., and Perron, Y. G. (1963). *J. Amer. Chem. Soc.* **85**, 643.
Wolff, E. C., and Arnstein, H. R. V. (1960). *Biochem. J.* **76**, 375.
Woodward, R. B. (1966). *Science* **153**, 487.
Woodward, R. B., Heusler, K., Gosteli, J., Naegeli, P., Oppolzer, W., Ramage, R., Ranganathan, S., and Vorbrüggen, H. (1966). *J. Amer. Chem. Soc.* **88**, 852.
Yanofsky, C. (1960). *Bacteriol. Rev.* **24**, 221.
Yura, T., and Vogel, H. J. (1957). *Biochim. Biophys. Acta* **24**, 648.

Chapter 10

BIOLOGICAL REACTIONS OF CEPHALOSPORINS AND PENICILLINS

CYNTHIA H. O'CALLAGHAN and P. W. MUGGLETON

I. The Action of β-Lactamases on Penicillins and Cephalosporins

A. Introduction

Following the discovery that some strains of *Staphylococcus, Bacillus,* and *Escherichia* were resistant to benzylpenicillin because they were able to destroy the antibacterial activity of the molecule, a large amount of work was done with enzymes from these and, later, from many other bacteria. For many years, their only known substrates were penicillins, and so they were known as penicillinases. They are now known to hydrolyze some cephalosporins as well and although some of these enzymes were then designated cephalosporinases, they are better referred to in general as β-lactamases.

Beta-Lactamases have been found in *Staphylococcus aureus, S. epidermidis, Bacillus cereus, B. licheniformis,* and various *Mycobacterium* spp. among gram-positive organisms. Strains of *Escherichia coli,* various *Proteus* spp., *Klebsiella aerogenes, Enterobacter cloacae, Pseudomonas aeruginosa,* and other gram-negative organisms also possess such enzymes. In many instances there is a strong correlation between the resistance of an organism to a β-lactam antibiotic and its ability to elaborate a β-lactamase able to destroy that antibiotic.

The different enzymes can be distinguished by their differing abilities to hydrolyze a range of penicillin or cephalosporin substrates. As more penicillins and then cephalosporins became available, increasing numbers of distinct profile types have been detected; it was also found that some bacteria can make more than one β-lactamase. These differ from each other in chemical, physical, and enzymological properties and can also be distinguished by their susceptibility to a range of potential competitive inhibitors. No β-lactamase so far described is exclusively a penicillinase or a cephalosporinase; an enzyme with very high activity against a penicillin usually has detectable activity against at least one cephalosporin, and the reverse is also true.

Beta-Lactamases (E.C. 3.5.2.6)* are here defined as enzymes of bacterial origin which hydrolyze the C–N bond in the β-lactam ring of a penicillin or cephalosporin. Units of β-lactamase activity are defined as that amount of β-lactamase which hydrolyzes 1 μmole of benzylpenicillin in 60 minutes at 30°C and pH 7 (Pollock and Torriani, 1953).

Substrate profile is defined as the relative activities of an enzyme against a number of different substrates. In order to make comparisons as meaningful as possible and to identify one enzyme when it has been investigated by several groups of workers, the activity against all substrates tested is being increasingly

* "Recommendations for Enzyme Nomenclature," Elsevier Publishing Co. (1965).

related to the activity against benzylpenicillin, which is given an arbitrary value of 100 for this purpose.

B. Occurrence of β-Lactamases and Their Relationship to Bacterial Resistance to β-Lactam Antibiotics

The first indication that an organism may produce a destructive enzyme is often the observation that the minimum inhibitory concentration (MIC) is very dependent on the size of inoculum used. This suggests that a destructive enzyme may be implicated in its resistance to that antibiotic. In some cases, this interpretation of the inoculum effect is too simple; similar effects can be obtained by the selection of mutants which are resistant by a different mechanism. In addition, not all β-lactamase-producing organisms elaborate sufficient quantities of enzyme to interfere with the inhibitory effect of the antibiotic and conversely, others with a high intrinsic resistance make no detectable enzyme.

Some bacteria possess a permeability barrier which may act to make the organism more resistant because the antibiotic is kept away from the site at which it acts. On the other hand, such a barrier may prevent the antibiotic reaching the cellular location of the β-lactamase and so prevent its rapid degradation. Some β-lactamases may be entirely endoenzymes which are not excreted into the growth medium; others are exoenzymes and comparatively high concentrations are found in culture supernatants where they are likely to effect the rapid destruction of a susceptible antibiotic. Some organisms, e.g., B. cereus, can produce both endo- and exoenzymes.

An enzymic component in the cell wall to which a penicillin or cephalosporin binds, and from which it cannot be recovered intact, may also be regarded as a special type of β-lactamase. This type of enzyme, however, is different in not being able to bring about the rapid destruction of large amounts of substrate, which can be observed with the more obvious β-lactamases.

Some bacteria make acylases, which are able to remove the 7- or 6-N-acyl group from some cephalosporins and penicillins. The ability of the enzyme to cleave a penicillin or a cephalosporin in this way depends entirely on the nature of the acyl group; the most easily removed ones are those which are substituted acetic acids which do not have a charged substituent. A number of organisms can deacylate benzylpenicillin or analogous cephalosporins, but so far no organism has been found which can remove the α-aminoadipoyl side chain from cephalosporin C. There have been occasional reports of organisms producing such enzymes, but none of these has been substantiated on fuller investigation. Some bacteria can make both an acylase and a β-lactamase; however, acylases act very slowly in comparison with β-lactamases, and when both are present simultaneously, acylases are generally masked by β-lacta-mases.

Cephalosporins with an acetoxymethyl group at C-3 can be deacetylated both by microorganisms and by body tissues. The reaction is usually rapid and the resulting product, the corresponding deacetylcephalosporin, is of lower antibacterial activity. The enzymic stability of deacetylcephalosporins relative to their parent compound is also changed, being more stable to some enzymes and less stable to others. Deesterification can also occur when a cephalosporin has other ester groups on the 3-methyl position. However, should the carbon atom adjacent to the carbonyl group in the acyl moiety of that ester have one or two substituents, then the rate of hydrolysis is markedly reduced.

C. Products of β-Lactamase Hydrolysis

The enzymic hydrolysis of the β-lactam ring of the penicillins occurs as follows.

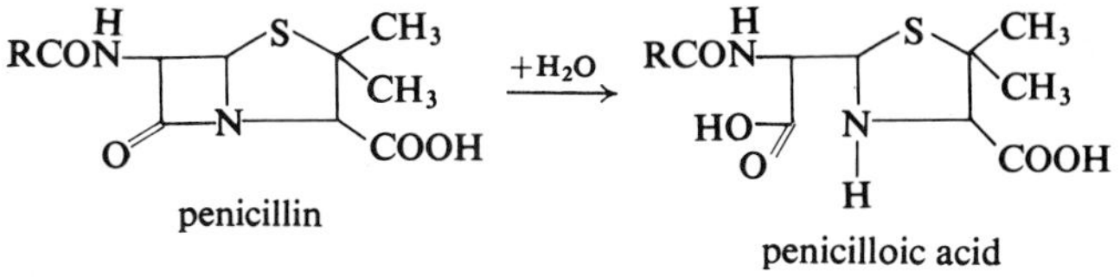

The reaction was discovered by Abraham and Chain (1940), but the identity of the product was not determined until 1949 (Abraham et al., 1949). Penicillin has one acidic group but the corresponding penicilloic acid has two strongly acidic functions so that this increase in acidity can be used to estimate the rate of hydrolysis. Analogous penicilloic acids are produced from all penicillins regardless of the nature of the 6-acylamino group, and with all β-lactamases regardless of their source or detailed characteristics.

The situation with the cephalosporins is more complicated. Hamilton-Miller et al. (1970) suggested that the enzymic hydrolysis of cephalosporin C proceeded as follows.

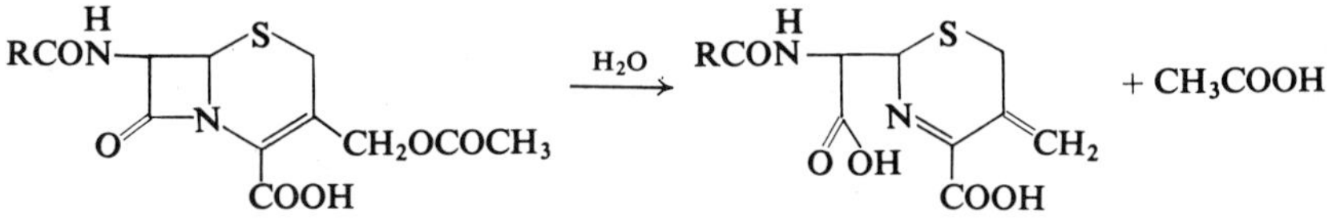

Both cephalosporin C and its deacetyl derivative give this type of product, but the compound with the exocyclic methylene group at C-3 is not very stable; the reaction proceeds rapidly but on longer incubation the initial product decomposes further.

Cleavage of the β-lactam ring affects the stability of the 3-methyl substituent. Compounds such as cephalosporin C or cephalothin lose one molecule of acetic acid from the C-3 acetoxymethyl as the β-lactam ring is opened, with the consequent formation of two extra equivalents of acid (Sabath et al., 1965). Hydrolysis of quaternary compounds such as cephaloridine is also accompanied by expulsion of the C-3 methyl substituent, but this gives rise to one equivalent of a base in addition to the formation of one molecule of acid from the lactam ring. Other groups able to accept an electron and leave the C-3 methyl position, such as azide (O'Callaghan et al., 1972), are released quantitatively and free azide ion accumulates at exactly the same rate as the loss of antibacterial activity and loss of ultraviolet absorption in the 260 nm range. Probably all groups able to accept an electron are expelled in this way. It is still a matter for speculation as to what happens to a substituent at this position when it does not readily leave the molecule, as in cephalexin or cefazolin.

D. *Methods of Determining and Measuring* β-*Lactamase Activity*

The methods employed to detect β-lactamase activity in a bacterial culture and to determine its substrate specificity have varied widely, depending on the purposes of the tests and the equipment available. The concentration of either the hydrolysis products or the residual unchanged penicillin or cephalosporin can be estimated to determine the rate of reaction, using methods based on the biological, physical, or chemical properties of the compounds.

Biological methods are based on the loss of antibacterial activity which occurs when the β-lactam ring is ruptured and the decrease in antibacterial activity can be measured by any suitable bioassay procedure.

Several physical properties show changes associated with β-lactam hydrolysis and assay methods based on these include the measurement of changes in optical rotation, infrared absorption (Holt and Stewart, 1965), ultraviolet absorption for cephalosporins only (O'Callaghan et al., 1969), and pH (Wise and Twigg, 1950; Benedict et al., 1945; Jeffery et al., 1961).

The products of hydrolysis may be estimated chemically by such methods as the iodometric method of Perret (1954) or by determination of the carbon dioxide evolved (Henry and Housewright, 1947; Abraham and Newton, 1956). Residual penicillin can be estimated chemically with hydroxylamine (Staab et al., 1946). The methods have been reviewed in detail by Hamilton-Miller et al. (1963) and Citri and Pollock (1966).

These methods can all be used quantitatively to determine rate of hydrolysis. Some can be adapted for use as rapid screening methods to determine either the enzyme production of a large number of bacterial strains or the susceptibility of a large number of penicillin or cephalosporin compounds to one or more enzymes.

There are advantages and disadvantages with all the methods and the one chosen is governed largely by the investigator's purpose. The iodometric assay is fairly rapid and accurate but has the disadvantage that the required substrate concentration is very high. A method based on ultraviolet absorption works well with one-hundredth of the concentration needed for iodometric assays, but is limited to a narrow concentration range and to cephalosporins. Extrapolation to cephalosporins of a method suitable for measuring penicillins, and even to one cephalosporin from another, may not be possible without considerable modification. For example, the hydroxylamine method used for penicillin assay does not extrapolate readily to all cephalosporins and cannot be used under highly reducing conditions because the ferric chromophore is unstable under conditions of low oxygen tension. Microbiological methods for detecting penicillins and cephalosporins are very sensitive but are not rapid, usually requiring overnight incubation, although large numbers can be done simultaneously. The type of enzyme preparation being investigated is also very important. A purified isolated enzyme may have a different activity profile from that of the intact living cell from which it was derived. Enzymes which are excreted into the medium may be examined as crude culture supernatants, but endoenzyme preparations must be made from disrupted whole cells.

In many organisms, the β-lactamase is inducible and the cells will not exhibit their full enzyme-producing potential unless they have been grown in the presence of a suitable inducer. Instability of enzyme or substrate under various conditions may also complicate the assay. It is obvious that the experimental conditions used will be of major importance and will have considerable influence on the interpretation of results. In many instances it is impossible to correlate the results from different groups of workers who have used different substrates, methods, and types of enzyme preparation.

E. Effect of β-Lactamases from Different Microorganisms on Penicillins and Cephalosporins

Although the products of β-lactamase hydrolysis do not depend on the source of the enzyme, different bacterial species produce enzymes with very different substrate specificities. Some substrates are resistant to enzymes from widely different species, but this can be due either to very low enzyme substrate affinity or to very high affinity combined with extremely low speed of reaction.

1. STAPHYLOCOCCAL β-LACTAMASE

a. SENSITIVITY OF PENICILLINS AND CEPHALOSPORINS. Many strains of
S. aureus can destroy large amounts of benzylpenicillin, by means of β-lactamase activity. Richmond (1963) found that these organisms can make three
distinct but similar β-lactamases. Before benzylpenicillin was in widespread use,
some 10% of strains of *S. aureus* could inactivate it. Fifteen years of intensive
and widespread use of benzylpenicillin resulted in a high incidence of β-
lactamase-producing staphylococci in hospitals; infection of patients with these
organisms became a real hazard and threatened to diminish greatly the
usefulness of the penicillins in use up to that time. All penicillins which can be
made by fermentation have a 6-acylamido group of the general structure
R–CH$_2$–CONH, and all of these are susceptible to hydrolysis by staphylococcal β-lactamase.

The isolation of the penicillin nucleus, 6-amino penicillanic acid (6-APA)
(Batchelor *et al.*, 1959, 1961) permitted the preparation of analogs with more
complex 6-acylamido groups, which could not be made by biosynthesis.
Methicillin, the first penicillin resistant to staphylococcal β-lactamase, was
described in 1960 (Rolinson *et al.*, 1960; Brown and Acred, 1960). Soon after
the introduction of methicillin, the isoxazole penicillins were also found to
have almost total resistance to staphylococcal β-lactamase (Gourevitch *et al.*,
1961; Nayler *et al.*, 1962), and in addition to being some five times more active
than methicillin, they could also be given by mouth. Other enzyme-resistant
penicillins were synthesized, for example, ancillin (Dolan *et al.*, 1962), quinacillin (Richards *et al.*, 1963), nafcillin (Yurchenco *et al.*, 1962; Smith and White,
1963), and these compounds also had very low affinities for the β-lactamase.
Structures of the penicillins are shown in Table I.

Table I

6-AMINOPENICILLANIC ACID (6-APA) AND SOME OF ITS DERIVATIVES

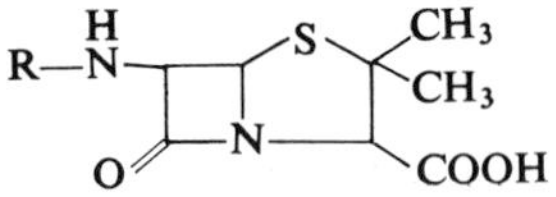

(General structure of a penicillin)

Side chain R (6-acyl group)	Name
1. H–	6-Aminopenicillanic acid
2. C$_6$H$_5$–CH$_2$CO–	Benzylpenicillin
3. C$_6$H$_5$–OCH$_2$CO–	Phenoxymethylpenicillin
4. C$_6$H$_5$–CH(NH$_2$)CO–	Ampicillin

Side chain R (6-acyl group)	Name
5. Structure: 2-chlorophenyl isoxazole with $-CO-$ and $-CH_3$, ring $N-O$	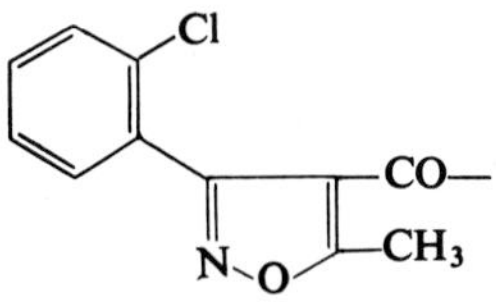 Cloxacillin
6. Structure: benzene ring with two OCH_3 groups and $-CO-$	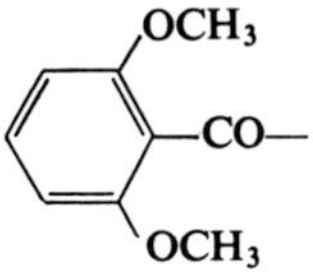 Methicillin
7. Structure: quinoxaline with $-CO-$ and $-COOH$, ring N	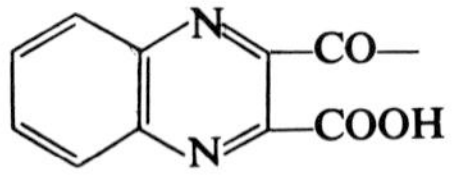 Quinacillin
8. Structure: naphthalene with $-CO-$ and OCH_2CH_3	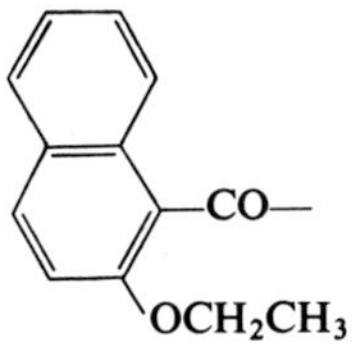 Nafcillin
9. Structure: benzene ring with C_6H_5 and $-CO-$	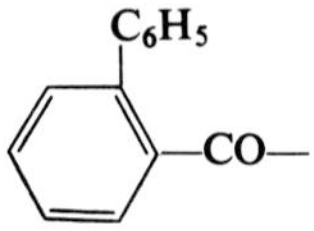 Ancillin
10. $C_6H_5-CH(CO_2H)CO-$	Carbenicillin
11. $C_6H_5-CH(NHOSO_2H)CO-$	α-Sulphamoylphenylacetamido-penicillanic acid
12. $C_6H_5-CH(NHCONHN=NH-NH_2)CO-$	α-Guanoureidophenylacet-amidopenicillanic acid
13. Structure: thiophene with $-CH-CO$ and $COOH$	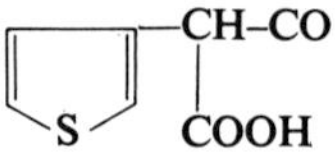 α-Carboxy-3-thienylacetamido-penicillanic acid
14. $HO-$ (phenyl) $-CH(NH_2)CO-$	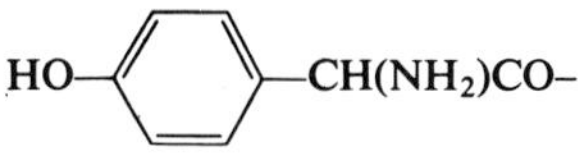 α-Amino-4-hydroxyphenyl-acetamidopenicillanic acid
15. (cyclohexadienyl) $-CH(NH_2)CO-$	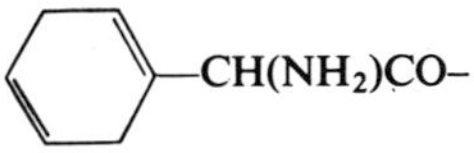 α-Aminocyclohexa-1,3-dienyl-acetamidopenicillanic acid

Comparison of the acyl groups of penicillins resistant to staphylococcal β-lactamase shows that in all cases they are derived from acids in which the α-carbon atom is substituted with a bulky group or is contained in an aromatic ring. This high degree of substitution probably means that the enzyme is prevented from approaching the penicillin sufficiently closely to bind firmly to it and bring about its rapid hydrolysis. The resistant penicillins have a very low affinity for staphylococcal β-lactamase, but they are not completely resistant to it under all conditions. Provided the substrate concentration is very high, about 0.06 M (≈ 20 mg/ml), then some hydrolysis can occur (Eriksen and Erichsen, 1964). Such concentrations are greatly in excess of those which could be obtained in a patient and this small degree of hydrolysis of the enzyme-resistant penicillins under these extreme conditions is not therapeutically relevant.

There are now many reports of strains of S. aureus resistant to methicillin and the isoxazole penicillins (Jevons et al., 1963; Seligman and Hewitt, 1966; Chabbert and Pillet, 1967; Zygmunt et al., 1968). These organisms do not possess a new kind of β-lactamase able to hydrolyze the hitherto enzyme resistant penicillins; although they almost always have a β-lactamase, their resistance is intrinsic. They are usually of phage type III and serotype 18 and grow more slowly than other strains of S. aureus at 37°C, growing better at 30°C.

Penicillins which have only a small substituent adjacent to the amide link in the 6-acylamido group, such as in ampicillin or carbenicillin, are still susceptible to hydrolysis because the degree of steric hindrance is inadequate. As the steric hindrance increases, so does the resistance of the penicillins. A more detailed account of structure–activity relationships of penicillins with regard to their resistance to staphylococcal β-lactamase has been written by Doyle and Nayler (1964).

In 1956, when deep concern was being felt about the increase in the incidence of strains of staphylococci resistant to benzylpenicillin, Newton and Abraham described cephalosporin C. It is highly resistant to staphylococcal β-lactamase, but its low level of activity against all strains of staphylococci is a great disadvantage. Changes in the 7-acylamido group have given compounds with much higher intrinsic activity against β-lactamase-producing staphylococci while retaining the original high resistance to staphylococcal β-lactamase.

In the penicillin series, changes in the 6-aminoacyl substituent bring about dramatic changes in resistance to β-lactamases, and the enzyme-resistant properties appear to depend wholly on the configuration of this substituent. In the case of the cephalosporins, the ring system must also greatly influence the enzymic hydrolysis. The picture is further complicated by the presence of two sites in the molecule which can be altered chemically, and changes in both side chains give compounds with altered enzyme susceptibility and changed antibacterial properties. Conversion of cephalosporin C to the deacetyl compound, or to cephalosporin C_A by the replacement of the acetoxy group at the C-3 methyl with pyridine, greatly affect the rate of hydrolysis, relative to that of benzylpenicillin (Crompton *et al.*, 1962; Jago, 1964). So far, no cephalosporin has been found to be as sensitive to staphylococcal β-lactamase as benzylpenicillin although lactonization of deacetylcephalosporin C increased the sensitivity of the compound some 1600-fold, making it only six times more resistant than benzylpenicillin.

The stability of the more active cephalosporins, cephalothin, and cephaloridine to staphylococcal β-lactamase has been qualitatively examined by various investigators (Barber and Waterworth, 1964; Benner *et al.*, 1965; Ridley and Phillips, 1965; Hewitt and Parker, 1968) who concluded from qualitative studies that cephalothin retains the almost total enzyme resistance of cephalosporin C but that cephaloridine is rather less resistant.

It is very difficult to distinguish between enzyme sensitivity effects and intrinsic resistance by such methods. Hamilton-Miller and Ramsay (1967) showed quantitatively that cephalothin is inactivated at about 0.01 % of the rate of benzylpenicillin and cephaloridine at about 0.1 %. The difference in susceptibilities between the two compounds must be due to the different effects of acetoxy and of pyridine at the C-3 methyl position; this is similar to the change seen by Crompton *et al.* (1962) when cephalosporin C was converted to cephalosporin C_A.

While the presence of a pyridine ring at the 3-methyl position may account for the decrease in enzyme resistance with these two examples, it cannot be assumed that all quaternary groups at position 3 will have the same effect. Many analogs of cephaloridine have now been synthesized (e.g., Spencer *et al.*, 1967), and it is clear that different substituents on the pyridine ring have a marked effect on the stability of the compounds to staphylococcal β-lactamase. Should the 3-methyl substituent be isonicotinamide, for example, the cephalosporin (known as cephalonium) is more stable than cephalothin, but other substituents in the pyridine ring may increase the susceptibility of the cephalosporins. However, while these differences between cephalosporin analogs are clearly detectable, they are trivial compared with the much greater susceptibility of benzylpenicillin.

Changes in the 7-acylamido group, while maintaining acetoxy in the 3-methyl position, also have some effect on the lactamase stability of the resulting cephalosporins although, again, the changes are insignificant in comparison with the difference between the penicillins and benzylpenicillin. The orally absorbed cephalosporins, cephaloglycin and cephalexin, have a high stability to staphylococcal β-lactamase (Wick and Boniece, 1965; Muggleton *et al.*, 1969); although small α substituents in the 7-acyl group do not generally affect β-lactamase stability, some larger α substituents may have an adverse effect.

Recently, three new cephalosporins have been described (Table II, Nos.

Table II

7-AMINOCEPHALOSPORIN ACID (7-ACA) AND SOME OF ITS DERIVATIVES

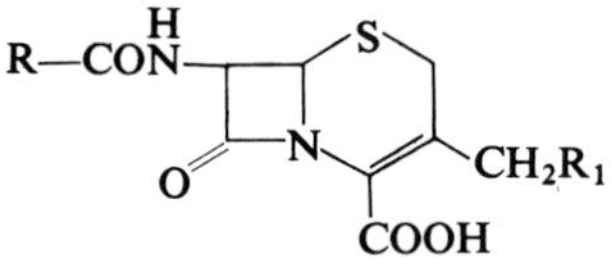

(General structure of a cephalosporin)

Side chain R (7-acyl group)	Side chain R_1 (3 substituent)	Cephalosporin
1. $HO_2CCH(NH_2)(CH_2)_3CO-$	$-OCOCH_3$	Cephalosporin C
2. $HO_2CCH(NH_2)(CH_2)_3CO-$	$-OH$	Deacetoxy-cephalosporin C
3. $HO_2CCH(NH_2)(CH_2)_3CO-$	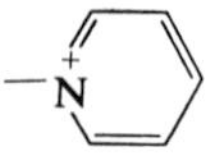	Cephalosporin C_A (pyridine)
4. $HO_2CCH(NH_2)(CH_2)_3CO-$	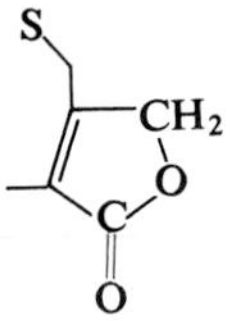	Cephalosporin C_C
5. 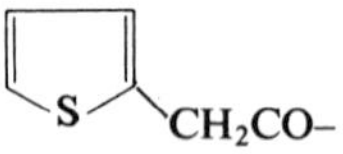	$-OCOCH_3$	Cephalothin
6. 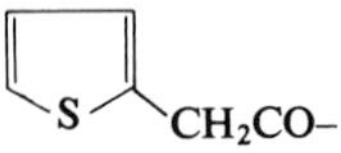	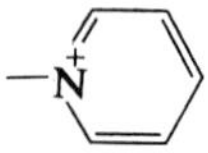	Cephaloridine
7. 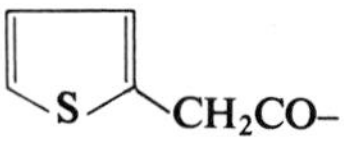	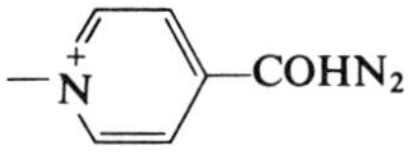 $-COHN_2$	Cephalonium
8. $C_6H_5CH_2CO-$	$-OCOCH_3$	Cephaloram
9. $C_6H_5CH(NH_2)CO-$	$-OCOCH_3$	Cephaloglycin
10. $C_6H_5CH(NH_2)CO-$	$-H$	Cephalexin
11. 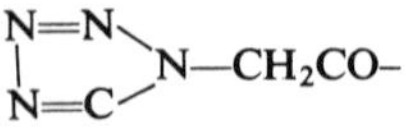	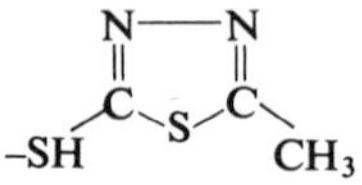	Cefazolin
12. $N{\equiv}C-CH_2CO-$	$-OCOCH_3$	7-Cyanacetamido-cephalosporanic acid

Side chain R (7-acyl group)	Side chain R_1 (3 substituent)	Cephalosporin
13. (pyridine ring)—SCH$_2$CO–	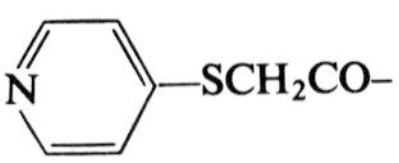 –OCOCH$_3$	Cephapirin
14. (2,6-dimethoxyphenyl, OCH$_3$)—CO– (OCH$_3$)	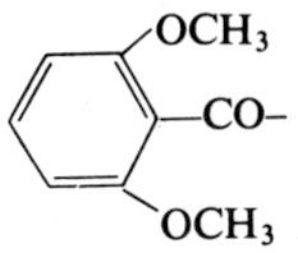 –OCOCH$_3$	2,6-Dimethoxybenz-amidocephalo-sporanic acid
15. (o-chlorophenyl isoxazole, Cl ... N–O ... CH$_3$)—CO–	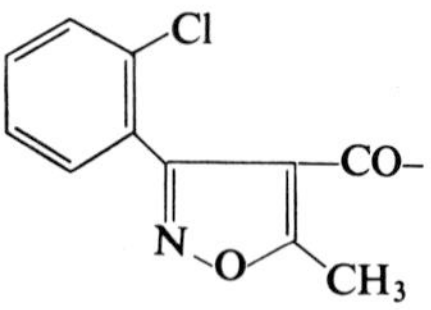 –OCOCH$_3$	3(o-chlorophenyl)-5-methylisoxazole-4-carboxamido-cephalosporanic acid
16. C$_6$H$_5$CH–CO | COOH	–OCOCH$_3$	α-Carboxyphenyl-acetamidocephalo-sporanic acid

11–13). Their 7-acyl groups are all derived from simple substituted acetic acids, and they are almost completely stable to staphylococcal β-lactamase.

b. INHIBITION. The β-lactamase-resistant penicillins have a very low affinity for the enzyme, but they can be inactivated under some conditions. When incubated with it at very high concentrations, i.e., 0.06 M (≈ 20 mg/ml), methicillin and cloxacillin irreversibly inactivate staphylococcal β-lactamase, but they cannot prevent decomposition of benzylpenicillin when a mixture is exposed to the enzyme (Gourevitch et al., 1962). In contrast to these penicillins, cephalosporins have a very high affinity for the enzyme and also very low rates of hydrolysis. In such a case, there is the possibility that such compounds may act as competitive inhibitors for the enzyme and prevent the hydrolysis of benzylpenicillin. This may result in some synergy between a cephalosporin and benzylpenicillin, and such effects have been observed in vitro (Crawford and Abraham, 1957; Hamilton-Miller and Ramsay, 1967; Hamilton-Miller, 1967; Sabath, 1968) with benzylpenicillin and some cephalosporins with some strains of S. aureus at concentrations which might be attained in vivo. The amount of synergy seen is small and variable from one strain to another. It tends to diminish when the time of incubation is increased (Moat et al., 1961). Jago (1964) showed a synergistic effect in vivo between benzylpenicillin on the one hand and either cephalosporin C or C_A on the other, with one strain of *S. aureus*.

From what little is known about the cephalosporins giving rise to this effect, it seems likely that the essential structure is the fundamentally β-lactamase-resistant cephalosporin ring system and that the 7- and 3-substituents have only slight modifying influences.

c. INDUCTION. In addition to benzylpenicillin, many of the β-lactamase-resistant penicillins and all the cephalosporins tested so far induce β-lactamase in enzyme-producing strains of *S. aureus* although different quantities of the various compounds are needed to produce the same effect. Enzyme resistance does not appear to be an absolute prerequisite for induction. It seems likely that the basic structure needed for a substance to induce staphylococcal β-lactamase is the β-lactam ring and that the various substituents in the 6-, 7-, or 3' positions have only minor modifying influences.

Induction of β-lactamase does not appear to occur to any significant extent *in vivo*. Eyckmans and Hook (1966) have found that mice with an experimental staphylococcal infection in the peritoneum showed no significant increase in penicillinase activity 6 hours after administration of benzylpenicillin although it could induce β-lactamase in this strain *in vitro*. Induction of β-lactamase occurred *in vivo* if the mice were leukopenic; conversely, *in vitro* induction was inhibited in the presence of leukocytes.

2. GRAM-POSITIVE, AEROBIC SPORING BACILLI

Although, with the exception of *Bacillus anthracis*, these bacteria are of little clinical importance, they are very widespread and can have a considerable nuisance value as contaminants, particularly when they make β-lactamases. For example, penicillin fermentations can become contaminated with members of this group and heavy losses then ensue, and they can grow on the charcoal columns used in the extraction of cephalosporin C from fermentation broth and inactivate the antibiotic.

a. RESISTANCE OF PENICILLINS AND CEPHALOSPORINS. The work on inactivation of benzylpenicillin and its analogs and early work on the inactivation of cephalosporin C and derivatives by *B. cereus* was done before it was realized that this organism made more than one β-lactamase. In 1956, Abraham and Newton found that a purified preparation from *B. cereus* 569, although highly active against benzylpenicillin, had no detectable activity against cephalosporin C. Later, Crompton *et al.* (1962) observed that a crude enzyme preparation from the same strain appeared to contain two β-lactamases, one of which is much more active than the other against cephalosporins. Other workers (Sabath and Abraham, 1966b; Kuwabara, 1970; Pollock, 1965; Pechere and Zanen, 1962) also showed that *B. cereus* produced more than one enzyme.

Because the two enzymes are produced at different rates, substrate profiles varied from one experiment to another and from one laboratory to another.

There is some doubt as to how many types of enzyme *B. cereus* 569 actually produces. Pollock (1965) has described an exoenzyme which he termed the alpha enzyme and a cell-bound enzyme known as the gamma enzyme, which have now been shown to be interconvertible (Rudzik and Imsande, 1970). Kuwabara and Abraham (1967) and Kuwabara (1970) have also purified two exoenzymes from *B. cereus*; enzyme I appears to be identical with Pollock's alpha enzyme, while enzyme II requires zinc as cofactor for activity (Sabath and Abraham, 1966a; Sabath and Finland, 1968) and is lost during purification if no zinc is present.

Kuwabara and Abraham (1969) have also described two cell-bound enzymes which appear to be similar in many respects to the exoenzymes previously purified. Cell-bound enzyme II has much in common with Pollock's gamma enzyme, and the differences between the two may only be due to the presence or absence of zinc. Citri and Kalkstein (1967) found the gamma enzyme to be very sensitive to iodine; Kuwabara and Abraham found this to be true of their enzyme II but only in the absence of zinc.

Enzymes I and II, both cell bound and cell free, have been purified and their activities compared against a selection of penicillins and cephalosporins. The rate of hydrolysis of benzylpenicillin was given an arbitrary value of 100; the rates of hydrolysis of the other substrates were related to this and are shown in Table III.

The substrate profile of enzyme I, both free and cell bound, has much in common with the substrate profile of staphylococcal β-lactamase in that penicillins derived from highly sterically hindered acids and most cephalosporins are resistant to attack. The only substrates resistant to enzyme II are those cephalosporins which have no leaving group on the C-3 methyl. There are sufficient resemblances between free and cell-bound enzyme I to suggest that they are very alike and may be different versions of the same enzyme; free and cell-bound enzyme II may be similarly related. The exoenzymes are present in the supernatant fluids in comparatively large amounts, but both cell-bound enzymes are found in very much smaller quantities. Differences in substrate profile may thus easily be found with different preparations of β-lactamase from *B. cereus*.

Other organisms in this group produce β-lactamases with substrate specificities not unlike those of enzyme I from *B. cereus*. *Bacillus licheniformis* produces an extracellular β-lactamase (Pollock, 1961) which, in substrate profile, has much in common with *B. cereus* lactamase I.

b. INHIBITION. Enzyme I from *B. cereus* is inhibited competitively to some extent by cephalosporin C, which is highly resistant to it (Abraham and Newton, 1956) and also by cloxacillin. It is likely that other penicillins and

Table III

MAXIMUM RATES OF HYDROLYSIS AND MICHAELIS CONSTANTS FOR DIFFERENT
PENICILLINS AND CEPHALOSPORINS WITH BOTH CELL-BOUND AND
EXTRACELLULAR β-LACTAMASE I AND β-LACTAMASE II[a]

Enzyme	Substrate	Extracellular V_{max}[b] (Relative)	Cell bound V_{max}[b] (Relative)
β-Lactamase I	Benzylpenicillin	100	100
	Phenoxymethylpenicillin	102	98
	Ampicillin	100	101
	Penicillin N	38	31
	Methicillin	<1.0	<1.0
	Oxacillin	<2.6	<2.6
	Cephalosporin C	<0.1	<0.1
	Cephalothin	<0.1	<0.1
	Cephaloridine	<0.1	<0.1
	Cephaloglycin	<0.1	<0.1
	Deacetylcephalosporin C	<0.1	<0.1
	Deacetylcephalosporin C lactone	30	30
	Deacetoxycephaloglycin[c]	<0.1	<0.1
β-Lactamase II	Benzylpenicillin	100	100
	Ampicillin	64	75
	Methicillin	89	111
	Oxacillin	89	112
	Cloxacillin	89	83
	Quinacillin	10[d]	9[d]
	Cephalosporin C	80	75
	Cephalothin	89	67
	Cephaloridine	41	56
	Cephaloglycin	50	67
	Deacetylcephalosporin C	<0.5[e]	<0.5[e]
	Deacetylcephalosporin C lactone	<0.5	<0.5
	Deacetoxycephaloglycin[c]	<0.5	<0.5

[a] Kuwabara and Abraham (1969).
[b] Values of V_{max} were obtained from Lineweaver–Burk plots—usual substrate concentration, 10.0 mM.
[c] Cephalexin.
[d] Relative rate of hydrolysis with substrate concentrations, 3.0 mM.
[e] Relative rate of hydrolysis with substrate concentrations, 1.0 mM.

cephalosporins not hydrolyzed by this enzyme may also inhibit it to some extent.

Enzyme II is not active against cephalosporins with no leaving group at position 3. One of these, deacetylcephalosporin C, is a weak competitive inhibitor for enzyme II (Kuwabara, 1969), and deacetoxycephaloglycin (cephalexin) is a mild noncompetitive inhibitor for this enzyme. This could occur if cephalexin complexed zinc.*

c. INDUCTION. The enzyme produced from *B. cereus* 569 is inducible with benzylpenicillin (Pollock, 1950). Crompton *et al.* (1962) found that enzyme I is induced by benzylpenicillin, methicillin, cephalosporin C, cephalosporin C_A, deacetylcephalosporin C, cephaioram, and N-α-phenoxypropionyl-7-amino cephalosporanic acid although the amounts of each compound needed for maximal induction varied 100-fold between benzylpenicillin (the best) and cephalosporin C. These induction results are probably relevant only to enzyme I. It appears that the essential structure for an inducer is a β-lactam-containing compound or one which may have some conformational similarity such as a peptidoglycan (Ozer *et al.*, 1970).

Little is known about the abilities of other penicillins or cephalosporins to induce β-lactamase II in *B. cereus* since most of the later work was done with strain 569/H in which the enzyme is constitutive.

3. BACTEROIDES

Some strains of *Bacteroides* have been shown to possess a β-lactamase. In 1968, Pinkus *et al.* showed that 16 out of 40 strains examined could inactivate benzylpenicillin. It seemed likely that only one type of enzyme was produced which inactivated ampicillin less rapidly than benzylpenicillin. If sufficient enzyme were present, some hydrolysis of cloxacillin could also be demonstrated.

4. MYCOBACTERIA

Several species of *Mycobacteria*, including strains of *Mycobacterium tuberculosis*, can inactivate benzylpenicillin by means of a β-lactamase (Kasik, 1965) although the role of this enzyme in mycobacterial resistance has not been established in relation to the permeability barrier which also exists in these organisms. Some differences between β-lactamase from different species occur and *M. tuberculosis*, which is more sensitive to benzylpenicillin than is *M. smegmatis*, produces only about one-thirtieth the amount of β-lactamase on a dry cell weight basis (Mishra and Kasik, 1970).

a. RESISTANCE OF PENICILLINS AND CEPHALOSPORINS. Penicillins and cephalosporins with nonsterically hindered groups are, in general, sensitive to β-lactamases from all species of mycobacteria. Conversely, penicillins with heavily sterically hindered groups are resistant. There is more variation between different cephalosporins with *M. smegmatis* enzyme although increases in resistance are obtained when the acyl group is heavily substituted (Kasik and

* E. P. Abraham, personal communication.

Peacham, 1968). The cephalosporin analogous to methicillin is more sensitive to β-lactamase from *M. smegmatis* than is methicillin.

b. INHIBITION. The penicillins which are resistant to β-lactamases from *M. smegmatis* can bring about inhibition of the enzyme action on benzylpenicillin, cephalosporin C, cephaloridine, and cephalothin. However, resistant cephalosporins with related acyl groups are not able to inhibit the enzyme; this is consistent with their lower affinities. There was insufficient variation in the 3 position of the cephalosporins tested here to determine what effect, if any, could be attributed to different leaving groups at position 3'. The inhibitory effect of dicloxacillin on the β-lactamase of *M. tuberculosis* has been demonstrated *in vivo*, and in its presence, mice were protected from a lethal challenge of *M. tuberculosis* by benzylpenicillin (Kasik *et al.*, 1966).

c. INDUCTION. None of the mycobacterial β-lactamases described to date is inducible.

5. GRAM-NEGATIVE ORGANISMS—GENERAL

There have been numerous reports of β-lactamase activity in many species of gram-negative organisms. Enzyme-producing strains of *Escherichia, Klebsiella, Enterobacter, Aerobacter, Citrobacter, Hafnia, Shigella, Salmonella,* and *Pseudomonas* have all been widely studied in these species. The picture which has emerged is very complex. Many gram-negative organisms can produce one or more β-lactamases, which vary from strain to strain and from species to species, differing from each other in several characteristics. Sometimes the differences manifested, which are usually first seen as differences in substrate specificity and in sensitivity or otherwise to competitive inhibitors, are clear cut to the extent that it has been suggested they may be of value taxonomically (Dunmore, 1969; Slocombe and Sutherland, 1970; Fleming *et al.*, 1970).

In contrast, there are also β-lactamases mediated by transferable R factors. Because of this, the same kind of β-lactamase activity may be found in widely differing organisms, even of different species. Thus, the enzyme of the type mediated by R_{TEM} has been found to be naturally occurring in a strain of *Pseudomonas aeruginosa*. It may readily be transferred from this species to *E. coli* and back again (Sykes and Richmond, 1970; Fulbrook *et al.*, 1970).

Other β-lactamases, clearly distinguishable from R_{TEM} have been found associated with other R factors (Egawa *et al.*, 1967; Evans *et al.*, 1968; Yamagishi *et al.*, 1969).

The many different kinds of β-lactamase elaborated by gram-negative organisms have been reviewed by Sawai *et al.* (1968) and Smith *et al.* (1969). The overall picture, however, remains confused, and it is not always possible to relate to each other the enzymes described by different authors. This is because the various studies were done with different purposes in mind, which led to the use of enzyme preparations of differing degrees of purity, from cell suspensions or culture supernatants to highly purified material, together with different permutations of substrates and assay methods. Much remains to be done before a clear picture of β-lactamases among gram-negative bacteria emerges.

6. ENTEROBACTERIACEAE

a. CLASSIFICATION. In an attempt to bring some order into a confused situation, Jack and Richmond (1970a) investigated 46 clinical isolates selected on the basis of their resistance to ampicillin but excluding *Pseudomonas* strains. The factors examined were substrate profile against benzylpenicillin, ampicillin, and cephaloridine, sensitivity to inhibition by *p*-chlormercuribenzoate (*p*-CMB) and cloxacillin, reaction with an antiserum to purified TEM enzyme, and electrophoretic mobility in starch gel at pH 8.5.

From the results obtained, they concluded that the β-lactamases produced by the organisms they had examined fell into eight categories, ranging from an enzyme that is almost totally a cephalosporinase in its substrate profile to one almost entirely a penicillinase. Three of the eight categories were mediated by genes carried on transmissible R factors. The properties found are summarized in Table IV.

It is possible that, had a larger number of substrates been used and a wider range of inhibitors tested against organisms selected on a basis other than resistance to ampicillin, more differences might have been seen. The enzyme mediated by another R factor (Sawai *et al.*, 1968) may represent a ninth category and further classes may well be described in the future. However, three major classes are immediately apparent. These are as follows: (1) Enzymes which are much more active against cephalosporins (as represented by cephaloridine) than penicillins (types 2 and 5 in the table). They are resistant to *p*-CMB and inhibited by cloxacillin. (2) Those which are equally active against penicillins and cephalosporins, sensitive to *p*-CMB, and not inhibited by cloxacillin nor anti-TEM serum (types 3, 4 and 8). (3) Those which are equally active against penicillins and cephalosporins, resistant to *p*-CMB but comparatively sensitive to cloxacillin and to neutralization by anti-TEM serum (types 1, 6, and 7).

The differentiation of the classes by resistance or otherwise to inhibition is dependent on the amount of inhibitor used. Although class 1 enzymes are not inhibited by *p*-CMB at $M \times 10^{-5}$, exposure to this substance at $M \times 10^{-4}$ inactivates them by about 30%. Similarly, although both classes 1 and 3 are inhibited by cloxacillin, class 1 enzymes are very much more sensitive to this inhibitor than are class 3. Thus, when used at similar activities, e.g., 2 units, class 1 enzymes (e.g., P99) and class 3 enzymes (e.g., TEM) are inhibited by $0.5\ \mu M$ and $500\ \mu M$ cloxacillin, respectively.

Table IV

Properties of the Eight Types of β-Lactamase Detected among the Enteric Bacteria[a]

Enzyme type	Type species (if any)	Substrate profile (hydrolysis of benzylpenicillin = 100)			Sensitivity to			Chromatographed on	Mobility (cm/hour)
		Benzylpenicillin	Ampicillin	Cephaloridine	Anti-TEM serum	pCMB	Cloxacillin		
1	E. coli TEM	100	150	180	+	R	S	DEAE	−1.6
2	Aerobacter cloacae P99	100	0	8000	−	R	S	CM	+0.1
3	E. coli 53	100	120	150	−	S	R	CM	+0.1
4	None	100	125	60	−	S	R	DEAE	−1.0
5	None	100	0	350	±	R	S	CM	+0.7
6	None	100	160	15	±	R	S	DEAE	−0.2
7	None	100	170	0	−	R	S	DEAE	−0.6
8	None	100	170	70	−	S	R	DEAE	−0.6

[a] From Jack and Richmond (1970a).

As the inhibition obtained both with p-CMB and with cloxacillin is a matter of degree, it is clearly necessary to define the concentration of the inhibitor and conditions of experiment before using these factors to assign an enzyme to a particular category.

Enzyme inhibitors such as p-CMB, depending as they do on the presence of a heavy metal, may produce equivocal results when used to arrest the course of an enzymic hydrolysis. Penicillins, cephalosporins, and particularly their breakdown products, interfere with inhibition of the enzymes by mercury; in the presence of these antibiotics, a much higher concentration of inhibitor is needed to inactivate the enzymes than is effective in their absence and the amount required is proportional to the substrate concentration present.

A wide range of different enzymes exists in the *Enterobacteriaceae*, but these may all be closely related. Minor variations in β-lactamase structure have been found within a single species, for example in *S. aureus* (Richmond, 1965) and *B. licheniformis* (Pollock, 1965). In 1969, Ambler and Meadway showed that, despite having different substrate profiles, isoelectric points, and amino acid compositions, the enzymes from *B. licheniformis* and *S. aureus* have similar underlying amino acid sequences. It is not inconceivable that many of the β-lactamases found in gram-negative organisms may share some basic sequences; minor variations in structure could well account for the differences in properties found in the various enzymes, particularly those with very similar molecular weights. Amino acid analyses on one enzyme from each of the three major classes (Jack and Richmond, 1970b), based on a histidine content of one residue per mole, are given in Table V.

Although the amino acid compositions of enzymes from the different classes are not identical, considerable similarities are obviously present. Many of the β-lactamases reported in the literature can be assigned to one of these eight categories with some confidence, and some of them, such as *E. cloacae* P99 (Fleming *et al.*, 1963), *E. cloacae* 214 (Hennessey, 1967), *K. aerogenes* 418 (Hamilton-Miller, 1963), *E. coli* TEM (Datta and Kontamicha-lou, 1965), *E. cloacae* 53 (Smith, 1963), were included in the screen. Others can be identified comparatively easily, such as the R-factor-mediated lactamase of Egawa *et al.* (1967) or the categories described by Sawai *et al.* (1968) in their survey of many species of gram-negative organisms.

It does not mean, however, that other categories do not exist. Classification into these three major classes is used for convenience. Nor does it mean that all organisms producing a particular enzyme will produce the same amounts of it. The level of expression of a β-lactamase gene may vary greatly from one strain to another.

b. Sensitivity of Penicillins and Cephalosporins. Most workers have used benzylpenicillin as their reference compound when comparing the relative sensitivities of penicillin substrates and this allows comparisons to be made fairly readily. On this basis, some extrapolation is usually possible from one worker to another. The position with regard to the cephalosporins is more complex; cephalosporin C was first used as the reference cephalosporin because it is highly sensitive to most β-lactamases from gram-negative bacteria but reference to benzylpenicillin is now favored by most workers.

Table V

AMINO ACID ANALYSES OF PURIFIED PREPARATIONS OF
β-LACTAMASES ISOLATED FROM ENTERIC BACTERIA

Amino acid	Sources of enzyme preparations			
	E. coli TEM	214	53	D31[a]
Lys	10	9	10	9
His	1	1	1	2
Arg	4	5	5	5
Cys	0	0	1	0
Asp	17	16	14	12
Thr	10	10	10	9
Ser	7	7	10	8
Glu	14	16	13	16
Pro	8	8	5	8
Gly	8	8	11	11
Ala	10	12	12	14
Val	7	8	8	8
Met	2	2	2	2
Ile	5	5	5	8
Leu	11	12	11	11
Tyr	5	2	4	5
Phe	8	4	5	4
Try	?	?	?	?
Enzyme type[b]	1	2	3	5
Strain No.[c]	1	21	2	16

[a] The analysis of enzyme from strain D31 is reported in Lindstrom et al. (1970). The analyses are based on a histidine content of 1 residue/mole, except for strain D31 where the total number of residues is adjusted to similar values to those used for the other three enzymes.
[b] Enzyme type refers to Table 5 in Jack and Richmond (1970a).
[c] Jack and Richmond (1970a).

The susceptibilities of both the penicillins and cephalosporins appear to depend primarily on the nature of the substituent at positions 6 and 7, respectively. One feature which emerges clearly is that both penicillins and cephalosporins in which the acyl substituent has the general structure R–CH$_2$–CO– (e.g., benzylpenicillin and cephalothin) will almost certainly be sensitive to hydrolysis by all three classes of enzymes. Many cephalosporins tested have acetoxy at the C-3 methyl; this is readily converted to hydroxy by esterases found in citrus peel (Jeffery *et al.*, 1961) and mammalian tissues (O'Callaghan and Muggleton, 1963). Although the cephalosporin thus formed has a poor leaving group on the methyl position, there is little change in susceptibility to enzymes from gram-negative bacteria, susceptibility of the cephalosporin being due primarily to the structure of the 7-acylamido group.

Steric effects on the sensitivity of the substrate to hydrolysis are greater with the gram-negative enzymes and when the acyl group is changed to R–CHX–CO–, then changes in susceptibility occur even when the substituent is very small. Rates of hydrolysis depend much more on the type of enzyme being used and, to a lesser extent, on the nature of the group on the α-carbon atom. Ampicillin, with an α-amino group on the acyl moiety, is resistant to enzymes from class 1 but is sensitive to those in classes 2 and 3. Penicillins like ampicillin but in which the α-amino group itself is substituted (Table I, Nos. 11 and 12) are slightly more resistant than ampicillin to enzymes of class 3.* Carbenicillin, which also has a small α substituent but which, however, is negatively charged instead, is resistant to enzymes from classes 1 and 3, but not to those of class 2.

Cephalosporins with a small α substituent in the 7-acyl group behave rather differently from the corresponding penicillins. Once the 7-acyl group has introduced a degree of enzyme resistance, this is then strongly mediated by the substituent on the C-3 methyl. For example, cephaloglycin, with the same 7-acyl group as ampicillin, is resistant to the enzymes of class 1, but cephalexin is not. Both compounds are comparatively resistant to enzymes from classes 2 and 3. A similar situation exists with α-carboxyphenylacet-amidocephalosporanic acid (i.e., carbenicillin analog) and its deacetoxy derivative. In general, most cephalosporins with an α substituted 7-acyl-amido group, and a leaving group on the methyl at position 3, are compara-tively resistant to enzymes of class 1; their susceptibility increases when the 3′ substituent cannot readily be lost. The effects of enzymes in classes 2 and 3 are at present less predictable although many substances with small α substitu-ents have some resistance to hydrolysis by them. It seems to be immaterial whether the acyl substituent is charged or not. The nature of the 3′ substituent appears to have less influence with classes 2 and 3 than it does with class 1 enzymes.

When the α-carbon atom becomes more sterically hindered so that it is, for instance, included in an aromatic ring system (ArCO–), then resistance to hydrolysis increases further. Penicillins like cloxacillin or methicillin are in this category. They are resistant to hydrolysis by enzymes of classes 1 and 3 and are comparatively resistant to class 2; although measurable amounts of

* K. E. Price, personal communication.

cloxacillin are hydrolyzed by a strain of *Klebsiella aerogenes* in this class (Jack and Richmond, 1970a) (Strain No. 19), this was only about 1% of the amount of benzylpenicillin hydrolyzed under the same conditions.

Cephalosporins with sterically hindered 7-acyl groups are generally resistant to enzymes from all three classes. The nature of the nucleus has an influence in this case, as exemplified by a comparison between cloxacillin, which is hydrolyzed by the strain of *K. aerogenes* referred to above, and the analogous cephalosporanic acid, which is not. Increase in the amount of substitution adjacent to the side-chain α-carbon atom tends to increase the enzyme stability of the compounds. Stability is greatest and most consistent to enzymes from class 1; it is generally least and also least predictable for enzymes of class 2, with class 3 being intermediate.

The changes in enzyme resistance which occur when the structures of the 7-acyl groups change from one to another within a type is usually very much less than when changes are made from one type to another (Table VI). If cephalosporins are being compared, it is essential to keep the 3 substituent constant while investigating the effects of changing the 7-acylamido group.

c. COMPETITIVE INHIBITION OF THE ENZYMES. Effective competitive inhibitors are also resistant to the enzymes, but the converse is not always the case, particularly with enzymes from classes 2 and 3. Generally speaking, enzymes in class 1 are very efficiently inhibited by most compounds which are resistant to their action, whether these are penicillins or cephalosporins. Cloxacillin and methicillin are the best-known examples of effective inhibitors for this class (Bach *et al.*, 1967; Bornside, 1968; Hamilton-Miller and Smith, 1964; Hamilton-Miller *et al.*, 1964; Huber *et al.*, 1968).

Other penicillins in which the α-carbon atom is substituted, e.g., ampicillin or carbenicillin, are also inhibitors for class 1. The structure of the side chain is clearly of considerable importance in determining the amount of inhibition that occurs. The nucleus itself, 6-APA, has also been reported to inhibit β-lactamases (Walton, 1964). Enzymes from class 3 are inhibited by the same penicillins that inhibit class 1 enzymes, but much larger concentrations are required to be effective. For any inhibition of class 1 and class 3 enzymes to occur, it is essential that the amide link in the 6 position be heavily sterically hindered or even that it should be absent altogether, as in 6-APA. Enzymes from class 2 are most resistant to inhibition, and so far, no good competitive inhibitor for them is known.

Cephalosporins with the same acyl groups as cloxacillin and methicillin are also good inhibitors for class 1 enzymes although the position again is complicated by the nature of the 3' substituent. If their 3-methyl substituent is acetoxy, then inhibition is good (O'Callaghan *et al.*, 1967). Should the acetoxy group be converted, for example, by mammalian esterases, to the corresponding deacetyl compound, then the inhibiting activity is lost (O'Callaghan *et al.*,

Table VI

RESPONSE OF DIFFERENT TYPES OF PENICILLIN AND CEPHALOSPORIN STRUCTURE TO HYDROLYSIS BY THREE TYPES OF β-LACTAMASE FROM *Enterobacteriaceae*

6- or 7-Acyl group	3 Substituent in cephalosporin	Susceptibility to hydrolysis by			Ability to inhibit		
		Group 1	Group 2	Group 3	Group 1	Group 2[b]	Group 3
R–CH₂–CO	None[a]	+++	+++	+++	–	–	–
	Leaving	+++	+++	+++	–	–	–
	Nonleaving	+++	+++	++	–	–	–
R–CH–CO	None[a]	–	+++	++	++	–	–
|	Leaving	–	++	+	++	–	–
X	Nonleaving	++	+++	++	–	–	–
Ar–CO	None[a]	–	+	–	+++	–	+
	Leaving	–	–	–	+++	+V, (T)	–
	Nonleaving	+++	–	–	–	+V, (T)	–

[a] That is, the compound is a penicillin.
[b] V = variable (not all compounds of the type able to inhibit); T = transient.

1969). Other derivatives of these compounds with good leaving groups at the 3-methyl, such as pyridine or azide, are also effective inhibitors for group 1. If the group at 3 is not a leaving group, then the cephalosporins, although themselves highly stable to the enzyme, are unable to afford more than traces of inhibitory action.

Enzymes in class 2 are most refractory to inhibition and no good inhibitor for them is available yet among the cephalosporins either. Such information as exists suggests that the active center is of a different conformation from that in class 1 enzymes. With class 1, as exemplified by *E. cloacae* P99, it appears that the more three dimensional the acyl substituent becomes, the more efficient is the inhibition obtained; 1-adamantoylcarboxamido-cephalosporanic acid is an extreme example of this kind of three-dimensional acyl group and is a very good inhibitor for *E. cloacae* P99 enzyme, but although it is stable to class 2 enzymes, it has no inhibiting effect on them at all. Cephalosporanic acids with planar 7-acyl groups give some transient inhibition of class 2 enzymes. This increases along the series benzamido $< p$-R-benzamido $<$ α-naphthamido and, contrary to the class 1 case, the absence of a leaving group at 3 in the small series investigated gives variable results and may, in one case at least, be a positive advantage (O'Callaghan and Morris, 1972).

Enzymes in class 3 can be inhibited by cloxacillin or methicillin although concentrations considerably greater than those which will inhibit class 1 enzymes are necessary. The corresponding cephalosporanic acids, however, are ineffective as inhibitors for class 3 enzymes, partial inhibition having been obtained with cephalosporins in isolated cases only. This is in contrast to inhibitors of class 1 enzymes where the nature of the nucleus is immaterial. Extrapolation suggests that a good inhibitor for class 3 will probably have a planar 7-acyl group although many cephalosporins of this type fail to inhibit class 3 enzymes. The nature of the best type of 3-methyl substituent required to go with this hypothetical ideal 7-acylamido group is at present obscure.

The structures, and the enzyme resistance and inhibitory effect that they generally confer on penicillins and cephalosporins, are summarized in Table VI although it is emphasized that, where resistance and inhibition are shown, many exceptions to these generalizations are known.

d. INDUCTION OF β-LACTAMASE. The earliest reports of β-lactamase activity in gram-negative organisms showed that the enzymes found in *E. coli*, *Klebsiella*, and *Aerobacter* were constitutive. However, some species of *Proteus* have β-lactamases inducible by 100 μg/ml of benzylpenicillin, methicillin, or cephalothin (Ayliffe, 1964). Other penicillins such as ampicillin (Bornside, 1968), cloxacillin, and quinacillin also induce β-lactamase in these species (Ayliffe, 1965) although the enzyme production is often masked because some of the inducers can act as enzyme inhibitors, making it difficult to detect the enzyme produced.

Inducible enzymes have also been observed in several strains of *E. cloacae* (Hennessey, 1967), and for maximal enzyme production the concentration of inducer used needs to be much larger than that used for similar induction in gram-positive organisms.

Other gram-negative species, said not to produce an inducible β-lactamase, may in fact do so if sufficiently large concentrations of inducer are used. At least one organism has been described which can make two lactamases, one constitutive and one inducible (Hennessey, 1967).

The range of penicillins and cephalosporins used as inducers with both the *Proteus* and *Enterobacter* species has been very limited so that no conclusions can be drawn about the best substituents on either ring system to make the compound a good inducer. Even between different strains of the same species, there is considerable variation in the increase in enzyme produced by different inducers.

7. PSEUDOMONAS AERUGINOSA

a. SENSITIVITY OF PENICILLINS AND CEPHALOSPORINS. Jago *et al.* (1963) found that a laboratory strain of *P. aeruginosa* hydrolyzed cephalosporin C more rapidly than benzylpenicillin. Sabath and Abraham (1964) and Sabath *et al.* (1965) showed that the hydrolytic activity of this organism on both substrates was almost certainly due to one enzyme. It appears to be cell bound, and disrupted cells have a much greater activity than intact cells or culture supernatants. All strains of *Pseudomonas* tested so far produce this enzyme in varying amounts (Sykes and Richmond, 1971). Sabath and Abraham (1964) showed that growing cells can destroy large amounts of benzylpenicillin; indeed, they do not start rapid multiplication until the amount present has fallen to less than 50 μg/ml.

Cephalosporin C, cephaloram, cephalothin, and cephaloridine were all more rapidly hydrolyzed than benzylpenicillin, while methicillin and cloxacillin were stable. It was concluded that this β-lactamase must play an important part in the resistance of strains of *P. aeruginosa* to β-lactam antibiotics (Sabath *et al.*, 1965) although this may be an oversimplification. Carbenicillin, a penicillin having good activity against strains of *P. aeruginosa*, is resistant to the enzyme, as are the newer penicillins with anti-*Pseudomonas* activity (Price *et al.*, 1969, 1971).

A second enzyme was detected in one clinical isolate by Newsome *et al.* (1970) which had a substrate profile quite distinct from that of the first enzyme and which cannot be induced. It is highly active against carbenicillin and α-sulfamoylpenicillin but has much less activity against cephalexin.

In addition to these two enzymes, some strains of *P. aeruginosa* harbor an R-factor-mediated β-lactamase (Fulbrook *et al.*, 1970; Sykes and Richmond,

1970). This has the same substrate profile as the β-lactamase in *E. coli* R_{TEM} and is indistinguishable from TEM enzyme in its reaction with antiserum prepared against purified TEM enzyme. The amount of β-lactamase associated with this R factor depends on the host strain, but in each case it has the same substrate specificity (see Section I,E,6,b for the characteristics of TEM enzyme). The substrate profiles of these three enzymes are given in Table VII.

b. COMPETITIVE INHIBITION OF *P. aeruginosa* β-LACTAMASE. It has also been observed with the *P. aeruginosa* enzymes, as with others of gram-negative origin, that it is necessary for a penicillin to have a sterically hindered acyl

Table VII

SUBSTRATE PROFILES OF THREE LACTAMASES IN *Pseudomonas aeruginosa*

Substrate	Inducible enzyme	Carbenicillin-active enzyme[a]	R-Factor-mediated enzyme
Benzylpenicillin	100	100	100
Ampicillin	2	180	150
Cephaloridine	400	40	130
Cephalexin	140	8	5
Carbenicillin	10	150	10
Cloxacillin	0	12	0
Methicillin	0	6	15
α-Carboxyphenylacetamidocephalosporanic acid	<1	<1	<1
α-Sulphamoylphenylacetamidopenicillanic acid	<1	N.T.	64
α-Guanoureidophenylacetamidopenicillanic acid	5	N.T.	60

[a] N.T. = not tested.

group before competitive inhibition is seen. The Sabath and Abraham enzyme is strongly inhibited by cloxacillin and methicillin (Sabath and Abraham, 1964; Sabath, 1968; Fraher and Jawetz, 1968; Jago *et al.*, 1963). It is also inhibited by carbenicillin, which has a negatively charged, α-substituted 7-acylamido group, but not by ampicillin, a penicillin with a positively charged side chain. The newer penicillins with activity against *P. aeruginosa* (see Table I, 10–15 inclusive), will probably be able to inhibit this enzyme as well.

Sterically hindered cephalosporins, analogous to the inhibitory penicillins, are also competitive inhibitors of the Sabath and Abraham enzyme, provided that they have a leaving group at position 3. Should they lack such a group, then the competitive inhibition effect is much reduced. The substrate and inhibition profiles of the enzyme as outlined here are very close to those of class 1 enzymes in the *Enterobacteriaceae*. The enzyme active against carbenicillin (Newsome *et al.*, 1970) is more difficult to inhibit with cloxacillin, but some inhibition does occur. This enzyme does not appear to correspond to either of the other two classes of enzymes of the *Enterobacteriaceae*.

The R-factor-mediated enzyme identified with the TEM enzyme is inhibited by the same compounds when it is found in *P. aeruginosa* as it is when present in *E. coli* (see Section I,E,6,c).

c. INDUCTION. Sabath *et al.* (1965) found that the β-lactamase first described by them is present only in negligible amounts in whole cells or culture supernatant when the organism is grown in the absence of an inducer. Benzylpenicillin or cephalosporin C are good inducers, but maximum enzyme production is not obtained unless the inducer is at a concentration of 4–10 mg/ml. This is 10,000-fold more than the amount required to induce maximum enzyme production in *B. cereus*. Most of the inducers are sensitive to the enzyme and the large amounts required may be due partly to their destruction by the enzyme they induce.

The enzyme is also induced by cephalosporins such as cephaloridine under the same conditions as benzylpenicillin. Low concentrations of carbenicillin induce small amounts of enzyme but higher concentrations cannot be tested since they cause lysis. The property of induction appears to depend on the presence of the β-lactam ring rather than on the substituents attached to either the penicillin or cephalosporin nucleus.

The other two enzymes, i.e., R_{TEM} mediated and the enzyme active against carbenicillin, are not inducible.

F. Summary of Structure–Activity Relationships

From the structure–activity relationships detailed above, some broad rules may be deduced. It is clear that a penicillin with a $-CH_2-$ group next to the amide link will be sensitive to attack by β-lactamase from various sources. When this group is substituted, a degree of resistance is introduced which depends to a large extent on the size, charge, and nature of the substituent. Should this α-carbon atom be included in a heavily substituted aromatic ring system, as in cloxacillin or methicillin, then resistance to some enzymes will increase. This is not to say that all such structures will be certain to confer resistance to all β-lactamases, e.g., cloxacillin is susceptible to *B. cereus* enzyme II and *Enterobacteriaceae* class 2. Doyle and Nayler (1964) have comprehensively reviewed the relationship between the type and degree of steric hindrance in the 6-acylamido group in penicillins and their enzyme stability.

Broadly speaking, the same generalizations about structure can be made for the 7-aminoacyl group of the cephalosporins. The cephalosporin nucleus is naturally resistant to staphylococcal and *B. cereus* I enzymes, but variations between analogs do occur although these are trivial in comparison with the resistance of the cephalosporins as a whole to these enzymes. The presence of $-CH_2-$ next to the amide link is almost always accompanied by sensitivity to the enzymes from gram-negative organisms, and this decreases as steric hindrance is introduced. The 3-methyl substituents in cephalosporins also have an effect on enzyme resistance; they can be broadly classified into those which can readily accept an electron and leave the molecule, e.g., acetoxy as in cephalosporin C, and those which cannot, e.g., hydrogen as in cephalexin.

Not all enzyme-resistant penicillins and cephalosporins can act as enzyme inhibitors although there is a close correlation between resistance and inhibition with *B. cereus* β-lactamase I, class 1 of the *Enterobacteriaceae* and the inducible enzyme of *P. aeruginosa*. It is true to say that all resistant and inhibiting compounds known so far have the types of structures outlined above; however, by no means all compounds with these structures are inhibitory or even resistant.

The effect of the two different ring systems is most apparent with the staphylococci. Almost all cephalosporins are highly resistant and some may competitively inhibit staphylococcal β-lactamase, whereas resistance in penicillins is very dependent on the 6-acylamido group and penicillins cannot act as competitive inhibitors. Some differences are seen with mycobacteria, which have enzyme(s) which are inhibited by penicillins but not by cephalosporins. With enzymes from gram-negative bacteria, although some differences between penicillins and cephalosporins do occur, the effect of the different nucleus in these molecules is usually much less than that of the acyl group. Some aspects of the conformational changes in the enzyme brought about by interaction between the enzyme and substrate have been discussed by Citri and Zyk (1965).

The relationship between structure and ability to induce β-lactamases is not at all clear. Those strains which produce inducible enzyme do so to a greater extent in the presence of most penicillins and cephalosporins so far tested. There seems to be no correlation between the susceptibility of a β-lactam antibiotic and its ability to induce an enzyme although a resistant enzyme-inhibiting inducer may well mask the enzyme it induces. Induction does not depend on whether the major substrates for the enzyme are penicillins or cephalosporins; members of either group will induce such enzymes as are inducible, albeit at different rates. Too little is yet known to predict which 7-acyl groups and 3 substituents of the cephalosporins will make a good inducer.

G. Clinical Implications of β-Lactamases

The possession of a β-lactamase is generally accepted as a major factor in the resistance of many bacterial species to β-lactam antibiotics, and the relationship between resistance and enzyme production has been reviewed by Smith *et al.* (1969). Ability to hydrolyze benzylpenicillin undoubtedly plays a major part in the resistance of strains of *S. aureus* to this antibiotic.

Although the semisynthetic penicillins are very resistant to hydrolysis by staphylococcal β-lactamase, they have lower intrinsic antibacterial activity against non-lactamase-producing strains than has benzylpenicillin. However, they do maintain a fairly constant level of activity against staphylococci, whether the strains are enzyme-producing or not, and are clinically highly effective in cases where benzylpenicillin cannot be used.

Cephaloridine is sufficiently resistant to staphylococcal β-lactamase to be able to protect mice infected experimentally with β-lactamase-producing strains of *S. aureus* (Muggleton *et al.*, 1964) where benzylpenicillin is totally ineffective. Cephalothin, despite its almost complete β-lactamase resistance, is less effective in animals challenged with a lactamase-producing strain than it is in animals infected with a non lactamase producer (O'Callaghan and Kirby, 1970). Foord (1967) found that the therapeutic effectiveness of cephaloridine in *S. aureus* infections was independent of the penicillin resistance of the infecting organism.

At first it seemed as if the new penicillins and cephalosporins had solved the problem of infection by penicillin-resistant staphylococci, but strains with intrinsic resistance to methicillin and cloxacillin not obviously connected with β-lactamase production are now known. These strains generally possess a β-lactamase, but enzyme-free mutants of them can be obtained, which maintain the high intrinsic resistance of the parent strains. In the presence of methicillin or cloxacillin they grow comparatively slowly on agar, with an optimal temperature of 30°C, to produce colonies with very variable morphology and heterogeneous resistance. The same type of growth occurs with cephalothin and cephaloridine. There is usually a marked cross-resistance between cephalothin and methicillin, but cephaloridine, although more susceptible to staphyloccal β-lactamase than cephalothin, is more active against this type of *S. aureus*.

For some time, the pathogenicity of the methicillin-resistant strains was in doubt and their incidence did not increase very rapidly. They are unevenly distributed and very few cases have been reported until recently in the United States; many more have occurred in some European countries. There is now no doubt that at least some of the organisms are pathogenic (Jessen *et al.*, 1969), though 10- to 1000-fold less than methicillin-sensitive strains, in experimental infections (Wick and Preston, 1970). Further discussion may be found in Chapter 11.

Not all gram-negative organisms owe their resistance to β-lactam antibiotics to their possession of a β-lactamase. Some species have a high intrinsic resistance and no β-lactamase. Repeated exposure to sublethal antibiotic concentrations in the laboratory will increase the intrinsic resistance of all strains, but this is never accompanied by an increase in, or the acquisition of, a β-lactamase. In addition, not all gram-negative organisms which have a β-lactamase make enough of it to affect their *in vitro* sensitivity.

The resistance of *P. aeruginosa* to β-lactam antibiotics has been attributed to possession of an inducible enzyme (Sabath and Abraham, 1964), but other factors must also be involved. The very large increase in sensitivity of these organisms to penicillins such as carbenicillin or α-sulfaminobenzylpenicillin is much more than would be expected from only a tenfold increase in resistance to the enzyme (Table VII). Similarly, the *Pseudomonas* enzyme which inactivates carbenicillin and increases the resistance of the organism many fold, only inactivates carbenicillin at 150% of the rate of benzylpenicillin. The corresponding cephalosporin derivative is stable to both enzymes but, nevertheless, has very poor antibacterial activity against strains of *P. aeruginosa*. The lower activity of the cephalosporin compounds against *P. aeruginosa* may be because they are intrinsically less active, or less able to penetrate the cells, or both.

The location of a β-lactamase within the cell can modify the enzyme–substrate interaction (Neu, 1968, 1969) although the evidence so far available does not readily distinguish between enzyme type and enzyme location and, indeed, there may be a strong correlation between them. There are also permeability barriers in some organisms preventing either the enzyme leaving the cell or the antibiotic entering it, which will thus affect the rate of hydrolysis. Organisms such as *E. cloacae*, which produce an exoenzyme, very rapidly inactivate high concentrations of compounds such as cephaloridine, and MIC's of the order of 4 mg/ml are recorded for *E. cloacae* with cephaloridine. At this concentration the antibiotic can kill the cells before it is inactivated, but growth occurs without interruption in the presence of only slightly lower amounts which are very rapidly destroyed. In contrast, an organism such as *P. aeruginosa*, with a cell-bound enzyme, is also inhibited by 4 mg/ml of cephaloridine. In the presence of lower concentrations, however, no growth occurs and the cells slowly inactivate the antibiotic over a period of some hours. Only when almost all of the cephaloridine has been hydrolyzed does growth occur.

It is therefore apparent that, although β-lactamase is an important factor in the susceptibility of bacteria to β-lactam antibiotics, other factors will also have considerable influence and the final state of resistance will depend on all of them. Consequently, much of the classical biochemical investigation of the β-lactamases using purified enzymes and substrate concentrations too high to be therapeutically feasible may have little relevance to what actually happens clinically when a crude enzyme in an intact living cell encounters comparatively low substrate concentrations. In order to express the functional efficiency of the enzyme under these conditions, Pollock (1965) introduced the concept of physiological efficiency, which was defined as the specific activity (micromoles of substrate metabolized per microgram of enzyme protein per hour) at enzyme saturation divided by the k_m (molarity) for any particular substrate. Thus, although two enzymes may have very similar V_{max} values for a given substrate, there may be large differences between the k_m values, resulting in widely divergent physiological efficiencies of the two enzymes and thus very different effects in infections.

H. Therapeutic Application of β-Lactamase Inhibition

The degree of inhibition of the β-lactamases of staphylococci by cephalosporins such as cephalothin is not very high and tends to be variable from strain to strain. It is unlikely to have any useful clinical application with these organisms since the enzyme-inhibiting compounds are active in their own right. Some inhibition of β-lactamases of mycobacteria has been observed *in vivo* with cloxacillin (Kasik *et al.*, 1966). The practical usefulness of such therapy would probably be small, partly because of the length of time treatment must be continued in tuberculosis.

Penicillins and cephalosporins resistant to β-lactamases from gram-negative organisms usually have low antibacterial activity against the species producing them. Effective activity can be produced by mixing an enzyme-susceptible antibiotic having good activity with an inactive but highly enzyme-inhibitory one. In view of the variety of enzyme types which are encountered among gram-negative organisms and the variety of structures needed to inhibit them, it is not surprising that clinical opinion on the likely therapeutic usefulness of a mixture of this sort is divided. The inhibition of gram-negative β-lactamases *in vivo* has been demonstrated with *Proteus morganii* NCTC 235 (O'Callaghan *et al.*, 1967; O'Callaghan and Muggleton, 1967) and a strain of *Hafnia** with obvious synergy occurring between the active antibiotic and the enzyme inhibitor. The magnitude of the synergy depends on the numbers of organisms in the challenge, the amount of β-lactamase produced by the organism used, and the ability of the inhibitor to suppress the β-lactamase activity. *In vivo* tests with organisms of high virulence, or which produce a β-lactamase less susceptible to the inhibitor, were not successful (Hamilton-Miller *et al.*, 1964).

There have not been very many attempts to apply the principle of enzyme inhibition to treatment of β-lactamase-producing gram-negative infections in man. Sabath *et al.* (1967) treated 17 incidents of significant bacteriuria due to β-lactamase-producing organisms with either benzylpenicillin or ampicillin together with either cloxacillin or nafcillin as the enzyme inhibitor. The urine of these patients either became sterile or the bacterial counts were markedly

---

* C. H. O'Callaghan, unpublished results.

reduced during this therapy in 12 of the episodes, but bacteriuria recurred after cessation of therapy and the original organism was found in six cases. Good *in vitro* synergy has been seen with this type of mixture and strains of *P. aeruginosa* (Sabath, 1968), but very large amounts of enzyme inhibitor are needed. Although sufficient inhibitor can substantially reduce the amount of active antibiotic needed to inhibit the growth of the organisms, it is unlikely such concentrations could be attained clinically (Fraher and Jawetz, 1968).

Other workers have had poor results and Riff *et al.* (1970) found that treatment with a combination of hetacillin and dicloxacillin was ineffective. Although 12 of their 13 hetacillin-resistant isolates produced β-lactamase *in vitro*, the combination showed synergy with only four, and they concluded that therapy with a combination of a hydrolyzable and a nonhydrolyzable penicillin had little usefulness.

Despite the lack of therapeutic success attained so far, the idea of inhibiting β-lactamases where these are responsible for antibiotic resistance remains an attractive one. The ultimate aim would be to devise a penicillin or cephalosporin active against a broad spectrum of bacteria and at the same time being resistant to, or inhibiting the formation or activity of, the β-lactamases they produce.

II. Mode of Action of Penicillins and Cephalosporins Against Bacteria

A. Cell Wall Structure and Biosynthesis

Bacteria are completely enclosed in a cell wall, which gives them shape and form and protects them from harmful influences such as osmotic shock. Penicillin interferes with the synthesis of the rigid component of cell walls, which is known variously as mucopeptide, murein, or peptidoglycan. As the cells grow under the influence of penicillin, with a progressively disordered cell wall structure, the bacteria increasingly lose their osmotic barrier. Because the cell membrane becomes unable to contain the high osmotic pressure of the cell contents, the cells ultimately burst.

Synthesis of bacterial cell walls has been described in detail by Strominger *et al.* (1967). This takes place in three distinct stages which occur at three different sites in the cell. In the first stage, the uridine nucleotide precursors, UDP-acetyl-muramyl-pentapeptide and UDP-acetylglucosamine, are synthesized in the cytoplasmic region of the cell. At the second stage, these uridine nucleotide precursors are utilized, together with other substrates in the cell membrane, to introduce new disaccharide-pentapeptide units into the growing peptidoglycan of the cell wall, via a membrane-bound phospholipid. This step varies somewhat from one bacterial species to another; for instance, in *S. aureus*

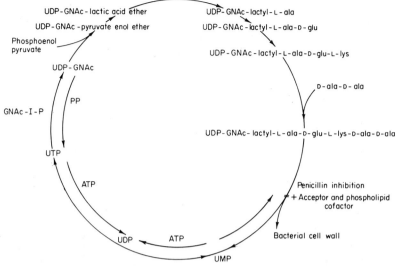

Fig. 1. Biosynthesis of the uridine nucleotide precursors of the cell wall in the cytoplasm (Strominger *et al.*, 1967).

a pentaglycine chain is added to the ε-amino group of lysine and an amide to the α-carbonyl group of glutamic acid. Ultimately, a complete subunit of peptidoglycan is synthesized and transferred to the growing peptidoglycan with a release of *P-P*-phospholipid. (See Fig. 1.)

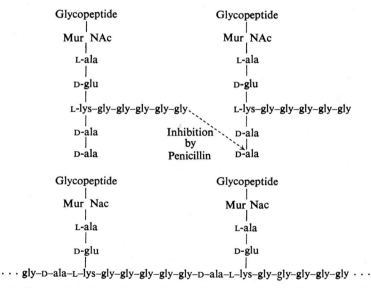

Fig. 2. Closure of glycine bridges in *S. aureus* by transpeptidation (Strominger, 1967).

The third stage of cell wall synthesis is the crosslinking of the linear peptidoglycan strands which takes place outside the cell membrane. The crosslinking is effected by a transpeptidation in which two linear peptidoglycan strands interact with each other, forming a peptide bridge, with the elimination of D-alanine. No additional energy source is required at this stage. (See Fig. 2.)

B. Mechanism of Action of Penicillins and Cephalosporins

Most of the work investigating the mechanism of action of β-lactam antibiotics has been carried out with benzylpenicillin (Ott and Godzeski, 1967; Burdash et al., 1968; Chang and Weinstein, 1964; Hugo and Russell, 1962; Russell and Fountain, 1970). In 1945, Duguid first suggested that penicillin interfered with cell wall synthesis and Park and Johnson (1949) observed the accumulation of uridine nucleotides in S. aureus exposed to penicillin. These were thought to be precursors of the peptidoglycan of the cell wall. Collins and Richmond (1962) suggested that penicillin might be a stereoanalog of N-acetylmuramic acid and that it exerted its effect by preventing the addition of N-acetylmuramic acid or its peptide to a cell wall polymer.

It is now known that penicillin does not affect the first two stages in cell wall synthesis but that it is the third stage which is specifically inhibited by penicillins and cephalosporins (Martin, 1964; Wise and Park, 1965; Tipper and Strominger, 1965). It was then postulated more specifically that penicillin might be a structural analog of the end of the peptide chain because its action is limited to this stage of the synthesis. When molecular models of benzylpenicillin and D-alanyl-D-alanine were compared, it was found that they had a similar conformation. The highly reactive CO–N bond in the β-lactam ring of penicillin occupies a spatial position analogous to that of the CO–N bond in D-alanyl-D-alanine. Having observed this conformational similarity, Tipper and Strominger (1965) suggested that if the transpeptidase formed an acyl intermediate with the end of the pentapeptide, eliminating D-alanine, it could also react with penicillin, forming an analogous penicilloyl intermediate, and thereby become inactivated. In these circumstances, the transpeptidase may be looked upon as a special type of β-lactamase.

In gram-negative organisms such as E. coli, there is also a carboxypeptidase involved in the terminal peptidoglycan synthesis; this enzyme removes the D-alanine residue from the second strand and presumably thereby limits the size of the oligomers. No such enzyme has been found in S. aureus and the oligomers are much larger in that organism. The carboxypeptidase is also inhibited by penicillins and cephalosporins, but the reaction is reversible and the enzymic activity can be recovered by treating the enzyme–penicillin complex with a β-lactamase (Izaki, 1967). The concentrations of penicillin required to inhibit the carboxypeptidase are very much less than those needed to inhibit the growth of the organism. The concentrations which are needed to inhibit the transpeptidase, on the other hand, are comparable with those which prevent bacterial growth. It therefore seems likely that the primary effect of penicillin is inhibition of the transpeptidase.

C. Killing Action of β-Lactam Antibiotics

Penicillin binds irreversibly to bacteria in that intact penicillin cannot be recovered once it has been bound, and Cooper (1956) showed that the amount bound is related to the degree of inhibition obtained. There is a close correlation between the avidity of the binding with a penicillin or a cephalosporin and the degree of inhibition that will result (Edwards and Park, 1969). However, Rogers (1967a) showed that most of the penicillin bound to staphylococci has no effect on their growth, and Pennington and O'Grady (1967) found that inhibition of the cross-linking reaction itself is not necessarily lethal. The effects of bound penicillin can be removed from the cell by treatment with added β-lactamase. If this removal is effected within 100 minutes, the cells are able to resume their normal growth, suggesting that despite the almost immediate action of penicillin on the cell wall mucopeptide synthesis, the cells remain viable for some considerable length of time. Cells saturated with penicillin in this way are extremely sensitive to the addition of further small amounts of penicillin; this may be reacting with freshly uncovered active sites or it may be acting in some other way, being possibly better able to enter the cell once the cell wall becomes disorganized and more permeable.

Rogers (1967b) suggested that, in growing cells, there is an equilibrium between mucopeptide synthesis and the lytic enzymes which are necessary to open part of the cell wall to permit insertion of fresh mucopeptide, thus allowing the cells to grow. In the presence of penicillin, cell wall synthesis is inhibited by the lytic enzymes, the mucopeptidases, function normally, resulting in increasing permeability of the cells and ultimately their lysis. The actual time of cell death will depend on a complex of factors, including avidity of binding, activity or muramidases, and osmolality of the surrounding medium.

D. Structure–Activity Relationships

Although it is now certain that penicillin, in inhibiting the transpeptidase responsible for cell wall biosynthesis is acting as an antimetabolite, the irreversible covalent binding by which it is attached to the receptor site is much firmer than is the case with most antimetabolites (Albert, 1960), which are usually only held by reversible physical binding. Classically, antimetabolites are thought to be structures as similar as possible to that of the normal substrate, but only the configuration of the 6-amide bond and the amide portion of the β-lactam ring of the penicillin molecule has a structural similarity to the end of the peptide chain. Nevertheless, provided stereospecific requirements of the enzyme are met in some part of the molecule, marked differences in structure elsewhere are immaterial, and in some cases, may even be advantageous. However, some penicillins and cephalosporins in which the acyl groups are amino acids often have poor antibacterial activity.

Although most penicillins and cephalosporins investigated so far appear to have similar modes of action, there are large differences in their activities. High antibacterial activity probably depends on the spatial arrangements of certain atoms in the side chains with regard to the ring systems. In contrast to the large number of side chains with high activity, very little change can be tolerated in the nucleus of a penicillin or a cephalosporin before antimicrobial activity is markedly reduced or lost altogether. It is not known, however, whether loss consequent on conformational changes is due to the altered compounds having lost their affinity for the binding site or becoming unable to penetrate cell walls, or both. Structure–activity relationships are discussed in much more detail in Chapter 12.

Permeability of cell walls to penicillins and cephalosporins must play a not inconsiderable part in the sensitivity of bacteria to them. Treatment of cells with ethylenediaminetetraacetic acid (EDTA) potentiates the activity of many antibacterial agents, including penicillin, presumably by rendering the cells more permeable by chelation of magnesium (see Review, Russell, 1970). EDTA can enhance the activity of cephalexin against *E. coli* under some conditions (Russell and Fountain, 1970) and also that of carbenicillin and cephaloridine against *P. aeruginosa*,* but here the effect is sporadic and very dependent on the strain used.

Correlations have been made between the lipophilic character of the penicillin or cephalosporin and its activity against *S. aureus* and *E. coli* (Biagi *et al.*, 1970), the more lipophilic compounds being found to be more likely to be active against *S. aureus* only, and the more hydrophilic compounds to be active against *E. coli* as well. This is attributed to the higher lipid content of the *E. coli* cell walls which would tend to retain lipophilic substances and prevent their passing through and reaching their site of action.

* C. H. O'Callaghan, unpublished results.

E. Effect on Cell Morphology

1. SPHEROPLAST FORMATION

The most obvious manifestation of the effect of cell wall inhibitors on bacteria is the production of aberrant forms, both microscopically and macroscopically. Penicillin induces the formation of spheroplasts in many species; these structures have little or no cell wall and so are osmotically fragile. They are stable only in media of high osmolality. They will revert to the parent form when the antibiotic is removed (Lederberg, 1956), but if serially subcultured in the presence of antibiotic in media of high osmolality, they develop into L forms which are devoid of mucopeptide and which may not revert to the parent form (Kleineberger-Nobel, 1960). The most usual way of stabilizing spheroplasts is to induce their formation in a nutrient medium which contains 0.33 M sucrose (i.e., 11.4%, w/v). Magnesium is also essential (Hugo and Russell, 1962) and this is added at 0.25% w/v magnesium sulfate heptahydrate. The concentration of antibiotic required obviously depends on the minimum inhibitory concentration of the particular penicillin or cephalosporin for the particular organism, but all penicillins and nearly all cephalosporins so far tested produce spheroplasts under the appropriate conditions. When antibiotics are used under conditions of low osmolality, as in nutrient broth when MIC measurements are carried out, then the antibiotic causes the organisms to lyse.

Bacteria must be actively dividing before cell wall synthesis inhibitors can be effective. If the organisms are exposed to penicillins or cephalosporins in media in which they cannot grow, then the antibiotics are unable to exert any killing effect upon them (Hobby et al., 1942; Lambin and Bernard, 1967). The existence of live bacteria with no increased penicillin resistance, known as "persisters," during antibiotic treatment is attributed to those particular cells being in a resting state and thus being temporarily insensitive to penicillin. Pennington and O'Grady (1967) showed that cell wall synthesis in S. aureus may be interrupted by penicillin and restored after several hours exposure without affecting the viability of the cells.

2. FORMATION OF FILAMENTS

Another effect of exposure to penicillins and cephalosporins in normal nutrient media is the formation of very elongated cells in cultures of such organisms as E. coli and P. mirabilis. Such filaments are apparently normal in every way except that they do not divide into cells of normal length but continue to elongate until they may be as much as 50 times longer than the parent cells. This effect has been shown to occur with ampicillin (Rye and Wiseman, 1967) and cephalexin (Muggleton et al., 1969; Fujii et al., 1969).

The concentrations at which organisms become filamentous are very dependent on the antibiotic and the organism. Cephaloridine and ampicillin produce such forms over a very narrow concentration range around the MIC, but cephalexin can induce them over a very much larger range. When these filaments are resuspended in non-antibiotic-containing medium, they rapidly revert to normal morphology with cross walls being formed at the correct intervals along the length of the filament. If, however, the exposure to cephalexin is of sufficiently long duration, weak places form in the sides of the filaments and they burst without generalized lysis occurring. Filamentous forms are also produced when bacteria such as *Proteus vulgaris* are grown on solid media in the presence of cephalothin (Burdash et al., 1968). Growth of the organism appears in macroscopically distinct rings on the agar around a cephalothin-containing disc and microscopical examination of the organisms from the different zones shows the presence of many aberrant morphological forms. The innermost zone contains very variable forms, with many large irregular bodies; outside this zone is one in which the organisms occur mainly as filamentous forms. Benzylpenicillin also gives rise to this kind of aberrant morphology (Fleming et al., 1950). When the organisms are exposed to higher concentrations of antibiotic, they form spheroplasts and lyse without many filamentous forms being produced. Although the formation of filaments precedes spheroplast formation, the two steps are not necessarily sequential; filaments are formed at all pH values but spheroplasts are not formed above pH 7.5 (Grula and Grula, 1962).

It is not possible to investigate every penicillin and cephalosporin in the painstaking detail which was used to elucidate the mode of action of benzylpenicillin. Comparisons have been made of the secondary effect these compounds produce, such as spheroplast formation, in comparison with the effects of benzylpenicillin. In practically every case, the same manifestations have occurred, although under varying conditions of concentration, and it has been concluded that penicillins all act in the same way (Hugo and Russell, 1960) and that cephalosporins act in the same way also (Russell and Fountain, 1970).

F. Other Effects of Penicillins and Cephalosporins

It is possible that penicillins and cephalosporins have more than one activity inside the bacterial cell. Cephaloridine has some inhibitory activity against organisms such as *Mycoplasma pneumoniae*; although this is insufficient to be useful, it is of the same order as the activity of benzylpenicillin against, for example, *E. coli*. As *Mycoplasma* spp. do not have cell walls, cephaloridine must be exerting its effect against some other system in this species. Other cephalosporins have some anti-*Mycoplasma* activity, and one group of compounds is much more effective than cephaloridine. These have a dimethyldithiocarbamate group at the 3-methyl position; the nature of the 7-acylamido group is largely immaterial (Fallon, 1970).

These cephalosporins could not induce spheroplasts themselves; they inhibited the formation of spheroplasts by benzylpenicillin and also inhibited the growth of preformed spheroplasts (Fountain and Russell, 1969). Sodium dimethyldithiocarbamate acts in the same way and it thus appears possible that if one of the substituents of a cephalosporin has some antimicrobial activity in its own right, this may override the more usual mode of action expected of a cephalosporin.

III. Serum Binding of Penicillins and Cephalosporins

Reversible binding to serum proteins occurs to some extent with all penicillins and cephalosporins and decreases the antibacterial activity seen *in vitro*. However, the significance of serum binding *in vivo* is uncertain. Although the available antibacterial activity of the antibiotic will be reduced considerably if it is strongly bound to serum protein, the bound complex may well act as a reservoir. The binding may thus permit a more favorable equilibrium between tissues and plasma to be established and to be maintained for a longer period. This in turn may delay excretion which might otherwise be too rapid to permit the antibiotic to act to its fullest potential.

Several methods can be used to determine the extent of binding, but often the results obtained are very variable. The simplest method is comparison of the dose–response curves obtained in plate assay of solutions of the compound in buffer and in serum, but if the two dose–response lines are not parallel, as is often the case, the value obtained will depend on the concentration used (Scholtan and Schmidt, 1962). Other methods commonly used are ultrafiltration through Visking tubing, either under positive pressure or by centrifugation (Abraham and Chain, 1940) and equilibrium dialysis (Abraham *et al.*, 1941). Values for several penicillins and cephalosporins are given in Table VIII. It is evident that the values reported for different methods and by different groups of workers show considerable variation.

In general, penicillins with bulky, nonpolar 6-acylamido groups are more strongly bound than those with smaller, more polar acyl groups. The degree of binding generally increases with the size and steric complexity of the side chain (Price, 1970). The variability of the results obtained for different compounds

Table VIII

SERUM BINDING OF PENICILLINS AND CEPHALOSPORINS

Compound	Percentage binding	Method of determination	Reference
Benzylpenicillin	35	Equilibrium dialysis	Richards *et al.* (1963)
	41	Visking ultrafiltration	Nishida *et al.* (1969)
	59	Visking ultrafiltration	Rolinson and Sutherland (1965)
	50	Agar diffusion	a
Cephaloram	29	Agar diffusion	a
Phenoxymethylpenicillin	80	Visking ultrafiltration	Rolinson and Sutherland (1965)
Ampicillin	18	Visking ultrafiltration	Rolinson and Sutherland (1965)
Cephaloglycin	24	Agar diffusion	a
	43	Ultrafiltration	a
Cephalexin	26	Agar diffusion	a
	12	Agar diffusion	Nishida *et al.* (1969)
	15	Ultrafiltration	Kind *et al.* (1969)
	40	Ultrafiltration	b
Cloxacillin	94	Ultrafiltration	Rolinson and Sutherland (1965)
5-Methyl-3-(*o*-chlorophenyl)isoxazole-4-carboxamido-cephalosporanic acid	<10	Agar diffusion	a
Methicillin	49	Ultrafiltration	Rolinson and Sutherland (1965)
2,6-Dimethoxybenzamidocephalosporanic acid	<10	Agar diffusion	a
Carbenicillin	49	Membrane filtration by centrifugation	English (1969)

Compound		Method	Reference
α-Carboxyphenylcephalosporanic acid	<10	Agar diffusion	a
Quinacillin	20	Equilibrium dialysis	Richards et al. (1963)
Nafcillin	87	Ultrafiltration	Rolinson and Sutherland (1965)
Ancillin	75	Dialysis	Dolan et al. (1962)
α-Sulphaminopenicillanic acid	56	Agar diffusion	c
α-Guanoureidopenicillanic acid	25	Agar diffusion	c
α-Carboxythienyl-3-acetamido penicillanic acid	45	Ultrafiltration	Sutherland et al. (1971)
α-Amino-4-hydroxyphenylacetamidopenicillanic acid	17	Ultrafiltration	Sutherland and Rolinson (1971)
Cephalosporin C	20	Agar diffusion	a
Cephalothin	56	Ultrafiltration	Sidell et al. (1963)
	65	Ultrafiltration	Nishida et al. (1969)
Deacetylcephalothin	16	Agar diffusion	a
Cephaloridine	31	Ultrafiltration	Nishida et al. (1969)
	20	Ultrafiltration	Kind et al. (1969)
Cephalonium	15	Agar diffusion	a
Cefazolin	29	Agar diffusion	a
	74	Ultrafiltration	Nishida et al. (1970)
7-Cyanoacetamidocephalosporanic acid	<10	Agar diffusion	a
Cephapirin	47	Agar diffusion	Chisholm et al. (1970)

[a] C. H. O'Callaghan, unpublished results.
[b] P. Acred, personal communication.
[c] K. E. Price, personal communication.

when different methods have been used, or even the same methods by different workers, makes comparisons between a penicillin and an analogous cephalosporin difficult. Derivatives of 7-ACA are often, but not always, bound to a lesser extent than 6-APA derivatives. If the cephalosporin has a highly polar group in position 3, then the amount of binding dependent on the nature of the 7-acylamido group will be reduced. As with the other properties of cephalosporins, serum binding is dependent on the interaction between the 7-acyl group and the 3-methyl substituent. The ultimate degree of attachment of cephalosporins to serum proteins will probably depend on the overall polarity of the molecule.

IV. Allergy to Penicillins and Cephalosporins

Some kind of reaction, said to be allergic, has been reported in a high proportion of patients who receive one or other of the penicillins. In some areas, such as the United States, as many as 10% of patients are said to be penicillin sensitive. While it is doubtful if more than a small proportion of these are true allergic reactions involving reaginic antibodies, very unpleasant episodes of the true allergic type do occur and give rise to classical skin allergies of both the immediate and delayed type, to serum-sickness-like reactions and to anaphylactic reactions which may result in death (Fellner, 1968; Idsøe et al., 1968).

With the advent of the cephalosporin antibiotics it seemed that these were non-cross-allergenic with the penicillins and that cephalosporin C, cephalothin, or cephaloridine could be given to patients who were penicillin sensitive. The early promise of these cephalosporins was partly, but not entirely, fulfilled. A recent survey* has indicated that, while about 90% of penicillin-allergic patients will tolerate cephaloridine, about 10% react to the cephalosporin antibiotic also, even though it may be their first experience of it. Some degree of cross allergy must, therefore, exist in some individuals. In addition, some cases of primary allergy to the cephalosporins have been reported in patients not known to be penicillin hypersensitive.

A. Penicillin Allergy

Considerable evidence now exists that the induction of allergy to the penicillins may be mainly, or at least partly, brought about by contaminants of higher molecular weight which become chemically associated by covalent

* R. D. Foord, personal communication.

linking with breakdown products of the penicillin. Batchelor *et al.* (1967) showed that penicilloylated protein in benzylpenicillin could act as a potent antigen in guinea pigs or rabbits, both IgM and IgG antibodies being produced. The protein contaminant was believed to have come from mycelial residues from the penicillin fermentation process and which had come through the purification process in trace amounts. Removal of the high molecular weight impurity resulted in a marked reduction in the antigenicity of the penicillin. Similar observations were made on humans (Knudsen *et al.*, 1967). Volunteers with a previous history of penicillin allergy were given cutaneous sensitivity tests with commercial penicillin (presumably containing penicilloylated protein as a contaminant) and a specially purified penicillin in which such a contaminant was absent. Of 21 immediate reactions in 20 volunteers, 11 were with the commercial but not with the purified penicillin. One was with the purified product only. The remaining 9 persons reacted to both but gave a more marked reaction with the commercial product in one, with the more purified product in 3 and equal reactions in 5. Similar conclusions were drawn from tests on penicillin-allergic human patients by Stewart (1967a). The process which he described for separating his pure penicillin and proteinaceous polymer, involving prolonged dialysis, has subsequently been abandoned due to the possibility of artefacts arising during the process. The higher molecular weight substances are more readily and much more rapidly separated by chromatography on Sephadex.

More antigenic still was 6-aminopenicillanic acid (6-APA) which had been produced by removal of the side chain by *E. coli* acylase. Remaining trace contamination with the *E. coli* enzyme was incriminated as the source of protein which became penicilloylated by association with breakdown products of the penicillin. The breakdown of 6-APA cannot yield penicillenic acid. Its high degree of antigenicity in unpurified form, therefore, seems certain to be due to contamination by *E. coli* enzyme residues. When highly purified its antigenicity is much diminished although, on allowing solutions of 6-APA to stand, breakdown products, which probably form small polymers, can still elicit an allergic reaction in a previously sensitized animal (Batchelor *et al.*, 1967). More recent studies have confirmed the high antigenicity of the penicilloylated *E. coli* protein residue from the 6-APA production process. This substance forms the most potent antigen for raising, in rabbits, the antisera for passive cutaneous anaphylaxis tests in guinea pigs. Such tests afford a valuable control method for testing batches of penicillin in order to minimize the possibility of their being contaminated by potentially dangerous, proteinaceous material.

Also present in penicillin may be varying amounts of nonprotein polymer and these also may be antigenic. The means by which they arise are not fully understood but they are produced in solutions of penicillin which are allowed to stand under conditions which favor the breakdown of the penicillin. The breakdown is increased in rate by elevated temperature, falling pH, and high concentration. Various breakdown pathways have been identified but those which result in the formation of penicilloic acid appear to be the most import-ant since relatively low molecular weight polymers are formed which have penicilloyl antigenic specificity. The presence of these polymers appears to increase the chance of a previously sensitized animal or human reacting to the penicillin. As a result of this finding, it is evident that solutions of penicillin

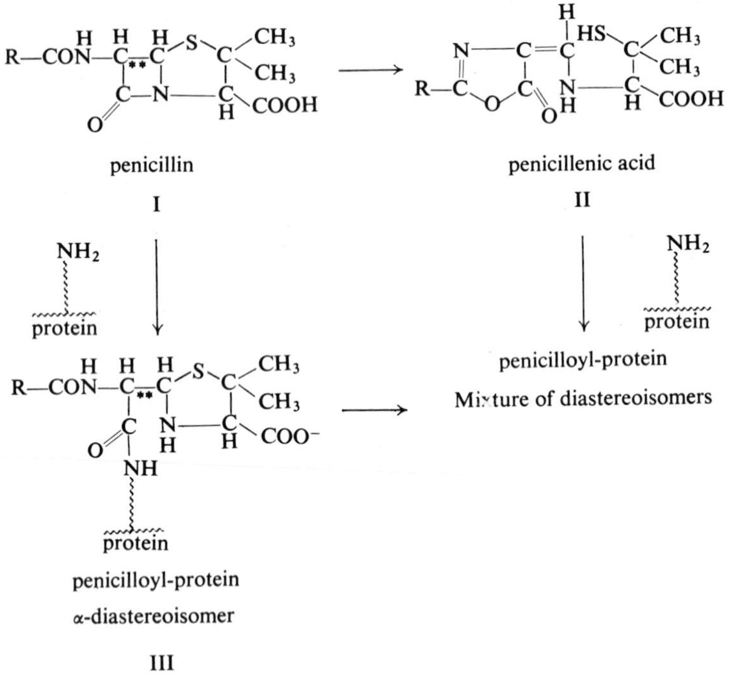

Fig. 3. Formation of penicilloyl–protein (Schwartz, 1969). (Reproduced by permission of the copyright owners.)

should not be prepared long before injection into the patient. The addition of a buffer to reduce the fall in pH which accompanies penicillin breakdown and which accelerates it has also been suggested.

The breakdown of penicillin and the formation of macromolecules with penicilloyl determinants has been extensively studied. Several pathways exist by which these may be formed *in vivo* (Schneider and de Weck, 1969). These include a direct reaction between penicillin itself and suitable carriers (proteins and even simple amines). Evidence for this was obtained by studying the reac-tion of 6-(2,4-dinitrophenyl)aminopenicillanic acid with amines. (See Fig. 3.) This compound, although incapable of forming a penicillenic acid, penicilloylates amines and is capable of eliciting the formation of specific antibody (Schneider and de Weck, 1966). Schneider and de Weck (1967) have also shown that proteins are not necessarily involved in the formation of an antigenic macromolecule with benzylpenicilloyl specificity. Similar complexes with polysaccharides such as inulin or dextran, although unstable, can also act as antigens at least in experimental animals. A recent review (Schwartz, 1969) summarized the chemical aspects of penicillin allergy and gives a good account of the available data to that time.

Earlier work on penicillin allergy suggested that penicillins given orally were unlikely to induce allergy since a dissociation of the protein–penicilloyl complex would be likely to occur in the gastrointestinal tract. Moreover, it seemed unlikely that such macromolecular structures, even if they survived the action of digestive enzymes, would be absorbed intact. The fact that anaphylactic shock could be elicited in patients believed to have a preexisting allergy to penicillin by giving penicillin orally (Fox, 1965) was not inconsistent with this view. However, the more recent finding that the high incidence of allergic reactions due to ampicillin given orally (Shapiro et al., 1969; Willis and Phair, 1970) may be reduced by purifying the substance so as to remove contaminants (Knudsen et al., 1970) seems to show that protein complexes can be absorbed from the gastrointestinal tract and cause allergic reactions. These protein contaminants in ampicillin may arise from the E. coli enzyme used in the 6-APA process or, apparently, from proteins of mycelial origin which have survived the chemical process for the production of 6-APA (Knudsen and Dewdney, 1970).

It is evident that allergy to the penicillins is by no means a simple and easily understood matter, and the continuing researches of a number of groups of workers have produced a sizeable amount of data relevant to the problem. The review by de Weck et al. (1968) shows that, whereas penicillenic acid, a highly reactive degradation product which readily appears in solutions undergoing degradation, is probably the major cause of penicillin allergy, other determinants may be formed which can play a greater or lesser part. Further, there is some evidence that antigenic determinants which may form in vitro may be of less importance in the in vivo situation. There is no doubt, however, that covalent linkages between the penicillin-derived determinant and some carrier molecule are necessary to take part in the final allergic reaction. Simple binding such as is encountered between intact antibiotics and tissue proteins and which is usually reversible is not capable of eliciting an antibody response. The covalently linked molecules may, however, be very small, and de Weck and his team have shown that simple dimers of the penicillin molecule may be sufficient to elicit allergic-type reactions in highly sensitized animals or in man. It seems that the dimer most likely to be implicated is penicillenic acid disulfide.

Studies by Pedersen-Bjergaard (1967b) in humans have confirmed that the penicilloyl radical appears to be of major importance in penicillin allergy since patients allergic to penicillin show a specificity to the radical in cutaneous and serological tests. He points out, however, that penicilloyl-allergic patients often tolerate penicillin therapy without any clinically manifest allergic reaction. The intramuscular administration of commercial penicillin in therapeutic doses gave rise to low and slowly increasing penicilloyl concentration in the body. Oral treatment with commercial penicillins also produced signs of exposure to penicilloyl compounds and intravenous injection of high doses gave considerable penicilloyl specific reactions as shown by Prausnitz–Kustner tests. When the same experiments were done with highly purified penicillins, a much lower degree of reactivity was found and the contamination of the commercial penicillins with penicilloylated macromolecules was therefore assumed. Pedersen-Bjergaard's final conclusion seems to sum up present thinking on the practical aspect of penicillin allergy. His results call attention to the importance of using pure penicillin preparations, but he adds that such preparations will hardly be able to prevent all penicillin allergic reactions with specificity for the penicilloyl radical as penicilloyl derivatives may be formed *in vivo* from penicillin. Schneider and de Weck (1970) have added to the nomenclature by defining intrinsic and extrinsic penicilloyl-specific immunogenicity. They have designated sensitization to penicillins due to conjugation reactions formed *in vivo*—"intrinsic immunogenicity" and to contaminants in the penicillin such as penicilloylated protein impurities, polycondensation products or penicillenic acid disulfide—"extrinsic immunogenicity." Schneider and de Weck, in their belief that the intrinsically formed products have considerable importance in penicillin allergy contribute to the belief that cleaning up the penicillin administered to patients will not solve the penicillin allergy problem.

The possibility that the side chain of the penicillins may have a marked effect in their allergenic properties has been believed by some workers. However, de Weck (1962) in studies with benzylpenicillin, phenoxymethylpenicillin, allylmercaptomethylpenicillin, phenoxyethylpenicillin, and 2,6-dimethoxyphenylpenicillin concluded, from experiments in rabbits, that the side chain plays little, if any, role in the *specificity* of antibodies produced to the injection of the penicillins. It did, however, have a sigifincant effect on the *reactivity* and *immunogenicity* of the various penicillins. Feinberg (1968b), reporting later studies with benzylpenicillin, methicillin, phenethicillin, and propicillin, showed that the side chain did have a marked effect on the immunogenicity of the substances, benzylpenicillin and methicillin being found to be immunogenic while phenoxyethylpenicillin and phenoxypropylpenicillin were hypoimmunogenic. These properties were directly correlated with their degree of conversion to penicillenic acid in solution. Feinberg concludes that an extension of his observation may help in the design of hypoallergenic penicillins.

The detection of penicillin allergy in patients has been a matter for debate for a number of years and various solutions for skin testing have been investigated. There is no doubt that solutions of intact benzylpenicillin, without penicilloyl determinant, are of no value. Benzylpenicillin polylysine (BPL) at a concentration of 1×10^{-6} M of the conjugate appears to remain the best test solution for use in evaluating by the wheal and flare reaction in humans (Levine and Price, 1964). In a considerable study involving 218 patients with histories of penicillin allergy, Levine and Zolov (1969) concluded that skin tests with BPL were valuable predictive tests for immediate (including anaphylactic) and accelerated urticarial reactions to penicillins. They used scratch tests first followed, if negative, by the intradermal injection of 0.005 ml into the deltoid region of the arm. Tests were read after 15 minutes.

In summary, therefore, it seems likely that all penicillins are cross-allergenic and that while a high degree of purity, particularly in respect of protein contamination, is a desirable objective, even highly purified penicillins may give rise to allergic reactions, particularly in previously sensitized persons. Breakdown products which form covalently linked associations with penicilloyl specificity appear to be the most incriminated in allergic reactions, and their presence should be kept at a minimum by not allowing solutions of penicillin to stand before injection. Even so, formation of intrinsic penicilloyl specific antigens *in vivo* cannot be eliminated. On present evidence it seems that a nonallergenic penicillin is an impossibility.

B. Cephalosporin Allergy

Much speculation about the allergenicity of the cephalosporins has arisen by extrapolation of data obtained with the penicillins, e.g., Stewart (1967a) and Feinberg (1968a). This is natural when one considers that the two molecular nuclei have many features in common and that the cephalosporins, like many of the penicillins, are produced semisynthetically from a mold fermentation process. That they are not, in general, cross-allergenic is evident from the fact that much cephalosporin antibiotic is prescribed for patients because they have a previous history of penicillin allergy, notwithstanding which allergic reactions to the cephalosporins are relatively uncommon (e.g., Cohen *et al.*, 1966).

There is, however, direct evidence that common antibodies between the penicillins and cephalosporins can be formed. Abraham *et al.* (1968) studied the immunogenicity of cephalothin and its cross-reactivity with penicillin in a series of 174 adult patients who received either cephalothin or benzylpenicillin intravenously. The patients who received cephalothin had a higher incidence of anticephalothin antibody than did controls. A high incidence of anticephalothin antibodies in the patients who received the benzylpenicillin indicated cross-allergenicity. Conversely, patients who received cephalothin developed a high incidence of antipenicillin antibody and antipenicillin antibody titers which preexisted in the patients increased during the injections with cephalothin. Treatment of the sera with 2-mercaptoethanol indicated that the antipenicillin and anticephalothin antibodies resided mainly in the IgM immunoglobulin fraction. Evidence for the cross-reactivity was obtained by hemagglutination tests on the sera using antibiotic-sensitized erythrocytes. Despite these findings, cases of hemolytic anemia due to cephalothin administration are extremely rare and one must assume that cephalothin alone or cephalothin plus anticephalothin antibody complex is insufficiently bound to erythrocytes *in vivo* for this to be of any practical consequence.

In a study of rabbits, Brandriss *et al.* (1965) showed that cephalothin and benzylpenicillin formed cross-reacting antibodies. These were most evident in hemagglutination studies but were less convincing in passive cutaneous anaphylaxis (PCA) tests. The suggestion was made that cephalothin and 6-APA become antigenic *in vivo* through direct conjugation of the β-lactam carbon to native protein. Cephalothin, of course, cannot form any intermediate *in vitro* corresponding to penicillenic acid.

Stewart (1962) reported that penicillin-sensitive patients failed to react to skin tests with cephalosporin C. In contrast, Grieco (1967) found that a patient who exhibited an anaphylactic reaction to oral penicillin gave a positive skin reaction to cephalothin, cephaloridine, and 7-ACA as well as to the penicillins. The patient was not, however, given any of the cephalosporin drugs in therapeutic amounts so that whether or not he would have reacted is unknown. Girard (1968) studied 36 patients allergic to benzylpenicillin and demonstrated reaginic antibodies to cephalosporins in about one-third of them. Evidence for a significant degree of immunological cross-reactivity was recorded, based on hemagglutination and inhibition of hemagglutination studies. This author concludes that more clinical data is required to assess whether the immunological cross-reactivity measured in this way represents a potentially dangerous situation. Other authors have reported allergic episodes following the injection of cephalothin into penicillin hypersensitive patients (Rothschild and Doty, 1966; Thoburn, 1966; Kabins *et al.*, 1965; Scholand *et al.*, 1968). The latter authors described a severe anaphylactic reaction on first exposure to cephalothin in a patient who gave a positive prick test reaction to penicilloyl polylysine. Pedersen-Bjergaard (1967a) found that in the Prausnitz–Kustner test, commercial cephalothin gave a cross-reaction with penicillin in a number of human sera with reagin specificity to the penicillin radical. This could have been explained by the gross contamination of the cephalothin with penicillin but the amounts needed would have been far beyond the bounds of possibility in the cephalothin sample. Some degree of cross-allergy is therefore supposed.

Further evidence for a degree of immunological cross-reactivity between cephalothin and related compounds and benzylpenicillin was forthcoming from laboratory tests done by Japanese workers (Shibata *et al.*, 1966). Passive cutaneous anaphylaxis, quantitative precipitin reactions, and hapten inhibition tests were used. They concluded that cephalothin and related compounds would be potent antigens under physiological conditions through irreversible bonding to proteins and that strong cross-reactions occur between penicillin and cephalothin in these antigenicity tests. These findings appear to be in some conflict with the majority of clinical findings in which cephalothin, or cephaloridine, can apparently be given safely to penicillin-sensitive patients. Stewart (1967b) draws attention to this. He postulates a degree of overlap between antibodies reacting with all the penicillin haptenes and the cephalosporins but, in effect, questions their relevance. He felt that further study of this problem would be rewarding in that it might give some clue to the nature of allergy to antibiotics in man.

Cases of primary sensitivity to cephaloridine have also been reported (Mitchell, 1965).

A detailed laboratory study on the immunogenicity of cephalothin, cephaloridine, and penicillin was reported by Batchelor *et al.* (1966). They showed that the two cephalosporins they studied formed protein conjugates with which they were able to stimulate the production of hemagglutinating, precipitating, and guinea pig skin-sensitizing antibodies in the rabbit. They found a high degree of cross-reaction with the benzylpenicilloyl determinant group but only very limited cross-reaction with the haptenic determinant of the penicillin nucleus 6-APA. These workers thought that both the side chains and the nuclei played a part in determining the antigenic specificity. They concluded that more clinical evidence is required before the extent to which these results may be related to penicillin allergic human patients is known. They felt, however, that cephalothin or cephaloridine should be given with caution to such patients.

Cephaloridine is prepared from 7-ACA derived from cephalosporin C by chemical removal of the 7-acyl side chain. No commercial process has yet been developed for the side-chain removal involving the use of enzymes from bacterial or other sources. Protein contamination from this source is thus avoided. In addition, the cephaloridine manufacturing process involves chemical treatment—including treatment with nitrosyl chloride—which makes it unlikely that protein of mycelial origin can remain either. If such a protein contaminant from the *Cephalosporium acremonium* were to be found in a cephalosporin, it would be present in cephalosporin C. A protein-like material was separated from a batch of crude cephalosporin C by chromatography on Sephadex; this material was found to be highly antigenic in rabbits when injected in a suitable repeated dose schedule with complete Freund's adjuvant.* Antisera from the rabbits gave strongly positive reactions in hemagglutination tests using erythrocytes coated with the protein and also gave strongly positive

* P. W. Muggleton *et al.*, unpublished results.

passive cutaneous anaphylaxis tests in guinea pigs injected with the homologous antigen. The same antisera were also tested with purified cephalosporin C, cephaloridine, cephalexin, benzylpenicillin, and ampicillin. No cross-reactions were found, even with purified cephalosporin C. Moreover, antisera produced in rabbits against cephaloridine or benzylpenicillin failed to agglutinate erythrocytes coated with the crude cephalosporin C protein and hemagglutination titers with cephaloridine-coated erythrocytes were not reduced when protein was added. It therefore seems that the mycelial protein from *Cephalosporium acremonium*, although antigenic, cannot act as a carrier for the cephalosporin antibiotics or their breakdown products.

Although apparently devoid of contaminating protein (none has ever been detected in any commercial batch despite strenuous attempts to do so),* cephaloridine readily breaks down in aqueous solution and the breakdown products polymerize to form small polymers (perhaps only dimers) which have sulfur–sulfur linkages. Polymer formation is increased in rate by raising the pH above neutrality and by raising the temperature. The breakdown is accompanied by a loss of antibacterial activity, and UV spectrophotometry shows that the β-lactam ring is opened. The precise chemical mechanisms involved are not yet known but they involve the discharge of pyridine from the 3' position on the molecule.

Cephaloridine polymers have been isolated and extensively studied. They appear to be no more toxic than cephaloridine and, when injected into susceptible animals, they have not been shown to produce signs of nephrotoxicity nor to give specific toxic reactions in other organs. However, Stewart (1969) claimed to have found large amounts of polymers in commercial material and that such polymers caused nephrotoxicity. The polymers are highly antigenic and, when injected into rabbits with Freund's complete adjuvant, produce hemagglutinating and passive cutaneous anaphylaxis-sensitizing antibodies to much the same extent as the parent cephaloridine. Common haptenic groups obviously exist since there is a marked cross-reaction between the two antisera.

Many workers have seen a degree of cross-reaction between antisera raised in rabbits to cephaloridine and benzylpenicillin. This is particularly noticeable in hemagglutination and hemagglutination inhibition tests and, curiously, is more marked in the anticephaloridine sera than in the antipenicillin sera. One could argue that this might mean that treatment with cephaloridine was more likely to give rise to penicillin sensitization rather than the other way round. Clinical experience with cephaloridine, now very extensive, has failed to show that it can sensitize to penicillin in man.

Using hemagglutination, hemagglutination inhibition and PCA tests, cross-reactions between the various cephalosporins have been studied.*

* P. W. Muggleton *et al.*, unpublished results.

Complete cross-reaction between cephalothin and cephaloridine was found and cephalosporin C was also cross-reactive. Thus far the evidence seems that with the cephalosporins, as with the penicillins, the side chain confers little specificity to the antigenicity (or haptenic potency) of the molecule. It is surprising, therefore, to find no cross-reaction in any of the tests with cephalexin. It was possible that with this substance there might have been both cross-reaction with the other cephalosporins (on account of their common nucleus) and with ampicillin (on account of their common side chain). Whereas antiserum to ampicillin could readily be raised in rabbits (giving positive hemagglutination and PCA reactions against ampicillin), no positive reactions were obtained in the PCA tests with these antisera when cephalexin was used as the antigen, nor were positive hemagglutination titers obtained with erythrocytes "coated" with cephalexin. Not too much conclusion can be drawn from the lack of hemagglutination, however, as so far it has not been possible to demonstrate that cephalexin is bound onto red cells. Conversely, attempts to raise antisera to cephalexin have been completely unavailing despite injecting rabbits with cephalexin in complete Freund's adjuvant and boosting repeatedly. The rabbit sera failed to react in either the hemagglutination or PCA tests with either cephalexin, cephaloridine, benzylpenicillin, or ampicillin. It can only be concluded that cephalexin is a very poor antigen; hopefully, this may mean that it will be of very low sensitizing potency in man also.

In contrast to these findings with cephalexin, Mashimo (1969) found cross-reactivity between conjugates of ampicillin and cephalexin with bovine gamma globulin when he did agar diffusion tests against antiserum raised to a complex of benzylpenicillin with human gamma globulin. He concluded that ampicillin and cephalexin antigens react with the antibenzylpenicillin antibody by the same mechanism and that this is related to the fact that they have a common side chain. Mashimo points out, however, that the cross-reactivity is not as strong as with other cephalosporins.

Cefazolin has recently been studied from the point of view of its antigenicity (Mine et al., 1970). Protein conjugates of cefazolin-produced antibodies in rabbits could be demonstrated by both specific precipitation tests and also hemagglutination tests. The authors report minimal cross-reactivity between cefazolin and benzylpenicillin and also between it and cephaloridine or ampicillin. They think that the different N-acyl side chain of cefazolin is responsible for this low degree of cross-reactivity.

C. Penicillins, Cephalosporins, and the Direct Coombs' Test

About 10% of patients, without a history of penicillin allergy, who receive therapeutic doses of penicillin show a positive direct Coombs' test. Occasionally, this may be associated with a hemolytic anemia (Nesmith and Davis, 1968). Remission is usually rapid when the antibiotic is withdrawn (Lyon, 1968). There is frequently cross-reaction between penicillin and cephalothin. Gralnick and McGinniss (1967) reported that sera from patients who had never received cephalothin agglutinated red blood cells coated with either penicillin or cephalothin in an indirect Coombs' test (antibiotic coated cells plus serum plus antiglobulin reagent) and in a direct Coombs' test (antibiotic coated cells plus serum) also. Almost identical titers were obtained with the two antibiotics. Other cases of Coombs' positive reactions associated with cephalothin therapy have been reported (e.g., Gralnick et al., 1967), and occasionally it has been associated, although not conclusively, with a hemolytic anemia (e.g., Molthan et al., 1967).

Cephaloridine has also been associated with positive reactions in the direct Coombs' test (York et al., 1968; Perkins et al., 1968), and laboratory investigations have been carried out with a number of cephalosporins (cephalothin, cephaloridine, cephalexin, cephaloglycin, and cefazolin). Kosakai and Miyakawa (1970) showed that sera from healthy donors would agglutinate red cells coated with all the cephalosporins listed when mixed, in an indirect test with antiglobulin serum. The titers obtained varied with samples of antiglobulin serum from different suppliers.

Herz et al. (1969) showed that human erythrocytes, treated with cephalothin, lost acetylcholinesterase activity irreversibly. The effect was dependent on temperature and concentration of the antibiotic. Cephaloridine and cephaloglycin did not have the same inactivating effect. Ferrone et al. (1968) also showed this effect of cephalothin and associated it with the effect of the antibiotic in the Coombs' test in that both phenomena may be a reflection of injury to the cell membrane. This author emphasizes, however, that his observations concern only in vitro phenomena and may not apply in vivo. Certainly there is little evidence that the reaction between cephalosporins and erythrocytes is associated with hemolytic disease. The phenomenon appears to constitute more of a nuisance in the cross-matching of blood for transfusion purposes than a hazard to the patient.

References

Abraham, E. P., and Chain, E. B. (1940). *Nature* **146**, 837.
Abraham, E. P., and Newton, G. G. F. (1956). *Biochem. J.* **63**, 628.
Abraham, E. P., Chain, E. B., Fletcher, C. M., Florey, H. W., Gardner, A. D., Heatley, N. G., and Jennings, M. A. (1941). *Lancet* **ii**, 177.
Abraham, E. P., Baker, W., Boon, W. R., Calam, C. T., Carrington, H. C., Chain, E. B., Florey, H. W., Freeman, G. G., Robinson, R., and Sanders, A. G. (1949). *In* "The Chemistry of Penicillin" (H. T. Clarke, J. R. Johnson, and R. Robinson, eds.), Chapter 2. Princeton Univ. Press, Princeton, New Jersey.
Abraham, G. N., Petz, L. D., and Fudenberg, H. H. (1968). *Clin. Exp. Immunol.* **3**, 343.
Albert, A. (1960). *In* "Selective Toxicity." Methuen, London.

Ambler, R. P., and Meadway, R. J. (1969). *Nature* **222**, 24.

Ayliffe, G. A. J. (1964). *Nature* **201**, 1032.

Ayliffe, G. A. J. (1965). *J. Gen. Microbiol.* **40**, 119.

Bach, J. A., Buono, N., Chisholm, D., Price, K. E., Pursiano, T. A., and Gourevitch, A. (1967). *Antimicrob. Ag. Chemother.* **1966**, 328.

Barber, M., and Waterworth, P. M. (1964). *Brit. Med. J.* **2**, 344.

Batchelor, F. R., Doyle, F. P., Nayler, J. H. C., and Rolinson, G. N. (1959). *Nature* **183**, 257.

Batchelor, F. R., Chain, E. B., Hardy, T. L., Mansford, K. R. L., and Rolinson, G. N. (1961). *Proc. Roy. Soc. Ser. B* **154**, 498.

Batchelor, F. R., Dewdney, J. M., Eston, R. D., and Wheeler, A. W. (1966) *Immunology* **10**, 21.

Batchelor, F. R., Dewdney, J. M., Feinberg, J. G., and Weston, R. D. (1967). *Lancet* i, 1175.

Benedict, R. G., Schmidt, W. H., and Coghill, R. D. (1945). *Arch. Biochem.* **8**, 337.

Benner, E. J., Bennett, J. V., Brodie, J. L., and Kirby, W. M. M. (1965). *J. Bacteriol.* **90**, 1599.

Biagi, G. L., Guerra, M. C., Barbaro, A. M., and Gamba, M. F. (1970). *J. Med. Chem.* **13**, 511.

Bornside, G. H. (1968). *Appl. Microbiol.* **16**, 1507.

Brandriss, M. W., Smith, J. W., and Steinman, H. G. (1965). *J. Immunol.* **94**, 696.

Brown, D. M., and Acred, P. (1960). *Lancet* ii, 568.

Burdash, N. M., Ehrlich, M. A., Ehrlich, H. G., and Parish, J. T. (1968). *J. Bacteriol.* **95**, 1956.

Chabbert, Y. A., and Pillet, J. (1967). *Nature* **213**, 1137.

Chang, T. W., and Weinstein, L. (1964). *Science* **143**, 807.

Chisholm, D. R., Leitner, F., Misiek, M., Wright, G. E., and Price, K. E. (1970). *Antimicrob. Ag. Chemother.* **1969**, 244.

Citri, N., and Kalkstein, A. (1967). *Arch. Biochem. Biophys.* **121**, 720.

Citri, N., and Pollock, M. R. (1966). *Advan. Enzymol. Relat. Subj. Biochem.* **28**, 237.

Citri, N., and Zyk, N. (1965). *Biochim. Biophys. Acta* **99**, 407.

Cohen, P. G., Romansky, M. J., and Johnson, A. C. (1966). *Antimicrob. Ag. Chemother.* **1965**, 894.

Collins, J. F., and Richmond, M. H. (1962). *Nature* **195**, 142.

Cooper, P. D. (1956). *Bacteriol. Rev.* **20**, 28.

Crawford, K., and Abraham, E. P. (1957). *J. Gen. Microbiol.* **16**, 604.

Crompton, B., Jago, M., Crawford, K., Newton, G. G. F., and Abraham, E. P. (1962). *Biochem. J.* **83**, 52.

Datta, N., and Kontamichalou, P. (1965). *Nature* **208**, 239.

de Weck, A. L. (1962). *Int. Arch. Allergy Appl. Immunol.* **21**, 38.

de Weck, A. L., Schneider, C. H., and Gutersohn, J. (1968). *Int. Arch. Allergy Appl. Immunol.* **33**, 535.

Dolan, M. M., Bondi, A., Hoover, J. R. E., Tumilowicz, R., Stewart, R. C., and Ferlauto, R. J. (1962). *Antimicrob. Ag. Chemother.* **1961**, 648.

Doyle, F. P., and Nayler, J. H. C. (1964). *Advan. Drug. Res.* **1**, 1.

Duguid, J. P. (1945). *Edinburgh Med. J.* **53**, 401.

Dunmore, R. T. (1969). *Can. J. Med. Technol.* **31**, 91.

Edwards, J. R., and Park, J. T. (1969). *J. Bacteriol.* **99**, 459.

Egawa, R., Sawai, T., and Mitsuhashi, S. (1967). *Jap. J. Microbiol.* **11**, 173.

English, A. R. (1969). *Antimicrob. Ag. Chemother.* **1968**, 482.

Eriksen, K. R., and Erichsen, I. (1964). *Acta Pathol. Microbiol. Scand.* **62**, 399.

Evans, J., Galindo, E., Olarte, J., and Falkow, S. (1968). *J. Bacteriol.* **96**, 1441.

Eyckmans, L., and Hook, E. W. (1966). *J. Bacteriol.* **91**, 997.

Fallon, R. J. (1970). *J. Appl. Bacteriol.* **33**, 744.

Feinberg, J. G. (1968a). *Int. Arch. Allergy Appl. Immunol.* **33**, 439.

Feinberg, J. G. (1968b). *Int. Arch. Allergy Appl. Immunol.* **33**, 444.

Fellner, M. J. (1968). *Arch. Dermatol.* **97**, 503.

Ferrone, S., Zanella, A., Mercuriali, F., and Pizzi, C. (1968). *Eur. J. Pharmacol.* **4**, 211.

Fleming, A., Voureka, A., Kramer, J. R. H., and Hughes, W. H. (1950). *J. Gen. Microbiol.* **4**, 257.

Fleming, P. C., Goldner, M., and Glass, D. G. (1963). *Lancet* ii, 1399.

Fleming, P. C., Charlebois, M., and Dunmore, R. T. (1970). *Postgrad. Med. J., Suppl.* **46** 51.

Foord, R. D. (1967). *Postgrad. Med. J. Suppl.* **43**, 63.

Fountain, R. H., and Russell, A. D. (1969). *J. Appl. Bacteriol.* **32**, 312.

Fox, A. M. (1965). *Brit. Med. J.* **2**, 206.

Fraher, M. A., and Jawetz, E. (1968). *Antimicrob. Ag. Chemother.* **1967**, 711.

Fujii, R., Konno, M., and Ubukata, K. (1969). *Proc. Symp. Clinical Evaluation Cephalexin,* p. 19. Royal Society of Medicine, London.

Fulbrook, P. D., Elson, S. W., and Slocombe, B. (1970). *Nature* **226**, 1054.

Girard, J.-P. (1968). *Int. Arch. Allergy Appl. Immunol.* **33**, 428.

Gourevitch, A., Hunt, G. A., Pursiano, T. A., Carmack, C. C., Moses, A. J., and Lein, J. (1961). *Antibiot. Chemother.* **11**, 780.

Gourevitch, A., Pursiano, T. A., and Lein, J. (1962). *Nature* **195**, 496.

Gralnick, H. R., and McGinnis, M. H. (1967). *Nature* **216**, 1026.

Gralnick, H. R., Wright, L. D., and McGinnis, M. H. (1967). *J. Amer. Med. Ass.* **199**, 725.

Grieco, M. H. (1967). *Arch. Intern. Med.* **119**, 141.

Grula, E. A., and Grula, M. M. (1962). *J. Bacteriol.* **83**, 981.

Hamilton-Miller, J. M. T. (1963). *Biochem. J.* **87**, 209.

Hamilton-Miller, J. M. T. (1967). *Nature* **214**, 1333.

Hamilton-Miller, J. M. T., and Ramsay, J. (1967). *J. Gen. Microbiol.* **49**, 491.

Hamilton-Miller, J. M. T., and Smith, J. T. (1964). *Nature* **201**, 999.

Hamilton-Miller, J. M. T., Smith, J. T., and Knox, R. (1963). *J. Pharm. Pharmacol.* **15**, 81.

Hamilton-Miller, J. M. T., Smith, J. T., and Knox, R. (1964). *Nature* **201**, 867.

Hamilton-Miller, J. M. T., Richards, E., and Abraham, E. P. (1970). *Biochem. J.* **116**, 385.

Hennessey, T. D. (1967). *J. Gen. Microbiol.* **49**, 277.

Henry, R. J., and Housewright, R. D. (1947). *J. Biol. Chem.* **167**, 559.

Herz, F., Kaplan, E., and Sevdalian, D. A. (1969). *Acta Haematol.* **41**, 94.

Hewitt, J. H., and Parker, M. T. (1968). *J. Clin. Pathol.* **21**, 75.

Hobby, G. L., Meyer, K., and Chaffee, E. (1942). *Proc. Soc. Exp. Biol. Med.* **50**, 281.

Holt, R. J., and Stewart, G. T. (1965). *Biochim. Biophys. Acta* **100**, 23.

Huber, F. M., Caltrider, P. G., and Noble, S. (1968). *Can. J. Microbiol.* **14**, 349.

Hugo, W. B., and Russell, A. D. (1960). *J. Bacteriol.* **80**, 436.

Hugo, W. B., and Russell, A. D. (1962). *Biochem. Pharmacol.* **11**, 829.

Idsøe, O., Guthe, T., Willcox, R. R., and de Weck, A. L. (1968). *Bull. W.H.O.* **38**, 159.

Izaki, K. (1967). *Fed. Proc. Fed. Amer. Soc. Exp. Biol.* **26**, 388, Abstract 735.

Jack, G. W., and Richmond, M. H. (1970a). *J. Gen. Microbiol.* **61**, 43.

Jack, G. W., and Richmond, M. H. (1970b). *FEBS Lett.* **12**, 30.

Jago, M. (1964). *Brit. J. Pharmacol. Chemother.* **22**, 22.

Jago, M., Migliacci, A., and Abraham, E. P. (1963). *Nature* **199**, 375.

Jeffery, J. D'A., Abraham, E. P., and Newton, G. G. F. (1961). *Biochem. J.* **81**, 591.

Jessen, O., Rosendal, K., Bulow, P., Faber, V., and Eriksen, K. R. (1969). *N. Engl. J. Med.* **281**, 627.

Jevons, M. P., Coe, A. W., and Parker, M. T. (1963). *Lancet* **i**, 904.
Kabins, S. A., Eisenstein, B., and Cohen, S. (1965). *J. Amer. Med. Ass.* **193**, 159.
Kasik, J. E. (1965). *Amer. Rev. Resp. Dis.* **91**, 117.
Kasik, J. E., and Peacham, L. (1968). *Biochem. J.* **107**, 675.
Kasik, J. E., Weber, M., Winberg, E., and Barclay, W. R. (1966). *Amer. Rev. Resp. Dis.* **94**, 260.
Kind, A. C., Kestle, D. G., Standiford, H. C., Freeman, P., and Kirby, W. M. M. (1969). *Antimicrob. Ag. Chemother.* **1968**, 405.
Kleineberger-Nobel, E. (1960). *In* "The Bacteria" (I. C. Gunsalus and R. Y. Stanier, eds), Vol. 1, p. 361. Academic Press, New York.
Knudsen, E. T., and Dewdney, J. M. (1970). *Brit. Med. J.* **ii**, 206.
Knudsen, E. T., Robinson, D. P. W., Croydon, E. A. P., and Tees, E. C. (1967). *Lancet* **i**, 1184.
Knudsen, E. T., Dewdney, J. M., and Trafford, J. A. P. (1970). *Brit. Med. J.* **i**, 469.
Kosakai, N., and Miyakawa, C. (1970). *Postgrad. Med. J. Suppl.* **46**, 107.
Kuwabara, S. (1969). Ph.D. Thesis, Oxford Univ.
Kuwabara, S. (1970). *Biochem. J.* **118**, 457.
Kuwabara, S., and Abraham, E. P. (1967). *Biochem. J.* **103**, 27C.
Kuwabara, S., and Abraham, E. P. (1969). *Biochem. J.* **115**, 859.
Lambin, S., and Bernard, J. (1967). *Postgrad. Med. J.* **43**, 42.
Lederberg, J. (1956). *Proc. Nat. Acad. Sci. U.S.A.* **42**, 574.
Levine, B. B., and Price, V. H. (1964). *Immunology* **7**, 542.
Levine, B. B., and Zolov, D. M. (1969). *J. Allergy* **43**, 231.
Lindstrom, E. B., Boman, H. G., and Steele, B. B. (1970). *J. Bacteriol.* **101**, 218.
Lyon, L. J. (1968). *J. Mt. Sinai Hosp. New York* **25**, 258.
Martin, H. H. (1964). *J. Gen. Microbiol.* **36**, 441.
Mashimo, K. (1969). *Proc. Symp. Clinical Evaluation Cephalexin*, p. 97. Royal Society of Medicine, London.
Mine, Y., Nishida, M., Goto, S., and Kuwahara, S. (1970). *J. Antibiot.* **23**, 195.
Mishra, R. K., and Kasik, J. E. (1970). *Int. Z. Klin. Pharmakol. Ther. Toxikol.* **3**, 73.
Mitchell, J. H. (1965). *Lancet* **ii**, 511.
Moat, A. G., Ceci, L. N., and Bondi, A. (1961). *Proc. Soc. Exp. Biol. Med.* **107**, 675.
Molthan, L., Reidenberg, M. M., and Eichman, M. F. (1967). *N. Engl. J. Med.* **277**, 123.
Muggleton, P. W., O'Callaghan, C. H., and Stevens, W. K. (1964). *Brit. Med. J.* **ii**, 1234.
Muggleton, P. W., O'Callaghan, C. H., Foord, R. D., Kirby, S. M., and Ryan, D. M. (1969). *Antimicrob. Ag. Chemother.* **1968**, 353.
Nayler, J. H. C., Long, A. A. W., Brown, D. M., Acred, P., Rolinson, G. N., Batchelor, F. R., Stevens, S., and Sutherland, R. (1962). *Nature* **195**, 1264.
Nesmith, L. W., and Davis, J. W. (1968). *J. Amer. Med. Ass.* **203**, 27.
Neu, H. C. (1968). *Biochem. Biophys. Res. Commun.* **32**, 258.
Neu, H. C. (1969). *Appl. Microbiol.* **17**, 783.
Newsome, S. W. B., Sykes, R. B., and Richmond, M. H. (1970). *J. Bacteriol.* **101**, 1079.
Newton, G. G. F., and Abraham, E. P. (1956). *Biochem. J.* **62**, 651.
Nishida, M., Yokota, Y., and Matsubara, T. (1969). *J. Antibiot.* **22**, 381.
Nishida, M., Matsubara, T., Murakawa, T., Mine, Y., Yokota, Y., Kuwahara, S., and Goto, S. (1970). *Antimicrob. Ag. Chemother.* **1969**, 236.
O'Callaghan, C. H., and Kirby, S. M. (1970). *Postgrad. Med. J.*, Suppl. **46**, 9.
O'Callaghan, C. H., and Morris, A. (1972). In preparation.
O'Callaghan, C. H., and Muggleton, P. W. (1963). *Biochem. J.* **89**, 304.
O'Callaghan, C. H., and Muggleton, P. W. (1967). *J. Gen. Microbiol.* **48**, 449.

O'Callaghan, C. H., Muggleton, P. W., Kirby, S. M., and Ryan, D. M. (1967). *Antimicrob. Ag. Chemother.* **1966**, 337.

O'Callaghan, C. H., Muggleton, P. W., and Ross, G. W. (1969). *Antimicrob. Ag. Chemother.* **1968**, 57.

O'Callaghan, C. H., Kirby, S. M., Morris, A., Waller, R. E., and Duncombe, R. E. (1972). *J. Bact.* (in press.)

Ott, J. L., and Godzeski, C. W. (1967). *Antimicrob. Ag. Chemother.* **1966**, 75.

Ozer, J. H., Lowery, D. L., and Saz, A. K. (1970). *J. Bacteriol.* **102**, 52.

Park, J. T., and Johnson, M. (1949). *J. Biol. Chem.* **179**, 585.

Pechere, J. F., and Zanen, J. (1962). *Nature* **195**, 805.

Pedersen-Bjergaard, J. (1967a). *Acta Allergol.* **22**, 299.

Pedersen-Bjergaard, J. (1967b). *Acta Allergol.* **22**, 466.

Pennington, J. H., and O'Grady, F. (1967). *Nature* **213**, 34.

Perkins, R. L., Mengel, C. E., and Saslaw, S. (1968). *Proc. Soc. Exp. Biol. Med.* **129**, 397.

Perret, C. J. (1954). *Nature* **174**, 1012.

Pinkus, G., Veto, G., and Braude, A. I. (1968). *J. Bacteriol.* **96**, 1437.

Pollock, M. R. (1950). *Brit. J. Exp. Pathol.* **31**, 739.

Pollock, M. R. (1961). *J. Gen. Microbiol.* **26**, 239.

Pollock, M. R. (1965). *Biochem. J.* **94**, 666.

Pollock, M. R., and Torriani, A. M. (1953). *C. R. Acad. Sci. Paris* **237**, 276.

Price, K. E. (1970). *Advan. Appl. Microbiol.* **2**, 17.

Price, K. E., Chisholm, D. R., Leitner, F., Misiek, M., and Gourevitch, A. (1969). *Appl. Microbiol.* **17**, 881.

Price, K. E., Leitner, F., Misiek, M., Chisholm, D. R., and Pursiano, T. A. (1971). *Antimicrob. Ag. Chemother.*, **1970**, 17.

Richards, H. C., Housely, J. R., and Spooner, D. F. (1963). *Nature* **199**, 354.

Richmond, M. H. (1963). *Biochem. J.* **88**, 452.

Richmond, M. H. (1965). *Biochem. J.* **94**, 584.

Ridley, M., and Phillips, I. (1965). *Nature* **208**, 1076.

Riff, L., Olexy, V. M., and Jackson, G. G. (1970). *Antimicrob. Ag. Chemother.* **1969**, 405.

Rogers, H. J. (1967a). *Biochem. J.* **103**, 90.

Rogers, H. J. (1967b). *Nature* **213**, 31.

Rolinson, G. N., and Sutherland, R. (1965). *Brit. J. Pharmacol. Chemother.* **25**, 638.

Rolinson, G. N., Stevens, S., Batchelor, F. R., Cameron-Wood, J., and Chain, E. B. (1960). *Lancet* **ii**, 564.

Rothschild, P. D., and Doty, D. B. (1966). *J. Amer. Med. Ass.* **196**, 372.

Rudzik, M. B., and Imsande, J. (1970). *J. Biol. Chem.* **245**, 3556.

Russell, A. D. (1970). *In* "Inhibition and Destruction of the Microbial Cell." Academic Press, London.

Russell, A. D., and Fountain, R. H. (1970). *Postgrad. Med. J. Suppl.* **46**, 43.

Rye, R. M., and Wiseman, D. (1967). *J. Pharm. Pharmacol.* **19**, 45.

Sabath, L. D. (1968). *Antimicrob. Ag. Chemother.* **1967**, 210.

Sabath, L. D., and Abraham, E. P. (1964). *Nature* **204**, 1066.

Sabath, L. D., and Abraham, E. P. (1966a). *Antimicrob. Ag. Chemother.* **1965**, 392.

Sabath, L. D., and Abraham, E. P. (1966b). *Biochem. J.* **98**, 11C.

Sabath, L. D., and Finland, M. (1968). *J. Bacteriol.* **95**, 1513.

Sabath, L. D., Jago, M., and Abraham, E. P. (1965). *Biochem. J.* **96**, 739.

Sabath, L. D., Elder, H. A., McCall, C. E., and Finland, M. (1967). *N. Engl. J. Med.* **277**, 232.

Sawai, T., Mitsuhashi, S., and Yamagishi, S. (1968). *Jap. J. Microbiol.* **12**, 423.

Schneider, C. H., and de Weck, A. L. (1966). *Helv. Chim. Acta* **49**, 1707.

Schneider, C. H., and de Weck, A. L. (1967). *Immunochemistry* **4**, 331.
Schneider, C. H., and de Weck, A. L. (1969). *Int. Arch. Allergy Appl. Immunol.* **36**, 129.
Schneider, C. H., and de Weck, A. L. (1970). *Immunochemistry* **7**, 157.
Scholand, J. F., Tennenbaum, J. I., and Cerilli, G. J. (1968). *J. Amer. Med. Ass.* **206**, 130.
Scholtan, W., and Schmidt, J. (1962). *Arzneim. Forsch.* **12**, 741.
Schwartz, M. A. (1969). *J. Pharm. Sci.* **58**, 643.
Seligman, S. J., and Hewitt, W. L. (1966). *Antimicrob. Ag. Chemother.* **1965**, 387.
Shapiro, S., Slone, D., Siskind, V., Lewis, G. P., and Jick, H. (1969). *Lancet* **i**, 969.
Shibata, K., Atsumi, T., Horiushi, Y., and Mashimo, K. (1966). *Nature* **212**, 419.
Sidell, S., Burdick, R. E., Brodie, J., Bulger, R. J., and Kirby, W. M. M. (1963). *Arch. Int. Med.* **112**, 21.
Slocombe, B., and Sutherland, R. (1970). *Antimicrob. Ag. Chemother.* **1969**, 78.
Smith, J., and White, A. (1963). *Antimicrob. Ag. Chemother.* **1962**, 354.
Smith, J. T. (1963). *Nature* **197**, 900.
Smith, J. T., Hamilton-Miller, J. M. T., and Knox, R. (1969). *J. Pharm. Pharmacol.* **21**, 337.
Spencer, J. L., Siu, F. Y., Flynn, E. H., Jackson, B. G., Sigal, M. V., Higgins, H. M., Chauvette, R. R., Andrews, S. L., and Bloch, D. E. (1967). *Antimicrob. Ag. Chemother.* **1966**, 573.
Staab, F. W., Ragan, E. A., and Brinkley, S. B. (1946). Abstracts of Papers. *109th Meeting Amer. Chem. Soc. April, Atlantic City, New Jersey* p. 3B.
Stewart, A. G. (1962). *Lancet* **i**, 509.
Stewart, G. T. (1967a). *Lancet* **i**, 1177.
Stewart, G. T. (1967b). *Postgrad. Med. J.* **43**, 31.
Stewart, G. T. (1969). *Antimicrob. Ag. Chemother.* **1968**, 128.
Strominger, J. L. (1967). *In* "Antibiotics" (D. Gottlieb and P. D. Shaw, eds), Vol. 1, p. 705. Springer-Verlag, New York.
Strominger, J. L., Izaki, K., Matsuhashi, M., and Tipper, D. J. (1967). *Fed. Proc. Fed. Amer. Soc. Exp. Biol.* **26**, 9.
Sutherland, R., and Rolinson, G. N. (1971). *Antimicrob. Ag. Chemother.* **1970**, 411.
Sutherland, R., Burnett, J., and Rolinson, G. N. (1971). *Antimicrob. Ag. Chemother.* **1970**, 390.
Sykes, R. B., and Richmond, M. H. (1971). *Lancet* **2**, 342.
Sykes, R. B., and Richmond, M. H. (1970). *Nature* **226**, 952.
Thoburn, R. (1966). *J. Amer. Med. Ass.* **198**, 345.
Tipper, D. J., and Strominger, J. L. (1965). *Proc. Nat. Acad. Sci. U.S.A.*, **54**, 1133.
Walton, R. B. (1964). *Science* **143**, 1438.
Wick, W. E., and Boniece, W. S. (1965). *Appl. Microbiol.* **13**, 2.
Wick, W. E., and Preston, D. A. (1970). *Proc. Int. Congr. Chemother., 6th* **1**, 428.
Willis, R. R., and Phair, J. P. (1970). *Arch. Int. Med.* **125**, 312.
Wise, E. M., and Park, J. T. (1965). *Proc. Nat. Acad. Sci. U.S.A.* **54**, 75.
Wise, W. S., and Twigg, G. H. (1950). *Analyst* **75**, 106.
Yamagishi, S., O'Hara, K., Sawai, T., and Mitsuhashi, S. (1969). *J. Biochem. (Tokyo)* **66**, 1.
York, P. S., Landes, R. R., and Seay, L. S. (1968). *J. Amer. Med. Ass.* **206**, 1086.
Yurchenco, J. A., Hopper, M. W., and Warren, G. H. (1962). *Antibiot. Chemother.* **12**, 534.
Zygmunt, W. A., Harrison, E. F., Browder, H. P., and Tavormina, P. A. (1968). *Appl. Microbiol.* **16**, 1174.

Chapter 11

BIOLOGICAL EVALUATION

WARREN E. WICK

I. Introduction

A. Historical

During the first few years of clinical use, benzylpenicillin was extremely efficient for therapy of severe staphylococcal infections. However, by 1950, approximately 80% of hospital-acquired *Staphylococcus aureus* infections were found to be caused by penicillin-resistant cultures of the organism. To counter this, bacteremic staphylococcal infections were often treated with antibiotics such as erythromycin and chloramphenicol until 1955, when vancomycin was introduced. Considerable improvement in curing rate was noted with vancomycin therapy, but the occurrence of fever, chills, and phlebitis was frequent following intravenous administration of this antibiotic. A new antibiotic that was clinically acceptable and was not degraded by staphylococcal penicillinase was needed.

Study of cephalosporin antibiotics was encouraged by evidence that the ring system of cephalosporin C was quite stable to penicillinase (Crompton *et al.*, 1962) and that activity against gram-negative bacteria might be attained. Procedures for biological evaluation of cephalosporin compounds were therefore designed to detect broad-spectrum antibacterial activity.

B. Background for Biological Evaluation

Methodology for biological evaluation of antibacterial agents has evolved both by plan and as a result of experimental observations. Fleming's (1929) serendipitous discovery of penicillin led to ideas for methods to use when searching for new antibiotics. The observation that the activity of Prontosil® was due entirely to release, in the body, of sulfanilimide (Fuller, 1937) resulted in development of procedures for evaluation of sulfa drugs. Stability of antibiotics under test conditions was emphasized by Bohonos *et al.* (1954). They showed that, because of instability, oxytetracycline appeared more active *in vitro* than chlortetracycline, yet the latter antibiotic was more active *in vivo*. These early observations, along with many others, made it evident that activities of new antibiotics are not compelled to fit established criteria, i.e., a new antimicrobial agent may possess unique properties that must be considered during biological evaluation.

Chemical structures of the cephalosporins possess a β-lactam ring in common with the penicillins; a major difference is the presence of the six-membered dihydrothiazine ring in place of the five-membered thiazolidine ring in the penicillins. Crompton *et al.* (1962) showed that the ring system of the cephalosporins was stable to penicillinase. In addition, a hypothesis has been advanced that the dissimilarity of the ring structures could influence the occurrence of cross-allergenicity between cephalosporin and penicillin antibiotics. Unique reactions by cephalosporin antibiotics may also be anticipated in that they have three primary chemically active sites rather than two as found in the penicillins.

Utilizing the three primary chemically active sites present in 7-amino-cephalosporanic acid (7-ACA), it has been possible to synthesize many unique cephalosporin derivatives. Chemical reactivity of the β-lactam compounds may make certain derivatives more labile in biological tests. Both the penicillin and the cephalosporin antibiotics are subject to enzymatic inactivation by amidases and β-lactamases. In addition, certain of the cephalosporin antibiotics, in which the acetyl groups of 7-ACA have not been replaced, are susceptible to deacetylation. Deacetylcephalosporin antibiotics still possess biological activity, but may have a different level of activity than the parent antibiotics from which they are derived. Therefore, physical–chemical characteristics of each cephalosporin antibiotic must be studied and considered during biological evaluation of the compound.

II. Methodology

A. *In vitro Antimicrobial Activity*

In determining the activity of an antibiotic against any genus of microorganisms, it is important that the strains tested be, in fact, different. For this reason large numbers of clinical isolates of pathogenic bacteria have been employed during evaluation of cephalosporin antibiotics. Some workers have used stock strains from private collections and isolates from clinical investigators located in different areas of the world. Other investigators have been careful to identify each isolate of a bacterial genus as a strain by phage typing, antigenic analysis, or drug-susceptibility spectra. Certain bacterial, fungal, or yeast cultures for which clinical isolates were not readily available, have been obtained from commercial culture collections.

Once a series of cephalosporin derivatives is produced, *in vitro* screening procedures may be employed to select those compounds with a significant antibacterial spectrum. The necessary tests are done by broth- or agar-dilution susceptibility testing methods and by the gradient plate technique.

Dilution susceptibility tests have been performed by preparing a twofold concentration series of the antibiotic with either broth in tubes or agar in petri plates. Each tube in the broth-dilution test is usually inoculated so that it contains 10^4–10^5 organisms/ml. Agar-dilution plates are inoculated by "spotting" or streaking a specified number of organisms on the agar surface. This is done with a calibrated loop or with an inoculating device similar to the

Steers' replicator (Steers *et al.*, 1959). Results from the tests are usually determined after overnight incubation at 37°C. The lowest antibiotic concentration that prevents growth of the organism, the minimal inhibitory concentration (MIC), is the measure of susceptibility.

The gradient plate screening method used by Godzeski *et al.* (1963) was essentially that described by Bryson and Szybalski (1952). Antibiotic is incorporated in the agar medium employed to pour the bottom layer, with the petri plate tilted. The plate is then returned to a horizontal position, and agar media without antibiotic is used to overlay the first layer. Diffusion of antibiotic from the bottom layer provides a gradient of antibiotic concentrations on the surface of the agar. Each plate is inoculated by streaking from properly diluted bacterial suspensions, across the antibiotic gradient. After overnight incubation, bacterial growth is visible along the streak to a point of inhibition by the antibiotic. The MIC is determined by measuring the distance of growth of the test organism and calculating from the original concentration of antibiotic employed in the bottom agar layer, i.e., an MIC of 50 μg/ml is determined for an organism which grew half-way across the surface of a plate containing 100 μg/ml of antibiotic.

An antibiotic is usually considered to possess bactericidal activity if >99% of the bacteria used to inoculate an *in vitro* test are killed. Bactericidal action may be partial, i.e., the number of surviving organisms are reduced; or complete, where the growth medium is sterilized (Naumann, 1966). To detect bactericidal activity for cephalosporin antibiotics, several methods are employed. These include procedures involving liquid media with subculture and the cellophane transfer technique.

There have been several variations of methods employed for determining bactericidal activity using liquid media with subsequent subculturing. Most techniques are extensions of the broth-dilution test. In one method, a loop transfer is made from each clear tube in the MIC series to a tube of antibiotic-free broth. After overnight incubation, the absence of growth in the transfer tube indicates bactericidal activity in the original tube. The lowest concentration of antibiotic in the original MIC series from which no growth is obtained, the minimal bactericidal concentration (MBC), is the measure of bactericidal activity. In other methods, bactericidal activity is detected by determining changes in viable cell counts during the incubation of broth-dilution MIC tests. Counting of viable cells is accomplished either by plating methods or by streaking, with a loop, a known volume from the clear tubes in the MIC series to antibiotic-free agar plates.

Barber and Waterworth (1964) tested for bactericidal activity using the cellophane transfer technique of Chabbert (1957). Filter paper strips impregnated with antibiotic are placed on the agar surface of petri plates. The paper is removed after the antibiotic has diffused into the agar. Bacteria are then seeded on the surface of a cellophane disc placed on the agar. The antibiotic passes from the agar through the cellophane and kills the bacteria. After contacts of varying time duration, the cellophane disc is transferred to a second plate containing a nutrient agar. Following incubation, the number of colonies that grow on the surface of the disc is counted. Each colony represents a viable surviving organism, and the number of survivors is compared with the number of bacteria used to inoculate the cellophane disc.

B. Microbiological Assays

Assays employed for cephalosporin antibiotics include the disc–plate, the cylinder–plate, the agar well, and the superposition tube methods. For the first three procedures, petri plates are prepared with agar inoculated with either *Bacillus subtilis* strain ATCC 6633 or *Sarcina lutea* strain PCI-1001-FDA. Standard solutions of antibiotic are prepared to have a series of $\log_2$ concentrations. Paper discs (6 mm) are saturated from the solutions and placed on the surface of the seeded agar plates. Measured volumes of the solutions (usually 0.1 ml) are transferred either to wells cut in the agar or to stainless steel cylinders that have been previously placed on the agar surface. The antibiotic diffuses from the disc, cylinder, or well into the surrounding agar, inhibiting growth of the test organism, and a zone of inhibition becomes visible after incubation. Following overnight incubation, diameters of inhibition zones are measured. The diameter of a zone is dependent on antibiotic concentration in the solution used. A standard curve is plotted relating the varied zone diameters to the several antibiotic concentrations employed. Values for zone diameters produced by antibiotic in a specimen can be obtained by interpolating from the standard curve.

The superposition assay is a one-dimensional diffusion method (Shimizu and Nishimura, 1970). Melted agar (50°C) containing 5% defibrinated rabbit blood is inoculated with *Streptococcus hemolyticus* D. Aliquots (1 ml) of inoculated agar are transferred to 7 × 80-mm tubes (agar height of 40 mm) and the agar is allowed to solidify. Standard antibiotic solutions are prepared in a series of $\log_2$ concentrations, and 0.5-ml amounts of the solutions are pipetted to surfaces of the agar tubes. The antibiotic diffuses in one dimension (down) for distances depending on the antibiotic concentration. Inhibition of bacterial growth by the antibiotic in turn stops hemolysis of the red blood cells, and red bands of various widths can be observed in the agar just below the interfaces of the agar and antibiotic solutions. A standard curve is plotted relating the width of the bands to the several antibiotic concentrations used. Values for widths of bands produced by antibiotic in specimens can be obtained by interpolating from the standard curve.

C. Stability of Cephalosporins to β-Lactamases

Biological reactions of cephalosporin antibiotics are detailed in Chapter 10. However, for evaluation, certain experiments were required in order to assess the stability of an antibiotic to enzymatic degradation. For this, cultures of bacteria that produce β-lactamases, such as *Bacillus cereus, S. aureus,* and *Enterobacter* sp. are employed. Penicillinases are produced by cultures of the first two organisms, but the enzyme preparation from *Enterobacter* sp. had greater affinity for the cephalosporins than penicillins (Fleming *et al.*, 1963). Thus, the latter enzyme was classified as a cephalosporinase.

Antibiotic solutions are incubated with either live bacteria, ultrasonically disrupted cell suspensions, or partially purified enzyme preparations. After incubation for various intervals the extent of degradation of an antibiotic by an enzyme can be determined by either microbiological assay (Wick *et al.*, 1960) or the iodometric method of Perret (1954). An *in vivo* method (Wick *et al.*, 1962), quantitatively estimating the therapeutic activity of β-lactam antibiotics in the presence of penicillinase, was also used. *Streptococcus pyogenes* strain C203 is employed as an indicator organism. β-Lactamases are injected subcutaneously into groups of 10 mice 30 minutes after the animals have been infected intraperitoneally with *S. pyogenes.* Twofold concentrations of antibiotic, given in single subcutaneous doses, are administered 1 hour after infection to groups of mice that received β-lactamase and to mice receiving no enzyme. The ED_{50} values are usually calculated after 7 days. The resistance of the cephalosporin antibiotic to *in vivo* inactivation by β-lactamase is noted by comparing the differences in the amounts of antibiotic required for therapeutic effects in the presence or absence of the enzyme.

D. Physical–Chemical Stability

Knowledge of the stability of an antibiotic in solution is imperative for accurate evaluation of new compounds. Of particular importance is stability during incubation of an antibiotic incorporated in broth or agar media used for susceptibility testing and in stored solutions, such as serum specimens, urine samples, and standard assay solutions.

Stability of each of the cephalosporin antibiotics is estimated by microbiological assay of solutions of the compound. The assay procedures used are those described above. A specific amount of antibiotic is dissolved in various diluents such as broths, buffers, water, serum, blood, or urine. These solutions are stored or incubated for different time periods. At various intervals, aliquots are withdrawn and assayed immediately for residual antibiotic content.

E. Binding of Antibacterial Activity by Serum

Godzeski and his associates (1963) questioned the meaning of serum inactivation of antibiotics. They stated that the entire concept of serum inactivation is based on the fact that an MIC value is elevated in the presence of serum. However, the binding demonstrated is dependent on the microorganism used for the test. In addition, even though bound physically or chemically to a serum component, an antibiotic may still be very active against some bacteria.

Regardless of the value, the amount of serum binding is usually determined for new antibiotics.* The necessary tests are based on results obtained in media with or without added serum.

Elevation of MIC values when serum is added to media is one method of expressing binding. A second method for estimating the percentage of antibacterial activity bound by sera is to compare serum and buffer curves from microbiological assays (Wick, 1967; Naumann, 1967; Griffith and Black, 1970). Finally, Bennett and Kirby (1965) have described a modified ultrafiltration method for determining serum protein binding. Some detailed discussion will be found in Chapter 10.

F. Experimental Bacterial Infections in Animals

Experiments designed to predict the probable use of a new cephalosporin for therapy of bacterial infections in humans have been performed in mice, rats, and monkeys (Boniece et al., 1962; Muggleton et al., 1964, 1969; Wick and Boniece, 1965; Nishimura et al., 1965; Wick, 1967; Saslaw and Carlisle, 1968, 1969, 1970; Saslaw et al., 1970; Nishida et al., 1970; Chisholm et al., 1970; Kradolfer et al., 1970; Ryan, 1970).

One of the most useful tools of the antibiotic scientist is determination of the effective dose—50% (or ED_{50}) of an antibiotic in the therapy of experimental infections of mice. Groups of eight to ten mice are challenged with a specific number of bacteria by either intraperitoneal or intravenous injection. Twofold dilution concentrations of the antibiotic are then administered orally or subcutaneously to five groups of mice at various times after infection. Times of treatment vary with the investigator, but most commonly the mice have been treated with from one to three doses starting within 1 hour post infection. The mice are then observed for a specific period (usually 7 days), deaths are

---

* The author's experience with hundreds of active compounds has been convincing that the importance of the degree of serum binding is dependent on the toxicity of the antibiotic. In other words, the capacity of human serum to bind a compound can be overcome by increasing the dosage of a safe antibiotic.

recorded, and ED_{50} values have been calculated by probit analysis or by the method of Reed and Muench (1938).

An experimental urinary tract infection in rats, with *E. coli* as the test organism was used (Muggleton *et al.*, 1969; Ryan, 1970). The implantation of a length of nylon suture into the urinary bladder, along with a challenge dose of the infecting organism, produced an ascending infection that remained as a persistent heavy infection if not treated.

Saslaw and his associates (1968, 1969, 1970) use adult monkeys (*Macaca mulatta*: 3.0–4.2 kg) for their experiments with staphylococcal and streptococcal infections. Base line observations, including physical examinations, hematological and bacteriological studies are made for 2 weeks prior to intravenous bacterial infection. Therapy with the experimental antibiotics is initiated after laboratory findings prove that an acute infection is well established and are continued for a period of 10 days. All infected monkeys will normally die if left untreated.

G. Preliminary Immunological Studies

Dissimilarity in the chemistry of the ring structures in penicillins and cephalosporins could preclude the occurrence of cross-allergenicity between the two antibiotics. Details of more precise immunological studies are discussed elsewhere (Chapter 10). Preclinical studies have been performed on cephalothin (Wick, 1962) and on cephaloridine (Muggleton *et al.*, 1964).

An observation by a technician in Dr. Allen Ley's blood typing laboratory led to his report that red blood cells (rbc) incubated in solutions of benzylpenicillin could be agglutinated in the presence of certain human sera (Ley *et al.*, 1958). Soon after, Josephson (1960) modified Ley's technique for sensitizing red cells with penicillin to prove that he had developed penicillin antibodies in rabbits.

Josephson's methods were employed to develop rbc-agglutinating antibodies to benzylpenicillin. For rabbit sensitization, penicillin was dissolved in saline and an equal volume of Freund's complete adjuvant was added. The first week, small amounts of this antigen preparation were injected into each footpad of the rabbit and intradermally into 16 other areas. Repeated injections of penicillin in adjuvant were made at 2, 3, and 4 weeks. One week after the last injection, serum was collected.

The method for detection of antibodies consisted of dissolving benzylpenicillin in Alsever's solution. To this was added an equal volume of fresh normal rabbit blood. This combination was incubated for 1 hour at 37°C, and the resulting antibiotic-sensitized red cells were washed three times with saline. In the test, one drop of a 2% suspension of the sensitized red cells was added to 0.3 ml of dilutions of serum from immunized animals. The test was incubated at 37°C for 2 hours after which time the endpoint was determined by observing the degree of hemagglutination. Penicillin antisera were also cross-checked with red cells that had been similarly treated with other unrelated antibiotics to check the specificity of the antibodies.

A second immunological method is easily performed, i.e., the absorption technique. By adding penicillin to the specific antiserum and incubating for 1 hour at 37°C, the antibodies were overwhelmed, or "absorbed," and hem-agglutination was no longer possible. Absorption with other antibiotics would not occur.

Penicillin, or a degradation product thereof, is considered to be a hapten incapable of eliciting antibodies unless it is combined with a protein to form a "complete" antigen, or haptane. These complete conjugated antigens are then capable of stimulating antibody production. Rabbits were immunized as above with conjugated antigens of cephalothin or penicillin with egg white albumin. Antibodies formed to these antigens could be titered by the precipitin reaction. However, since egg white albumin is antigenic by itself, the precipitin reaction was controlled with horse serum albumin.

Another method was utilized to measure the degree of cross-reaction between penicillins and cephalothin. This was the passive-cutaneous-anaphylaxis (PCA) test in guinea pigs. The procedure involves an injection of a small volume of the antiserum intradermally. After 5–6 hours, 0.5 ml of the conju-gated antigen, combined with an equal volume of 0.5% Evan's blue dye is injected into the vein located between the toes of the lightly anesthetized guinea pig. A large blue area occurs at the site of the intradermal injection, indicating an anaphylactoid reaction.

H. Development of Bacterial Resistance

The appearance of organisms resistant to an antibiotic following its use in therapy has been a recurrent problem. Whether or not these resistant isolates are "developed" or "selected" *in vivo* is an ageless question. Certainly, the rapid one-step increase in resistance *in vitro*, as occurs with streptomycin, may also occur *in vivo*. However, when laboratory-induced resistance occurs slowly, i.e., more than one transfer is required, the appearance of resistant organisms during therapy may be a selection from a heterogeneous cell popula-tion. Kayser (1966) postulated that only one cell in 10^{40} is capable of mutating to produce progeny by *in vitro* multistep transfers, with significant increase in resistance to penicillin, and in doing so, will lose virulence. The chance of that cell, or its progeny, surviving both antibiotic and natural body defenses for more than two to three generations is negligible. *Staphylococcus aureus* cultures that were lyophilized many years prior to the discovery of penicillin have been shown to produce penicillinase and are therefore resistant to some penicillins. None of the *S. aureus* mutants that are made resistant to penicillin by laboratory exposure produce penicillinase, and resistance to the antibiotic is by other mechanisms. On the other hand, all benzylpenicillin-resistant *S. aureus* cultures isolated from infections do produce penicillinase and are resistant to certain penicillins because of hydrolysis of these antibiotics by the enzyme.

In view of the above, certain definitions of resistant bacteria should be employed. For example, bacteria made resistant in the laboratory to one macrolide antibiotic always exhibit *"cross-resistance"* to other macrolides, whereas, those organisms isolated from infections that are resistant to a macrolide antibiotic may or may not show "multiple-resistance" to other antibiotics of the same family type. Thus, the terms "cross" and "multiple" can differentiate between "developed" and natural ("selected") resistance. Cross-resistance can be studied in the laboratory by susceptibility testing of cultures made resistant by serial transfer in the presence of an antibiotic. Multiple-resistant organisms are detected by comparing MIC values for natural isolates with a multitude of antibiotics.

I. Antibiotic in Serum or Urine

The concentration of a compound in body fluids of the larger animals used by pharmacologists and toxicologists is determined by the same procedures employed for humans. However, such experiments are normally deferred until effectiveness has been established in smaller experimental animals, such as the mouse. Information concerning the fate of an antibiotic in the mouse is desirable in order to more accurately interpret experimental results in larger animals.

Peak serum concentrations range from 2 to 4 μg/ml when 250 mg of phenoxymethyl penicillin is administered orally to humans. Administration of 20 mg/kg was required in order to obtain equal concentrations of penicillin in mouse serum. Giving this amount (20 mg/kg) seemed to be a logical approach for comparing antibiotic levels attained with new cephalosporin derivatives. Peak concentrations could be determined by assaying heart blood, but a mouse could not be bled from the heart more than once. Thus, a different procedure was used (Wick and Boniece, 1965). This method permitted bleeding of the same mouse several times and eliminated any possibility of error due to delay in collecting and assaying serum. To determine antibiotic levels, a disc–plate assay (described earlier) is utilized. After administration of the antibiotic, a mouse is bled at intervals from the orbital sinus. The blood is collected in a heparinized hematocrit tube, which is allowed to fill by capillary action. Paper discs (6 mm) are saturated with the blood or dilutions thereof and immediately placed on seeded assay plates. Urine is also assayed as soon as it is collected.

J. Detection of Metabolites

Perhaps the best way to study the fate of antibiotics *in vivo* is to employ radiocarbon-labeled compounds. Methodology for this has been described (Sullivan and McMahon, 1967; Sullivan *et al.*, 1969a, b). Studies of this nature are not usually performed until an antibiotic is recommended for clinical trial. Therefore, initial information concerning metabolism, both *in vitro* and *in vivo*, is obtained by chromatographic procedures. If the metabolite is biologically active, bioautographs of paper chromatograms that have been developed in various solvent systems are prepared (Miller, 1962; O'Callaghan and Muggleton, 1963; Wick, 1964; Muggleton *et al.*, 1964; Hoehn and Pugh, 1968; Shimizu and Nishimura, 1970; Wick *et al.*, 1971). For metabolites having little or no biological activity, other analytical procedures are used (Kukolja, 1968).

K. Disc-Susceptibility Studies

Selection of an antibiotic for therapy of bacterial infections is often dependent on knowledge of the susceptibility of the infecting organism. Usually, it is possible to determine susceptibility by *in vitro* tests. When these tests are properly standardized, the results obtained correlate well with the response to therapy observed in clinical practice (Ryan *et al.*, 1970).

The necessary *in vitro* susceptibility tests used to measure an antibiotic's ability to inhibit bacterial growth are done by either diffusion or dilution methods. Disc-diffusion methods are usually preferred over dilution procedures for routine testing because of their simplicity and because they can be performed rapidly. In diffusion methods, filter paper discs (usually 6 mm in diameter) are impregnated with an antibiotic and placed on agar that has been uniformly inoculated with the test organism. A concentration gradient of the antibiotic forms by diffusion from the disc to inhibit the susceptible bacteria. The basis for judging susceptibility may be the actual size of a zone of inhibition or the mere presence or absence of a zone, depending upon the test.

Two standardized disc-diffusion methods have been described. In the United States, a technique designed by Bauer *et al.* (1966), known as the Bauer–Kirby (or Kirby–Bauer) disc method, is used in many hospitals. A second standardized method is described in a preliminary report of a working group of the International Collaborative Study (ICS) on standardization of antibiotic susceptibility sponsored by the World Health Organization (Ericsson, 1964). This method is referred to as the ICS disc method.

Investigators working with cephalosporin antibiotics used the two standardized methods described above and a third less accurate technique known as the TSA method. This nonstandardized procedure represents the test in which a zone of inhibition, regardless of size, indicates qualitative susceptibility of the pathogen. Use of the first two methods which specify measurement of zones of inhibition provides the most precise estimate of bacterial susceptibility.

To serve as guides for therapy, *in vitro* tests must predict probable *in vivo* effectiveness of an antibiotic. The range of zone diameters for predictive purposes is determined by correlation of zone diameters with MIC values in the light of clinical experience with the antibiotic. Experimentally determined zone diameters and MIC values are plotted, and the points fall along a least squares line, the "regression line." Thus, zone diameter is a measure of MIC, and the two are inversely related. Clinical evidence provides information as to the degree of susceptibility (MIC) of bacterial pathogens that have responded to therapy. The zone diameter corresponding to that MIC value can then be interpolated from the regression line. Regression lines for cephalosporin antibiotics have been calculated by several investigators (Sherris *et al.*, 1967; Ericsson, 1967; Wick, 1969; Washington and Yu, 1970; Matsen *et al.*, 1970; Foz, 1970; Wick *et al.*, 1971).

III. Biological Properties of Cephalosporin Antibiotics from a Laboratory Standpoint

A. Cephalothin

Cephalosporin C itself has a low order of antibacterial activity. This biologically produced compound exhibits activity about equivalent to benzylpenicillin against gram-negative bacilli, but is considerably less active against gram-positive bacteria. A synthetic chemical program based on modification of the cephalosporin nucleus, 7-ACA, has yielded many new cephalosporin antibiotics. The generic name cephalothin was assigned to 7-(thiophene-2-acetamido)cephalosporanic acid (Fig. 1), (Boniece *et al.*, 1962; Chauvette *et al.*, 1962). Cephalothin exhibits *in vitro* activity against both gram-positive and gram-negative bacteria. The antibiotic has no known activity against yeast, fungi, or viruses. Cephalothin is not absorbed in humans after oral administration, and must be given parenterally.

Fortunately, cephalothin is highly active against penicillinase-producing staphylococci, an activity that, alone, would have warranted a clinical trial of the antibiotic. All strains of *S. aureus* tested were inhibited by <1 μg/ml of cephalothin (Boniece *et al.*, 1962). However, early *in vitro* studies with gram-negative bacteria yielded conflicting results. Boniece *et al.* (1962) noted that relatively light inocula were required for detection of gram-negative bacilli susceptible to cephalothin. Godzeski *et al.* (1963) discussed the differences in

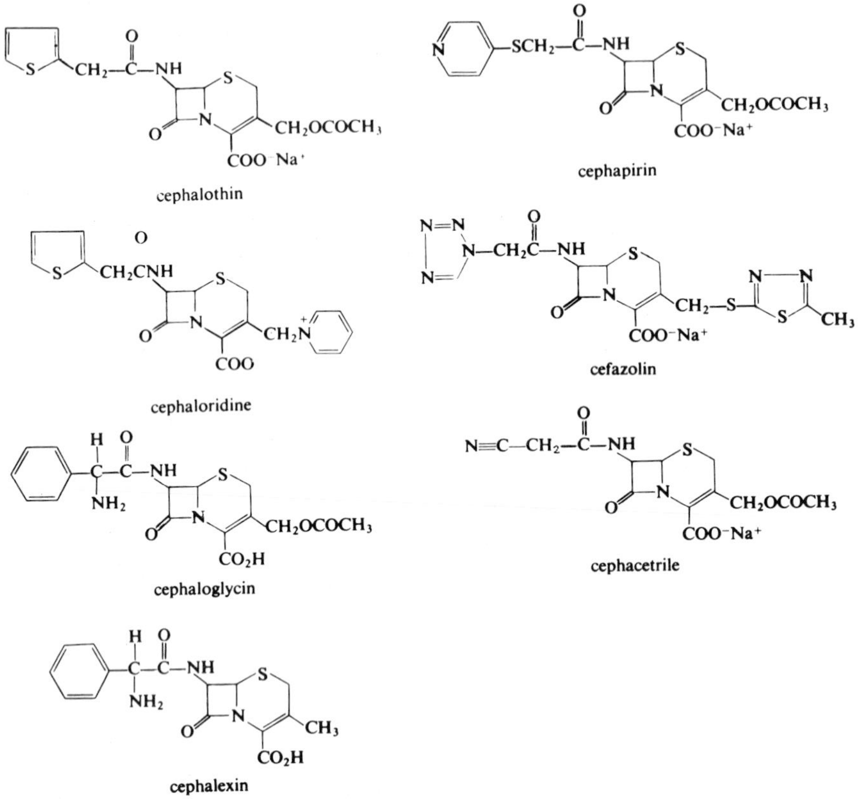

Fig. 1. Chemical structures of cephalosporin antibiotics.

activity observed with various *in vitro* test methods. Klein *et al.* (1964) found that cephalothin had little antibacterial activity against gram-negative organisms, when tested by their inocula-replication procedure. These latter authors noted that other investigators (Anderson and Petersdorf, 1963; Walters *et al.*, 1963), using broth-dilution methods, did demonstrate activity of cephalothin against gram-negative bacteria.

Cephalothin is partially converted to deacetylcephalothin after parenteral administration to man, and the metabolite accounts for one-third of the antibiotic activity excreted in the urine (O'Callaghan and Muggleton, 1963; Lee et al., 1963). Wick (1964) found that this degradation of cephalothin was of greater magnitude in vitro. He showed that the instability of cephalothin in trypticase soy broth had an adverse effect on MIC values for cephalothin after the 12th hour of incubation at 37°C. This phenomenon is particularly important when testing susceptibility of gram-negative organisms. More recently, a study has confirmed that MIC values determined by the broth-dilution procedure increase commonly over the period 12–24 hours and that greater stability of endpoints with the agar-dilution method is an advantage over the broth-dilution technique (Sherris et al., 1967). Barber and Waterworth (1964) used the agar-dilution method with nutrient agar and found that cephalothin had activity similar to that of ampicillin against most strains of Enterobacteriaciae, with greater activity against some strains of Proteus and Klebsiella sp.

Several modified methods for testing bacterial susceptibility to cephalothin have been recommended as a result of in vitro studies. These include the reduction of initial inocula to 10^3 bacteria/ml when enriched broth media are employed (Boniece et al., 1962); using the gradient–plate method (Godzeski et al., 1963); determination of endpoints at 12 hours instead of after overnight incubation, when inocula of 10^5 bacteria/ml and enriched broths are used (Wick, 1964); and using 10^4–10^5 bacteria/ml inocula and substituting nutrient broth, if overnight determinations are desired (Naumann, 1966; Ronald and Turck, 1967). Perhaps the best approach is to employ the agar-dilution method described in a preliminary report of a working group of the International Collaborative Study (ICS) on standardization of antibiotic susceptibility testing sponsored by the World Health Organization as recommended by Sherris et al. (1967), and by Wick (1969).

Regardless of the difficulties with initial susceptibility testing, sufficient data are now available to describe the antimicrobial spectrum of cephalothin. In vitro, cephalothin inhibits almost all isolates of Staphylococcus aureus, Staphylococcus albus, Streptococcus pyogenes (Group A), Streptococcus sp. (Viridans Group), Diplococcus pneumoniae, Clostridium sp., Listeria monocytogenes, Corynebacterium diphtheriae, Actinomyces sp., Bacillus subtilis, Neisseria gonorrheae, Proteus mirabilis, Klebsiella pneumoniae, Salmonella sp., and Shigella sp. (Weinstein and Kaplan, 1970). Many strains of Escherichia coli and Citrobacter sp. (75%), Paracolobactrum sp. (60%), and Haemophilus influenzae (50%) are also susceptible to the antibiotic. Most isolates of Proteus morgani, Proteus rettgeri, Proteus vulgaris, Pseudomonas sp., Herellea sp., Serratia sp., Providentia sp., Bacteroides sp., Enterobacter sp., and many of the enterococci (Group D streptococci) are unaffected by cephalothin. Anticipated per cent susceptibilities of commonly isolated bacterial pathogens are shown in Tables I and II.

The antimicrobial activity of cephalothin is somewhat variable with changes in pH of test media. Studies with isolates of *E. coli* and *S. aureus* showed that MIC values were elevated only slightly as the pH of broth was increased from 5.0 to 8.0 (Godzeski *et al.*, 1963). Variations in MIC values for cephalothin are more dependent on inoculum size or media employed than pH (Boniece

Table I

ANTICIPATED PERCENT SUSCEPTIBILITY OF SOME COMMONLY ISOLATED GRAM-POSITIVE
BACTERIAL PATHOGENS AND TREPONEMA TO FOUR CEPHALOSPORIN ANTIBIOTICS[a]

Organism	Estimate of percent susceptible to			
	Cephalothin	Cephaloridine	Cephaloglycin[b]	Cephalexin
Staphylococcus aureus (penicillin sensitive)	~100	~100	~100	~100
Staphylococcus aureus (penicillin resistant)	~100[c]	~100	~100	~100
Staphylococcus aureus (methicillin resistant)	50[d]	60	?	10
Streptococcus pyogenes (group A)	100	100	100	100
Streptococcus sp. (viridans group)	100	100	100	100
Streptococcus sp (group D)	50	40	40	20
Diplococcus pneumoniae	100	100	100	100
Bacillus sp.	100	100	e	e
Clostridium sp.	100	100	e	e
Cornyebacterium diphtheriae	100	100	e	e
Treponema pallidum	~100	~100	e	~100

[a] Susceptibility is based on the probability of obtaining MIC values ≤8 μg/ml by the ICS agar dilution method. Isolates of certain genera will be much more susceptible than those from others.

[b] With cephaloglycin, the activity of deacetylcephaloglycin must also be considered.

[c] Many *S. aureus* isolates that have been reported as resistant have been incorrectly identified enterococci (group D streptococci).

[d] Because of the heterogeneity of methicillin-resistant *S. aureus* cultures, the MIC values from susceptibility tests are variable, and clinical significance of the MIC values are difficult to predict.

[e] Isolates of these genera are probably susceptible. However, there is not sufficient data currently available to make a positive estimate, with the antibiotic indicated.

et al., 1962; Wick, 1964; Turck *et al.*, 1965; Naumann, 1966; Ronald and Turck, 1967).

Cephalothin exhibits bactericidal activity against both gram-positive and gram-negative bacteria. Naumann and Fedder (1970) summarized the bactericidal activity of four cephalosporin antibiotics. With nutrient broth and inocula of 10^5 bacteria/ml, the partial bactericidal concentrations of cephalothin were equal to, or only slightly higher than, the bacteriostatic levels. Total sterilization of the broth media required more antibiotic. Wick (1964) demonstrated bactericidal activity by making viable cell counts from tubes in the MIC series, and

Table II

ANTICIPATED PERCENT SUSCEPTIBILITY OF SOME COMMONLY ISOLATED GRAM-NEGATIVE BACTERIAL PATHOGENS TO FOUR CEPHALOSPORIN ANTIBIOTICS[a]

Organism	Estimate of percent susceptible to			
	Cephalothin	Cephaloridine	Cephaloglycin[b]	Cephalexin
Bordetella pertussis	100	100	c	c
Brucella spp.	d	d	d	d
Escherichia coli	85	90	85	85
Citrobacter sp. (*E. Freundii*)	<50[d]	<50[d]	<50[d]	<50[d]
Hemophilus influenzae	>60	>60	c	e
Herellea sp.	<10	<10	<10	<10
Klebsiella pneumoniae	~100	~100	~100	~100
Enterobacter sp.	<10	<10	40[f]	<10
Neisseria sp.	~100	~100	~100	~100
Pasteurella sp.	~100	~100	~100	~100
Proteus mirabilis	~100	~100	~100	~100
Proteus sp. (indole-positive)	<10	<10	30[f]	<10
Pseudomonas sp.	~0	~0	~0	~0
Salmonella sp.	~100	~100	~100	~100
Serratia sp.	<10	<10	<10	<10
Shigella sp.	~100	~100	~100	~100
Vibrio sp.	~100	~100	~100	~100

[a] Susceptibility is based on the probability of obtaining MIC values ≤32 μg/ml by the ICS agar dilution method. Isolates of certain genera will be much more susceptible than those from others.

[b] With cephaloglycin, the activity of deacetylcephaloglycin must also be considered.

[c] Isolates of these genera are probably susceptible. However, there is not sufficient data currently available to make a positive estimate, with the antibiotic indicated.

[d] Resistant isolates have been reported, but there is insufficient data to predict susceptibility.

[e] MIC values for cephalexin that have been reported to date for *H. influenzae* are quite high (4–16 μg/ml). However, susceptibility tests are difficult to perform, and there is currently insufficient data to indicate what the MIC values mean.

[f] Because cephaloglycin is quite stable to cephalosporinase, some isolates of these genera may be susceptible. However, deacetylcephaloglycin is less active than cephaloglycin against these organisms.

by loop transfer to antibiotic-free broth. He reported complete bactericidal activity against 23 of 40 gram-negative bacilli with concentrations of 10 μg/ml of cephalothin. Turck *et al.* (1965) found that all of 50 isolates of *E. coli* were inhibited by 25 μg/ml of cephalothin, and the antibiotic was bactericidal against all but two cultures. At 100 μg/ml, a concentration readily attainable in urine, cephalothin was bactericidal against all of the *E. coli* cultures. Barber and Waterworth (1964), using the cellophane transfer technique of Chabbert (1957), demonstrated bactericidal activity of cephalothin on staphylococci. Other investigators who performed initial studies with cephalothin also reported bactericidal activity (Klein *et al.*, 1964; Walters *et al.*, 1963; Perkins and Saslaw, 1966).

Binding of cephalothin by serum was initially discussed by Godzeski *et al.* (1963). They showed that cephalothin MIC values were elevated for some organisms, but not others, when 50% dog, rat, or human serum was added to growth media. Klein *et al.* (1964) reported the median MIC values for two staphylococcal assay organisms in broth containing 50% human serum were two or five times greater than when determined in broth without serum. Binding of cephalothin by serum proteins has been reported to range from 40 to 65%. Sidell *et al.* (1963) reported the binding as 40%, whereas Kind *et al.* (1969), by an ultrafiltration method, found the binding to be as high as 65%.

Penicillinase has little effect on cephalosporin C (Crompton *et al.*, 1962); however, Abraham and Newton (1961) have suggested that some organisms produce a β-lactamase, cephalosporinase, that degrades cephalosporin compounds. Fleming *et al.* (1963) studied the distribution of cephalosporinases and penicillinases in over 1000 isolates of *Enterobacteriaceae* and other related organisms. These studies led to the classification of gram-negative bacteria on the basis of their ability to hydrolyze cephalosporin C: *Group I*—organisms that consistently produced cephalosporinase were the *Enterobacter* sp., *Serratia* sp., *Hafnia* sp., *Pseudomonas* sp. and *Proteus morganii*. *Group II*— organisms that did not produce the enzyme were *Salmonella* sp., *Klebsiella* sp., and *Proteus mirabilis*. *Group III*—organisms that did or did not produce cephalosporinase included *Proteus vulgaris*, *Proteus rettgeri*, *Escherichia coli*, and *Shigella* sp.

Early studies showed that cephalothin is active against both benzylpenicillin-sensitive and -resistant *S. aureus* cultures, indicating that the antibiotic is not susceptible to hydrolysis by penicillinase. Purified penicillinase from *S. aureus* and *B. cereus* has little effect on cephalothin, if any (Chang and Weinstein, 1964; Godzeski *et al.*, 1963). β-Lactamases elaborated by *Klebsiella* sp. have a greater affinity for penicillins than cephalosporins, while enzymes produced by some species of *Proteus* and *Escherichia* degrade cephalosporins more rapidly (Hamilton-Miller, 1964). Ott and Godzeski (1967) also reported rapid enzymatic inactivation of cephalothin by β-lactamase from *Enterobacter* sp. (Table III). Thus, it appears that no gram-positive pathogens are resistant to cephalothin because of β-lactamase, but elaboration of cephalosporinase by certain gram-negative bacilli is a major reason these organisms are resistant to the antibiotic.

Cephalothin is active in therapy of experimental bacterial infections in mice.

The ED_{50} values (Table IV) for gram-positive cocci are indicative of a very effective antibiotic. However the ED_{50} values against gram-negative bacilli are quite high, when compared with other antibiotics (Table IV). Boniece

Table III
β-LACTAMASE ACTIVITY OF *Enterobacter* SP.[a]

Antibiotic	Minimal inhibitory level (μg/ml)	Rate of hydrolysis by β-lactamase
Cephalothin	>200	Rapid
Cephaloridine	>200	Rapid
Cephalexin	>200	Rapid
Cephaloglycin	>200	Very Slow
Benzylpenicillin	>200	Slow
Oxacillin	>200	None
Methicillin	>200	None

[a] From Ott and Godzeski (1967).

Table IV
ACTIVITY OF FOUR CEPHALOSPORINS IN EXPERIMENTAL BACTERIAL INFECTIONS IN MICE

Organism	ED_{50} by subcutaneous therapy[a]		ED_{50} by oral therapy[a]	
	Cephalothin	Cephaloridine	Cephaloglycin	Cephalexin
Streptococcus pyogenes	1.7	0.038	3.6	1.8
Diplococcus pneumoniae type I	11.2	0.065	29.2	58.5
Staphylococcus aureus				
Benzylpenicillin sensitive	1.7	2.6	1.68	0.475
Benzylpenicillin resistant	15.8	<1.2	7.8	3.7
Klebsiella pneumoniae	14.7	5.2	14.7	5.2
Escherichia coli	78.0	8.2	23.5	8.2
Salmonella typhosa	118.0	18.0	11.6	14.5
Shigella flexneri	63.0	<5.0	15.5	15.6
Proteus mirabilis	35.0	10.2	12.9	22.1

[a] ED_{50} value expressed as milligrams per kilogram × two treatments (1 and 5 hours post infection).

et al. (1962) found a straight-line relationship, in experimental gram-negative infections, between cephalothin ED_{50} values and the number of LD_{50} doses of the challenge. In other words, as the strength of the bacterial challenge increased, more cephalothin was required for therapy. In Japan, Nishimura *et al.* (1965) showed that in mice cephalothin was 11–40 times less active than chloramphenicol or tetracycline, respectively. Finally, in England, O'Callaghan and Muggleton (1963) investigated the formation of metabolites from cephalosporin compounds, mainly because of the erratic results they had obtained with cephalothin in their mouse protection studies.

In general, the mouse data correlated well with early clinical evidence of successful cephalothin therapy of human infections caused by gram-positive cocci. However, response in humans against gram-negative infections was much better than could be predicted by early *in vitro* tests, or by ED_{50} results in mice. The reason for high MIC values with established susceptibility testing procedures was explained by Wick (1964). An attempt was made to explain variations in mouse protection experiments on the basis of *in vivo* metabolism of cephalothin (O'Callaghan and Muggleton, 1963). Since a great percentage of the administered antibiotic was excreted as the parent compound and since the metabolite, deacetylcephalothin, still possessed biological activity (Wick, 1966), metabolism was not the explanation.

Regardless of early difficulties with *in vitro* and *in vivo* test methods, cephalothin is now a proven effective agent against susceptible gram-negative infections. An explanation for the lack of correlation between mouse experiments and human therapy is the rapid excretion of cephalothin by the mouse. Usual dosage schedules for therapy of mouse infections do not simulate human therapy. For the latter, antibiotic concentrations are maintained by repeated dosage. Experimental infections normally are treated only one or two times. If one antibiotic is excreted from the mouse more rapidly than a second, the infecting organisms are exposed a shorter time to the first antibiotic and longer to the second. Once an antibiotic is no longer present in the animal, a few organisms can recover to kill the host. Since the bacteria are exposed to the more slowly excreted antibiotic longer, that antibiotic will appear the more active. When equal amounts (20 mg/kg) of several antibiotics were given to mice, cephalothin was excreted in 30 minutes, compared with 1–3 hours for other compounds. These included chloramphenicol, tetracycline, kanamycin, ampicillin, streptomycin, etc. However, the single dose ED_{50} value of 125 mg/kg of cephalothin for an *E. coli* infection was reduced to 7.8 mg/kg when cephalothin concentrations were maintained by five hourly doses (Wick and Boniece, 1967). The latter dosage correlated better with results in human therapy. Unrecognized at the time was the fact that the mouse data was predicting the probable safety of cephalothin in patients with renal insufficiency by showing the rapid excretion of the antibiotic.

Therapy with cephalothin, of experimental infections in animal species other than mice, was not done until after the clinical efficacy of the antibiotic was already well established. Comparing the effects of antibiotics in life-threatening infections is not possible in man. However, an excellent model for such comparisons is the rhesus monkey (Saslaw and Carlisle, 1968, 1969).

These investigators found cephalothin to be effective in controlling severe lethal staphylococcal or streptococcal infections in monkeys. One advantage of this model is that these animals can be observed as individuals, and that the clinical progress of infection and therapy can be followed as it is in man. Although these experiments were not used to predict the efficacy of cephalothin, the model is established as a valuable tool for evaluating newer cephalosporins and other new antibiotics.

Table V

ABSORPTION OF BENZYLPENICILLIN ANTIBODIES WITH VARIOUS
PENICILLIN AND CEPHALOSPORIN COMPOUNDS

Benzylpenicillin rabbit antiserum "absorbed" with 1 mg/ml of	Hemagglutination titer[a]
Benzylpenicillin (K salt)	0
Phenoxymethylpenicillin (K salt)	0
2-Thienylmethylpenicillin (K salt)	0
Benzylpenicillenic acid (K salt)	0
Benzylpenicilloic acid	1:2
Benzylpenillic acid	1:16
6-Aminopenicillanic acid (6-APA)	1:32
7-Aminocephalosporanic acid (7-ACA)	1:32
Cephalothin (K salt)	1:32
Cephalothin (Na salt)	1:32
Nonabsorbed rabbit antiserum (control)	1:32
Normal rabbit serum (control)[b]	0

[a] Hemagglutination titers of absorbed antisera with benzylpenicillin-sensitized rabbit red blood cells.

[b] Normal serum from immunized rabbits was obtained prior to immunizing the animals.

Before administering cephalothin for the first time to penicillin-allergic patients, clinicians desired some laboratory evidence showing lack of cross-allergenicity between the two antibiotics. Antibodies to benzylpenicillin were developed in rabbits by the procedures of Josephson (1960). These antibodies were detected with hemagglutination techniques, using penicillin-sensitized rabbit red blood cells. The antibodies did not agglutinate cells coated with other unrelated antibiotics, indicating specificity for penicillin. Attempts to sensitize red cells with cephalothin were not successful at the time; therefore, the absorption procedure was utilized. Data presented in Table V show that benzylpenicillin, phenoxymethylpenicillin, 2-thienylmethylpenicillin, and benzylpenicillenic acid completely absorbed the benzylpenicillin antibodies; on the other hand, 6-APA, 7-ACA, and cephalothin did not, indicating no reaction occurred between the antibodies and the latter compounds.

Antibodies produced by penicillin conjugated antigens can be detected by the precipitin reaction. Conjugated antigens were prepared by combining cephalothin or penicillin with either egg white or horse serum albumin. The

Table VI

PRECIPITIN REACTIONS WITH SERUM FROM RABBITS IMMUNIZED WITH
BENZYLPENICILLIN OR CEPHALOTHIN CONJUGATED WITH EGG WHITE ALBUMIN

Rabbit antiserum to	Precipitin reaction with antigen[a,b]						
	Egg	Horse	PEN + egg	PEN + horse	CET + egg	CET + horse	Saline
PEN + Egg	++++	----	++++	++++	+++[c]	----	----
CET + Egg	++++[c]	----	+++	----	++[c]	----	----

[a] Reaction did not occur with penicillin or cephalothin alone.

[b] PEN = benzylpenicillin; CET = cephalothin; egg = egg white albumin; horse = horse serum albumin.

[c] Expected positive reactions; because egg white albumin was part of the conjugated antigen and is antigenic by itself.

Table VII

PASSIVE-CUTANEOUS-ANAPHYLAXIS IN GUINEA PIGS, WITH RABBIT ANTISERA

0.1 ml intradermal antiserum to	Antigen with Evans-blue dye intraveneously[a]					
	PEN + egg	PEN + horse	CET + egg	CET + horse	Egg	Horse
Normal rabbit serum	−	−	−	−	−	−
PEN + egg	++++[b,c]	++++	++++[c]	−	++++[c]	−
CET + egg	++++[c]	−	++++[c]	−	++++[c]	−
PEN only	++++	++++	−	−	−	−

[a] PEN = benzylpenicillin; CET = cephalothin; egg = egg white albumin; horse = horse serum albumin.

[b] Positive reaction indicated by large blue area surrounding intradermal injection site.

[c] Expected positive reaction; because egg white albumin was part of the conjugated antigen and is antigenic by itself.

egg white conjugates were used for immunization of rabbits to produce penicillin–egg and cephalothin–egg antisera. Results from precipitin reactions with these antisera are shown in Table VI. Since egg white albumin is antigenic by itself, the reactions were controlled with either horse serum albumin alone or combined with the antibiotics. The data indicated there were no cross-reactions between the two antibiotics.

Another method was available to ascertain a lack of cross-reaction between the conjugated antibodies prepared with penicillin or cephalothin. This was the PCA, or passive-cutaneous-anaphylaxis test performed with guinea pigs. The results (Table VII) from PCA tests were identical to those for the precipitin reactions (Table VI), giving additional evidence of no cross-allergenicity between cephalothin and penicillin. Further discussion is given in Chapter 10.

B. *Cephaloridine*

The second clinically useful cephalosporin derivative, 7-[α-(2-thiophene)-acetamido]-3-(1-pyridylmethyl)-3-cephem-4-carboxylic acid betaine, was given the generic name cephaloridine (Muggleton *et al.*, 1964; Wick and Boniece, 1965). Cephaloridine, like penicillins and other cephalosporins, interrupts cell wall synthesis of susceptible bacteria. The antibiotic is not sufficiently absorbed following oral administration to man, so cephaloridine must be given parenterally.

Cephaloridine is made from cephalothin by replacing the acetoxy group with pyridine (Fig. 1). Without taking into consideration the instability of cephalothin under *in vitro* test conditions, cephaloridine at first appeared considerably more active *in vitro*. However, the qualitative spectrum of antibacterial activity of cephaloridine is almost identical to that described for cephalothin (Tables I and II). There are differences in the degree of activity against specific bacterial genera. *In vitro*, cephaloridine is approximately twice as active against gram-positive cocci, *Neisseria*, and *E. coli*, but is less active than cephalothin against *Proteus mirabilis*. The two antibiotics have approximately equal activity against the rest of the *Enterobacteriaceae*.

In retrospect, cephaloridine was developed because of misinterpretations of the *in vitro* and *in vivo* activities of its predecessor, cephalothin. However, certain benefits that were found during clinical trial, such as lack of pain on injection and longer sustained concentrations in the body, made development worthwhile.

When the acetoxy group of cephalothin is replaced with pyridine, the resulting compound, cephaloridine, is more stable both *in vitro* and in the body. The stability of cephaloridine was demonstrated by chromatographic studies, biological assays, and physicochemical methods (Muggleton *et al.*, 1964; Wick and Boniece, 1965). Because the pyridine is not easily removed from cephaloridine, the difficulties in susceptibility tests described for cephalothin were not encountered. With cephaloridine, broth-dilution endpoints can be determined after usual overnight incubation. Urine specimens, both animal and human that were examined by chromatograms and bioautograms, showed that no other microbiologically active metabolites were present and that cephaloridine was excreted unchanged (Muggleton *et al.*, 1964; Sullivan and McMahon, 1967).

Staphylococcal penicillinase from one strain of *S. aureus* had no effect on rates of degradation of cephaloridine, while *B. cereus* penicillinase slowly degraded the antibiotic (Wick and Boniece, 1965). This inactivation of cephaloridine was much slower than that observed with benzylpenicillin. Benner *et al.* (1965) reported increases in cephaloridine MIC values for certain *S. aureus* isolates, when inocula sizes were increased. Naumann (1967) suggested that these high MIC values were due to the use of inocula about 100-fold greater than those used by other workers. However, three types of staphylococcal penicillinase have been described (Richmond, 1965), and one of these enzymes may slowly inactivate cephaloridine. There is no evidence that the slow inactivation of the antibiotic as observed *in vitro* is significant when cephaloridine is used for therapy of staphylococcal infections in man.

Muggleton and associates (1964) were unable to induce hypersensitivity to cephaloridine in rabbits or guinea pigs injected repeatedly for 3 months. Patients that were hypersensitive to penicillin were given injections of cephaloridine without showing untoward reactions, i.e., cephaloridine did not readily cause hypersensitivity nor was there any cross-allergenicity with penicillins.

Cephaloridine was highly effective in protecting mice against experimental infections, including those with penicillin-resistant staphylococci, and gram-negative bacilli (Muggleton *et al.*, 1964). Indeed, the activity of cephaloridine against gram-positive bacteria approached that of benzylpenicillin (Wick and Boniece, 1965). Thus, like the initial *in vitro* studies, early animal experiments suggested that cephaloridine was more active than cephalothin. However, Wick and Boniece (1967) explained that usual dosage schedules for treatment of experimental infections in mice do not simulate human therapy. They showed that the antibiotic that was excreted slowly (cephaloridine) appeared superior in therapy of mouse infections to the rapidly excreted cephalothin. Comparisons in humans of the activity of these two agents has shown little differences in their degree of antibacterial effectiveness for therapy of infections in humans (Weinstein and Kaplan, 1970).

C. Cephaloglycin

The zwitterion of 7-(D-α-aminophenylacetamido)cephalosporanic acid is generically called cephaloglycin (Wick and Boniece, 1967). This antibiotic is structurally related to cephaloridine and cephalothin, differing from the latter in the substitution of phenylglycine group for the 2-(2-thienyl)acetamido group attached to the cephalosporanic acid nucleus, and in the formation of the zwitterion (Fig. 1).

Cephaloglycin is commercially available as the dihydrate. *In vitro*, the antibiotic exhibits an antibacterial spectrum similar to that of other cephalosporins (Tables I and II). Cephaloglycin is administered orally to man and is indicated for use in treating bacterial infections of the urinary tract.

Like ampicillin as a penicillin, cephaloglycin as a cephalosporin exhibits increased activity against gram-negative bacilli. However, unlike ampicillin, cephaloglycin is stable to penicillinase and is only slowly degraded by cephalosporinase (Ott and Godzeski, 1967). Of the clinically useful cephalosporin derivatives, cephaloglycin is the most stable to inactivation by β-lactamases (Table III). Basically, *in vitro* gram-negative activity of the antibiotic is excellent, even to the extent of inhibiting growth of some cephalosporinase-producing *Enterobacter* sp. and some of the indole-positive *Proteus* sp.

Table VIII
DETECTION OF THE ACTIVITY OF CEPHALOSPORINS WITH *Streptococcus pyogenes*

Cephalosporin[a]	Oral ED_{50} (mg/kg $\times$ 2)	MIC (μg/ml)	Peak serum conc. (μg/ml)
Cephalothin	26	0.1	0.1
Cephaloridine	1.0	0.008	0.5
Cephaloglycin	3.9	0.2	3.8
Cephalexin	1.2	0.5	18.0

[a] Antibiotics were administered orally to mice at 1 and 5 hours post infection.

Detection of the oral absorption of cephaloglycin (and later cephalexin) was based on a combination of experimental data (Wick and Boniece, 1965). The results of the experiments are presented in Table VIII. Cephaloglycin, when administered orally to mice infected with streptococci, had an oral therapeutic ED_{50} value of 3.9 mg/kg as compared with 26 and 1.0 mg/kg for cephalothin and cephaloridine, respectively. Oral administration of either cephalothin or cephaloridine to humans had produced no significant concentrations of these antibiotics in serum. Thus, the excellent ED_{50} value for cephaloridine in mice had to be ascribed to the minute quantities of the antibiotic required for inhibition of the infecting organism, rather than oral absorption. On the other hand, cephaloglycin was less active than cephalothin *in vitro*, yet was almost ten times more active *in vivo*. The difference in ED_{50} values between cephalothin and cephaloglycin could be attributed to absorption of the latter antibiotic. Peak cephaloglycin concentrations of 3.8 μg/ml in mouse blood confirmed this conclusion. Additional experiments with mice showed that cephaloglycin was orally effective against other organisms, both gram-positive and gram-negative (Table IV).

Stability of cephaloglycin is dependent on pH, degrading very rapidly in basic media and remaining stable under acid conditions. Because of this stability pattern, susceptibility tests for staphylococci and gram-negative bacilli that are performed in broths at pH 7.0 or above should be read after 12 hours of incubation (Wick and Boniece, 1965). Broth-dilution MIC values can be determined after the usual overnight incubation, when the media is acidified (Ronald and Turck, 1967). Several clinical investigators reported the *in vitro* activity of cephaloglycin (Ronald and Turck, 1967; Boyer and Andriole, 1968; Applestein *et al.*, 1968; Eyckmans *et al.*, 1968; Braun *et al.*, 1968; Mössner *et al.*, 1969; Naumann and Fedder, 1970). When the tests were performed in nutrient broth or acidified media, the antibiotic exhibited good gram-positive activity and excellent inhibition of gram-negative bacilli.

Esterases can remove the acetyl group from the C-3 methyl position of 7-ACA to yield deacetyl cephalosporins (Newton and Hamilton-Miller, 1967). This was shown to occur with cephalothin by action of tissue esterases or bacterial enzymes in the intestine (Lee *et al.*, 1963; O'Callaghan and Muggleton, 1963). The same deacetylation reaction was expected with cephaloglycin.

Although deacetylation of cephaloglycin *in vivo* was expected, two experiments suggested that the reaction would occur slowly. First, cephaloglycin was deacetylated much slower than cephalothin in mouse-liver homogenates. In addition, chromatographic studies of mouse urine showed that cephaloglycin by oral administration was deacetylated to about the same degree as cephalothin by injection. Therefore, an assumption was made that, like injected cephalothin, deacetylation in humans would not be of great significance with orally administered cephaloglycin.

Prediction of the degree of deacetylation of orally administered cephaloglycin in man proved to be erroneous. Carefully controlled studies, by microbiological assay procedures and chromatographic techniques, have shown that the antibiotic activity of serum and urine specimens from humans receiving cephaloglycin is from 2 to 10% parent antibiotic. The remainder of the biological activity (90–98%) is due to the active metabolite deacetylcephaloglycin (Wick, 1968; Shimizu and Nishimura, 1970; Wick *et al.*, 1971).

In vitro studies performed during the clinical trial of cephaloglycin were done with the parent antibiotic. Since the antibiotic present in the greatest amount in body fluids is deacetylcephaloglycin, MIC values for the metabolite were needed to correlate with MIC values for cephaloglycin. Preparation of crystalline deacetylcephaloglycin by Kukolja (1968) made this correlation possible. Deacetylcephaloglycin exhibited approximately equal *in vitro* activity to cephaloglycin against staphylococci but was about fourfold (range, two- to eight-fold) less active against other gram-positive cocci and gram-negative bacilli (Wick *et al.*, 1971). This *in vitro* correlation was confirmed by therapeutic experiments in experimental mouse infections. Additional studies are needed to assess the contribution the small amount of cephaloglycin makes to successful therapy that seems to be mostly due to the biologically active metabolite, deacetylcephaloglycin.

D. Cephalexin

Deacetyoxycephaloglycin, or cephalexin, is 7-(D-α-amino-α-phenylacet-amido)-3-methyl-3-cephem-4-carboxylic acid (Wick, 1967; Ryan et al., 1969). Cephalexin differs in structure from cephaloglycin by substitution of the acetoxy group with a hydrogen atom (Fig. 1). Both cephaloglycin and cephalexin are absorbed from the gastrointestinal tract, but the slight change in structure apparently accounts for the difference in pharmacological properties of the two antibiotics. Cephaloglycin is metabolized mostly to deacetyl-cephaloglycin in man. Cephalexin is excreted in urine unchanged (Sullivan et al., 1969b).

The antibacterial spectrum of cephalexin is similar to that of cephalothin and cephaloridine (Tables I and II); however, more cephalexin is required for in vitro inhibition of susceptible organisms. Foz (1970) studied the suscepti-bility to cephalexin of a large number of bacterial isolates by an agar-dilution procedure similar to the method used by the ICS committee sponsored by WHO (Ericsson, 1964). His results are summarized in Table IX. Although these data were obtained with bacteria isolated in a particular geographical area, the degrees of susceptibilities are quite representative of those by other investi-gators (Griffith and Black, 1968; Perkins et al., 1968; Braun et al., 1968; Kind et al., 1969; Thornhill et al., 1969; Leigh et al., 1970; Naumann and Fedder, 1970).

As with cephaloglycin, detection of the oral absorption of cephalexin was based on a combination of experimental data (Table VIII). Cephalexin was also less active than cephalothin against the streptococcus in vitro, but more active in vivo. The 18-μg/ml blood level in mice with 20 mg/kg confirmed the oral absorption of the antibiotic. Activities of cephalexin and other orally administered antibiotics against a variety of bacterial infections in mice were compared (Wick, 1967; Muggleton et al., 1969). The amounts of cephalexin required for in vitro inhibition of the bacteria were higher than those for the other antibiotics examined. However, in vivo activity of cephalexin was equal to or better than the comparison antibiotics. The difference between in vitro and in vivo activity was attributed to the excellent absorption of cephalexin.

Ryan (1970) was able to control experimental urinary tract infections in rats with 32 mg/kg of cephalexin. He explained that the test model used was a severe test and that the amount of compound needed to eradicate an infection accordingly would be high. Likewise, Saslaw and his associates (1968, 1969,

1970) were successful in treating severe life-threatening staphylococcal and streptococcal infections in monkeys. Their data showed that cephalexin given orally was as effective as the parenterally administered cephalosporins in the therapy of these severe infections.

Serum inactivation or protein binding of cephalexin is low. Standard curves, obtained with *S. lutea* microbiological assays by use of 6-mm discs saturated

Table IX

SUSCEPTIBILITY OF 787 BACTERIAL ISOLATES TO CEPHALEXIN[a]

Organism	Number of isolates	Percent susceptible to ≤16 μg/ml cephalexin
Staphylococcus aureus (penicillin sensitive)	19	100
Staphylococcus aureus (penicillin resistant)	78	100
Staphylococcus aureus (oxacillin resistant)	18	0
Staphylococcus epidermidis (penicillin sensitive)	23	100
Staphylococcus epidermidis (penicillin resistant)	24	100
Staphylococcus epidermidis (oxacillin resistant)	2	0
Streptococcus pyogenes (group A)	6	100
Streptococcus sp. (group D)	54	0
Diplococcus pneumoniae	14	100
Escherichia coli	197	93
Citrobacter freundii	16	43
Klebsiella pneumoniae	108	91
Enterobacter aerogenes	7	57
Enterobacter cloacae	14	0
Serratia marcescens	4	0
Proteus mirabilis	92	94
Proteus sp. (indole positive)	80	9
Pseudomonas sp.	17	0
Salmonella sp.	14	100

[a] From Foz (1970). Susceptibility tested by the agar-dilution procedure, with Mueller–Hinton agar.

in either pH 7.0 buffer or human serum were identical (Wick, 1967). This lack of a difference in the curves indicated no loss of antibacterial activity in human serum. Under identical conditions, the decrease in activity of cephalothin, cephaloglycin, and cephaloridine was 45, 24, and 15%, respectively. Griffith and Black (1970) found that protein binding of cephalexin in human serum was 9% at concentrations above 1 μg/ml, and 41% at 0.2 μg/ml. Naumann and Fedder (1970) also found that the amount of cephalexin bound to serum proteins varied with concentration. They estimated the degree of binding of cephalexin was between that found for cephalothin and cephalori-

dine. Serum binding of cephalexin by an ultrafiltration method was 15%
(Kind et al., 1969).

Stability data for cephalexin have been reported. Loss of biological activity
after 24 hours of incubation in either pH 7.0 buffer or human sera was 0–7%
at 4°C, 15–32% at 25°C, and 50–55% at 37°C (Wick, 1967). Naumann and
Fedder (1970) found similar 24-hour degradation, and extended their studies
for 15 days. After 15 days, antibiotic remaining in pH 7.0 phosphate buffer
was 85, 70, and 10% at −15, 4, and 20°C, respectively. These values were
approximately the same for cephalexin in human serum. Recent studies at
−70°C showed no significant change in assay values for 1 mg/ml saline or
serum cephalexin solutions over a 6-month period. When urine or serum
specimens and standard solutions for assay were stored, the stability of the
antibiotic was considered.

Because of the difficulties encountered with cephalothin and cephaloglycin,
the stability of cephalexin was determined for another reason—susceptibility
testing. Rates of degradation for cephalexin in trypticase–soy, brain–heart
infusion, and nutrient broths when incubated at 37°C, were 1.5, 2.0, and
0.9%/hour, respectively (Wick and Boniece, 1967). The first two broths are
buffered to maintain pH 7.2–7.4, while nutrient broth pH ranges are 6.5–6.8.
Thus, cephalexin appeared slightly more stable in acidic media but not enough
to affect MIC values. Braun et al. (1968) showed that the susceptibility of an
E. coli strain was not affected by differences in media pH of 5.5–8.0. However,
the MIC values for cephaloglycin increased up to 32-fold at higher pH. Since
cephalexin does not possess an acetyl group, it is not deacetylated like cephalothin or cephaloglycin. However, the remainder of the cephalexin molecule is
similar to cephaloglycin. Because cephalexin is more stable in solution,
susceptibility testing during evaluation of cephalexin was not a great problem
as it was with cephalothin and cephaloglycin.

Peak cephalexin concentrations in mouse blood of 18 μg/ml with a 20
mg/kg dose accurately predicted the peak serum concentration in man given
500 mg (Griffith and Black, 1968; Wick, 1969). Studies in dogs showed that up
to 80% of orally administered cephalexin was excreted within 6 hours (Welles
et al., 1970). Thus, it was no surprise that up to 100% of cephalexin is absorbed
from the gastrointestinal tract of humans.

E. Cefazolin

A new cephalosporin derivative of clinical interest is 7-[1-(1H)tetrazolyl-
acetamido] - 3 - [2 - (5 - methyl - 1,3,4 - thiadiazolyl)thiomethyl]- 3 - cephem - 4-
carboxylic acid, generically called cefazolin (Fig. 1). The antibiotic is equally
active in vitro to cephalothin against gram-positive organisms and has slightly

greater activity than cephaloridine toward gram-negative bacteria (Nishida et al., 1970).

The antibacterial spectrum of cefazolin is similar to the four related antibiotics previously described. Strains of *S. aureus* are slightly less susceptible to cefazolin than to cephaloridine. However, gram-negative bacteria were more susceptible *in vitro* to cefazolin than cephaloridine. A marked difference in viable cell counts during incubation of bacteria with cefazolin was noted during 8 hours of incubation. Accordingly, cefazolin is considered to be bactericidal.

Binding of cefazolin to human serum proteins, as determined by the ultrafiltration method, was about equal to that for cephalothin, and more than cephaloridine. However, the antibiotic did not seem so firmly bound as to affect *in vivo* activity, for the ED_{50} values obtained against experimental mouse infections with cefazolin and cephaloridine were comparable.

Cefazolin has received considerable clinical trial in Japan as an injectable antibiotic. The role of this cephalosporin antibiotic for therapy in humans is dependent on the results of these clinical trials. Of particular interest is the amount of pain occurring after injections and the excretion rate in patients with renal insufficiency.

F. Cephapirin

Preliminary experimental studies for BL-P1322, 7-(pyrid-4-yl-thioacetamido)cephalosporanate, have been described (Chisholm *et al.*, 1970). This cephalosporin derivative has been given the generic name cephapirin (Fig. 1). Laboratory experience with the antibiotic compared favorably with cephalothin. The antimicrobial spectra of cephalothin and cephapirin were similar. Against most bacteria, the amounts of both antibiotics required for inhibition were about equal; however, cephapirin was more effective *in vitro* against strains of *Diplococcus pneumoniae*, *Enterobacter* sp., and *Mycobacterium tuberculosis*. Therapeutic efficacy of experimental bacterial infections in mice compared favorably with that of cephalothin. Concentrations of the two antibiotics in body fluids following subcutaneous administration to mice were comparable. Both compounds were equally bactericidal against *S. aureus*. The extent to which the compounds were bound to human serum proteins, as determined by comparing buffer and serum assay curves, was 65% for cephalothin and 44–50% for cephapirin.

G. Cephacetrile

A cephalosporin derivative, 7-cyanoacetamido-3-acetoxymethyl-3-cephem-4-carboxylic acid, sodium salt (Fig. 1), has been assigned the generic name cephacetrile (Kradolfer *et al.*, 1970). This compound appeared to be more active than cephalothin but less active than cephaloridine in therapy of experimental mouse infections. Urinary tract infections in rats also responded to treatment with the antibiotic. Toxicity studies in mice, rats, rabbits, guinea pigs, and dogs have proven the safety of this compound for clinical trial.

IV. Resistance to Cephalosporins by Staphylococci

There are two kinds of resistance to penicillins and cephalosporins with staphylococcal strains (Chabbert, 1968). The first is associated with hydrolysis by β-lactamases. Cephalosporin antibiotics are quite resistant to β-lactamase produced by staphylococci. However, cephaloridine is more labile to one of the three staphylococcal penicillinases than is cephalothin. β-Lactamase production occurs with a staphylococcal cell because of the presence of an extra-chromosomal factor, called an episome or plasmid. This plasmid can be lost but can also be infective via transfer to other cells by phage transduction. Cells containing plasmids can be cured by substances acting on DNA, such as acriflavin. Thus, it is possible to have resistance transfer in nature provided there are plasmid-donor and -receptor cells together, there are no substances in the environment which cure the donor cells, the proper phage is present, and optimal conditions for transduction exist. Evidently, the foregoing conditions for plasmid transfer in nature do not occur frequently. If they did, complete resistance to a new antibiotic that is susceptible to enzyme hydrolysis would occur almost immediately after its introduction.

A second type of resistance described by Chabbert (1968) is a chromosomal one. Cells with this type of resistance are responsible for so-called methicillin-resistant staphylococci. These natural-isolated cultures also have *multiple resistance* to the orally absorbed, penicillinase-stable penicillins, and to a lesser degree, the cephalosporins. Methicillin-resistant *S. aureus* cultures, because resistance is chromosomal and genetically transferred, contain two types of cells. One type is susceptible to β-lactamase-stable penicillins and cephalosporins, while the other type expresses varying degrees of resistance to these antibiotics. The latter cells represent only a small percentage of the total cell population of a culture. For this reason, these *S. aureus* strains are described as "heterogeneous-resistant" or "hetero-resistant" (Chabbert *et al.*, 1965; Seligman and Hewitt, 1966).

Within 2 years after the introduction of methicillin, *S. aureus* cultures resistant to the antibiotic were isolated (Barber, 1961; Jevons, 1961). Other workers have found similar strains (Barber, 1964; Kayser and Wiemer, 1965; Benner and Morthland, 1967; Chabbert, 1967). Concern was expressed that organisms resistant to therapy with antistaphylococcal agents might be selected by broad-scale use of certain antibiotics, including methicillin. However, Wick and Preston (1970) showed that clinically isolated hetero-geneous methicillin-resistant cultures already exhibit, to some degree, *multiple resistance* to all commonly used antibiotics except vancomycin. They stated that it seemed unlikely that curtailing the use of many of these antibiotics would have prevented the occurrence of these heterogeneous-resistant staphylococci.

Most of the heterogeneous-resistant strains that are obtained from patients also produce penicillinase, which means that some of one or both types of cells within the culture must contain plasmids. In addition, there is *multiple resistance* to other antibiotics that are unrelated to the penicillins or cephalo-sporins. To complicate the problem further, experiments in mice have shown that these methicillin-resistant staphylococci are less virulent than methicillin-sensitive strains (Kayser and Wiemer, 1965; Wick and Preston, 1970).

In vitro studies regarding these staphylococcal cultures are difficult to interpret because of the multiple modes of resistance. Induction of resistance from penicillin-sensitive cultures to cephalosporin antibiotics does not occur readily (Godzeski *et al.*, 1963; Naumann and Fedder, 1970). When resistant mutants are obtained by multistep passage in the presence of one cephalosporin, the organisms exhibit cross-resistance to other cephalosporin compounds. Ott and Godzeski (1967) have shown that oxacillin-resistant mutants are likely to demonstrate cross-resistance to the various cephalosporins; however, there were one way crosses in some instances. For example, cultures made resistant to oxacillin were highly resistant to cephalexin, while strains that were made resistant to cephalexin were not highly resistant to oxacillin. It is obvious then, that *in vitro* data obtained with these heterogeneous-resistant organisms are very complex and may not be dependable in trying to understand the clinical picture.

There is insufficient evidence to prove that heterogeneous-resistant staphy-lococci are responsible for wide-spread infections. Infection with methicillin-resistant *S. aureus* appears to be a hospital problem. Benner and Kayser (1968) stated that for 115 patients, at least 50% of the infections were not acquired until the patient had been hospitalized for 21 days or longer with chronic debilitating diseases. Wick and Preston (1970) found that virulence of methicillin-resistant strains was 10- to 1000-fold less than that of methicillin-sensitive cultures. This indication of lower virulence may explain why these heterogeneous-resistant cultures are isolated mainly from long hospitalized, debilitated patients and have not been the epidemiological problem as was the 80, 81 phage-type staphylococci. If these cultures appear in a hospital, proper monitoring and sanitary controls thereof would be the appropriate procedures to employ.

Regardless of the virulence of these heterogeneous-resistant strains, debilitated patients are subject to infection. Clinical and bacteriological failures have been reported for both penicillin-stable penicillins and cephalosporins (Benner and Kayser, 1968; Chabbert, 1968; Acar *et al.*, 1970). However, clinical failures with methicillin-sensitive cultures have also been reported (Kirby, 1965). Chabbert (1967) found the number of cells within a culture that were able to express resistance to the cephalosporins was 100 times less than for oxacillin. Thus, it would appear that successful therapy might occur more frequently with the cephalosporins than with the penicillinase-stable penicillins. However, there still exists a certain degree of resistance to both types of antibiotics. Therefore, therapy of infections with methicillin-resistant staphylococci may require combinations of antistaphylococcal agents. The subject of resistance is also discussed in Chapter 10.

V. Disc-Susceptibility Testing

The amount of antibiotic impregnated in filter paper discs is expressed as content of the disc, not concentration (Ryan *et al.*, 1970). For example, a 10-μg disc simply contains 10 μg of antibiotic. The content bears no relationship to either the MIC value of the test organism nor the amount of antibiotic attainable in serum.

The content of antibiotic chosen for discs is dependent on the response obtained using the disc-duffusion test. A 30-μg cephalothin disc has been selected on the basis of data obtained with discs containing 1, 2.5, 5, 10, 30, and 50 μg of the antibiotic (Boniece *et al.*, 1962). The purpose of this study with discs of varying content was to select one having enough antibiotic to detect all susceptible bacterial cultures, both gram-positive and gram-negative. The cephalothin disc data showed that there was no significant difference in results with 30- or 50-μg discs. However, statistical differences were found below the 30-μg level. Based on these results, these workers chose the 30-μg disc for use during the clinical trial of cephalothin.

The study reported above was performed using trypticase–soy agar inoculated by swabbing from undiluted broth cultures. Results were based on whether or not there was a zone of inhibition present for the test organism. This procedure was being used in most hospitals at the time cephalothin was presented for clinical trial. However, other methods were also in use, for which different media or diluted inocula were employed. Workers using these latter methods felt that 30 μg of cephalothin in the disc was excessive. Thus, in Europe, a 15-μg disc has been temporarily used for cephalothin, and later cephaloridine (Ericsson, 1967). Turck *et al.* (1965) found the 30-μg disc satisfactory, providing a zone diameter of 15 mm or greater was used to indicate susceptibility to cephalothin.

About the time of the clinical trial of cephalothin, emphasis was being placed on the need for standardization of susceptibility testing methods (WHO Technical Report Series No. 210, 1961; Bauer *et al.*, 1959; Turck *et al.*, 1963).

Table X

SUGGESTED INTERPRETATION OF ZONE DIAMETERS
OBTAINED WITH 30-μg CEPHALOSPORIN DISCS

Cephalosporin disc used	Quantitative disc procedure (Bauer–Kirby)— measured diameter of inhibition zone (mm)		
	Resistant	Intermediate susceptibility	Susceptible
Cephalothin	14 or less	15–17	18 or more
Cephaloridine	11 or less	12–15	16 or more
Cephalexin	9 or less	10–15	16 or more
	For urinary tract infections only:		
	Resistant	Susceptible	
Cephaloglycin	16 or less	17 or more	

Table XI

SUGGESTED INTERPRETATION OF ZONE DIAMETERS OBTAINED WITH A
30-μg CEPHALOTHIN DISC FOR DETERMINING SUSCEPTIBILITY TO
CEPHALOTHIN, CEPHALORIDINE, CEPHALEXIN, AND CEPHALOGLYCIN

Cephalothin disc representing	Quantitative disc procedure (Bauer–Kirby)— Measured diameter of inhibition zone (mm)		
	Resistant	Intermediate susceptibility	Susceptible
Cephalothin Cephaloridine Cephalexin	14 or less	15–17	18 or more
	For urinary tract infections only:		
	Resistant	Susceptible	
Cephaloglycin	14 or less	15 or more	

At least two standardized methods have evolved, the Bauer–Kirby and ICS single-disc methods (discussed earlier in this chapter). Using the Bauer–Kirby method, zone diameter categories for cephalothin were proposed by Sherris *et al.* (1967), for cephaloridine by Ryan *et al.* (1970), for cephalexin by Wick (1969, 1970), and for cephaloglycin by Wick *et al.* (1971). Confirmation of zone diameters selected have been reported by several investigators (Washington and Yu, 1970; Matsen *et al.*, 1970; Foz, 1970).

Recently the United States Supreme Court ruled that antibiotic discs were considered a drug rather than a laboratory tool. This action has given the Food and Drug Administration more jurisdiction over the package literature for antibiotic discs. The range of zone diameters for predictive purposes as determined by the Bauer–Kirby technique, approved for cephalothin, cephaloridine, and cephaloglycin, and recommended for cephalexin are presented in Table X.

Values for zone diameters shown in Table X are for discs with the individual cephalosporins. However, many laboratories prefer to use only one generic disc for testing. Cephalothin discs have been selected for this purpose in the case of the cephalosporins. Approved zone diameters for cephalothin discs for use with the Bauer–Kirby method to test susceptibility to cephalothin, cephaloridine, cephaloglycin, and cephalexin are shown in Table XI.

References

Abraham, E. P., and Newton, G. G. F. (1961). *Biochem. J.* **79**, 377.
Acar, J. F., Courvalin, P., and Chabbert, Y. A. (1970). *Abstracts Intersci. Conf. Antimicrob. Agents Chemother.*, 10th Oct. 1970.
Anderson, K. N., and Petersdorf, R. G. (1963). *Antimicrob. Ag. Chemother.* **1962**, 724.
Applestein, J. M., Crosby, E. B., Johnson, W. D., and Kaye, D. (1968). *Appl. Microbiol.* **16**, 1006.
Barber, M. (1961). *J. Clin. Pathol.* **14**, 385.
Barber, M. (1964). *J. Gen. Microbiol.* **35**, 183.
Barber, M., and Waterworth, P. M. (1964). *Brit. Med. J.* **2**, 344.
Bauer, A. W., Perry, D. M., and Kirby, W. M. M. (1959). *Arch. Int. Med.* 104.
Bauer, A. W., Kirby, W. M. M., Sherris, J. C., and Turck, M. (1966). *Amer. J. Clin. Pathol.* **45**, 493.
Benner, E. J., and Morthland, V. (1967). *New Engl. J. Med.* **277**, 678.
Benner, E. J., and Kayser, F. H. (1968). *Lancet* **2**, 741.
Benner, E. J., Bennett, J. V., Brodie, J. L., and Kirby, W. M. M. (1965). *J. Bact.* **90**, 1599.
Bennett, J. V., and Kirby, W. M. M. (1965). *J. Lab. Clin. Med.* **66**, 721.
Bohonos, N., Dornbush, A. C., Feldman, L. I., Martin, J. H., Pelcak, E., and Williams, J. H. (1954). *Antibiotics Ann.* (1953–54), p. 49.
Boniece, W. S., Wick, W. E., Holmes, D. H., and Redman, C. E. (1962). *J. Bacteriol.* **84**, 1292.
Boyer, J., and Andriole, V. (1968). *Yale J. Biol. Med.* **40**, 284.
Braun, P., Tillotson, J. R., Wilcox, C., and Finland, M. (1968). *Appl. Microbiol.* **16**, 1684.
Bryson, V., and Szybalski, W. (1952). *Science* **116**, 45.
Chabbert, Y. A. (1957). *Ann. Inst. Pasteur.* **93**, 289.
Chabbert, Y. A. (1967). *Postgrad. Med. J., Suppl.* **43**, 40.
Chabbert, Y. A. (1968). *Int. J. Clin. Pharmacol. Sonderheft Cephalosporine.* 28.
Chabbert, Y. A., Baudens, J. G., Acar, J. F., and Gerbaud, G. R. (1965). *Rev. Franc. Etudes Clin. Biol.* **10**, 495.
Chang, T. W., and Weinstein, L. (1964). *Antimicrob. Ag. Chemother.* **1963**, p. 278.

Chauvette, R. R., Flynn, E. H., Jackson, B. G., Lavagnino, E. R., Morin, R. B., Mueller, R. A., Pioch, R. P., Roeske, R. W., Ryan, C. W., Spencer, J. L., and Van Heyningen, E. M. (1962). *J. Am. Chem. Soc.* **84**, 3401.

Chisholm, D. R., Leitner, F., Misiek, M., Wright, G. E., and Price, K. E. (1970). *Antimicrob. Ag. Chemother.* **1969**, 244.

Crompton, B., Jago, M., Crawford, K., Newton, G. G. F., and Abraham, E. P. (1962). *Biochem. J.* **83**, 52.

Ericsson, H. (1964). Preliminary report of a working group of The International Collaborative Study sponsored by the World Health Organization. Karolinska Sjukhuset, Stockholm.

Ericsson, H. (1967). *Postgrad. Med. J., Suppl.* **43**, 46.

Eyckmans, L., Van Landuyt, H., and Verberckmoes, R. (1968). *Chemotherapy* **13**, 193.

Fleming, A. (1929). *Brit. J. Exp. Pathol.* **10**, 226.

Fleming, P. C., Goldner, M., and Glass, D. G. (1963). *Lancet* **1**, 1399.

Foz, A. (1970). *Presna Med. Mex. Suppl.* **9**, 1.

Fuller, A. T. (1937). *Lancet* **2**, 194.

Godzeski, C. W., Brier, G., and Pavey, D. E. (1963). *Appl. Microbiol.* **11**, 122.

Griffith, R. S., and Black, H. R. (1968). *Clin. Med.* **75**, 14.

Griffith, R. S., and Black, H. R. (1970). *Med. Clin. No. Amer.* **54**, 1229.

Hamilton-Miller, J. M. T. (1964). *Nature (London)* **214**, 1333.

Hoehn, M. M., and Pugh, C. T. (1968). *Appl. Microbiol.* **16**, 1132.

Jevons, M. P. (1961). *Brit. Med. J.* **1**, 124.

Josephson, A. S. (1960). *J. Exp. Med.* **111**, 611.

Kayser, F. H. (1966). *Z. Med. Mikrobiol. U. Immunol.* **153**, 31.

Kayser, F. H., and Wiemer, U. (1965). *Z. Hyg. Infekt-Krh.* **150**, 308.

Kind, A. C., Kestle, D. G., Standiford, H. C., and Kirby, W. M. M. (1969). *Antimicrob. Ag. Chemother.* **1968**, 361.

Kirby, W. M. M. (1965). *Ann. N.Y. Acad. Sci.* **128**, 443.

Klein, J. O., Eickhoff, T. C., Tilles, J. G., and Finland, M. (1964). *Amer. J. Med. Sci.* **248**, 640.

Kradolfer, F., Sackmann, W., Zak, O., Brunner, H., Hess, R., Konopka, E. A., and Gelzer, J. (1970). *Abstracts Intersci. Conf. Antimicrob. Agents Chemother.*, 10th Oct. 18–21, p. 7.

Kukolja, S. P. (1968). *J. Med. Chem.* **11**, 1067.

Lee, C. C., Herr, Jr., E. B., and Anderson, R. C. (1963). *Clin. Med.* **70**, 1123.

Leigh, D. A., Faiers, M. C., and Brumfitt, W. (1970). *Postgrad. Med. J. Suppl.* **48**, 69.

Ley, A. B., Harris, J. P., Brinkley, M., Liles, B., Jack, J. A., and Cahan, A. (1958). *Science* **127**, 1118.

Matsen, J. M., Koepcke, M. J. H., and Qui, P. G. (1970). *Antimicrob. Ag. Chemother.* **1969**, 445.

Miller, R. P. (1962). *Antibiot. Chemother.* **12**, 689.

Mössner, G., Bürker, U., Egetmeyer, K. A., and Maurer, H. (1969). *Arzneim.-Forsch. (Drug Res.)* **19**, 1049.

Muggleton, P. W., O'Callaghan, C. H., and Stevens, W. K. (1964). *Brit. Med. J.* **2**, 1234.

Muggleton, P. W., O'Callaghan, C. H., Foord, R. D., Kirby, S. M., and Ryan, D. M. (1969). *Antimicrob. Ag. Chemother.* **1968**, 353.

Naumann, P. (1966) *Arzneim.-Forsch. (Drug. Res.)* **16**, 818.

Naumann, P. (1967). *Postgrad. Med. J. Suppl.* **43**, 26.

Naumann, P., and Fedder, J. (1970). *Int. J. Clin. Pharmacol. Beiheft Oracef.* 6–23.

Newton, G. G. F., and Hamilton-Miller, J. M. T. (1967). *Postgrad. Med. J. Suppl.* **43**, 10.

Nishida, M., Matsubara, T., Murakawa, T., Mine, Y., Yokota, Y., Kuwahara, S., and Goto, S. (1970). *Antimicrob. Ag. Chemother.* **1969**, 236.

Nishimura, H., Nakajima, K., Tanaka, Y., and Isono, J. (1965). *Ann. Rep. Shionogi Res. Lab.* **15**, 217.

O'Callaghan, C. H., and Muggleton, P. W. (1963). *Biochem. J.* **89**, 304.
Ott, J. L., and Godzeski, C. W. (1967). *Antimicrob. Ag. Chemother.* **1966**, 75.
Perkins, R. L., and Saslaw, S. (1966). *An. Int. Med.* **64**, 13.
Perkins, R. L., Carlisle, H. N., and Saslaw, S. (1968). *Amer. J. Med. Sci.* **256**, 122.
Perret, C. J. (1954). *Nature* **174**, 1012.
Reed, L. J., and Muench, H. (1938). *Amer. J. Hyg.* **27**, 493.
Richmond, M. H. (1965). *J. Bact.* **90**, 370.
Ronald, A. R., and Turck, M. (1967). *Antimicrob. Ag. Chemother.* **1966**, 82.
Ryan, C. W., Simon, R. L., and Van Heyningen, E. M. (1969). *J. Med. Chem.* **12**, 310.
Ryan, D. M. (1970). *Postgrad. Med. J. Suppl.* **46**, 19.
Ryan, K. J., Schoenknect, F. D., and Kirby, W. M. M. (1970). *Hosp. Pract.* **5**, 91.
Saslaw, S., and Carlisle, H. N. (1968). *Amer. J. Med. Sci.* **256**, 136.
Saslaw, S., and Carlisle, H. N. (1969). *Amer. J. Med. Sci.* **257**, 395.
Saslaw, S., and Carlisle, H. N. (1970). *Appl. Microbiol.* **19**, 943.
Saslaw, S., Carlisle, H. N., and Sparks, J. (1970). *Amer. J. Med. Sci.* **259**, 143.
Second Report of the Expert Committee on Antibiotics (1961). WHO Health Organization Tech. Rep. Ser., No. 210, 1.
Seligman, S. J., and Hewitt, W. L. (1966). *Antimicrob. Ag. Chemother.* **1965**, 387.
Sherris, J. C., Rashad, A. L., and Lighthart, G. A. (1967). *Ann. N.Y. Acad. Sci.* **145**, 248.
Shimizu, K., and Nishimura, H. (1970). *J. Antibiot.* **23**, 216.
Sidell, S., Burdick, R. E., Brodie, J., Bulger, R. J., and Kirby, W. M. M. (1963). *Arch. Int. Med.* **112**, 21.
Steers, E., Foltz, E. L., Graves, B. S., and Riden, J. (1959). *Antibiot. Chemother.* **9**, 307.
Sullivan, H. R., and McMahon, R. E. (1967). *Biochem. J.* **102**, 976.
Sullivan, H. R., Billings, R. E., and McMahon, R. E. (1969a). *J. Antibiot.* **22**, 27.
Sullivan, H. R., Billings, R. E., and McMahon, R. E. (1969b). *J. Antibiot.* **22**, 195.
Thornhill, T. S., Levison, M. E., Johnson, W. D., and Kaye, D. (1969). *Appl. Microbiol* **17**, 457.
Turck, M., Lindemeyer, R. I., and Petersdorf, R. G. (1963). *Ann. Int. Med.* **58**.
Turck, M., Anderson, K. N., Smith, R. H., Wallace, J. F., and Petersdorf, R. G. (1965). *Ann. Int. Med.* **63**, 199.
Walters, E. W., Romansky, M. J., and Johnson, A. C. (1963). *Antimicrob. Ag. Chemother.* **1962**, 706.
Washington, J. A., and Yu, P. K. W. (1970). *Appl. Microbiol.* **19**, 589.
Weinstein, L., and Kaplan, K. (1970). *Ann. Int. Med.* **72**, 729.
Welles, J. S., Froman, R. O., Gibson, W. R., Owen, N. V., Small, R. M., and Anderson, R.C. (1970). *Int. J. Clin. Pharmacol., Beiheft Oracef.* **36**, 44.
Wick, W. E. (1962). Unpublished data, Lilly Res. Lab., Indianapolis, Indiana.
Wick, W. E. (1964). *J. Bact.* **87**, 1162.
Wick, W. E. (1966). *Antimicrob. Ag. Chemother.* **1965**, 870.
Wick, W. E. (1967). *Appl. Microbiol.* **15**, 765.
Wick, W. E. (1968). *Proc. Meeting Jap. Cephaloglycin Committee, 5th Tokyo.*
Wick, W. E. (1969). *Antimicrob. Ag. Chemother.* **1968**, 435.
Wick, W. E. (1970). *Int. J. Clin. Pharmacol., Beiheft Oracef.* **24**, 28.
Wick, W. E., and Boniece, W. S. (1965). *Appl. Microbiol.* **13**, 248.
Wick, W. E., and Boniece, W. S. (1967). *Proc. Int. Cong. Chemother. Vienna*, 717.
Wick, W. E., and Preston, D. A. (1970). *Proc. Int. Congr. Chemother., 6th Tokyo* **1**, 428.
Wick, W. E., Holmes, D. H., and Boniece, W. S. (1960). *Antibiot. Chemother.* **10**, 71.
Wick, W. E., Streightoff, F., and Boniece, W. S. (1962). *Antimicrob. Ag. Chemother.* **1961**, 588.
Wick, W. E., Wright, W. E., and Kuder, H. V. (1971). *Appl. Microbiol.* **21**, 426.

Chapter 12

STRUCTURE–ACTIVITY RELATIONSHIPS OF β-LACTAM ANTIBIOTICS

MARVIN GORMAN and CHARLES W. RYAN

> Had I been present at the creation
> I would have given some useful hints
> for the better ordering of the universe.
>
> *Alphonso The Learned*
> *1221–1284*

I. Introduction

The demonstration that penicillin, the antibiotic substance produced by *Penicillium notatum* during fermentation, possesses both therapeutic effectiveness and a low order of toxicity in humans (Florey and Florey, 1943) prompted massive efforts to develop both the chemistry and production of the effective new agent. With the selection of high-yielding strains and the study of variations in the production medium, a variety of closely related compounds were observed in the fermentation (Moyer and Coghill, 1946). Further purification and study demonstrated that the β-lactam antibiotics produced by the culture were not all biologically equivalent (Stewart, 1965). Differences in these natural penicillins were first observed in terms of their relative ability to inhibit a rapidly growing culture of a sensitive organism. Later, more subtle differences were noted, such as the degree of serum binding (Tompsett *et al.*, 1947), acid stability (Brandl and Margreiter, 1954), and relative reactivity toward β-lactam opening enzymes (Barber, 1947). The ability of various β-lactam antibiotics to exhibit a qualitative shift in the spectrum of organisms inhibited was first realized with the discovery of penicillin N (*1*) (also known as synnematin B and cephalosporin N) (Abraham *et al.*, 1954, 1955). While penicillin N had only a fraction of the gram-positive activity of other natural penicillins, it possessed greater activity against gram-negative organisms. Acylation of the free amino group reduced the gram-negative activity (Newton and Abraham, 1954), giving the first indication of the type of functionality necessary for increased gram-negative activity. Penicillin N was effective in the treatment of human infections, but its use was short lived because of the relatively weak order of activity (Thayer *et al.*, 1961).

While studying the problem of penicillin N isolation, Abraham and Newton observed a second antibiotic produced in their fermentation of Brotzu's *Cephalosporium* culture (see Chapter 1). This compound was isolated and named cephalosporin C (*2a*). Its structure indicated that it shared many of the chemical features of penicillin N but was radically altered in the sulfur-containing ring (Chapter 1). The *in vitro* antibacterial spectrum of cephalosporin C is shown in Table III. It possessed considerable gram-negative activity but with a somewhat different antibacterial spectrum when compared to penicillin N. In addition, the cephalosporin was quite stable to the action of penicillin β-lactamases. Thus, while cephalosporin C was less active than penicillin N in inhibiting a penicillin-sensitive streptococcus, it was more active than the penicillin against penicillin β-lactamase-producing strains of staphylococcus. These differences justified a search for, and evaluation of, other β-lactam compounds.

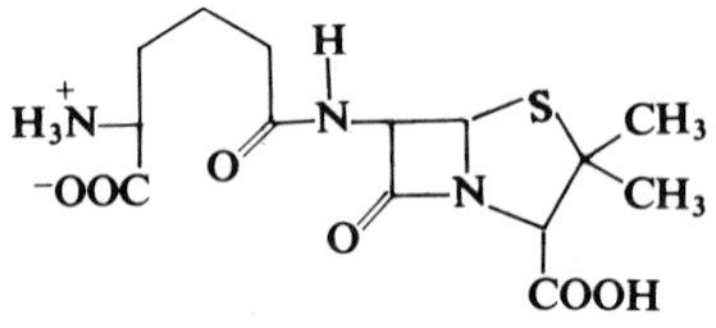

(1)

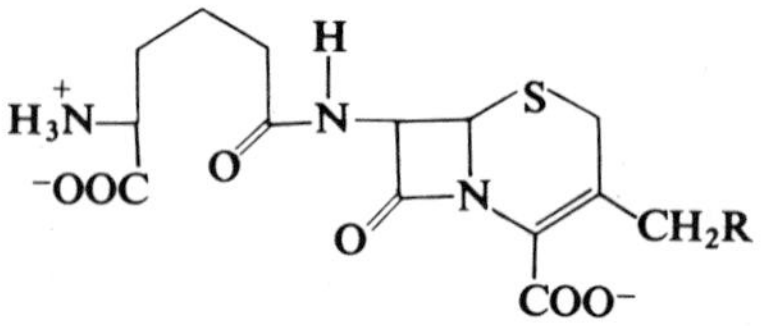

(2)

(2a) R = OCOCH$_3$

(2b) R = N

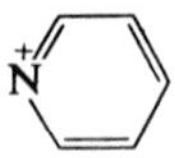

II. Sources of Antibiotics

Various changes and rearrangements were effected chemically as part of the structure elucidation of penicillin, but most of these did not produce new compounds with antibiotic activity. Modifications of cephalosporin C were more productive in that displacement of the acetoxyl (2a) moiety was possible (Chapter 4) with retention of activity; among other compounds, cephalosporin C$_A$ (2b) was obtained by direct reaction with pyridine (Hale et al., 1961) and showed an increase in potency, especially against gram-negative organisms (Table III).

Behrens and co-workers (1948) were able to show that the addition of various monosubstituted acetic acids to the Penicillium fermentation led to the

production of new penicillins. A number of new penicillanic acids were prepared and evaluated. Such studies led to phenoxymethylpenicillin (penicillin
V) which showed enhanced stability to acid and a somewhat shifted spectrum
of activity toward the gram-positive organisms (Price, 1969). This technique,
however, has not been successful when applied to the *Cephalosporium*
fermentation (Chapter 9).

Isolation of the penicillin nucleus (6-APA) (Batchelor *et al.*, 1959) from
a precursor-depleted fermentation of *P. chrysogenum* and reacylation of
synthetic 6-APA with a variety of acids by Sheehan and Henery-Logan (1959)
indicated the possibility of preparing large numbers of new penicillin derivatives. Many of these semisynthetic penicillins have found a place in the
armamentarium of infectious disease therapy (Butler, 1967).

The isolation of cephalosporin C (*2a*), which contained a new ring system
fused to the β-lactam, made obvious the importance of the cephalosporin
nucleus (7-ACA). Its availability (Chapter 2) was assured as a result of the work
of Morin and co-workers (1962). As described in Chapter 3 and below,
numerous derivatives have been prepared by direct acylation of the amino
function at C-7 and also through further modifications at other positions
around the molecules of the acylated compounds. Effectiveness of several of
these compounds, in terms of treatment of experimental infections, is presented elsewhere in this volume (Chapter 11). Pharmacology and related
studies are found in Chapter 13.

Another source of β-lactam compounds for evaluation is their preparation
by total synthesis (Chapter 6). While both the penicillin ring system and that
of the cephalosporins have been synthesized (Manhas and Bose, 1969),
relatively few new evaluable antibiotics have appeared from this source. The
general approach, however, offers the opportunity to observe the biological
effects of major changes in the molecular structure. A few recent examples of
new antibacterial β-lactam-containing compounds obtained by synthesis are
given later in the chapter.

III. Scope of this Review

This chapter will not attempt to catalog the large numbers of penicillins and
cephalosporins which have appeared in the scientific and patent literature over
the last 20 years. Our purpose is to examine changes in antibacterial properties
resulting from changes in structure. The reader is directed to two comprehensive reviews on this subject, one by Price (1969), covering the penicillins, and
the other by Sassiver and Lewis (1970), who review the cephalosporin literature.

IV. Factors Affecting Antibacterial Activity

A. Enzyme Inhibition

The mechanism of action of β-lactam antibiotics has been studied by Strominger and Tipper (1965), who have shown that inhibition of bacteria by these compounds likely occurs by reaction of the β-lactam with carboxypeptidase or transpeptidase enzymes important in cell wall synthesis. This irreversible acylation interferes with the synthesis of the cell wall in dividing cells, producing an osmotically unstable protoplast and eventually leading to destruction of the cell (Chapter 10). Strominger (1969) has proposed that the penicillins and cephalosporins resemble D-alanylalanine, which is a peptide fragment involved in bacterial cell wall synthesis. Polymerization of the building units of the wall requires cleavage of the alanylalanine bond, releasing free D-alanine.

The ability of several β-lactam antibiotics to block these reactions has been studied. The relative amounts of antibiotics needed to inhibit the growth of *Escherichia coli* were determined and those numbers correlated well with levels of the same compounds that would inhibit by 50% the glycopeptide transpeptidase. The D-alanine carboxypeptidase, however, was much more sensitive to the presence of the antibiotics (Butler, 1967; Strominger, 1969). The amounts of antibiotic were, for ampicillin, 3 μg/ml (growth), 3 μg/ml (transpeptidase), and 0.02 μg/ml (carboxypeptidase). For benzylpenicillin, values of 30, 3, and 0.02 μg/ml were found. For a β-lactamase-resistant penicillin, methicillin, the results were 1000, 1000, and 1 μg/ml while for a cephalosporin, cephalothin, the values 50, 50, and 1 μg/ml were obtained. Several factors in addition to that of enzyme inhibition are involved in the suppression of bacterial growth by β-lactam antibiotics.

B. Alkylating Ability

It has been suggested (Lawrence and Strominger, 1969) that reaction of the enzyme with penicillin occurs by sulfhydryl attack on the β-lactam to form a thioester (3). Conversion of the thioester to the corresponding amide or direct formation of the amide is also readily envisaged.

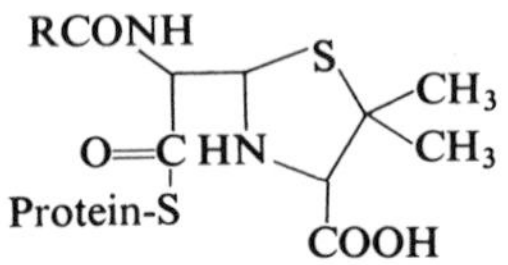

(3)

Wagner *et al.* (1969) have observed that penicillins react rapidly in aqueous solution with bifunctional mercaptoamines such as cysteine, under conditions where cephalosporins are stable. This finding is consistent with the lower intrinsic activity of the cephalosporin nucleus relative to the penicillin. The difference in ease of opening of the β-lactam of a cephalosporin or a penicillin is paralleled in the observation of the rates of hydrolysis of compounds such as (*4*) and (*5*) (Earle *et al.*, 1969). The four–five ring system (*4*) is much more rapidly destroyed in acid than is the corresponding four–six system (*5*). The

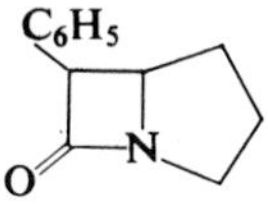

C_6H_5

C_6H_5

(4) 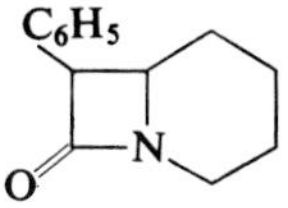   *(5)*

dihydro cephalosporins are devoid of biological activity and perhaps reflect this striking difference in ease of hydrolysis.

One may consider the ease of β-lactam ring opening in terms of strain on the β-lactam. Evidence for this strain is seen in the infrared spectrum of the carbonyl group of the β-lactam. Woodward and co-workers (Johnson *et al.*, 1949) have pointed out that a simple β-lactam carbonyl frequency is found at 1730 cm^{-1}, but in penicillins the band occurs at 1775 cm^{-1}. Morin and co-workers (1969) have attempted to use the position of the β-lactam carbonyl band in the infrared as a predictor of biological activity (Table I). As in the above example, the higher the IR frequency, the greater the predicted strain. Inhibition of a charged species resonance form (*6*) is responsible for this change in frequency. Simple amides which are capable of existing in a planar configuration have a carbonyl absorption at 1665 cm^{-1}.

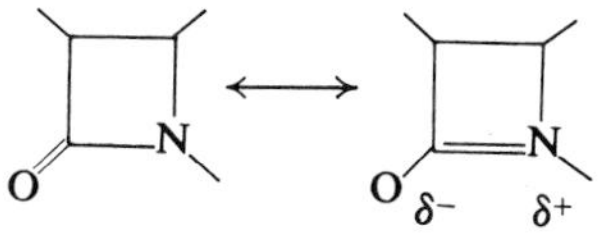

(6)

For a series of penicillins and cephalosporins shown in Table I, Morin *et al.* (1969) compared IR frequency with assay values against a penicillin-sensitive *Staphylococcus aureus* strain. The infrared frequencies of the antibiotic methyl esters (inactive as antibiotics) were measured and compared with assays obtained on the corresponding carboxylic acids. The ester lactam absorption seemed to predict the degree of activity, a useful correlation in terms of evaluating the antibiotic potential of compounds produced by complex chemical reactions which are more readily carried out on the ester. Some exceptions to

Table I

IR Frequency and Biological Activity of Some β-Lactam Compounds

Compound	β-Lactam frequency (cm^{-1}) $R = CH_3$	Bioassay $(units/mg)^a$ $R = H$
	1790	1800
	1795	140
	1792	300
	1785	25
	1784	6
	1780	15
	1776	4

Compound	β-Lactam frequency (cm^{-1}) R = CH$_3$	Bioassay (units/mg)[a] R = H
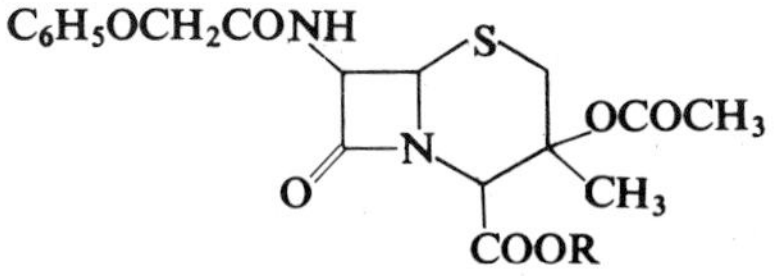 C$_6$H$_5$OCH$_2$CONH, S, OCOCH$_3$, CH$_3$, O, N, COOR	1780	low

[a] *Staphylococcus aureus* 209P (penicillin-sensitive).

the rule were noted, such as anhydropenicillin (Chapter 5) and penicillin sulfoxides (Chapter 5), which show quite strained β-lactams by IR measurement but do not possess much antibiotic activity.

Other physical methods contributing to the knowledge of properties of the β-lactam carbonyl–nitrogen bond include X-ray analysis (Chapter 7), which allows calculation of bond lengths and a measure of the pyramidal character of nitrogen in the β-lactam. In the case of the virtually inactive 2-cephems, the β-lactam is almost planar while in penicillins and active cephalosporins there is decreased amide resonance due to the nonplanar character of the nitrogen.

Hermann (1971) has correlated inductive effects on the β-lactam with the activities of several cephalosporins against gram-negative bacteria. The compounds (7), differing only in the functionality at the 3-methyl group, were studied by utilizing electronic structures established by molecular orbital calculations. He found that functions at the 3 position which were electron withdrawing, thus having a positive long-range inductive effect, possessed greater antibiotic activity toward gram-negative organisms. A positive correlation was obtained between the calculated inductive effect and bacterial inhibition (MIC values listed in Tables V and VI).

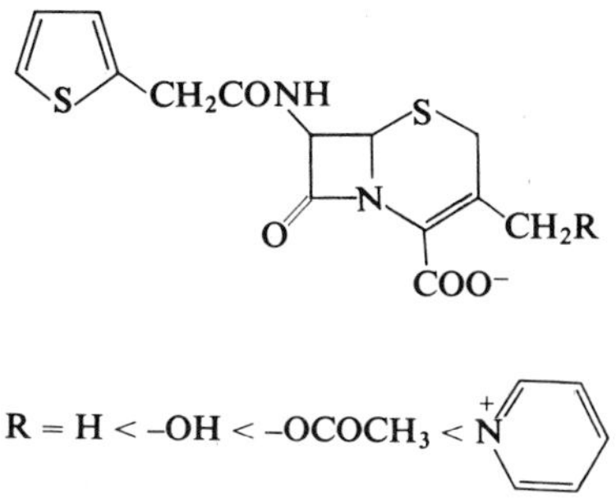

$$R = H < -OH < -OCOCH_3 < \overset{+}{N}$$

(7)

C. Permeability and Enzymic Affinity

Factors, other than ease of β-lactam ring opening, which contribute to inhibition of microorganisms by penicillins and cephalosporins include permeability differences, i.e., the ability of the compound to enter the cell wall and arrive at the enzyme which is to be inhibited. Once at the proper site, the affinity of the test compound for the active center on the enzyme will affect antibiotic activity. In Strominger's terms (1969), the degree to which the enzyme recognizes the β-lactam compound as resembling alanylalanine will affect the degree of inhibition of enzymic action.

While the composition of both gram-positive and gram-negative bacterial cell walls has been studied in detail, little is understood regarding the components of antibiotic structure which affect the binding affinity for transpeptidase or carboxypeptidase enzymes at the site of action. One may list several examples from the literature to illustrate these points. It has been shown that epimerization of the C-6 or C-7 positions of penicillins or cephalosporins respectively (8) results in virtual elimination of biological activity (Chapter 3).

RCONH H H S — O —N— COOH $\longrightarrow$ RCONH H H S — O —N— COOH

(8)

One recent report (Sawai *et al.*, 1970) claims that 6-epibenzylpenicillin retains a small percentage of antibiotic activity, but this is likely due to minor amounts of contamination with the normal isomer. Conversion of phenoxymethylpenicillin to its sulfoxides (Chapter 5) greatly reduces the antibacterial activity. A comparison of the α and β sulfoxides shows, however, that the α sulfoxide retains about five times as much gram-positive activity as the β compound (Spry, 1970). It would be difficult to attribute the changes in activity in these situations to either inductive effects on the β-lactam amide bond or to polarity differences which affect permeability into the cell. It is more reasonable to attribute these effects primarily to enzyme binding ability.

Several penicillins, as well as most cephalosporins, are relatively stable in the presence of staphylococcal β-lactamase. Kinetics of this enzymatic reaction have been analyzed in terms of both enzyme affinity and reaction rate. The results indicate a high affinity for benzylpenicillin and high reaction velocity. Lower affinity and high reaction rates were found for penicillins with bulky side chains such as phenoxyisobutylpenicillin. The highly resistant penicillins such as methicillin and oxacillin showed both a low affinity and slow β-lactam opening rate (Price, 1969). These latter compounds seem to act as competitive inhibitors of penicillin β-lactamase and protect the more reactive antibiotics against destruction by the enzyme. Perhaps similar kinetic considerations are also involved at the site of antibiotic action, but this remains to be shown.

So far we have explored differences in stability of various penicillins toward penicillin β-lactamase. Corresponding cephalosporin β-lactamase enzymes exist, particularly among gram-negative bacteria. O'Callaghan and associates (1969) have made a study of the interaction of cephalosporins with β-lactamases and can discern three types of responses which are qualitatively similar to those observed with the penicillins. Despite their low biological activity, the aroyl-substituted derivatives of 7-ACA were able to protect from destruction the highly susceptible cephalosporins such as those with arylacetamido side chains. Both *in vitro* and *in vivo* studies were carried out. β-Lactamases from *Aerobacter aerogenes* and *Proteus morganii* were much more reactive toward cephalosporins than toward penicillins, but methicillin was able to protect the very susceptible cephalosporins

Cell wall permeability appears to be partly responsible for the relative amounts of gram-positive and gram-negative activity of penicillins and cephalosporins. In a general sense structural changes which may affect permeability appear to cause similar qualitative alterations of activity for both the cephalosporins and penicillins. Differences in chemical reactivity and stability to β-lactamase action obscure the picture. Permeability appears to be mediated by side-chain polarity. As pointed out above, penicillin N is active against some non-penicillinase-producing gram-negative bacteria (Table III). Acylation of an α-amino group in the side chain changes polarity of the C-7 substituent by converting the basic nitrogen to a neutral species greatly diminishing gram-negative activity (Abraham *et al.*, 1954) but increasing activity against some gram-positive bacteria. Comparison of the activities of benzylpenicillin (*9a*)

(9a) $R = R_1 = H$

(9b) $R = H, R_1 = \overset{+}{N}H_3$

(9c) $R = \overset{+}{N}H_3, R_1 = H$

(9d) $R = H, R_1 = COOH$

(9e) $R = H, R_1 = NHSO_3H$

(9f) $R = OH, R_1 = \overset{+}{N}H_3$

(9g) $R = OH, R_1 = H$

with D-α-aminobenzylpenicillin (ampicillin) (*9b*) (Table V) and *p*-aminobenzylpenicillin (*9c*) shows this effect dramatically. It has also been discussed by both Price (1969) and Stewart (1965). In each of the foregoing situations a diminution of activity against susceptible gram-positive bacteria accompanies an increased inhibition of gram-negative bacteria, and acylation of each compound tends to reverse this effect (Tosoni *et al.*, 1958). If a carboxyl group (carbenicillin) (*9d*) or other acidic function (*9e*) is introduced in place of the amino group, the resulting compounds are much less active against gram-positive bacteria and show a change in gram-negative spectrum as exemplified by their inhibition of indole-positive *Proteus* sp. and *Pseudomonas* (Acred *et al.*, 1967; Barza *et al.*, 1971). A comparison of the reported biological activity for compound (*9f*) (Sutherland and Rolinson, 1971) with that of (*9g*) (Libby and Holmberg, 1945), a natural penicillin called penicillin X, shows that the effect of the polar phenolic function on overall activity is not nearly as dramatic as that of the amino group. The gram-positive activity of (*9g*) is somewhat less than (*9a*), while compound (*9f*) is similar in *in vitro* activity to ampicillin (*9b*). These differences in bacterial spectrum result from greater ability of the charged hydrophilic antibiotics to penetrate cell walls. They are also due to different resistance patterns toward β-lactamases produced by gram-negative bacteria. At least eight distinct classes of β-lactamases arising from gram-negative bacteria have been recognized (Jack and Richmond, 1970). A comprehensive discussion of β-lactamase involvement may be found in Chapter 10.

An analysis of relative antibiotic activities toward gram-positive and gram-negative bacteria expressed in terms of the lipophilic character of the β-lactam antibiotic (Biagi *et al.*, 1970) has recently appeared. These authors correlate a chromatographic value R_M, obtained by reversed phase thin-layer chromatography, with biological activities. They find that penicillins and cephalosporins which are most active against *Escherichia coli* are more hydrophilic than those which are active against *Staphylococcus aureus*. Their results are interpreted in terms of the variation in lipid content of the cell wall. The *E. coli*, like other gram-negative bacteria, has a greater lipid content and can, therefore, bind and prevent penetration by lipophilic compounds. *Treponema pallidum*, having no cell wall, more closely resembles *S. aureus* in its behavior.

Of the compounds discussed above, ampicillin (*9b*) possesses a value intermediate between the extremes of benzylpenicillin (*9a*) and carbenicillin (*9d*). The intermediate values for R_M would thus predict broad spectrum activity. It was found that gram-positive organisms grown under conditions which increased cellular lipid content (Hugo and Stretton, 1966) developed increased resistance to penicillins.

V. Evaluation

It will be readily apparent from data reported in Chapter 11 of this volume that when very large numbers of strains are tested against a single antibiotic, the minimal inhibitory concentration (MIC) values observed vary, not only from species to species, but from one strain or isolate to another. Consequently, when it is necessary to evaluate a large number of new antibiotics, selection of a few organisms representing both the gram-positive and gram-negative types must be made. In a continuing program, it is most important that all data be obtained with the same group of organisms if close comparisons are desired. Each laboratory tends to select a somewhat different group of cultures for their *in vitro* evaluation. In comparing compounds reported by different laboratories it is often possible only to establish trends or patterns of activity, as opposed to making judgements concerning close quantitative aspects of activity. The problem is somewhat lessened if appropriate standard compounds are included in the data supplied by various investigators.

VI. Test Methods

Methods of assaying for antibiotic activity have been reviewed by Grove and Randall (1955) and are elaborated in Chapter 11 of this volume. Most commonly, *in vitro* comparisons of antibiotics are carried out by one of two procedures. A disc–plate procedure (Boniece *et al.*, 1962) offers a simple, rapid method for comparing relative activities. With this technique a known concentration of test substance is placed on a paper disc, the disc is planted on an inoculated agar plate, and the plate is incubated. Diameter of the zone of inhibition is measured and compared with a standard substance for calculations of equivalent units of activity, or activity may be expressed simply in terms of zone diameter. Alternatively, a procedure whose results are often more informative involves the maintenance of a concentration gradient of the investigational compound in the agar onto which the test organisms are then streaked. MIC values in unit weight per milliliter are read directly after incubation is complete. This method has been described by Godzeski *et al.* (1963). A reference compound should be included when using either technique for determination of the relative biological activity of new substances.

Table II gives the variation of monthly MIC values obtained for cephalothin over a 2-year period, using the two test procedures described above and run in the Lilly laboratories. A key to the code letters for strains of bacteria used in these assays is provided by Chart 1, page 579. It is axiomatic that selection of the specific test organisms is dependent upon the goals of the research effort. It would be folly, for example, to utilize penicillin-resistant staphylococcus strains to select a new penicillin which is sensitive to β-lactamase. Occasionally, results obtained in these assays may be misleading because they may not predict a general trend, but rather an idiosyncratic response of a particular organism to a select compound. It is important that tentative conclusions gleaned from assays of this type be confirmed with tests on other strains of related bacteria (see Chapter 11).

Where possible in the ensuing discussion test data obtained in the Lilly Research Laboratories has been used if not contradictory to literature results reported on the same compounds by other workers. References are included

Table II

RANGE OF CEPHALOTHIN ASSAY VALUES OVER A 2-YEAR PERIOD[a]—MIC

Gram-positive *Staphylococcus* sp.					
Organism	V30	V41	V32	X400[b]	V84
Range (μg/ml)	0.2–0.3	0.2–0.5	0.2–0.6	10–>50[c,d]	0.1–0.4

Gram-negative microorganisms					
Organism	N9	N10	N26	X26[e]	X68	X514
Range (μg/ml)	9.0–19	12–21	10–18	0.8–13	2.3–5.0	1.0–2.1

[a] Disc–plate values: 800–940 units/mg *Bacillus subtilis*.
[b] Methicillin-resistant.
[c] >50 in 80% of tests.
[d] ">" denotes highest level tested.
[e] Range 0.8–2.6 with two higher values.

to the original preparations of the test antibiotics. Data obtained from reports of other laboratories is noted.

VII. Comparison of Penicillins and Cephalosporins

A. α-Aminoadipic Acid-Containing β-Lactam Compounds

While a number of penicillanic acids are produced in fermentations of *Penicillium* fungi, β-lactam antibiotics from other microorganisms are obtained as derivatives of α-aminoadipic acid (Chapter 9). Although these compounds have not been of clinical use per se, comparison of cephalosporin C and penicillin N has historical significance. Chemical modification of these naturally occurring substances has provided compounds which indicate the types of structural variation capable of producing more potent antibiotics. One example of this, already noted, is the conversion of cephalosporin C to cephalosporin C_A by reaction with pyridine. More recently, several streptomycetes have been shown to produce β-lactam antibiotics closely related to those produced by fungi (see Chapter 15). The first reported instance of β-lactam production by a streptomycete was the isolation of penicillin N in the Merck Laboratories (Miller *et al.*, 1962). Other β-lactams originating from *Streptomyces* species are those reported by Nagarajan *et al.* (1971) (Chapter 15). They include a cephalosporin having a C-3 carbamoyloxymethyl moiety, another which has a methoxyl in place of hydrogen at C-7, and a third having both of the foregoing substituents in the same molecule.

Table III indicates the antibiotic activity of β-lactam antibiotics which occur in nature as compared to cephalothin. Several derivatives prepared by reactions carried out at the 3-methyl position (see Chapter 4) are included to indicate trends observed in early work on these compounds by Abraham (Hale *et al.*, 1961). Both penicillin N and cephalosporin C have less than 1% of the activity of benzylpenicillin against a penicillin-sensitive staphylococcus (Flynn, 1967), but they show superior activity against gram-negative organisms, with penicillin N being more potent in several cases and cephalosporin C in others. The penicillin is more active against a penicillin-sensitive *S. aureus* (3055) where 1-mg/ml solutions of each produced zone diameters of 18 and 14 mm, respectively. The replacement of the acetoxyl function (cephalosporin C) on the 3-methyl group by a primary carbamate produces little change in *in vitro* antibacterial activity. Within the limits of the test these compounds appear equivalent. We shall see in Tables VII and VIII that the finding of approximate antibacterial equivalence with the naturally occurring antibiotics having 3-acetyloxymethyl and carbamoyloxymethyl function is found also for several semisynthetic derivatives possessing other amides at C-7 where the 3-methyl contains either aliphatic acyl analogs of acetyl groups or *N*-substituted carbamates. In the α-aminoadipic acid-containing antibiotics the presence of a methoxyl function at C-7 results in diminished activity against the gram-positive microorganisms. In contrast, a significant increase in inhibitory properties toward gram-negative bacteria is observed. The qualitative gram-negative bacterial spectrum of these methoxy substituted antibiotics is almost the same as for cephalosporin C.

The reaction of 7-ACA derivatives with nucleophiles has been studied extensively, and many examples of these products have been cited (see Chapter 4). The reaction of cephalosporin C with pyridine was reported by Hale *et al.* (1961). In contrast to most variations of structure, the resulting pyridinium betaine shows enhancement of both gram-positive and gram-negative activity.

A more common pattern observed when looking at new β-lactam antibiotic derivatives is a shift in antibacterial spectrum. For example, the 7-methoxyl cephalosporin C derivative in Table III shows a decrease in activity toward gram-positive organisms along with the increase in activity against the gram-negative bacteria. This shift in antimicrobial spectrum appears to be consistent with the correlations mentioned earlier concerning the differences in lipophilic character of the cell walls of various bacteria.

Table III
7-α-Aminoadipyl β-Lactam Derivatives

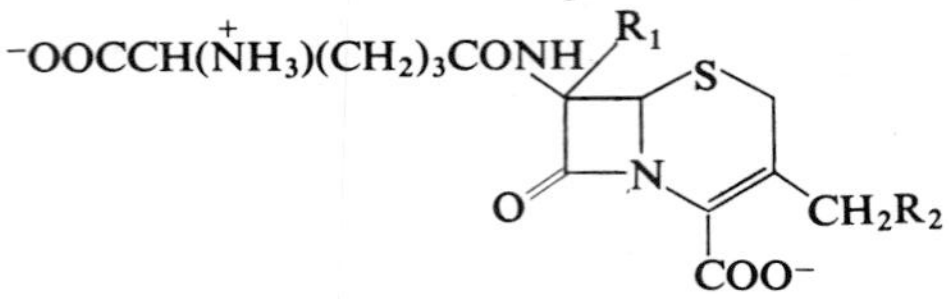

$^-OOCCH(\overset{+}{N}H_3)(CH_2)_3CONH$

Compound		S. aureus (MIC, µg/ml)			Gram-negative microorganisms (MIC, µg/ml)					Ref.
R₁	R₂	V32	V41	V48	N10	N9	X514	X26	X68	
-H	-OCOCH₃	39	40	36	67	85	25	38	45	a
-H	-OCONH₂	43	41	39	44	42	27	26	42	b
-OCH₃	-OCOCH₃	>200	>200	>200	33	16	9.3	8.1	13	b
-OCH₃	-OCONH₂	>200	130	130	10	11	15	19	18	b
-H	-H	>200	>200	>200	>200	>200	>200	>200	>200	c
-H	-OH	>200	>200	>200	130	150	100	74	170	d
-H	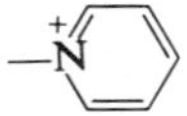 —N⁺(pyridinium)	12	9.0	8.0	26	22	—	23	>50	e
-H	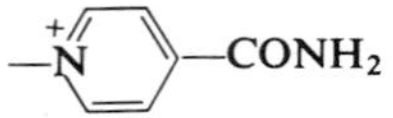 —N⁺(pyridinium)-CONH₂	11	9.0	6.0	19	16	—	16	21	f
-H	-SCOC₆H₅	14	13	12	>50	>50	>50	>50	>50	g
Penicillin N (I)		180	130	170	160	120	2.0	>200	140	h
Cephalothin (Table V)		0.5	0.4	0.4	6.4	8.8	1.0	0.8	2.4	i

a Newton and Abraham (1956).
b Nagarajan et al. (1971).
c Abraham and Newton (1956).
d Jeffery et al. (1961).
e Hale et al. (1961).
f Lilly Laboratories, unpublished work.
g Cocker et al. (1965).
h Abraham et al. (1954 and 1955).
i Chauvette et al. (1962).

These changes in biological spectrum of the α-aminoadipoyl derivatives are strongly suggestive of effects observed also with other 7-amido functions and have therefore been of great predictive value in structure–activity studies.

B. The β-Lactam Nucleus as an Antibiotic

The discovery of a procedure for the removal of α-aminoadipic acid from cephalosporin C and the work of Batchelor et al. (1959), which described methods for preparation of the penicillin nucleus, resulted in the availability of these substances for modification (Chapter 3). Data in Table IV shows that

Table IV

THE β-LACTAM NUCLEUS[a,b]

	Gram-positive			Gram-negative		
	SA	X12	X186	X45	X142	X161
6-APA	20[c]	24	40	21	23	21
7-ACA	Trace	16	15	—	—	—
7-ADCA	—	12	14	—	—	—

[a] Lilly Laboratories, unpublished results.
[b] Solution in buffer 1-mg/ml at pH 6.5.
[c] Zone diameter with 6-mm disc.

while these amino derivatives are relatively weak antibacterial agents, some biological activity is present. Both 7-ACA and 6-APA caused a lowering of the rate of alanine formation and of transpeptidation in E. coli, suggesting that they act by the same mechanism as their N-acyl counterparts (Izaki et al., 1968). While benzylpenicillin caused a sixfold decrease in alanine liberation by the enzyme at 7 μg/ml, a drop to half the control level was seen with the same concentration of 6-APA. No effect on transpeptidation was seen with 7-ACA or its deacetoxyl analog 7-ADCA, presumably due to the overall lower sensitivity of the test system to the cephalosporins (Strominger, 1969).

Rolinson and Stevens (1961) have observed inhibition of Corynebacterium species by 6-APA at levels of 1–5 μg/ml. Replacement of the cephalosporin 3-acetoxymethyl by a methyl group results in a decrease in antibacterial activity as shown by data in Table III for the α-aminoadipic acid derivatives and in Table IV for the 7-deacylated compound. The effect is quite general and will be observed repeatedly in other series of compounds which are discussed.

Table V

SOME CLINICALLY IMPORTANT COMPOUNDS

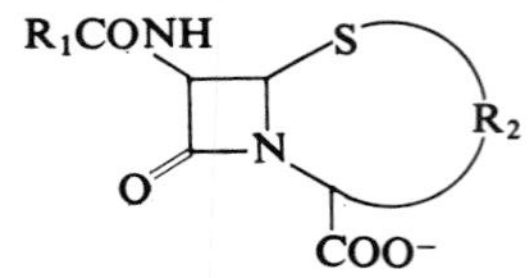

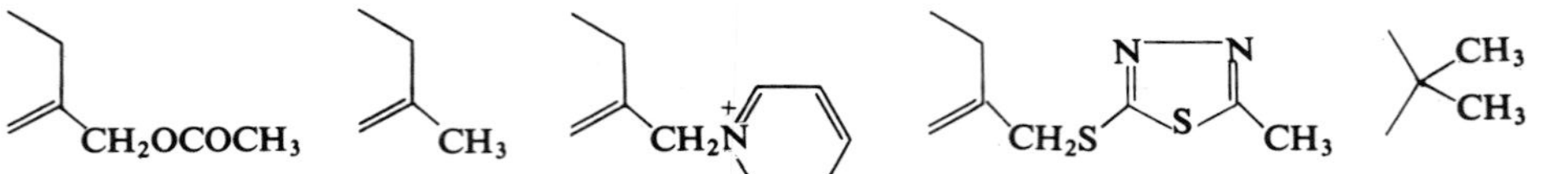

CH_2OCOCH_3 $R_2 = A$

(structure) CH_3 $R_2 = B$

(pyridinium) CH_2N^+ $R_2 = C$

(thiadiazole) CH_2S — CH_3 $R_2 = D$

$C(CH_3)_3$ $R_2 = E$

Compound		S. aureus (MIC, μg/ml)					Gram-negative microorganisms (MIC, μg/ml)							Ref.
R_1	R_2	V30	V32	V41	V84	X400[a]	N10	N9	X514	X26	X68	X99	X528	
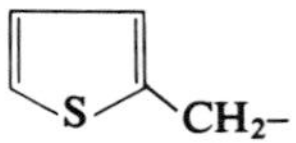 (2-thienyl-CH_2–)	A[b]	—	0.5	0.4	0.4	>20	6.4	8.8	1.0	0.8	2.4	>200	>200	c
	B	3.3	3.8	3.9	2.0	>20	>50	>50	—	16	>50	—	—	d
	C[e]	0.4	1.0	—	0.8	12	3.3	3.4	1.5	3.3	2.9	90	>200	f
	E	>20	>20	—	>20	>20	44	10	3.0	110	27	>200	>200	c
$C_6H_5CH_2$–	A	—	6.9	0.5	0.7	>20	27	43	6.9	1.0	8.1	>200	>200	g
	B	7.0	8.0	8.0	5.0	—	>50	>50	—	27	>50	—	—	d
	C	1.8	2.8	1.4	1.2	—	9.0	32	—	7.0	9.0	—	—	f
	E[h]	110	160	—	150	>20	52	21	6.2	110	48	>200	>200	
$C_6H_5OCH_2$–	A	—	—	0.2	0.2	>20	140	>200	110	6.2	110	>200	>200	c
	B	2.8	3.0	2.5	2.8	—	>50	>50	—	>50	>50	—	—	i
	C	0.3	0.2	0.2	0.2	—	38	>100	—	14	41	—	—	f
	E[j]	64	150	—	140	>20	>200	140	150	150	>200	>200	>200	k
$C_6H_5CH(\overset{+}{N}H_3)$–	A[l]	2.2	3.1	—	2.0	>20	3.5	3.3	1.0	1.0	3.5	68	>200	m
	B[n]	—	4.8	4.0	3.8	>20	9.7	10	6.0	6.6	6.4	80	>200	o
	E[p]	—	180	100	170	>20	6.3	3.3	0.6	110	22	8.8	>200	q

Structure	Form												Ref.
$C_6H_5CH(COOH)-$	A	—	6.2	8.0	9.3	>20	88	13	13	28	21	11	>200	r
	E^s	—	170	11	14	>20	8.8	4.7	1.5	>200	44	1.6	26	t
(2,6-dimethoxyphenyl, OCH_3, OCH_3)	A	—	18	>20	—	—	>200	>200	—	52	>200	—	—	u
	E^v	—	14	3.0	8.7	>20	>200	>200	>200	110	>200	>200	>200	w
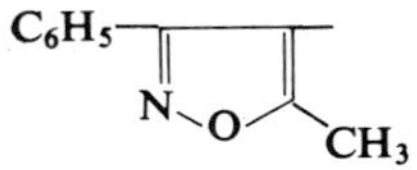 (C_6H_5 isoxazole, N–O, CH_3)	A	—	5.5	3.6	4.9	>20	110	86	>200	3.9	130	100	140	x
	E^y	—	16	0.5	0.5	>20	180	150	>200	29	>200	>200	>200	z
$NCCH_2-$	A^{aa}	—	0.6	0.7	0.8	>20	12	12	12	10	14	84	>200	bb
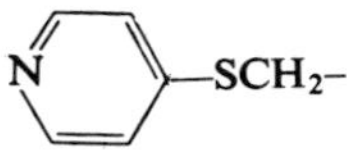 (pyridyl-SCH_2-)	A^{cc}	—	0.4	0.2	0.4	>20	17	15	1.4	3.1	3.9	>200	>200	dd
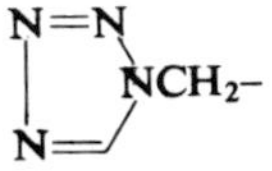 (tetrazolyl NCH_2-)	D^{ee}	—	0.6	0.6	0.5	>20	1.0	1.0	0.7	1.0	1.0	>200	>200	ff

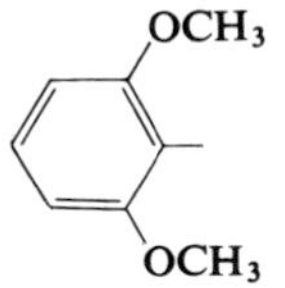

[a] Methicillin-resistant.
[b] Cephalothin.
[c] Chauvette et al. (1962).
[d] Stedman et al. (1964).
[e] Cephaloridine.
[f] Spencer et al. (1967).
[g] Chauvette et al. (1962).
[h] Penicillin G.
[i] Morin et al. (1963).
[j] Penicillin V.
[k] Behrens et al. (1948).

[l] Cephaloglycin.
[m] Spencer et al. (1966).
[n] Cephalexin.
[o] Ryan et al. (1969).
[p] Ampicillin.
[q] Doyle et al. (1962).
[r] Lewis et al. (1969).
[s] Carbenicillin.
[t] Acred et al. (1967).
[u] U.S. Patent 3,196,151.
[v] Methicillin.

[w] Rolinson et al. (1960).
[x] Lilly Laboratories, unpublished work.
[y] Oxacillin.
[z] Gourevitch et al. (1961).
[aa] Cephacetrile.
[bb] Knusel et al. (1971).
[cc] Cephapirin.
[dd] Chisholm et al. (1970).
[ee] Cefazolin.
[ff] Nishida et al. (1970).

C. Comparative Activity of Representative Penicillins and Cephalosporins

Comparison of the activity of penicillins and cephalosporins has been mentioned previously in this chapter and one may generalize that in non-β-lactamase-producing gram-positive bacteria the penicillin will be more inhibitory. Chauvette and co-workers (1962) commented on this fact very early while working with cephalosporins which, when directly compared in Oxford units of activity, were only about a fifth as active as the corresponding penicillin. They found that structural requirements for high activity were similar for side-chain amides of cephem and penam antibiotics. The difference in relative levels of inhibition has been attributed to a greater sensitivity of the enzymes at the site of action to inhibition by the penam as compared with the cephem (Izaki *et al.*, 1968) derivatives. Available evidence, cited earlier, attributes this intrinsic difference to a greater chemical reactivity of the β-lactam in the penicillin ring system.

The situation is more complex when comparing the activity of penicillanic and cephalosporanic acids toward gram-negative bacteria. The occurrence of β-lactamases is more common and their specificity has been shown to be more diverse in gram-negative organisms (Jack and Richmond, 1970). In Table V *Klebsiella* strain X26 appears to produce a penicillin β-lactamase since inhibition by the penicillins listed is uniformly poorer than for the cephalosporins, while less difference is evident when *E. coli* N10 is considered. Against many gram-negative organisms the MIC values are equivalent. Rarely, however, does the penicillin exhibit a superior level of activity. *Serratia marcescens* (X99) is one of these exceptions and generally responds to penicillins at lower MIC values than to cephalosporins, i.e., a penicillin (ampicillin) MIC of 8.8 μg/ml and a cephaloglycin MIC of 68 μg/ml are found for X99 (Table V).

Naito and co-workers (1968) have compared several derivatives of sydnone-3-acetamido-substituted penicillins and cephalosporins and find a broad spectrum of biological activity in both the penam and cephem compounds. Again, the penicillins are somewhat more active against gram-positive bacteria and less active against the gram-negative organisms used. Stedman *et al.* (1967) investigated a series of pyridylacetamidocephalosporanic and penicillanic acids which also conformed to these generalizations. However, Raap and Micetich (1968) found consistently higher activity for a series of substituted isothiazolylmethylpenicillins over the corresponding cephalosporins using strains of *E. coli* and several *Salmonella*. MIC values were determined with a twofold serial dilution technique.

The effects of penicillin β-lactamase-resistant penicillins are evident from the dramatic drop in MIC values with the resistant staphylococcus organisms cited when they are exposed to methicillin or oxacillin. Price (1969, p. 34) states that these compounds have only 2 and 10% respectively of the activity of penicillin G against sensitive staphylococci. *S. aureus* X400 is resistant to all penicillins including methicillin, and this strain whose resistance is not well understood (Benner and Kayser, 1968) is also resistant to most cephalosporin (Table V) antibiotics. See, however, Chapters 10 and 11 for extended discussion of this topic.

From data in Table V it can be seen that arylmethylene side chains such as benzyl and thienyl produce compounds possessing both potent gram-positive activity and moderate gram-negative bacterial inhibition. If the aromatic ring is separated from the acetamido function by oxygen (phenoxymethyl), gram-negative antibacterial action is greatly diminished and inhibition of the staphylococci improves somewhat. As mentioned previously, the presence of an α-amino function on the benzyl group greatly improves MIC values toward the gram-negative organisms. Note also the inhibition of *Pseudomonas* X528 when an α-carboxyl group is introduced into the benzyl penicillin. The general lower potency of the β-lactamase resistant penicillins is also observed when assessing their gram-negative activity.

D. Cephalosporins in Human Medicine

Four cephalosporanic acids have found a role in human medicine. They have been given the generic names cephalothin, cephaloridine, cephaloglycin, and cephalexin. The bacteriology and toxicology of these substances are discussed in Chapters 11 and 13, respectively. Three additional cephem derivatives have been reported to be under extensive investigation or on clinical trial. Two of these, cephacetrile, also known as CIBA 36278A-Ba (Knusel *et al.*, 1971; Kradolfer *et al.*, 1971), and cephapirin, called also BL-P1322 (Chisholm *et al.*, 1970), retain the acetoxymethyl function at C-3. The third antibiotic is called cefazolin (Nishida *et al.*, 1970) and represents the result of a thorough study of nucleophilic displacement at the 3 position by heterocyclic aromatic thiols. Examples of these displacement products are shown in Table XI, and they appear to have enhanced activity against gram-negative bacteria. Cefazolin has been reported to be metabolically stable, thereby overcoming the problem of metabolic deacetylation, a reaction which tends to produce an antibiotic with diminished gram-negative antibacterial activity (Ishiyama *et al.*, 1971) as illustrated by data for the compounds in Table VI. The three foregoing compounds are effective by parenteral administration. Gradient plate antimicrobial data presented in Table V allows a comparison of these newer substances with the other parenterally administered cephalosporins. In these evaluations, it would appear that cephalothin, cephacetrile, and

Table VI

3-Acetoxymethyl, 3-Hydroxymethyl Cephalosporins and Cephalosporin Lactones

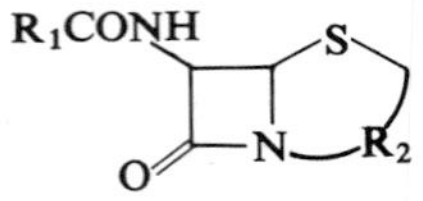

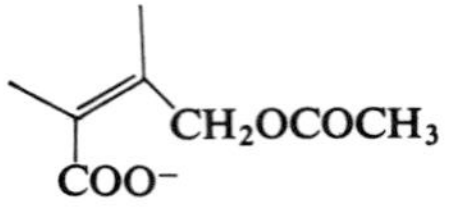

R₁CONH

$R_2 = A$: CH₂OCOCH₃ / COO⁻

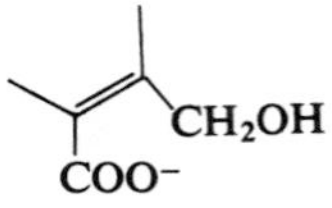

$R_2 = B$: CH₂OH / COO⁻

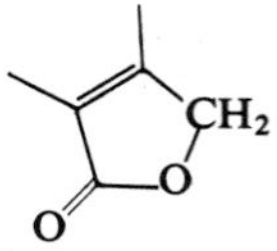

$R_2 = C$

Compound			S. aureus (MIC, μg/ml)					Gram-negative microorganisms (MIC, μg/ml)						Ref.
R_1	R_2		V30	V32	V41	V84	X400[a]	N10	N9	X514	X26	X68	N26	
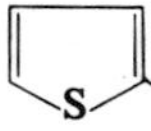 CH₂–	A		—	0.5	0.4	0.4	>20	6.4	8.8	1.0	0.8	2.4	—	b
	B		0.5	4.0	0.5	2.0	—	130	98	—	9.0	—	89	c
	C		4.9	4.6	3.9	1.8	—	46	>50	—	>50	>50	>50	c
C₆H₅CH₂–	A		—	6.0	0.5	0.7	>20	27	43	6.9	1.0	8.1	—	b
	B		0.5	1.5	0.5	1.0	—	>20	140	—	17	56	140	c
	C		1.0	9.0	2.0	8.0	—	>200	>200	—	95	>200	110	c

Compound												
C$_6$H$_5$SCH$_2$–	A	—	0.4	0.1	0.2	17	63	68	23	0.7	27	—	c
	B	—	0.5	0.4	0.2	>20	>200	>200	>200	>50	>200	—	c
	C	—	2.2	<1.0	0.3	>20	>200	>200	>200	110	>200	—	c
C$_6$H$_5$CH(NH$_3$)–⁺	A	—	3.1	2.2	2.0	>20	3.5	3.3	1.0	0.8	3.5	—	d
	B	3.4	2.8	—	1.3	>20	12	16	—	14	16	16	e
	C	>20	>20	—	>20	>20	>20	>20	>20	>20	>20	—	e
C$_6$H$_5$CH(OH)–	A	—	1.5	0.7	1.0	>20	5.6	3.0	0.7	2.1	1.9	—	f
	B	—	7.7	4.4	5.8	>20	48	19	12	13	18	—	g
	C	—	5.3	3.0	3.8	>20	>200	>200	>200	>200	>200	—	g

[a] Methicillin-resistant.
[b] Chauvette et al. (1962).
[c] Chauvette et al. (1963).
[d] Spencer et al. (1966).
[e] Kukolja (1968).
[f] U.S. Patent 3,167,549.
[g] Lilly Laboratories, unpublished work.

cephapirin are generally equivalent against the test organisms used, with cephalothin perhaps being slightly more potent. Cefazolin is similar to cephalothin against the staphylococcal strains shown but exceeds cephaloridine in its ability to inhibit gram-negative bacteria.

VIII. Cephalosporins Substituted at C-3

A. Deacetylcephalosporins and Cephalosporin Lactones

In both the penicillins and cephalosporins, a variety of acids can be used to yield new acyl derivatives for evaluation. By contrast, the dihydrothiazine ring of the cephalosporin, with its added functionality of a double bond and the attached acetoxymethyl grouping, offers a wider choice for modifications (Chapter 4) not available with penicillins. The effect of some of these changes has been commented upon previously; for example, removal of acetoxyl yields a 3-methyl cephem antibiotic which invariably possesses diminished antibacterial activity. In Table V this is demonstrated by the comparison of cephalexin and cephaloglycin. Two additional reactions, noted early in cephalosporin work (Chapter 1), are the deacetylation (Chapter 10) to the 3-hydroxymethyl cephem and lactonization to the tricyclic compounds indicated in Table VI. These reactions altered the microbiological activity of the products (Jeffery et al., 1961). Chauvette and associates (1963) reported that, for a representative series of cephalosporanic acids, the hydroxymethyl derivatives had about one-half of the activity of the parent antibiotics in a disc–plate assay with a penicillin-sensitive organism. The corresponding lactones in the same test were about as active as the acetoxymethyl compounds using a gradient–plate assay; little difference among the three derivatives was observed against resistant S. aureus in the absence of human serum. In the presence of serum the lactones were bound so extensively that no antibiotic effect was observed.

These authors also noted a decreased activity toward gram-negative bacteria with the deacetyl compound and the lactones appeared to be devoid of activity toward these organisms. Kukolja (1968) reported similar findings for the phenylglycyl derivatives. Table VI summarizes these results. It is of interest to note that significant gram-negative activity remains in deacetylcephaloglycin as compared to the other deacetylcephalosporins. This result again indicates the ability of the α-amino function to enhance gram-negative bacterial inhibition.

B. Acyloxymethyl- and Carbamoyloxymethylcephalosporins

Replacement of the acetoxyl moiety of cephalosporanic acids by closely related ester functions has been the goal of several laboratories (Kukolja,

Table VII

3-CARBAMOYLOXYMETHYL CEPHALOSPORINS

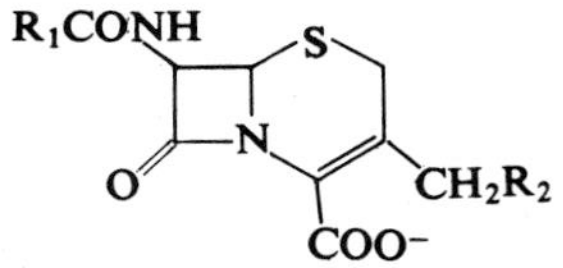

Compound		S. aureus (MIC, μg/ml)			Gram-negative microorganisms (MIC, μg/ml)							Ref.
R_1	R_2	V32	V41	V84	N10	N9	X514	X26	X68	X99	X528	
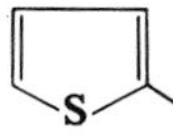 $\underset{S}{\text{thienyl}}CH_2-$	$-OCONH_2$	0.5	0.2	0.4	20	30	2.6	1.0	3.5	>50	>50	a
	$-OCONHCH_3$	0.5	0.5	0.3	15	7.4	2.5	0.6	3.7	>50	>50	b
	$-OCONHCH_2CH_2Cl$	0.7	0.5	0.4	8.5	6.4	2.2	0.4	3.6	>50	>50	b
	$-OCONHC_6H_5$	1.0	0.5	0.6	1.6	11	5.1	0.4	7.8	>50	>50	b
$C_6H_5CH(\overset{+}{N}H_3)-$	$-OCONH_2$	9.2	0.9	9.5	3.3	3.1	0.6	1.1	1.0	19	>200	a
	$-OCONHCH_3$	8.5	1.2	7.9	1.8	1.6	0.6	0.6	1.0	39	>200	c

[a] Lilly Laboratories, unpublished work.
[b] U.S. Patent 3,355,452.
[c] Belg. Patent 741,381.

1970; U.S. Patent 3,261,832; Van Heyningen, 1965), but its accomplishment has been a complicated task (Chapter 4). As noted above, the carbamate analog of cephalosporin C is a naturally occurring substance. This grouping has little effect on the antibacterial action when compared to cephalosporin C. This

Table VIII
3-ACYLOXYMETHYL CEPHALOSPORINS

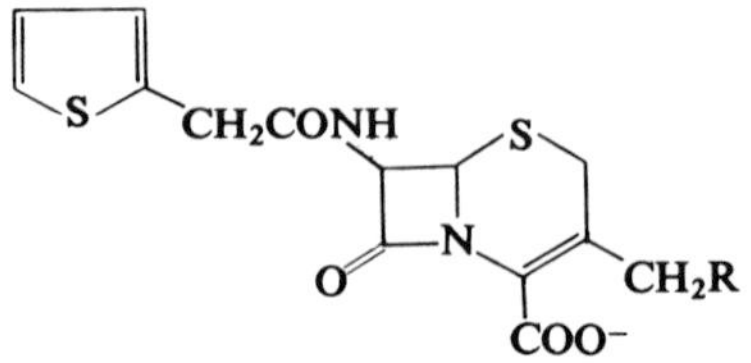

Compound	S. aureus (MIC, μg/ml)				Gram-negative microorganisms (MIC, μg/ml)					
R	V30	V32	V41	V84	N10	N9	X26	X68	N26	Ref.
–OCOCH₃	—	0.5	0.4	0.4	6.4	8.8	0.8	2.4	—	a
–OCOCH₂CH₃	0.5	0.5	—	0.4	12	6.7	5.5	8.1	9.4	b
–OCO(CH₂)₂CH₃	0.4	0.4	—	0.2	12	5.9	6.4	7.5	9.5	b
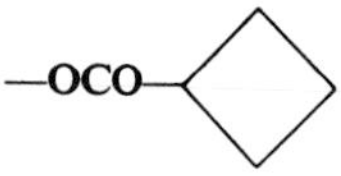 —OCO—⟨⟩	0.4	0.5	—	0.1	10	8.3	2.5	12	12	b
–OCOC₆H₅	0.1	0.1	0.1	0.1	41	18	0.5	43	37	c
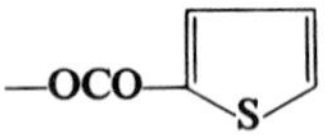 —OCO—⟨S⟩	6.0	6.0	3.0	6.0	96	53	7.0	54	63	c
–SCOCH₃	1.1	2.8	0.8	1.0	52	20	6.0	38	27	d
–SCOC₆H₅	0.7	10	—	1.5	27	18	0.6	14	—	e

[a] Chauvette et al. (1962).
[b] Kukolja (1970).
[c] Van Heyningen (1965).
[d] Lilly Laboratories, unpublished work.
[e] U.S. Patent 3,261,832.

similarity in activity is also true of substituted carbamates (U.S. Patent 3,355,452) which have been reported. Values are shown in Table VII for selected 3-carbamoyloxymethyl compounds.

The substitution of a phenyl for a methyl group in the 3-acyloxymethyl-cephalosporins pictured in Table VIII increases the activity of the compounds toward staphylococcus species. An increase in length of the aliphatic acyl function has little effect on antibacterial activity.

Conversely, the benzoyl esters show a diminished ability to inhibit gram-negative bacteria. The activity toward this latter group of microorganisms slowly decreases with increasing complexity of the aliphatic acyl functions.

Table IX
3-Aminomethyl and 3-Azidomethyl Cephalosporins

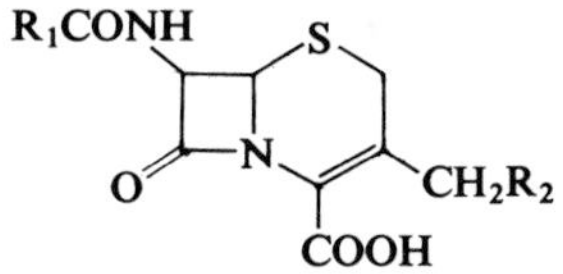

R_1CONH ... CH_2R_2 ... COOH

Compound		$S.\ aureus$ (MIC, μg/ml)			
R_1	R_2	663^a	604^a	3452^a	Ref.
C_6H_5CO-	$-N_3$	0.3	1.2	1.0	b
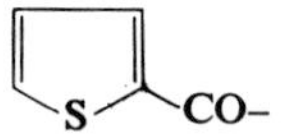 [thiophene]-CO-	$-N_3$	0.2	1.2	1.2	b
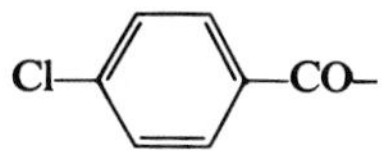 Cl-[phenyl]-CO-	$-N_3$	0.1	0.3	<0.5	b
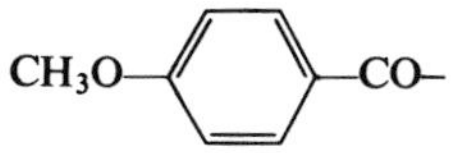 CH_3O-[phenyl]-CO-	$-N_3$	0.1	0.6	<0.5	b
$C_6H_5CH_2-$	$-NH_2$	0.2	1.2	0.3	c
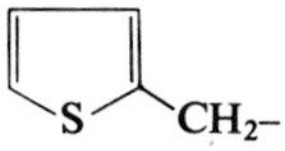 [thiophene]-CH_2-	$-NH_2$	0.1	2.5	>25	c
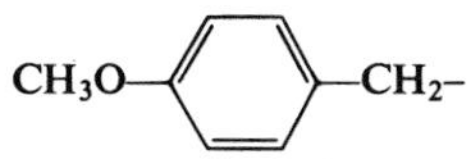 CH_3O-[phenyl]-CH_2-	$-NH_2$	0.3	>2.5	62	c
CH_3SCH_2-	$-NH_2$	<0.1	0.1	16	c

[a] Penicillin G resistant.
[b] U.S. Patent 3,546,219.
[c] Belg. Patent 634,644.

Several 3-acylaminomethyl (Belg. Patent 634,644) and 3-acylthiomethyl derivatives (U.S. Patent 3,261,832) have appeared in the patent literature. These latter groups appear to be equivalent to the aromatic acyloxy substituents, possessing potent activity against staphylococcus but having little effect

Table X
Thiocarbonic Acid Derivatives of 3-Methyl Cephalosporins

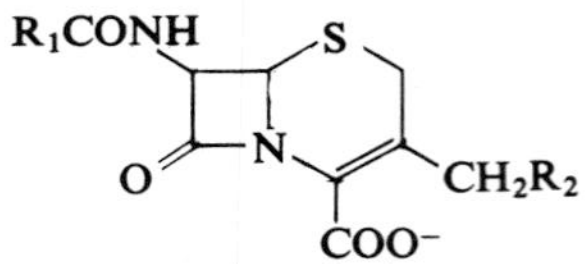

Compound		S. aureus (MIC, μg/ml)				Gram-negative microorganisms (MIC, μg/ml)					Ref.
R_1	R_2	V30	V32	V41	V84	N10	N9	X26	X68	N26	
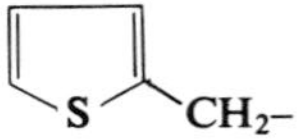	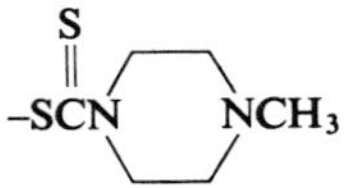	0.4	1.0	0.4	0.3	6	2	2	4	3	a
	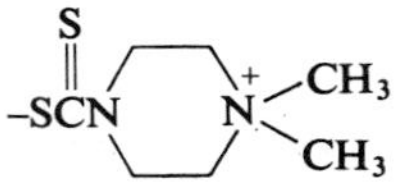	0.4	0.4	0.3	0.2	12	37	10	16	7	a
		0.6	0.7	0.5	0.5	34	21	14	17	27	b
	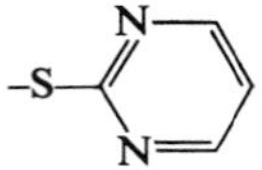	0.5	0.4	0.5	0.5	109	60	20	51	25	b

$\overset{S}{=}$ -SCOCH$_3$	0.7	1.0	0.6	0.6	106	78	6	67	83	[b]
$\overset{S}{=}$ -SCNHCH$_3$	1.5	1.2	1	1.2	69	>200	9	42	42	[a]
$\overset{S}{=}$ -SCN(CH$_2$CH$_3$)$_2$	0.6	0.6	0.2	0.4	100	85	13	130	79	[a]
benzothiazol-2-yl-S–	—	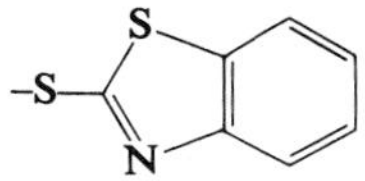 0.2	<0.1	0.2	36	26	3.0	8.2	—	[c]
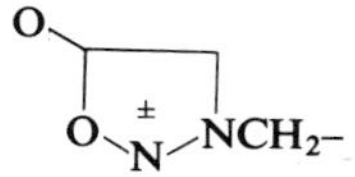 benzothiazol-2-yl-S–	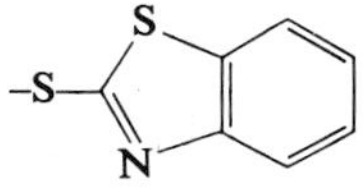 —	9.6	1.0	10.0	30	19	1.0	12	—	[d]

[a] Van Heyningen and Brown (1965).
[b] Van Heyningen (1967).
[c] Can. Patent 818,501.
[d] Lilly Laboratories, unpublished work.

Table XI

3-Heterocyclic Thioether Cephalosporins

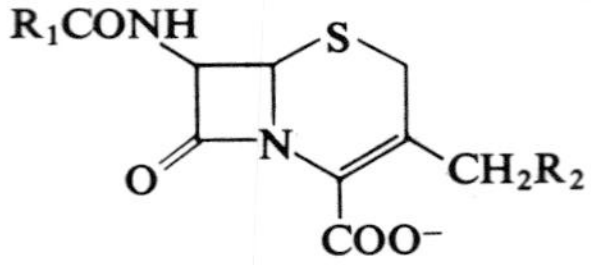

R₁CONH structure with S ring, CH_2R_2, COO^-, N, O

Compound		S. aureus (MIC, μg/ml)			Gram-negative microorganisms (MIC, μg/ml)						Ref.
R_1	R_2	V30	V32	V84	N10	N9	X514	X26	X68	N26	
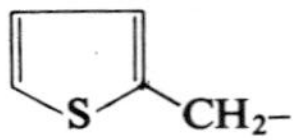 thiophene-CH_2-	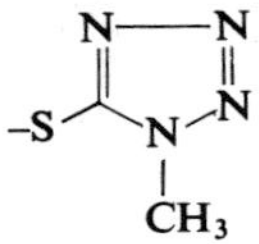 tetrazolyl ($N-CH_3$)	0.4	0.3	0.4	1.0	1.5	0.5	0.2	1.5	1.9	a
	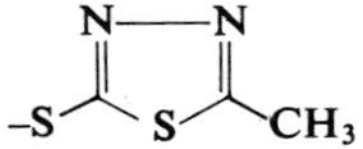 thiadiazolyl (S, CH_3)	0.1	0.3	0.2	5.7	5.1	—	0.7	2.9	6.2	a
	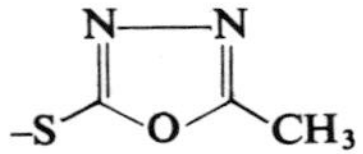 oxadiazolyl (O, CH_3)	0.4	0.3	0.3	20	44	—	5.0	13	10	a

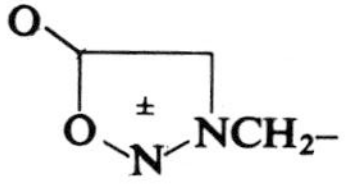	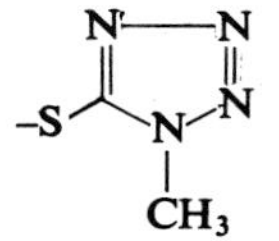	1.1	1.1	0.7	0.6	0.5	—	0.7	0.7	0.6	*b*
	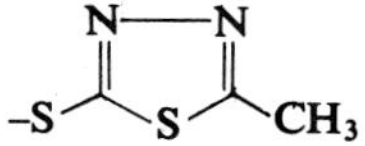	0.6	0.5	1.0	0.6	0.7	0.7	0.7	0.7	0.7	*b*
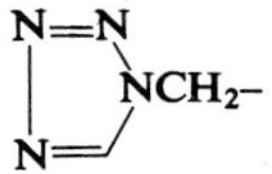	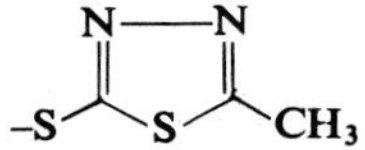	0.6	0.6	0.5	1.0	1.0	0.7	1.0	1.0	1.5	*c*
D-$C_6H_5CH(OH)$–	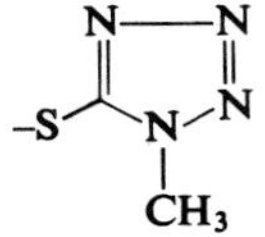	0.9	0.8	0.6	1.3	0.5	0.5	0.6	0.5	—	*d*
	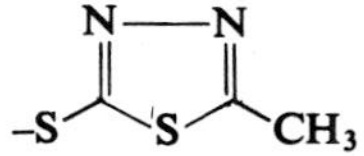	2.5	4.3	4.2	1.2	1.1	1.0	1.7	3.4	1.9	*d*

[a] U.S. Patent 3,516,997.
[b] U.S. Patent 3,530,123.
[c] Nishida *et al.* (1970).
[d] Neth. Patent 7,005,519.

on gram-negative bacteria. Table VIII illustrates the changing patterns of activity with variation in the 3-acylmethyl function.

C. Aminomethyl- and Azidomethylcephalosporins

Modification of the C-3 methyl with nonquaternized or non-acyl nitrogen has been limited by instability of the products (Chapter 4). Aminomethyl derivatives have shown little gram-negative activity but are quite active against gram-positive bacteria. Azidomethyl cephalosporins are quite potent (Neth. Patent 6,606,820), and a number of them have been evaluated. The phenyl-glyoxylyl side-chain derivatives in this series exhibit potent inhibition of gram-positive bacteria (U.S. Patent 3,546,219). Several members of these groups are shown in Table IX.

D. Cephalosporin Derivatives Formed by Reaction with Thiocarbonic Acid Derivatives

Table X lists examples of the types of compounds obtained by nucleophilic displacement of the acetoxyl function in cephalosporanic acids with derivatives of thiocarbonic acid. Such derivatives are the xanthates, thiocarbamates, isothioureas, and many others. The chemistry of these reactions is discussed in Chapter 4 and by Van Heyningen and Brown (1965) as well as in the patent literature (e.g., Belg. Patent 637,547). In general, these antibiotics, compared with the acetoxy compounds, are as active or more active against the *S. aureus* strains used. The nitrogen atom in the dithiocarbamates must be disubstituted to obtain good activity. Quaternized or protonated nitrogen in the derivatives resulted in enhanced activity as compared to basic or neutral substituents. Binding in the presence of human serum often decreased activity by a factor of 10 except where a charged amino function was present. Optimum activity against gram-negative bacteria was found in the piperazine-containing dithiocarbamates.

E. Nucleophilic Displacements with Heteroaromatic Thiols

The 3-acetoxymethyl function can be converted into a thioether substituent by several methods as described in Chapter 4. If a heterocyclic–aromatic thiol is used, the resulting compounds possess enhanced biological activity toward gram-negative bacteria as compared with the acetoxyl analogs, with little loss of gram-positive effectiveness being observed. One member of this series is presented in Table V as cefazolin. The structure and antimicrobial data for other representative cephalosporins of this type are recorded in Table XI. With arylacetamido functions at the C-7 position this series represents compounds which are most potent against gram-negative bacteria. As with other cephalosporins, no inhibition of *Pseudomonas* sp. is seen.

If the side-chain amide is a phenoxymethyl group, gram-negative activity is greatly diminished. Similar findings have been noted with 3-acetoxylmethyl-cephalosporins.

F. Nucleophilic Displacements with Pyridines

Cephalosporin C_A (Hale *et al.*, 1961) was obtained by chance reaction of cephalosporin C with aqueous pyridine. It had enhanced antibacterial activity and subsequently prompted detailed studies of the chemistry at C-3 in the cephem molecule (Chapter 4). This displacement reaction, when applied to cephalothin, yields a product which is called cephaloridine. The biological properties of the two substances are compared in Table V of this chapter as well as in more detail in Chapters 11 and 13. Table XII lists additional pyridinium-containing cephalosporins with their biological activities. The most potent members of the series are the compounds containing the 3-(4-carboxamido-pyridiniummethyl)-3-cephem with the 7-thiopheneacetamido or 7-phenyl-acetamido side chains (Spencer *et al.*, 1967). The 4-carboxamidopyridinium derivative containing a phenylthioacetamido function at C-7 still retains considerable potency against gram-negative bacteria, a rare occurrence with that particular 7-amido function (Chauvette *et al.*, 1963).

G. Ether and Thioether Cephalosporins

Listed in Tables XIII and XIV are a series of ether and thioether derivatives recently reported by several authors (Webber *et al.*, 1971; Murphy *et al.*, 1971). These papers describe the preparation of ethers and thioethers from deacetoxycephalosporins through a complex series of reactions (Chapter 4). The compounds generally were obtained with the 7-phenoxyacetamido group present and thus, from data presented in Table V, would not be expected to show gram-negative bacterial inhibition. All are potent inhibitors of penicillin resistant *S. aureus*. Since no clear superiority was noted with complex ethers or thioethers, additional efforts were concentrated on 3-methylthiomethyl and 3-methoxymethyl compounds with varied amide functions (Belg. Patents 719,710, 734,523) which could be prepared from the 3-acetoxymethyl compounds.

Table XII
Pyridinium Derivatives of Cephalosporins

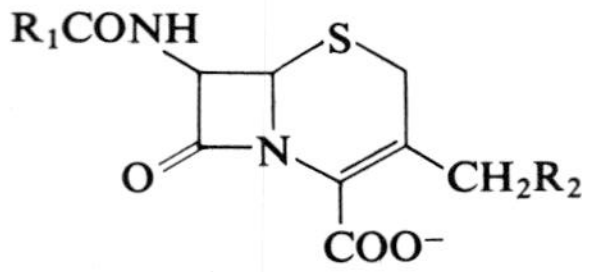

R₁CONH structure with S, N, O ring; substituents CH₂R₂ and COO⁻

Compound		S. aureus (MIC, µg/ml)[a]				Gram-negative microorganisms (MIC, µg/ml)[a]				
R₁	R₂	V30	V32	V41	V84	N10	N9	X26	X68	N26
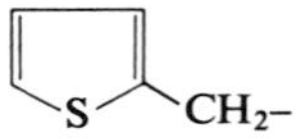 thiophene-CH₂-	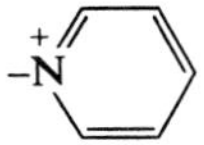 pyridinium	0.7	0.4	0.4	0.4	3.3	3.4	3.3	2.9	
	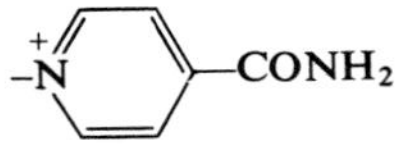 pyridinium-CONH₂	0.3	0.4	0.4	0.4	2.4	6	2.9	2.1	1.5
	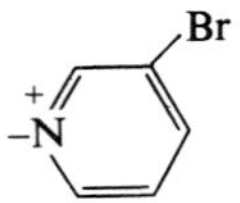 Br-pyridinium	0.1	0.1	<0.1	0.2	4.4	14	5	6	4.6

Substituent									
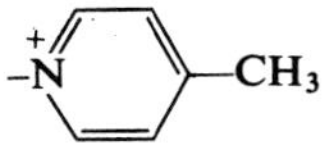 —CH₃ (pyridinium)	1.9	2.1	0.4	4.7	2.8	13	3.3	3.6	3.2
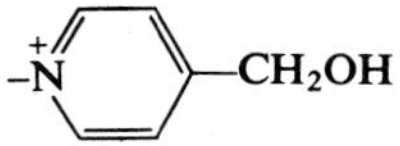 —CH₂OH (pyridinium)	2.9	3.1	1.8	2.5	4.1	17	5.0	5.0	4.4
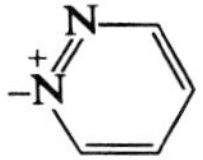 (pyridinium)	0.5	0.4	0.4	0.3	5	8	9	8	6
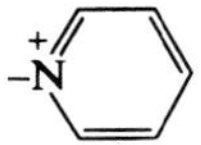 (pyridinium)	1.8	2.8	1.4	1.2	9	32	7	9	9
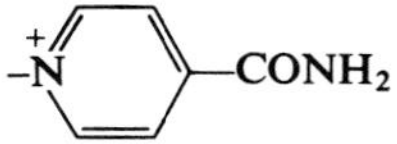 —CONH₂ (pyridinium)	1.6	1.8	1.1	1.5	27	19	8	16	16
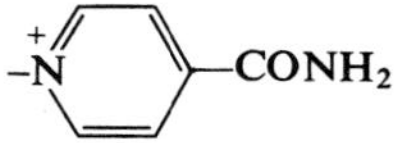 —CONH₂ (pyridinium)	2.9	3.2	0.9	2.9	4	10	7	6	4

$C_6H_5CH_2-$

$C_6H_5SCH_2-$

$D-C_6H_5CH(OH)-$

[a] Spencer et al. (1967).

Table XIII

7-Phenoxyacetamido-3-Alkoxymethyl
Cephalosporins

$C_6H_5OCH_2CONH$ ... CH_2R COO^-

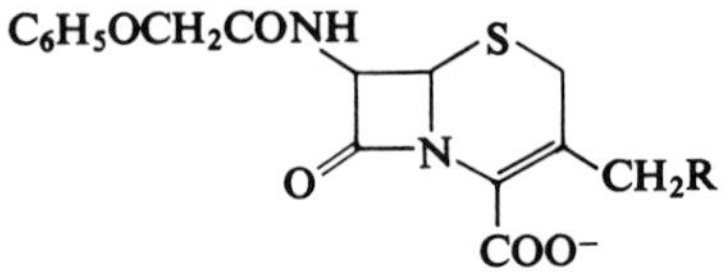

Compound	*S. aureus* (MIC, μg/ml)[a]		
R	V30	V32	V84
$-OCH_3$	<0.1	0.4	0.1
$-OCH_2CH=CH_2$	<0.1	<0.1	<0.1
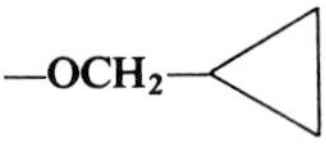 $-OCH_2-\triangleleft$	0.2	0.3	0.2
$-OCH_2C_6H_5$	0.4	0.4	0.4
$-OCH_2CH_2Br$	<0.1	0.1	<0.1
$-OCH_2CH_2CN$	0.1	0.1	0.3

[a] Webber *et al.* (1971).

Table XIV

7-Phenoxyacetamido-3-Alkylthiomethyl Cephalosporins

$C_6H_5OCH_2CONH$ ... CH_2R COO^-

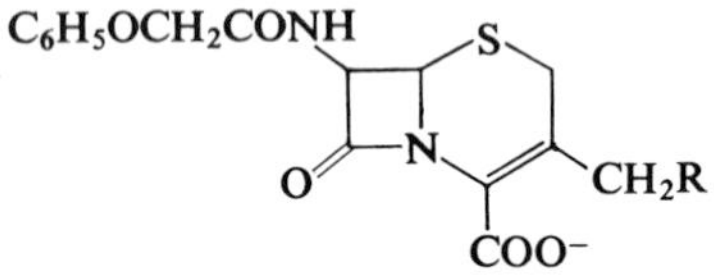

Compound	*S. aureus* (MIC, μg/ml)[a]			
R	V30	V32	V41	V84
$-SCH_3$	0.1	0.2	—	0.2
$-SCH_2CH=CH_2$	0.1	0.4	—	0.05
$-SCH_2CH(OH)CH_2OH$	—	0.6	0.4	0.1
$-SCF_3$	—	0.3	0.1	0.2
$-SC_6H_5$	—	<0.1	<0.1	<0.1
$-SCH_2C_6H_5$	0.9	1.4	—	0.5

[a] Murphy *et al.* (1971).

Table XV

3-Methoxymethyl Cephalosporins

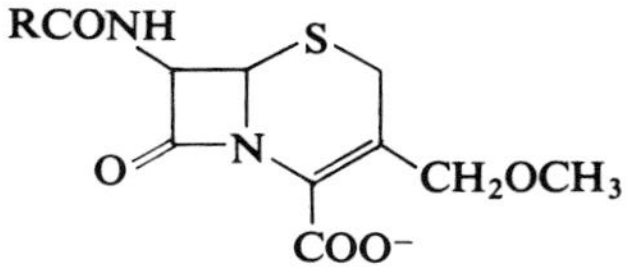

Compound	S. aureus (MIC, μg/ml)				Gram-negative microorganisms (MIC, μg/ml)					Ref.
R	V30	V32	V41	V84	N10	N9	X26	X68	N26	
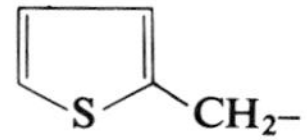 thiophene-CH$_2$–	0.4	0.5	—	0.5	39	>50	43	12	38	a
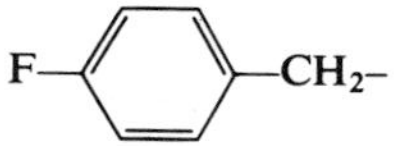 4-F-phenyl-CH$_2$–	0.3[b]	<0.1[c]	4[d]	2.5	16[e]	16[f]	62[g]	250[h]	—	i
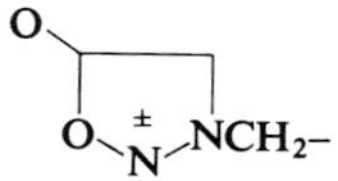 O=...N$^+$–O$^-$ NCH$_2$–	1.0	1.0	—	0.8	32	20	29	32	33	a
D-C$_6$H$_5$CH(NH$_3$)–	0.6	0.6	—	0.5	4.1	3.4	1.9	1.4	4.3	a
D-C$_6$H$_5$CH(OH)–	0.6	0.5	—	0.4	4.4	1.1	5.8	1.0	5.3	a
BrCH$_2$–	0.6[b]	0.3[c]	<0.5[d]	1[j]	120[e]	62[f]	31[g]	>250[h]	—	i
NCCH$_2$–	0.6[b]	0.2[c]	<0.1[d]	<0.5[k]	120[e]	62[f]	31[g]	>250[h]	—	i

[a] Webber et al. (1971).
[b] S. aureus 604.
[c] S. aureus 663.
[d] S. aureus 3452.
[e] E. coli 573.
[f] S. typhimurium.
[g] P. mirabilis.
[h] P. pyocanea.
[i] Belg. Patent 719,710.
[j] S. aureus 11092.
[k] S. aureus 11127.

Table XVI

3-Methylthiomethyl Cephalosporins

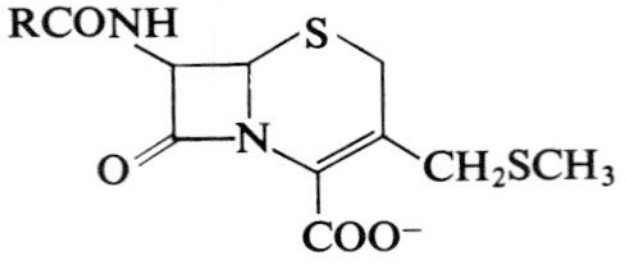

RCONH ... CH_2SCH_3 ... COO^-

Compound R	S. aureus (MIC, μg/ml)				Gram-negative microorganisms (MIC, μg/ml)					Ref.
	V30	V32	V41	V84	N10	N9	X514	X26	X68	
$C_6H_5CH_2-$	—	7.2	2.5	4.3	>50	>50	25	12	25	a
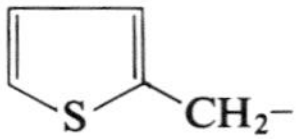 (thiophene)$S-CH_2-$	—	3.1	1.1	1.7	>50	38	16	17	18	a
$D\text{-}C_6H_5CH(NH_3)-$	0.8	1.4	—	1.0	3.6	3.9	—	1.8	1.4	a
$D\text{-}C_6H_5CH(OH)-$	2.7	6.6	—	0.6	7.7	4.9	1.4	9.8	1.4	a
$NCCH_2-$	>2.5[b]	2.5[c]	0.5[d]	4[e]	250[f]	250[g]	125[h]	—	—	i
$BrCH_2-$	>2.5[b]	>2.5[c]	16[d]	8[e]	16[f]	31[g]	31[h]	—	—	i

[a] Murphy et al. (1971).
[b] S. aureus 604.
[c] S. aureus 663.
[d] S. aureus 3452.
[e] S. aureus 11127.
[f] E. coli 573.
[g] S. typhimurium.
[h] P. mirabilis.
[i] Belg. Patent 734,523.

These series are listed and compared in Tables XV and XVI. Substantial activity against both gram-positive and gram-negative bacteria is seen for compounds having a D-phenylglycine or D-mandelic acid function attached to the 7-amino group. These ethers are usually equal or of slightly less activity than the corresponding acetoxyl derivatives, but are uniformly more potent than the 3-methyl-cephem series.

IX. Cephalosporins Substituted at C-2

It has been found possible to substitute C-2 in the cephalosporin sulfoxide esters under Mannich reaction conditions and then convert the resulting sulfoxides to the sulfide acids for evaluation as antibiotics (see Chapter 4). The 2-exomethylene has been prepared and has been reduced to the 2-α- and β-methyl derivatives (Wright et al., 1971). Addition of mercaptans to the exomethylene occurs readily and these products were evaluated (Kaiser et al., 1971). The compounds are reported in Table XVII; most are weaker antibiotics than the parent unsubstituted cephalosporins. The 2-methyl derivatives which are substituted by thioether groups are bound to human serum to the point where they are substantially less available as antibiotics.

Additional derivatives of this type have been reported from variations of the Woodward–Heusler (Woodward et al., 1966) total synthesis of cephalosporins (Chapter 6). The compounds shown below are examples recently reported by Professor Woodward (1970) in a Hanbury Memorial Award address. Compound (10) is inactive, but both compounds (11) and (12) are reported to show antibacterial activity.

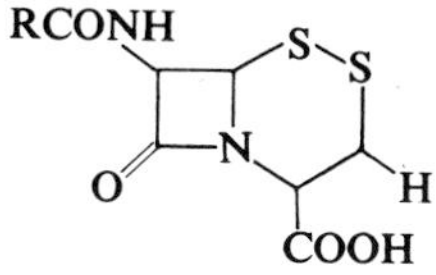

(10) 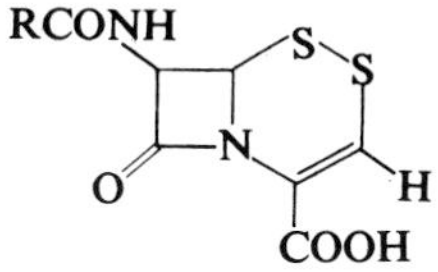   (11) 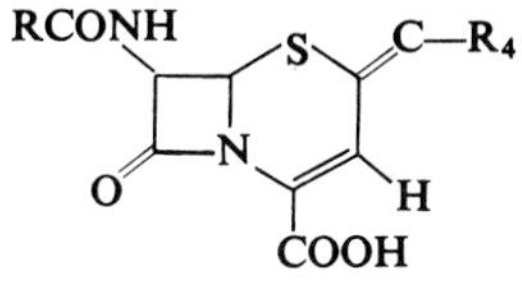   (12)

X. Cephalosporins Substituted at C-7

Table V indicates trends toward change in biological activity with change in acyl function at the amino group of penicillanic and cephalosporanic acids. Recent reviews by Price (1969) and Sassiver and Lewis (1970) discuss these effects for the penicillins and cephalosporins in detail. Tables XVIII–XXI contain examples of representative amide functions on the cephalosporanic acid nucleus with their resulting biological spectrum.

In Table XVIII are listed a series of α-substituted variations of benzyl cephalosporin. When the α function is a methyl, activity is diminished. In the penicillins activity is also lowered with this substitution. The effect of addition

Table XVII
2-SUBSTITUTED CEPHALOSPORINS

Compound			S. aureus (MIC, μg/ml)			
R_1	R_2	R_3	V30	V32	V84	Ref.

		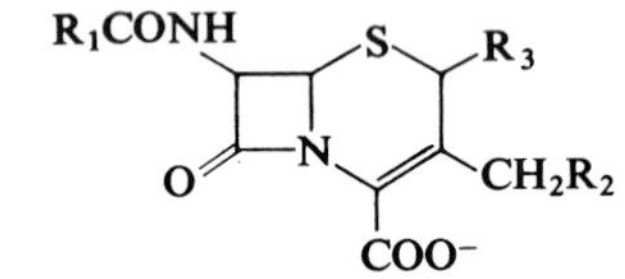				
$C_6H_5OCH_2-$	–H	β-CH$_3$	9.7	13	10	a
		α-CH$_3$	11	15	12	a
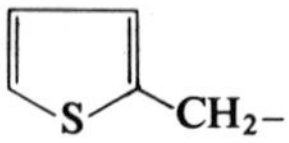 (thiophene)CH$_2-$	–OCOCH$_3$	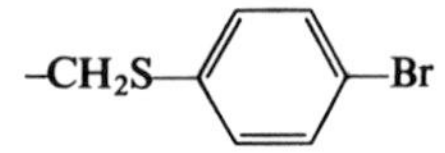 –CH$_2$S–(phenyl)–Br	0.6	0.6	0.6	b

		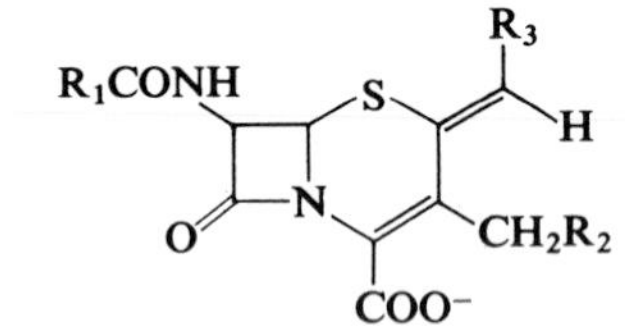				
$C_6H_5OCH_2-$	–H	–H	0.7	0.6	0.5	a
		–SCH$_3$	7.7	9.1	9.2	b
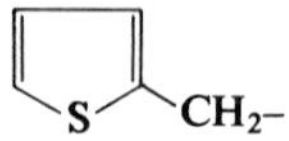 (thiophene)CH$_2-$	–OCOCH$_3$	–H	—	2.1	1.8	a
		–SCH$_2$C$_6$H$_5$	1.0	1.0	1.2	b
		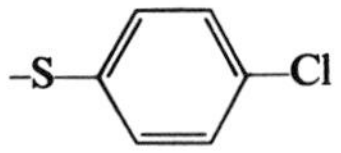 –S–(phenyl)–Cl	0.4	0.5	0.5	b

[a] Wright et al. (1971).
[b] Kaiser et al. (1971).

of an α substituent containing oxygen or nitrogen has been cited earlier. If the hydroxyl group is converted to an ether or ester, antibiotic activity is again diminished. If the α function is halogen, activity is lowered and is similar to that of the methyl substituent. Only the D isomer of these optically active

Table XVIII

α-Substituted Phenylacetamido Cephalosporins

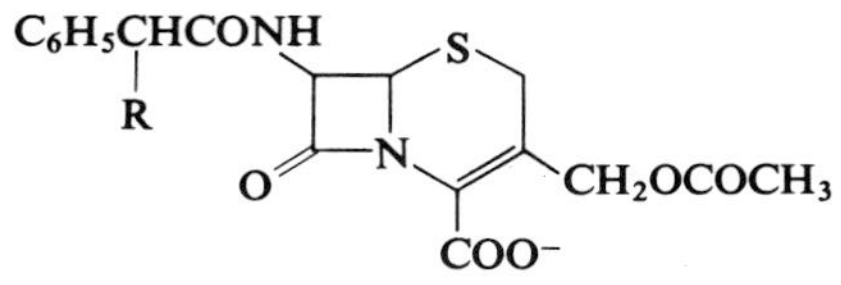

$C_6H_5CHCONH$
R

S
N
O
COO$^-$
CH_2OCOCH_3

Compound		S. aureus (MIC, μg/ml)				Gram-negative microorganisms (MIC, μg/ml)							Ref.
R	Epimer	V30	V32	V41	V84	N10	N9	X514	X26	X68	X99	N26	
-CH$_3$	DL	2.0	3.0	3.0	2.0	100	58	—	9.0	—	—	60	a
-OH	D	—	1.5	0.7	1.0	5.6	3.0	0.7	2.1	1.9	35	—	b
-NH$_3^+$	D	—	3.1	2.2	2.0	3.5	3.3	1.0	1.0	3.5	68	—	c
-NH$_3^+$	L	16	19	16	22	>200	69	—	46	84	—	89	c
-Cl	D	2.9	2.5	0.7	1.4	25	>50	—	26	—	—	26	d
-OCH$_3$	DL	0.1	0.2	0.1	0.1	57	27	—	—	28	—	39	d
-SCH$_3$	D	0.8	1.1	0.8	0.5	26	30	—	28	>50	—	26	d
-OCOCH$_3$	D	3.0	5.0	4.0	5.0	16	4.0	—	7.0	8.0	—	6.0	d

[a] Chauvette et al. (1963).
[b] U.S. Patent 3,167,549.
[c] Spencer et al. (1966).
[d] Takano et al. (1967).

Table XIX

7-HETEROAROMATIC-ACETAMIDO CEPHALOSPORINS

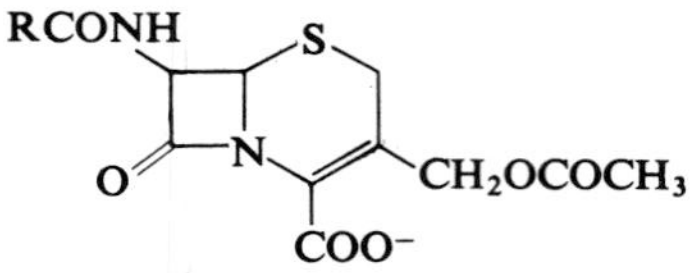

RCONH

CH$_2$OCOCH$_3$

COO$^-$

Compound R	S. aureus (MIC, μg/ml)				Gram-negative microorganisms (MIC, μg/ml)					Ref.
	V30	V32	V41	V84	N10	N9	X26	X68	N26	
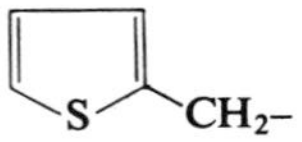 ⟨S⟩-CH$_2$–	—	0.5	0.4	0.4	6.4	8.8	0.8	2.4	—	a
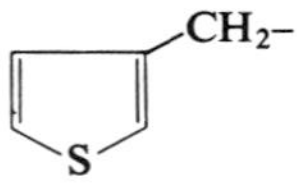 ⟨S⟩-CH$_2$–	0.8	0.8	0.7	0.6	12	5	0.4	3	6	a
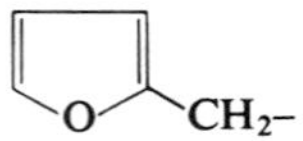 ⟨O⟩-CH$_2$–	1.0	1.0	1.0	1.0	160	76	3.4	3.9	8	a
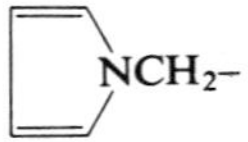 ⟨NCH$_2$–⟩	1.2	1.0	0.9	0.1	21	11	7.0	—	15	b
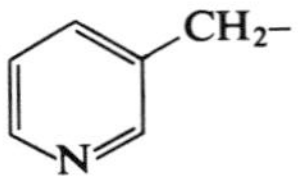 ⟨N⟩-CH$_2$–	2.3	2.8	0.8	0.8	50	86	7.0	6.0	24	c

Structure								Ref.
isothiazolyl–CH$_2$–	0.1^a	—	—	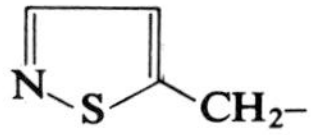 25^f	1.6^g	3.1^h	6.2^i	—	j
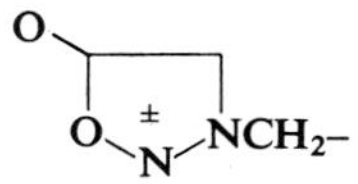 isoxazolone N–CH$_2$–	0.5	—	0.8^e	3.8	1.0	4.1	4.3	3.4	k
triazolyl N–CH$_2$–	—	0.7	—	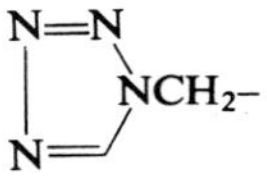 6.9	6.8	7.6	8.1	8.0	l
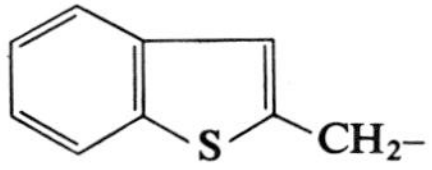 benzothienyl (S)–CH$_2$–	0.1	0.1	<0.1	62	67	3	67	61	a
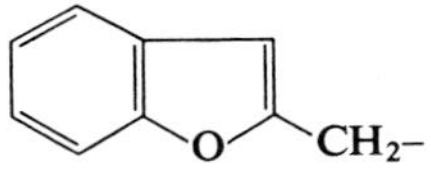 benzofuranyl (O)–CH$_2$–	0.1	0.1	0.1	86	62	6	56	56	a
indolyl (N–H)–CH$_2$–	0.2	0.2	0.1	>200	>200	5.0	—	100	m

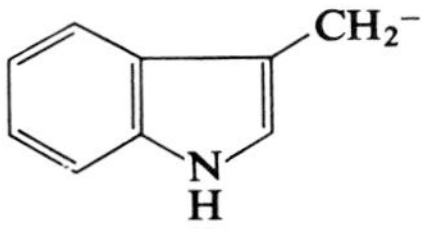

[a] Chauvette et al. (1962).
[b] U.S. Patent 2,218,318.
[c] Stedman et al. (1967).
[d] S. aureus (penicillin sensitive).
[e] S. aureus (penicillin resistant).
[f] E. coli
[g] S. enteritidis.
[h] S. typhosa.
[i] K. pneumoniae.
[j] Raap and Micetich (1968).
[k] Naito et al. (1968).
[l] U.S. Patent 3,468,874.
[m] U.S. Patent 3,360,515.

Table XX

7-Glycyl Cephalosporins

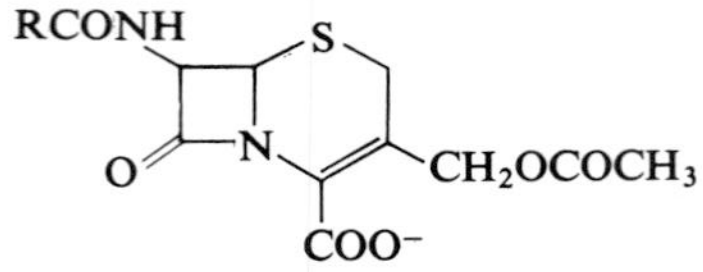

$$RCONH \ \text{—} \ \text{(cephem core)} \ \text{—} \ CH_2OCOCH_3, \ COO^-$$

Compound R	Epimer	S. aureus (MIC, µg/ml)				Gram-negative microorganisms (MIC, µg/ml)					Ref.
		V30	V32	V41	V84	N10	N9	X26	X68	N26	
$C_6H_5CH(NH_3)^+$—	D	—	3.1	2.2	2.0	3.5	3.3	0.8	3.5	—	a
$C_6H_5CH(NH_3)^+$—	L	16	19	16	22	>200	69	46	84	89	a
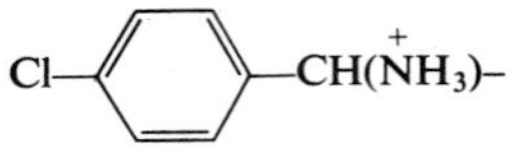 4-Cl-C₆H₄—$CH(NH_3)^+$—	DL	1.9	3.8	2.0	0.8	22	2.6	13	27	22	b
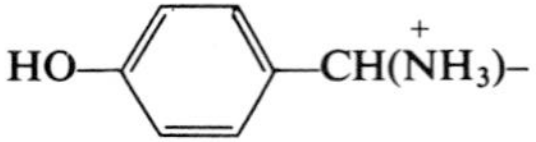 4-HO-C₆H₄—$CH(NH_3)^+$—	D	5.0[c]	0.1[d]	6.2[e]	2.5[f]	6.2[g]	6.2[h]	—	—	—	i
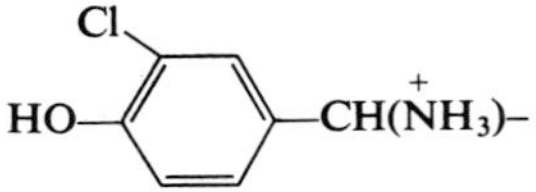 3-Cl-4-HO-C₆H₃—$CH(NH_3)^+$—	D	2.5[c]	0.1[d]	3.1[e]	1.2[f]	6.2[g]	3.1[h]	—	—	—	j

R group	Config.										Ref.
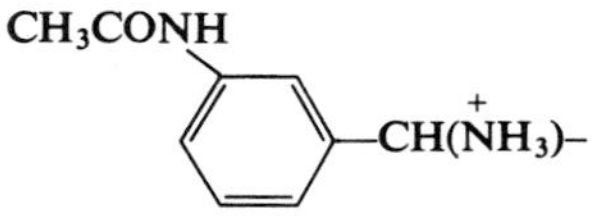 CH_3CONH—[phenyl, meta-$CH(\overset{+}{N}H_3)-$]	D	—	0.2[d]	—	2.5[f]	—	3.1[k]	—	—	—	l
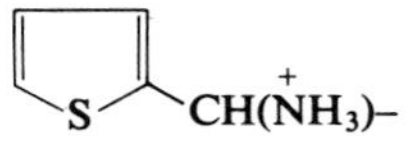 thiophen-2-yl-$CH(\overset{+}{N}H_3)-$	D	3.0	5.0	3.0	2.0	6.0	9.0	8.0	6.0	7.0	m
$C_6H_5CH(\overset{+}{N}H_2CH_3)-$	DL	4.9	6.0	3.2	4.6	32	24	9.0	16	19	b
$C_6H_5CH_2CH(\overset{+}{N}H_3)-$	D	>20	>20	11	10	>50	>50	>50	>50	>50	a
$C_6H_5CH(\overset{+}{N}H_3)CH_2-$	D	1.0	1.0	1.0	1.0	14	16	21	27	18	a
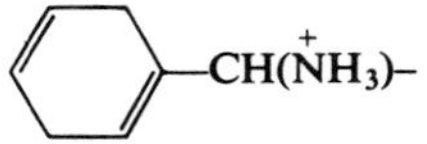 cyclohexadienyl-$CH(\overset{+}{N}H_3)-$	D	0.3[n]	3.1[o]	16[p]	—	9.4[q]	1.6[r]	—	—	—	s

[a] Spencer et al. (1966).
[b] Lilly Laboratories, unpublished work.
[c] S. aureus Smith.
[d] S. pyogenes.
[e] S. aureus BX-1633-2 (penicillin-resistant).
[f] D. pneumoniae.
[g] E. coli Juhl.
[h] S. enteritidis.
[i] U.S. Patent 3,489,752.
[j] U.S. Patent 3,489,751.
[k] S. typhosa.
[l] U.S. Patent 3,464,985.
[m] Kurita et al. (1966).
[n] S. aureus SC 1276.
[o] S. aureus SC 2399.
[p] S. aureus SC 2400 (penicillinase-producing).
[q] E. coli SC 2975.
[r] S. schottmuelleri SC 3850.
[s] Dolfini et al. (1971).

Table XXI

7-Substituted Phenyl, Phenoxy, and Phenylthioacetamido Cephalosporins

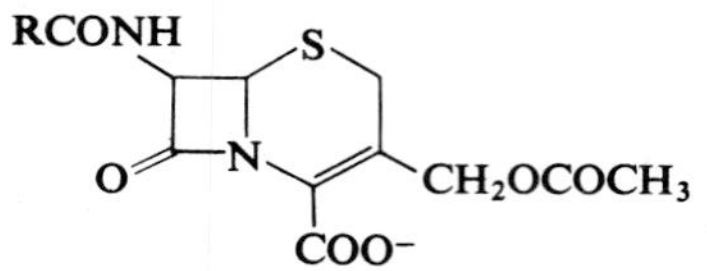

RCONH ... CH_2OCOCH_3, COO^-

Compound R	S. aureus (MIC, $\mu g/ml$)				Gram-negative microorganisms (MIC, $\mu g/ml$)					Ref.
	V30	V32	V41	V84	N10	N9	X514	X26	X68	
$C_6H_5CH_2-$										
H	—	6.0	0.5	0.7	27	43	6.9	1.0	8.1	a
p-Cl	0.5	0.6	0.6	0.5	100	94	44	28	24	a
p-OCH₃	0.3	0.4	0.3	0.2	110	108	28	20	28	a
p-CO₂H	3.8	5.1	—	1.0	30.5	—	—	10	1.0	b
$C_6H_5OCH_2-$										
H	—	—	0.2	0.2	140	>200	110	6.2	110	a
p-Cl	<0.1	<0.1	0.1	<0.1	>200	>200	>200	120	>200	a
p-OCH₃	0.3	0.4	0.3	0.2	160	150	140	150	130	a
p-CO₂H	12[c]	0.8[d]	—	—	3[e]	6[f]	—	—	—	b
$C_6H_5SCH_2-$										
H	—	—	0.1	0.2	63	68	23	0.7	27	a
p-Cl	0.2	0.3	—	0.2	>100	50	80	73	75	a
p-OCH₃	0.4	0.5	—	0.4	>100	>100	>100	>100	>100	a
p-CO₂H	6[c]	0.8[d]	—	—	1.6[e]	3[f]	—	—	—	b

[a] Chauvette et al. (1963).
[b] Lewis et al. (1969).
[c] S. aureus 11 (penicillinase-producing).
[d] S. pyogenes.
[e] S. typhosa.
[f] K. pneumoniae.

acids produces potent antibiotics. The L isomers are not only very weak antibiotics but are, with the phenylglycyl derivatives, also subject to ready cleavage by amidases (Sullivan *et al.*, 1969).

In Table XIX a series of heteroaromatic acetamido derivatives are shown. All members of this group are active against both the gram-positive and the gram-negative bacteria. The benz-analogs (benzthiophene versus thiophene, for example) generally have somewhat better gram-positive and less gram-negative activity as compared with the simple monocyclic heteroaromatic derivative.

Table XX lists some substituted variants of the phenylglycyl side chain, which are usually somewhat less active than the unsubstituted compound.

Table XXI shows the change in activity seen with substituted benzyl versus substituted phenoxymethyl and phenylthiomethyl derivatives. The latter group contains the most active gram-positive compounds while the first group contains compounds with somewhat less activity against staphylococcus.

XI. Miscellaneous Compounds with Diminished Activity

As long as the β-lactam ring is intact, the potential for an active antibiotic exists. However, most alterations other than the change of amide group or alterations of the dihydrothiazine ring in cephalosporins, as noted above, eliminate or greatly diminish activity. Because of the difficulties in rigorously excluding active starting compounds from evaluation of these substances, it is often difficult to define compounds as completely inactive. An additional complication in attempting to measure activity in compounds which retain traces of antibacterial effects is that in certain instances the active substances may no longer contain a β-lactam ring. In Chapter 5 are reported the results of experiments with anhydropenicillin which, on treatment with mercuric acetate, is converted to a product with some antibacterial activity. This substance (Wolfe *et al.*, 1969) is not a β-lactam compound but is an oxazolone related to penicillenic acid. Anhydropenicillin is not biologically active. All penicillins and cephalosporins in which the carboxyl function at C-4 is not intact are inactive; however, several esters and amides retain some antibiotic activity because they are capable of being cleaved *in vivo* (Daehne *et al.*, 1970). Change in the sulfur, either complete removal or oxidation to sulfone or sulfoxide, completely inactivates or greatly reduces activity. There is less activity in β-sulfoxides than in the α compounds. Change in the *gem*-dimethyl group of a penicillin does not destroy activity. Several modifications at this position were thought to be obtained by synthesis in very early work (Carpenter *et al.*, 1948). A penicillin with an ethyl group and hydrogen in place of the *gem*-dimethyl function is one example and is reported to be active. The acetoxy-substituted methyl derivatives (both α and β—Chapter 5) have recently been prepared by way of the sulfoxide ring expansion reaction reported in detail in Chapter 5. These products have some antimicrobial activity (Table I).

Several β-lactam compounds have been reported, such as compound (13) (Chapter 3), in which the stereochemistry has been maintained as it is in peni-

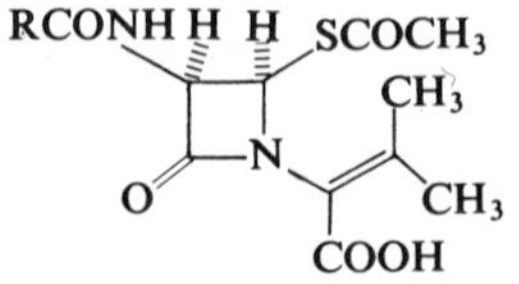

RCONH H H SCOCH₃

(structure of compound (13))

(13)

cillin. These substances still appear to retain a small portion of the antibiotic activity of penicillin and may find use when studying the reaction at the transpeptidase enzyme surface.

Additional compounds prepared from cephalosporins include the dihydro compound (Van Heyningen, 1967), which is inactive, and the Δ^2 double-bond isomers. The Δ^2 compounds retain some activity although it is much diminished, Of interest is the observation, in Table I, that a Δ^3-deacetoxycephalosporin with the phenoxymethyl side chain has only 25 Oxford units/mg of activity while the Δ^2 compound has 15 (penicillin V = 1400). Equilibration of the Δ^2 isomer to Δ^3 isomer under biological conditions cannot be excluded in this situation. It would appear that, to maintain useful levels of activity, few alterations from the structure of the natural penam or cephem nucleus are possible even though many changes of peripheral groups retain or enhance antimicrobial action.

XII. Conclusions

Modifications of the naturally occurring penicillins and cephalosporins have been studied in many laboratories and several thousand substances have been prepared and studied. The clinically useful antibiotics in these series, with the exception of benzyl- and phenoxymethylpenicillin, are partially synthetic materials and even the latter resulted from manipulation of the fermentation to produce a new compound. Recent papers (for example, the many papers on new penicillins and cephalosporins presented at the 1971 meeting of the Inter-science Conference on Antimicrobial Agents and Chemotherapy) indicate that these research efforts are not only continuing in the laboratory but show signs of producing new clinically successful antibiotics.

To date, certain penicillins, such as carbenicillin, are capable of inhibiting indole-positive *Proteus* and *Pseudomonas* species while no such cephalosporins have been reported. With these exceptions, inhibition at different concentrations occurs for the same organisms in both series of antibiotics as long as the β-lactam compounds are not destroyed by bacterial β-lactamases, thus supporting a common mechanism of action.

Final choice for clinical utility rests on optimizing many pharmacodynamic factors other than only the *in vitro* inhibition of bacteria.

The eventual importance of the new series of 7-methoxylcephalosporins which have inhibitory properties mainly toward gram-negative bacteria remains to be determined.

Acknowledgments

We wish to express our appreciation to Miss Barbara A. Kratochwill for her valuable aid in the preparation of this manuscript and to Miss Penny A. Guffin for her secretarial assistance.

CHART 1. Key to code letters of microorganisms

Gram-positive bacteria		Gram-negative bacteria	
V30	Penicillin-resistant *Staphylococcus aureus*	N9	*Shigella sonnei*
V32	Penicillin-resistant *S. aureus*	N10	*Escherichia coli*
V41	Penicillin-resistant *S. aureus*	N26	*E. coli*
V84	Penicillin-resistant *S. aureus*	X26	*Klebsiella pneumoniae*
X400	Methicillin-resistant *S. aureus*	X45	*Proteus vulgaris*
SA3055	Penicillin-sensitive *S. aureus*	X68	*Aerobacter aerogenes*
X12	*Bacillus subtilis*	X99	*Serratia marcescens*
X186	*Sarcina lutea*	X142	*Salmonella gallinarum*
		X161	*E. coli*
		X514	*Salmonella heidelberg*
		X528	*Pseudomonas aeruginosa*

References

Abraham, E. P., and Newton, G. G. F. (1956). *Biochem. J.* **62**, 658.

Abraham, E. P., Newton, G. G. F., and Hale, C. W. (1954). *Biochem. J.* **58**, 94.

Abraham, E. P., Newton, G. G. F., Olson, B. H., Schuurmans, D. M., Schenck, J. R., Hargie, M. P., Fisher, M. W., and Fusari, S. A. (1955). *Nature* **176**, 551.

Acred, P., Brown, D. M., Knudsen, E. T., Rolinson, G. N., and Sutherland, R. (1967). *Nature* **215**, 25.

Barber, M. (1947). *J. Pathol. Bacteriol.* **59**, 373.

Barza, M., Berman, H., Michaeli, D., Molavi, A., and Weinstein, L. (1971). *Antimicrob. Ag. Chemother.* **1970**, 341.

Batchelor, F. R., Doyle, F. P., Nayler, J. H. C., and Rolinson, G. N. (1959). *Nature* **183**, 257.

Behrens, O. K., Corse, J., Edwards, J. P., Garrison, L., Jones, R. G., Soper, Q. F., Van Abeele, F. R., and Whitehead, C. W. (1948). *J. Biol. Chem.* **175**, 793.

MARVIN GORMAN AND CHARLES W. RYAN

Belgium Patent 634,644.
Belgium Patent 637,547.
Belgium Patent 719,710.
Belgium Patent 734,523.
Belgium Patent 741,381.
Benner, E. J., and Kayser, F. H. (1968). *Lancet* **2**, 741.
Biagi, G. L., Guerra, M. C., Barbaro, A. M., and Gamba, M. F. (1970). *J. Med. Chem.* **13**, 511.
Boniece, W. S., Wick, W. E., Holmes, D. H., and Redman, C. E. (1962). *J. Bacteriol.* **84**, 1292.
Brandl, E., and Margreiter, H. (1954). *Osterr. Chem.-Ztg.* **55**, 11.
Butler, K. (1967). *In* "Kirk-Othmer Encyclopedia of Chemical Technology" (H. F. Mark, J. J. McKetta, and D. F. Othmer, eds.), 2nd ed., Vol. 14, pp. 652–707. Wiley (Interscience), New York.
Canada Patent 818,501.
Carpenter, F. H., Stacy, G. W., Genghof, D. S., Livermore, A. H., and duVigneaud, V. (1948). *J. Biol. Chem.* **176**, 915.
Chauvette, R. R., Flynn, E. H., Jackson, B. G., Lavagnino, E. R., Morin, R. B., Mueller, R. A., Pioch, R. P., Roeske, R. W., Ryan, C. W., Spencer, J. L., and Van Heyningen, E. M. (1962). *J. Amer. Chem. Soc.* **84**, 3401.
Chauvette, R. R., Flynn, E. H., Jackson, B. G., Lavagnino, E. R., Morin, R. B., Mueller, R. A., Pioch, R. P., Roeske, R. W., Ryan, C. W., Spencer, J. L., and Van Heyningen, E. M. (1963). *Antimicrob. Ag. Chemother.* **1962**, 687.
Chisholm, D. R., Leitner, F., Misiek, M., Wright, G. E., and Price, K. E. (1970). *Antimicrob. Ag. Chemother.* **1969**, 244.
Cocker, J. D., Cowley, B. R., Cox, J. S. G., Eardley, S., Gregory, G. I., Lazenby, J. K., Long, A. G., Sly, J. C. P., and Somerfield, G. A. (1965). *J. Chem. Soc.* 5015.
Daehne, W. v., Frederiksen, E., Gundersen, E., Lund, F., Morch, P., Petersen, H. J., Roholt, K., Tybring, L., and Godtfredsen, W. O. (1970). *J. Med. Chem.* **13**, 607.
Dolfini, J. E., Applegate, H. E., Bach, G., Basch, H., Bernstein, J., Schwartz, J., and Weisenborn, F. L. (1971). *J. Med. Chem.* **14**, 117.
Doyle, F. P., Fosker, G. R., Nayler, J. H. C., and Smith, H. (1962). *J. Chem. Soc.* 1440.
Earle, R. H., Hurst, D. T., and Viney, M. (1969). *J. Chem. Soc. C.* 2093.
Florey, M. E., and Florey, H. W. (1943). *Lancet* **1**, 387.
Flynn, E. H. (1967). *Antimicrob. Ag. Chemother.* **1966**, 715.
Godzeski, C. W., Brier, G., and Pavey, D. E. (1963). *Appl. Microbiol.* **11**, 122.
Gourevitch, A., Hunt, G. A., Pursiano, T. A., Carmack, C. C., Moses, A. J., and Lein, J. (1961). *Antibiot. Chemother.* **11**, 780.
Grove, D. C., and Randall, W. A. (1955). *In* "Assay Methods of Antibiotics, A Laboratory Manual." Medical Encyclopedia, New York.
Hale, C. W., Newton, G. G. F., and Abraham, E. P. (1961). *Biochem. J.* **79**, 403.
Hermann, R. B. (1971). Unpublished results.
Hugo, W. B., and Stretton, R. J. (1966). *J. Gen. Microbiol.* **42**, 133.
Ishiyama, S., Nakayama, I., Iwamoto, H., Iwai, S., Okui, M., and Matsubara, T. (1971). *Antimicrob. Ag. Chemother.* **1970**, 476.
Izaki, K., Matsuhashi, M., and Strominger, J. L. (1968). *J. Biol. Chem.* **243**, 3180.
Jack, G. W., and Richmond, M. H. (1970). *J. Gen. Microbiol.* **61**, 43.
Jeffery, J. D'A., Abraham, E. P., and Newton, G. G. F. (1961). *Biochem. J.* **81**, 591.
Johnson, J. R., Woodward, R. B., and Robinson, R. (1949). *In* "The Chemistry of Penicillin" (H. T. Clarke, J. R. Johnson, and R. Robinson, eds.), p. 440. Princeton Univ. Press, Princeton, New Jersey.

Kaiser, G. V., Ashbrook, C. W., Goodson, T., Wright, I. G., and Van Heyningen, E. M. (1971). *J. Med. Chem.* **14**, 426.

Knusel, F., Konopka, E. A., Gelzer, J., and Rosselet, A. (1971). *Antimicrob. Ag. Chemother.* **1970**, 140.

Kradolfer, F., Sackmann, W., Zak, O., Brunner, H., Hess, R., Konopka, E. A., and Gelzer, J. (1971). *Antimicrob. Ag. Chemother.* **1970**, 150.

Kukolja, S. (1968). *J. Med. Chem.* **11**, 1067.

Kukolja, S. (1970). *J. Med. Chem.* **13**, 1114.

Kurita, M., Atarashi, S., Hattori, K., and Takano, T. (1966). *J. Antibiot., Ser. A.* **19**, 243.

Lawrence, P. J., and Strominger, J. L. (1969). *Fed. Proc., Fed. Amer. Soc. Exp. Biol.* **28**, 473, Abstract 1207.

Lewis, A., Sassiver, M. L., and Shepherd, R. G. (1969). *Antimicrob. Ag. Chemother.* **1968**, 109

Libby, R. L., and Holmberg, N. L. (1945). *Science* **102**, 303.

Manhas, M. S., and Bose, A. K. (1969). *In* "Synthesis of Penicillin, Cephalosporin C and Analogs." Marcel Dekker, New York.

Miller, I. M., Stapley, E. O., and Chaiet, L. (1962). *Bacteriol. Proc.* **32**, Abstract A49.

Morin, R. B., Jackson, B. G., Flynn, E. H., and Roeske, R. W. (1962). *J. Amer. Chem. Soc.* **84**, 3400.

Morin, R. B., Jackson, B. G., Mueller, R. A., Lavagnino, E. R., Scanlon, W. B., and Andrews, S. L. (1963). *J. Amer. Chem. Soc.* **85**, 1896.

Morin, R. B., Jackson, B. G., Mueller, R. A., Lavagnino, E. R., Scanlon, W. B., and Andrews, S. L. (1969). *J. Amer. Chem. Soc.* **91**, 1401.

Moyer, A. J., and Coghill, R. D. (1946). *J. Bacteriol.* **51**, 57.

Murphy, C. F., Koehler, R. E., and Ryan, C. W. (1971). Unpublished results.

Nagarajan, R., Boeck, L. D., Gorman, M., Hamill, R. L., Higgens, C. E., Hoehn, M. M., Stark, W. M., and Whitney, J. G. (1971). *J. Amer. Chem. Soc.* **93**, 2308.

Naito, T., Nakagawa, S., Takahashi, K., Fujisawa, K., and Kawaguchi, H. (1968). *J. Antibiot.* **21**, 300.

Netherlands Patent 6,606,820.

Netherlands Patent 7,005,519.

Newton, G. G. F., and Abraham, E. P. (1954). *Biochem. J.* **58**, 103.

Newton, G. G. F., and Abraham, E. P. (1956). *Biochem. J.* **62**, 651.

Nishida, M., Matsubara, T., Murakawa, T., Mine, Y., Yokota, Y., Kuwahara, S., and Goto, S. (1970). *Antimicrob. Ag. Chemother.* **1969**, 236.

O'Callaghan, C. H., Muggleton, P. W., and Ross, G. W. (1969). *Antimicrob. Ag. Chemother.* **1968**, 57.

Price, K. E. (1969). *Advan. Appl. Microbiol.* **11**, 17.

Raap, R., and Micetich, R. G. (1968). *J. Med. Chem.* **11**, 70.

Rolinson, G. N., and Stevens, S. (1961). *Proc. Roy. Soc., Ser. B.* **154**, 509.

Rolinson, G. N., Stevens, S., Batchelor, F. R., Wood, J. C., and Chain, E. B. (1960). *Lancet* **2**, 564.

Ryan, C. W., Simon, R. L., and Van Heyningen, E. M. (1969). *J. Med. Chem.* **12**, 310.

Sassiver, M. L., and Lewis, A. (1970). *Advan. Appl. Microbiol.* **13**, 163.

Sawai, T., Saito, T., and Mitsuhashi, S. (1970). *J. Antibiot.* **23**, 488.

Sheehan, J. C., and Henery-Logan, K. R. (1959). *J. Amer. Chem. Soc.* **81**, 3089; United States Patent 3,157,617.

Spencer, J. L., Flynn, E. H., Roeske, R. W., Siu, F. Y., and Chauvette, R. R. (1966). *J. Med. Chem.* **9**, 746.

Spencer, J. L., Siu, F. Y., Flynn, E. H., Jackson, B. G., Sigal, M. V., Higgins, H. M., Chauvette, R. R., Andrews, S. L., and Bloch, D. E. (1967). *Antimicrob. Ag. Chemother.* **1966**, 573.

Spry, D. O. (1970). Unpublished results.

Stedman, R. J., Swered, K., and Hoover, J. R. E. (1964). *J. Med. Chem.* **7**, 117.

Stedman, R. J., Swift, A. C., Miller, L. S., Dolan, M. M., and Hoover, J. R. E. (1967). *J. Med. Chem.* **10**, 363.

Stewart, G. T. (1965). *In* "The Penicillin Group of Drugs." Elsevier, Amsterdam.

Strominger, J. L. (1969). *In* "Inhibitors: Tools in Cell Research" (Th. Bucher and H. Sies, eds.), pp. 187–207. Springer-Verlag, New York.

Strominger, J. L., and Tipper, D. J. (1965). *Amer. J. Med.* **39**, 708.

Sullivan, H. R., Billings, R. E., and McMahon, R. E. (1969). *J. Antibiot.* **22**, 27.

Sutherland, R., and Rolinson, G. N. (1971). *Antimicrob. Ag. Chemother.* **1970**, 411.

Takano, T., Hattori, K., Kurita, M., Atarashi, S., and Horibe, S. (1967). *J. Pharm. Soc. Japan* **87**, 1141.

Thayer, J. D., Field, F. W., Perry, M. I., Martin, J. E., Garson, W. (1961). *Antimicrob. Ag. Annu.* **1960**, 352.

Tompsett, R., Shultz, S., and McDermott, W. (1947). *Proc. Soc. Exp. Biol. Med.* **65**, 163.

Tosoni, A. L., Glass, D. G., and Goldsmith, L. (1958). *Biochem. J.* **69**, 476.

United States Patent 3,167,549.

United States Patent 3,196,151.

United States Patent 3,218,318.

United States Patent 3,261,832.

United States Patent 3,355,452.

United States Patent 3,360,515.

United States Patent 3,464,985.

United States Patent 3,468,874.

United States Patent 3,489,751.

United States Patent 3,489,752.

United States Patent 3,516,997.

United States Patent 3,530,123.

United States Patent 3,546,219.

Van Heyningen, E. M. (1965). *J. Med. Chem.* **8**, 22.

Van Heyningen, E. M. (1967). *In* "Advances in Drug Research" (N. J. Harper and A. B. Simmonds, eds.), Vol. 4, pp. 1–70. Academic Press, London.

Van Heyningen, E. M., and Brown, C. N. (1965). *J. Med. Chem.* **8**, 174.

Wagner, E. S., Davis, W. W., and Gorman, M. (1969) *J. Med. Chem.* **12**, 483.

Webber, J. A., Huffman, G. W., Koehler, R. E., Murphy, C. F., Ryan, C. W., Van Heyningen, E. M., and Vasileff, R. T. (1971). *J. Med. Chem.* **14**, 113.

Wolfe, S., Ferrari, C., and Lee, W. S. (1969). *Tetrahedron Lett.* 3385.

Woodward, R. B. (1970). *Pharm. J.* **205**, 562.

Woodward, R. B., Heusler, K., Gosteli, J., Naegeli, P., Oppolzer, W., Ramage, R., Ranganathan, S., and Vorbruggen, H. (1966). *J. Amer. Chem. Soc.* **88**, 852.

Wright, I. G., Ashbrook, C. W., Goodson, T., Kaiser, G. V., and Van Heyningen, E. M. (1971). *J. Med. Chem.* **14**, 420.

Chapter 13

PHARMACOLOGY AND TOXICOLOGY OF CEPHALOSPORINS

JOHN S. WELLES

I. Introduction

A. Selection of an Antibiotic

The selection of an antibiotic substance for use as a therapeutic agent in man is predicated not only on its antibacterial spectrum but also upon its characteristics of absorption, distribution, excretion, and metabolism, and its lack of toxicologic manifestations. Only a few of the multitude of antibacterial substances available as prospective antibacterial agents can be extensively studied in man. This emphasizes the importance of the pharmacologic and toxicologic studies in animals upon which the preclinical choices are made.

The story of the selection of cephalosporins as clinical therapeutic agents has been no exception. Four cephalosporin derivatives are now available for use in man in many parts of the world; they are cephalothin,* cephaloridine, cephaloglycin, and cephalexin. A review of the pharmacology and toxicology of these cephalosporins in animals and man may enable researchers to design animal studies that will reliably predict the clinical acceptance of derivatives for which no human data is yet available.

B. Toxicologic and Pharmacologic Properties of Cephalosporin C

This cephalosporin story had its beginning in the laboratory of E. P. Abraham at Oxford University. Abraham and his associates diligently pursued the isolation of cephalosporin C in order to obtain sufficient quantities, not only for a microbiologic evaluation but also for toxicologic and pharmacologic experiments in a few mice. Florey (1955) of this laboratory reported that mice tolerated a 5-gm/kg intravenous dose without apparent adverse effect. Approximately one-third of an intravenous dose was recovered in the urine, whereas only 1% of an oral dose was detectable. In a later report, Jago and Heatley (1961) stated that the cephalosporin C used in these initial studies was subsequently found to be only 75% pure. Nonetheless, the low order of acute toxicity and substantial urinary recovery of the parenterally administered antibiotic encouraged Abraham and his associates. Despite the weak antibacterial activity of cephalosporin C, they reasoned that it might be possible to modify the structure to achieve greater antibacterial activity and still retain the apparent safety.

O'Callaghan and Muggleton (1963) further investigated the fate of cephalosporin C in mice in conjunction with a study of various cephalosporin derivatives. Approximately 20% of the subcutaneously administered activity was

* Throughout this discussion the sodium salt of cephalothin is referred to as cephalothin.

recovered in the urine. Bioautographs of chromatograms of the urine revealed two microbiologically active spots, one of which was identified as the parent drug and the other as deacetylcephalosporin C (Table I). The same metabolite

Table I

THE CEPHALOSPORIN COMPOUNDS

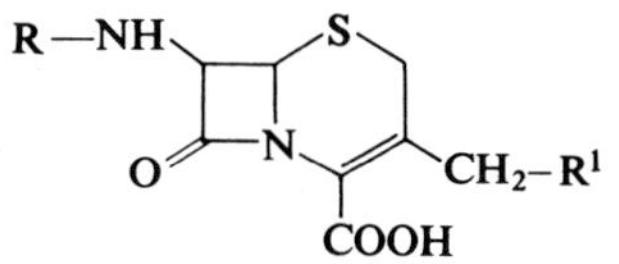

R	Compound	R^1
H_2N, $HOOC$ >CH(CH$_2$)$_3$—CO—	Cephalosporin C	—OCOCH$_3$
H_2N, $HOOC$ >CH(CH$_2$)$_3$—CO— H—	Deacetylcephalosporin C 7-Aminocephalosporanic acid	—OH —OCOCH$_3$
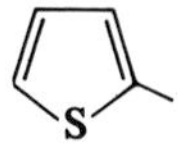 (thienyl)CH$_2$CO—	Cephalothin	—OCOCH$_3$
(thienyl)CH$_2$CO—	Deacetylcephalothin	—OH
(thienyl)CH$_2$CO—	Cephaloridine	$-\overset{+}{N}$(pyridinium)
$C_6H_5CH(NH_2)CO$ $C_6H_5CH(NH_2)CO$ $C_6H_5CH(NH_2)CO$	Cephaloglycin Deacetylcephaloglycin Cephalexin	—OCOCH$_3$ —OH —H
(tetrazolyl)NCH$_2$CO	Cefazolin	$-S$(thiadiazolyl)CH$_3$

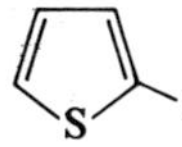

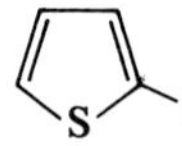

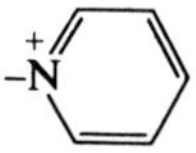

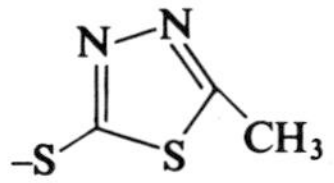

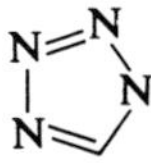

was detectable after the incubation of cephalosporin C with liver and kidney tissue of mice, rats, guinea pigs, and rabbits, but it was not detectable with tissue from monkey or man. None of the metabolite was detected in 24-hour urine collections from human volunteers that received a 1-gm intramuscular dose.

C. Preparation of Analogs of Cephalosporin C

The discovery of a practical method of cleavage of the aminoadipyl side chain of cephalosporin C by Morin *et al.* (1962) made large amounts of 7-aminocephalosporanic acid (Table I) available for the preparation of analogs of the naturally occurring antibiotic. Subsequently, many 7-acyl derivatives of 7-aminocephalosporanic acid were made and tested for *in vitro* antibacterial activity. Cephalothin (Table I), a compound prepared by Chauvette *et al.* (1962), was the first of the cephalosporin analogs to be intensively studied in animals and man. The cephalosporins (Section I, A) that have been approved for clinical use are introduced in this review in the order in which they became available to the clinician.

II. Toxicology of Cephalosporins in Therapeutic Use

A. Cephalothin

1. ANIMALS

Lee *et al.* (1963) administered cephalothin to mice, rats, guinea pigs, cats, and dogs. A summary of the toxicity of single doses is shown in Table II. A 5-gm/kg intravenous dose (LD_{50}) in mice caused clonic convulsions; all deaths occurred within 24 hours of drug administration. Convulsions were not observed when cephalothin was given by other routes. Oral administration of 10 gm/kg had no effect. Cephalothin had a similarly low order of acute toxicity in the other species, with the exception of the guinea pig, a species in which penicillin is also peculiarly toxic (Spector, 1957).

Rats, cats, and dogs were given daily subcutaneous or intramuscular doses of cephalothin. The daily administration of 500 mg/kg in growing rats, 400 mg/kg in dogs, and 200 mg/kg in cats caused no adverse reactions other than local effects of the repeated intramuscular injections in the dogs, i.e., evidence of pain and hardening of the muscle. Hematologic and blood chemistry data were normal. Renal function of the dogs, as determined by *p*-aminohippuric acid and creatinine clearance, was unaffected. Other than muscular fibrosis at the injection sites of the dogs, there was no histologic evidence of a drug effect in the tissues of any of the three species.

Pregnant rabbits were unaffected by 28 daily intramuscular doses of 200 mg/kg, and the progeny were normal (Lee and Anderson, 1963). More interest developed in the effect of cephalothin in the rabbit when it was discovered that cephaloridine caused renal injury in this species. Welles *et al.* (1966) gave equivalent doses to five rabbits for 30 days and examined the kidneys. Of the four surviving animals, two had normal renal tissue and two had slight nephrocalcinosis, which is a common finding in control rabbits. The animal that died (day 14) had evidence of moderate renal tubular necrosis.

Table II

ACUTE TOXICITY OF CEPHALOSPORIN DERIVATIVES—LD_{50}

Species	Route of administration	Antibiotic (gm/kg)			
		Cephalothin	Cephaloridine	Cephaloglycin	Cephalexin
Mouse	i.v.	≈5[a]	2.3[c,d]	>0.5[e]	
	i.p.	≈7[a]	9.6–12.5[c]	1.0–2.0[e,f]	0.4–1.6[g]
	s.c.	>7.5[a]	>7[d]	0.6[e]	
	p.o.	>10 LD_0[a]	>15[c]	>10 LD_0[f]	1.6–6.2[g]
Rat	i.v.	>4 LD_0[a]	1.3[c,d]		
	i.p.	≈6.3[a]	2.5–4.3[c]	1.6[e]	>3.7[g]
	s.c.	≈7.5[a]	3.2[d]	0.7[e]	
	p.o.	>10 LD_0[a]	>5 LD_0[d] 1.0–1.4[c]	>10 LD_0[f]	>5[g]
Guinea pig	s.c.	0.11–0.20[a]	0.55[c]	0.33[e]	
Cat	i.v.	>1.0[b]	>0.25 LD_0[d]		
	i.p.				>1.0[g]
	p.o.			>0.75 LD_0[e]	>1.0 LD_0[g]
Dog	i.v.	>1.0[b]	>1.0 LD_0[d]		
	i.p.				>1.0[g]
	p.o.			>0.75 LD_0[e]	>2.0 LD_0[g]

[a] Lee et al. (1963).
[b] Welles (unpublished).
[c] Atkinson et al. (1966a).
[d] Welles et al. (1966).
[e] Welles et al. (1971).
[f] Mineshita et al. (1970).
[g] Welles et al. (1970).

Perkins et al. (1968a) performed further subacute experiments in rabbits (3 weeks) and in monkeys (2 weeks). Daily intramuscular doses of 100, 200, or 500 mg/kg were given to both species with no changes in appearance or behavior. There were no significant changes in glomerular filtration rate nor were proteinuria or glycosuria observed. The renal tissue of the monkeys was normal. Slight histologic changes were found in the renal tissue of the rabbits, which consisted of minimal swelling or hydropic changes of the tubular epithelium in all of the 500-mg/kg group. A lesser effect was seen in the renal tissue of the rabbits on the 200-mg/kg dosage and no effect in those that received 100 mg/kg/day.

Cephalothin was administered intracerebrally to mice and intracisternally to rats (Welles *et al.*, 1966). In these intradural toxicity experiments, cephalothin was one-fifteenth as toxic as sodium benzylpenicillin in the mouse and one-eighth as toxic in the rat.

Perrelli and Tempesta (1968) investigated the cardiovascular effects of cephalothin in four species of animals. The minimum intravenous dose required to evoke a change in the cardiovascular parameters was 25–100 mg/kg in rats, 80–150 mg/kg in rabbits, and 100–125 mg/kg in cats and dogs. They observed a transient decrease in diastolic pressure in association with a lesser decrease in systolic pressure which was usually accompanied by a compensatory tachycardia. Cephalothin did not significantly alter the vascular effects of acetylcholine, histamine, or serotonin in cats and dogs. The response of the nictitating membrane to preganglionic stimulation was also unaffected in cats.

2. Man

Cephalothin has been the subject of many clinical investigations (e.g., Riley *et al.*, 1963; Griffith and Black, 1964; Heitler *et al.*, 1964; Weinstein *et al.*, 1964; Steinbrunn and Haemmerli, 1966), and it has been administered to thousands of patients. Pain and induration after multiple intramuscular injections have been frequently encountered as well as the occurrence of phlebitis during intravenous infusions. Most clinical investigators have concluded that cephalothin does not produce renal injury. Recently, Maynard (1969) and Benner (1970a) have both commented on the lack of nephrotoxicity of this antibiotic but have noted the accumulating evidence, in certain patients with impaired renal function, of serum concentrations that may cause further deleterious effects in the kidney. Maynard (1969) commented on the non-specificity of findings of tubular necrosis in these patients with renal insufficiency and observed that congestive heart failure, low cardiac output, or unrecognized hypertension may be contributory or totally responsible for the condition.

Most of the remaining adverse effects observed in patients were those associated with allergy; eosinophilia, drug fever, serum sickness, skin rashes, and in rare instances, anaphylaxis (Kabins *et al.*, 1965). Hemolytic anemia has also occurred during cephalothin therapy (Molthan *et al.*, 1967).

B. *Cephaloridine*

1. ANIMALS

The toxicity of cephaloridine in laboratory animals was extensively studied by Atkinson *et al.* (1966a, b) and Welles *et al.* (1966). A summary of the acute toxicity is given in Table II. The data of the two laboratories were in good agreement with the exception of the oral toxicity in rats. All Harlan rats survived a 5-gm/kg oral dose (Welles *et al.*, 1966), whereas the oral LD_{50} in rats of the PVG strain was 1.0–1.4 gm/kg (Atkinson *et al.*, 1966a). This discrepancy remains unexplained since the parenteral toxicity data were in close agreement. By the intravenous route, cephaloridine was two times as toxic as cephalothin in the mouse and three times as toxic in the rat. Deaths after intravenous administration occurred within a few minutes (Welles *et al.*, 1966) and were apparently the result of central nervous system toxicity. This correlates with the finding that intradurally, cephaloridine was 8–10 times as toxic as cephalothin in the mouse and rat. Deaths after subcutaneous or intraperitoneal administration of cephaloridine occurred 24–96 hours later. Renal tubular necrosis was the only significant histopathologic finding in the animals that succumbed as well as in some survivors.

Special studies were conducted by Atkinson *et al.* (1966a) to determine the acute parenteral dose which would produce renal lesions (nephrotoxicity) in 50% of the animals (ND_{50}). No renal changes were detected in dogs (1.5 gm/kg) or cats (1.0 gm/kg). The other species in the order of increasing susceptibility to nephrotoxic effects of cephaloridine were mice, rats, guinea pigs, monkeys, and rabbits. The ND_{50} in the rabbit was 90 mg/kg for the females and 140 mg/kg for the males.

Rats tolerated daily subcutaneous doses of 500 mg/kg for 5 months (Welles *et al.*, 1966). Effects were severe ulceration and necrosis at the injection site, slight depression of hemoglobin and hematocrit, and increased renal weight. There were no histologic changes in any of the tissues, including the kidney. A renal weight increase was also observed by Atkinson *et al.* (1966b) in a chronic rat study. Since a renal weight increase did not occur in rats that received an identical daily dose of cephalothin, this finding with cephaloridine may have been predictive of the renal injury observed on a higher dosage schedule. Kidneys of some rats after five daily doses of 1100 mg/kg contained a few regenerating tubules which represented evidence of renal injury and repair.

Muscular fibrosis at the injection sites was the only adverse effect of a 250 mg/kg/day regimen in dogs (Welles *et al.*, 1966). There were no alterations in hematology or blood chemistry, and there was no evidence of drug accumulation. Daily intravenous doses of 500 or 1000 mg/kg caused salivation, emesis, and anorexia in some dogs. Relaxation of the nictitating membrane and pupillary dilation were observed immediately after dosage. Renal function was unaffected and histopathologic findings were negative.

Cats that received repeated doses of cephaloridine did not fare as well as dogs. A daily 250-mg/kg intramuscular dose caused anorexia and death within 2 months. There were no adverse effects on auditory or vestibular function. Slight fatty metamorphosis of the liver was detected in cats on a 100-mg/kg/day regimen and a more severe fatty infiltration in those on the 250-mg/kg dose. Histologic findings in the other viscera were incidental to the treatment.

A daily intramuscular dose of 100 mg/kg in a monkey for 14 days did not impair renal function or produce histologic change in the renal tissue. A 200-mg/kg/day schedule caused a marked reduction in renal function and 500 mg/kg/day proved to be fatal within 4 days (Perkins et al., 1968a). Renal tissue changes were focal tubular necrosis and tubular regeneration.

With the knowledge of the susceptibility of rabbits to single doses of as little as 90 mg/kg of cephaloridine, Atkinson et al. (1966b) gave intramuscular doses of 15, 30, or 45 mg/kg for 2 months. The animals all survived. A dose-responsive renal weight increase was detected similar to that observed in rats on much higher doses. There were no drug-related histologic changes in the kidney tissue. Perkins et al. (1968a) gave rabbits daily intramuscular injections of 50, 100, 200, or 500 mg/kg for 3 weeks, during which time creatinine clearances were performed at various intervals. The 50- and 100-mg/kg regimens did not significantly alter the glomerular filtration rate, and there was no proteinuria or glycosuria. The 200-mg/kg/day dosage markedly reduced the glomerular filtration rate; all animals had proteinuria and one-half had glycosuria. A 500-mg/kg/day dose was lethal to all animals within 4 days. Histologic changes observed in renal tissue consisted of widespread areas of necrosis and hydropic degeneration in all animals of the 500-mg/kg group and some of the 200-mg/kg group. Focal cellular vacuolization and fragmentation of the proximal tubules were found in the renal tissue of the others.

Child and Dodds (1967) discovered that the severe nephrotoxic effect of a 12-gm/kg subcutaneous dose in mice could be completely prevented by the administration of a 100-mg/kg oral dose of probenecid. Probenecid offered a similar protection to the hen (Child and Dodds, 1967) and the rabbit (Fleming and Jaffe, 1967). Other compounds were also tested for the protective effect in mice. A number of compounds that were protective against the necrotizing effect of cephaloridine are actively secreted by the tubule, whereas others are not. Surprisingly, p-aminohippuric acid and p-aminosalicylic acid did not afford protection.

Comprehensive studies of the effect of cephaloridine on the renal function of anesthetized dogs and cats were performed by Child and Dodds (1966) before it was known that these two species were very resistant to renal injury by this antibiotic. Slight changes in glomerular filtration rate and effective renal plasma flow in dogs and cats receiving a cephaloridine infusion of 0.5 mg/kg/ minute were statistically significant but of no toxicological importance. Glucose reabsorption, urea clearance, and the maximum tubular capacity for p-aminohippuric acid excretion were also unaffected by cephaloridine administration.

Silverblatt et al. (1970) extended the knowledge of the nephrotoxic action of cephaloridine in the rabbit by in vivo fixation of renal tissues for light and electron microscopy. Changes in the uniformity and height of the brush border of the outermost proximal tubules were detected within 1 hour of a 200-mg/kg dose of cephaloridine. The mitochondria of these cells were less elongated and appeared more randomly aligned than normal. At 5–10 hours after the dose, the above changes were more widespread, many of the proximal tubular lumina were dilated, and epithelial changes were evident. Cells of the more distal elements of the proximal tubule had not undergone degeneration but contained large PAS-positive and PAS-negative droplets. In no instance, at this time interval or at more prolonged intervals when proximal tubular necrosis was widespread, was there evidence of injury to any other portion of of the nephron. The in vivo consequence of the renal changes observed histologically at 1 hour was demonstrated by the infusion of horse-radish peroxidase in normal rabbits and in rabbits that had been given a nephrotoxic dose of cephaloridine. At 1 hour, the peroxidase, a low molecular weight protein capable of being reabsorbed by the normal kidney, was present in all proximal tubules of the normal kidney but was absent in many proximal tubules of the cephaloridine treated animals. These investigators hypothesize that, as a consequence of the failure of injured cells of the proximal tubule to reabsorb filterable protein, the more distal uninjured elements are presented with an increased load. The presence of the PAS-positive droplets in the uninjured cells of the more distal elements of the proximal tubule were believed to be the result of a compensatory increase in protein absorption.

A 25-mg/kg intravenous dose of cephaloridine in anesthetized cats had no observed pharmacodynamic effect (Atkinson et al., 1966a). The superior cervical ganglionic blockade produced by a 100-mg/kg dose caused a fall in blood pressure that persisted for several minutes. Doses of 750 mg/kg had no effect on the electrocardiogram or on neuromuscular transmission.

2. MAN

The significance of the observed nephrotoxicity of cephaloridine in some animal species was not readily apparent in the early clinical investigations (Murdoch et al., 1964; Stewart and Holt, 1964; Benner et al., 1966; Cohen *et al.*, 1966; Holloway and Scott, 1966; Kislak *et al.*, 1966). Most patients had no adverse effects. The observed side effects were usually minor and of little clinical significance. They included phlebitis at the injection site, eosinophilia, rashes of various types, fever, nausea, vomiting, and mild transient leukopenia. Anaphylactic shock has occurred (Kaplan and Weinstein, 1967). Murdoch *et al.* (1964) observed central nervous system toxicity, nystagmus, and hallucinations after a 100-mg intrathecal dose.

Seriously-ill patients with reduced renal function have been treated without incident, but in a few, further deterioration of the renal function occurred (Cohen *et al.*, 1966; Holloway and Scott, 1966; Kislak *et al.*, 1966). In these instances, it was not possible to unequivocally state whether the observed deterioration represented the progression of the disease or an action of the antibiotic.

As an attempt to determine the effect of cephaloridine on normal kidneys, Linsell *et al.* (1967) collected urine from bronchitis patients that were receiving 6 gm/day of cephaloridine and examined it for hyaline casts. Cast production was increased during the treatment and returned to normal after the drug was withdrawn.

Foord (1970) and Benner (1970b) have recently reviewed the literature with regard to the clinical use of cephaloridine and commented specifically on the nephrotoxic potential in man. Both authors agree that a prolonged high serum concentration of cephaloridine can be deleterious to the kidney.

C. Cephaloglycin

1. ANIMALS

The effect of the administration of large doses of cephaloglycin to laboratory animals has been the subject of reports by Mineshita *et al.* (1970) and Welles *et al.* (1971). Parenterally administered cephaloglycin was markedly more toxic in mice and rats than either cephalothin or cephaloridine (Welles *et al.*, 1971) (Table II). Deaths occurred 2–4 days after drug administration. Mild to severe renal injury was detected in animals that succumbed. A 100-mg/kg intraperitoneal dose in rabbits caused slight renal tubular necrosis and 400 mg/kg produced severe necrosis.

Oral doses of 10 gm/kg had no observable effect on mice or rats (Mineshita *et al.*, 1970). Histologic examination of the tissues revealed minor focal necrosis of the liver in the mice and slight renal tubular necrosis in the rats. The oral LD_{50} of cephaloglycin in guinea pigs was 0.33 gm/kg, and in rabbits it was 0.2 gm/kg. Deaths in these two species occurred 2–6 days after the oral dose and were preceded by anorexia and diarrhea. Histologic findings in the renal tissue were negative. The effects were similar in nature to those observed by Somer (1955) in guinea pigs and by Gray and Lewis (1966) in rabbits after the oral administration of gram-positive antibiotics. They theorized that the toxic effects were the result of a profound alteration of the intestinal flora upon which these herbivores are vitally dependent.

Rats were given dietary concentrations of 0.5% for 1 year or 2% for 1 month, and dogs received daily oral doses of 250 mg/kg for 1 year or 750 mg/kg for 1 month. A daily dose of 2 gm/kg of cephaloglycin (2% diet) depressed rat weight gains about 10%. Some dogs on either of the above daily dosage regimens had transient anorexia. Hematology, blood chemistry, and histologic examination of the tissues revealed no drug effect. Administration of 1.0-gm/kg oral doses to pregnant rats during the period of organogenesis produced no adverse effects on dams or fetuses.

The intravenous administration of 20 mg/kg of cephaloglycin in anesthetized cats had no effect on blood pressure, electrocardiogram, or on normal responses of nictitating membrane, ileum, or uterus.

2. MAN

Clinical trials with cephaloglycin have been conducted by Boyer and Andriole (1968), Braun et al. (1968), Hogan et al. (1968), Landes et al. (1969), and Trafton and Lind (1969). Gastrointestinal intolerance manifested as diarrhea, nausea, or vomiting was the most frequent side effect. Allergic reactions were observed in low incidence.

D. Cephalexin

1. ANIMALS

A pattern of animal susceptibility different from that observed with the previously investigated cephalosporins emerged during the toxicity studies with cephalexin. Parenterally administered cephalexin was more toxic to the mouse than to the rat, dog, cat, or rabbit (Table II) (Welles et al., 1969, 1970). Although renal injury was detected in mice and rats that received lethal or sublethal doses, only slight changes were observed in the renal tissue of rabbits that were given 4 gm/kg intraperitoneally. This was surprising when one considers the relative susceptibility of the mouse and rabbit to the nephrotoxic effects of parenterally administered cephaloridine (Section II, B) and cephaloglycin (Section II, C). It is also noteworthy that toxic doses of cephalexin produced a diuresis, whereas toxic doses of cephaloridine resulted in oliguria.

Lethal or sublethal parenteral and oral doses in mice caused CNS depression, diuresis, anorexia, and weight loss. Animals died from 24 to 72 hours afterward. The lethality was peculiarly variable in this species; as much as a fourfold difference existed between LD_{50} values in different experiments. The viscera of animals that died were normal except for the kidney in which vacuolar degeneration and slight necrosis of the renal tubular epithelium were noted. These lesions were considered insufficient to have been the sole cause of death.

Rats were more resistant to the effects of the drug but large doses (2–5 gm/kg) produced signs of toxicity similar to those in mice; there was no evidence of renal injury in rats that received a 5-gm/kg oral dose.

An intraperitoneal dose of 1 gm/kg was lethal to 3 of 11 dogs. Adverse effects included, emesis, anorexia, and a water diuresis. Deaths occurred from 3 to 4 days after dosage, following prostration, partial paralysis, and apparent disorientation. Nausea was so severe in some instances that the animals were unable to retain food or water. All dogs survived if the water intake was maintained. Salivation and emesis were the only effects observed after a 2-gm/kg oral dose.

Diuresis and diarrhea were the only effects observed after a 4-gm/kg intraperitoneal dose in rabbits; one of six animals died 7 days later. Histologic examination of renal tissue revealed a slight vacuolar nephrosis.

Rats were given a diet containing 1 % cephalexin for 1 year, which resulted in daily doses as great as 1 gm/kg. The only drug-related effects were colonic and cecal enlargement and a leukocyte count 20 % less than control; both are common findings in rats receiving large daily doses of antibiotics. A 500-mg/kg/day oral dosage regimen in pregnant rats produced no teratogenic effects.

Dogs were given oral doses of 400 mg/kg for 1 year and monkeys were given the same regimen for 1 month. Conditioned salivation was observed in both species. Other observed effects were mild to moderate diarrhea in the monkeys and occasional emesis in the dogs. The hematology and blood chemistry as well as the histologic findings in these animals were normal.

A 500-mg/kg intraperitoneal dose of cephalexin in the anesthetized cat produced only a fleeting effect on blood pressure and heart rate. It was concluded that this antibiotic had no significant pharmacodynamic effect.

2. MAN

Cephalexin clinical trials have been conducted by various investigators (Griffith and Black, 1968; Braun et al., 1968; Kind et al., 1969; Levison et al., 1969, and Page et al., 1970). Griffith (1970) has summarized the data of various investigators who administered cephalexin to 1671 patients. In most instances the antibiotic was given as a daily oral dose of 4-gm/day or less. Side effects which occurred in 2 % of the patients were usually of a gastrointestinal nature, i.e., diarrhea, nausea, vomiting, and abdominal cramps. There were no apparent drug-related effects on hematology or blood chemistry.

III. Absorption, Distribution, and Excretion of Cephalosporins in Therapeutic Use

A. Cephalothin

1. ANIMALS

The absorption, distribution, and excretion of cephalothin was investigated in laboratory animals by Lee and Anderson (1963) and Lee et al. (1963). A 10-mg/kg intramuscular dose in dogs produced a mean peak blood serum concentration of 13 μg/ml. Cephalothin was poorly absorbed from the gastrointestinal tract. Disappearance from the blood was rapid. Based on serum concentrations of antibiotic activity from 20 minutes to 2 hours after a 10-mg/kg intravenous dose in dogs, the serum half-life of cephalothin was 22 minutes (Table III). A total of 78 % of the administered antibiotic was recovered in the urine within 5 hours. Renal excretion studies showed that cephalothin was secreted by the tubules. A cephalothin/creatinine clearance ratio of 1.8 was reduced to 1.0 by the administration of probenecid.

Only 0.04 % of a 10-mg/kg intramuscular dose of cephalothin was recovered in the bile of dogs during the first 6 hours after administration. The bile also represented a minor excretory pathway in the rat.

Cephalothin did not readily penetrate the meninges; 0.18–0.30 μg/ml was found in the cerebrospinal fluid of dogs that had received an intravenous dose of 25 mg/kg (Lee and Anderson, 1963). Perkins et al. (1968a) found similarly low concentrations of antibacterial activity in the brain of rabbits that received 250 mg/kg/day of cephalothin. The finding of a brain concentration of antibacterial activity equivalent to 2.5 μg/gm of tissue was in sharp contrast to concentrations of 869 μg/gm in the renal cortex and 215 μg/gm in the liver. Low levels were also detected in the aqueous humor (Lee and Anderson, 1963; Uwaydah and Faris, 1970).

Cephalothin readily passed the placenta (Lee and Anderson, 1963). Concentrations in the amniotic fluid and fetal serum of cephalothin-treated rabbits were 23.5 and 16 % of the blood serum concentration, respectively.

Kanyuck et al. (1971) investigated the penetration of radiocarbon-labeled cephalothin in the bone of rats. Within 15 minutes of a subcutaneous dose, the whole bone contained a concentration of radioactivity equivalent to 30 % of that in the circulating blood. The half-life of cephalothin in the bone was similar to that in the serum.

2. MAN

A 500-mg intramuscular dose of cephalothin in man resulted in a peak blood serum concentration of 10 μg/ml (Griffith and Black, 1964), which was similar

to that produced by a 10-mg/kg dose in the dog (Table III). Oral absorption
was poor. The serum half-life in man has been calculated as 30–50 minutes
(Kabins and Cohen, 1965; Kunin and Atuk, 1966; Naumann, 1966; and

Table III

PHARMACOLOGIC DATA OF CEPHALOSPORIN ANTIBIOTICS IN DOG (10 mg/kg)
AND MAN (500 mg)

Drug, species, and route of administration	Peak serum concentration (μg/ml)	Recovery of activity in urine (% dose)	Serum half-life (i.v.) (minutes)
Cephalothin			
Dog i.m.	13[a]	78[a]	22[a]
Man i.m.	10[b]	60–90[b]	30–50[c]
Cephaloridine			
Dog i.m.	21[d]	87[d]	32[d]
Man i.m.	15[e]	60–80[f]	90[f, g]
Cephaloglycin			
Dog p.o.	3[h]	12[h]	28[h]
Man p.o.	1–2[c]	25[c]	
Cephalexin			
Dog p.o.	17[i]	70[i]	86[i]
Man p.o.	15[c]	80–100[c]	36[j]
Cefazolin			
Dog i.m.	23[k]	80[k]	
Man i.m.	45[k]	82[k]	132[k]

[a] Lee *et al.* (1963).
[b] Griffith and Black (1964).
[c] Various investigators.
[d] Welles *et al.* (1966).
[e] Kislak *et al.* (1966).
[f] Kunin and Atuk (1966).
[g] Pryor *et al.* (1967).
[h] Welles *et al.* (1971).
[i] Welles *et al.* (1969).
[j] Kirby *et al.* (1971).
[k] Mineshita *et al.* (1970).

Tuano *et al.*, 1967). The latter investigators determined the required rate of an
intravenous infusion of cephalothin to attain a constant blood concentration.
They found that at a rate of 0.5 gm/hour a steady state was attained during the
third hour. The renal clearance of the antibiotic was nearly twice that of

creatinine: the clearance was markedly reduced by probenecid. A total of 60–90% of the administered antibacterial activity was recovered in the urine after a 500-mg intramuscular dose (Griffith and Black, 1964).

Significant concentrations of antibacterial activity were found in cord serum and amniotic fluid within 15 minutes after dosage (MacAulay and Charles, 1968). The antibiotic did not readily penetrate the normal meninges. Vianna and Kaye (1967) could not detect antibacterial activity in the cerebrospinal fluid of normal patients despite blood serum concentrations of 80–100 μg/ml. However, in patients with inflamed meninges, antibacterial concentrations were 0.16–0.31 μg/ml. Gump and Lipson (1968) detected activity in synovial fluid within 17 minutes of an intravenous dose of cephalothin.

B. Cephaloridine

1. ANIMALS

The absorption and excretion of cephaloridine in animals has been investigated by Child and Dodds (1966, 1967) and Welles *et al.* (1966). A 10-mg/kg intramuscular dose in dogs produced a peak serum concentration of 20 μg/ml (Welles *et al.*, 1966). Antibacterial activity was detectable in the serum for 6 hours. The half-life of cephaloridine in the blood serum after a 10 mg/kg dose was calculated to be 32 minutes, approximately 50% longer than cephalothin (Table III). The cephaloridine/creatinine renal clearance ratios varied from 0.9 to 1.0. A lack of an effect of probenecid on the renal clearance of cephaloridine was further proof that renal excretion of this antibiotic was solely the result of glomerular filtration in the dog. Child and Dodds (1966) came to the same conclusion in clearance experiments in cats, rabbits, and monkeys, but they were able to detect a small, but significant, tubular secretion of cephaloridine in the hen. A further investigation of the renal excretion of cephaloridine in dogs and rabbits by the stop-flow method was performed to determine if bidirectional tubular transport was occurring. There was no evidence of tubular reabsorption or secretion in either species.

Cephaloridine was widely distributed in various tissues, including the brain, of rats and rabbits after a 200-mg/kg subcutaneous dose (Welles *et al.*, 1966). Kidney tissue had the greatest concentration. It was observed in the rabbit, the species in which cephaloridine is more nephrotoxic, that the kidney/blood serum ratio of activity was 5 at 30 minutes and 30 at 4 hours, whereas in the rat, the ratios at the same times were 3 and 8, respectively. Cephaloridine was found in the aqueous humor and spinal fluid and it was readily transferred to the fetus.

Currie *et al.* (1966) determined the distribution of cephaloridine within the dog kidney. Isolated kidneys were perfused with nonrecirculating blood containing cephaloridine prepared with tritium-labeled pyridine. Radioautography of the tissue showed that the cephaloridine was well distributed in the medullary interstitial spaces, an important property for the treatment of renal disease, and was localized at the periphery of the proximal tubular cells.

2. MAN

Cephaloridine, like cephalothin, was readily absorbed from the intramuscular site and poorly absorbed from the gastrointestinal tract (Kislak *et al.*, 1966). A 500-mg intramuscular dose gave a peak blood serum concentration of 15 μg/ml. After equivalent doses, the plasma levels of cephaloridine measured at various times were usually twice those of cephalothin (Benner *et al.*, 1966). A serum half-life of approximately 90 minutes (Kunin and Atuk, 1966; Pryor *et al.*, 1967) was markedly longer than the 30- to 50-minute half-life of cephalothin (Table III). Renal excretion was considered to be largely the result of glomerular filtration but a 1.2-fold increase in cephaloridine serum concentration was found after probenecid administration (Tauno *et al.*, 1967). This appeared to indicate some tubular secretion. The constant infusion of 0.5 gm/hour resulted in a blood concentration which continued to rise through the third hour. In contrast, a similar infusion of cephalothin resulted in a constant serum concentration after 3 hours (Section III, A).

The urinary recovery of an intramuscular dose was 60–80% of that administered (Benner *et al.*, 1966; Kislak *et al.*, 1966). The role of the kidney in the overall elimination of this antibiotic was exemplified by a half-life of 23 hours in patients with little or no renal function (Kabins and Cohen, 1966). In one patient, assayable serum levels were present for 10 days after cephaloridine administration.

Biliary excretion was found to be a minor pathway of elimination. Acocella *et al.* (1968) found a biliary concentration of 10 μg/ml at a time when the serum concentration was 24 μg/ml.

Records (1969) was unable to detect antibacterial activity in the aqueous humor after a 1-gm dose of cephaloridine. However, levels of 7–28 μg/ml were found in the secondary aqueous humor that refills the eye following aspiration of the primary fluid. Cephaloridine concentrations in the spinal fluid of patients with uninfected meninges were 6–12% of those in the blood serum (Kabins and Cohen, 1966; Gonnella *et al.*, 1967).

The serum concentrations found in newborn infants were as great as 54% of the concentrations in the maternal serum (Barr and Graham, 1967; Arthur and Burland, 1969), indicating that cephaloridine readily passed the placenta.

C. Cephaloglycin

1. ANIMALS

The oral administration of 10 mg/kg of cephaloglycin to dogs gave a peak serum concentration of 3 μg/ml of antibacterial activity from 2 to 3 hours later. The level declined to 1 μg/ml by the sixth hour (Welles et al., 1971). All assay values were based on activity against Sarcina lutea, an organism which is equally sensitive to cephaloglycin and its microbiologically active metabolite (Section IV C). Thus, the activity represented the sum of the two substances. An intravenous dose of 10 mg/kg rapidly disappeared from the blood; the calculated half-life was 28 minutes, midway between that of cephalothin and cephaloridine (Table III). Following an intravenous dose, 65% of the activity was found in the urine, but after an oral dose, only 11% was recovered. Again, it should be reiterated that these recoveries represent cephaloglycin and its active metabolite. The renal clearance of cephaloglycin was determined in unanesthetized dogs that received a constant intravenous infusion of cephaloglycin and creatinine. Antibacterial activity was maintained at concentrations of 3–9 μg/ml. A cephaloglycin/creatinine clearance ratio of 1.38 was reduced to 1.15 by probenecid.

Antibacterial activity in the bile of rats and mice exceeded that in the circulating blood, but only 0.04–0.23% of a 200-mg/kg dose was recovered in the bile during a 24-hour period. The antibacterial activity in the tissues of mice was determined 4 hours after an oral dose of 200 mg/kg. The concentrations of activity in liver and kidney were 1.9 and 3.2 times greater than in the blood serum, respectively. Other tissues such as lung, spleen, heart, and skeletal muscle had approximately 40% of the activity of the blood serum.

2. MAN

Several clinical investigators reported the mean peak blood serum activity in the blood after a 500-mg dose as being in the range of 1–2 μg/ml (Griffith and Black, 1967; Boyer and Andriole, 1968; Pitt et al., 1968). Johnson et al. (1968) and Perkins et al. (1969) reported peak serum concentrations of 0.6–0.8 μg/ml, and Kunin and Brandt (1968) were unable to detect any activity. Some of the variation in the data of different laboratories was probably due to the assay organism and/or the conditions of the microbiologic assay. The activity in blood serum is due in part to cephaloglycin, but a large portion is due to the deacetylated metabolite (Section IV, C). Therefore, the reported activities determined by comparison with a cephaloglycin standard vary according to the relative sensitivity of the assay organism to the metabolite under the conditions of assay. Pitt *et al.* (1968) and Braun *et al.* (1968) found 25% of the orally administered activity in the urine. Most was due to the deacetyl metabolite (Shimizu and Nishimura, 1970; Griffith and Black, 1971). Urine concentrations of antibacterial activity after a 500-mg dose varied from 76 to 1330 μg/ml. Braun *et al.* (1968) reported that probenecid increased the serum concentration of antibacterial activity. Pitt *et al.* (1968) saw no increase with probenecid, but the duration of assayable activity was prolonged.

D. Cephalexin

1. ANIMALS

During the initial *in vivo* investigation of cephalexin, Wick (1967) found that a 20-mg/kg oral dose of cephalexin in mice gave a blood serum level of 18 μg/ml. This was in contrast to serum antibacterial concentrations of 4 μg/ml for cephaloglycin and 0.5 μg/ml for cephaloridine after equivalent oral doses. This excellent oral absorption was subsequently observed in other species as well.

A 10-mg/kg oral dose in the dog gave a peak serum concentration of 17 μg/ml (Welles *et al.*, 1969, 1970). The rapidity of oral absorption was demonstrated by the fact that antibacterial activity of the serum was the same within 1.5 hours of oral or intramuscular administration; thereafter, the levels of activity were higher for the oral dose.

Cephalexin was administered intraduodenally to dogs, and special experiments were performed in rats to determine the site of absorption in the gastrointestinal tract. It was concluded that the primary site of cephalexin absorption was in the duodenum and jejunum. However, absorption does occur in the lower tract since rectal administration of 10 mg/kg in dogs gave blood serum concentrations of 3–6 μg/ml.

Within 6 hours of intravenous or oral administration of cephalexin, the antibacterial activity in the urine represented 80 and 52% of the dose, respectively. The 24-hour recovery of an oral dose was 75%.

The blood serum disappearance of cephalexin was examined in various animal species after an intravenous dose of 10 mg/kg. Half-life values in dogs, mice, rats, and rabbits were 86, 26, 23, and 21 minutes, respectively. The difference between the renal clearance of cephalexin in the dog and rabbit correlated with the marked difference in half-life in the two species. Cephalexin was cleared at a rate of 0.7 times glomerular filtration rate in the dog and 3.1 times the glomerular filtration rate in the rabbit. After suppression of tubular secretion with probenecid, the clearance rate for both species was reduced to 0.4 times the glomerular filtration rate. It was concluded that cephalexin was secreted and reabsorbed by the tubules of both species with a much higher net excretion in the rabbit. A comparison of the half-life of 86 minutes in normal dogs with a half-life of 15.2 hours in nephrectomized animals demonstrated the dependence upon the kidney for cephalexin elimination. Only 0.2–0.3% of a 10-mg/kg oral dose in dogs and 5% of a similar dose in rats were recovered in the bile.

Cephalexin was detected in kidney, spleen, heart, lung, skeletal muscle, and bone of rats after oral dosage (Welles *et al.*, 1969, 1970; and Kanyuck *et al.*, 1971). No antibacterial activity was found in rat brain after a dose of 25 mg/kg and less than 3% of the serum concentration was found in dog brain after a 200-mg/kg dose. Similarly, low concentrations were found in the cerebro-spinal fluid of dogs. The antibiotic was found in aqueous humor, synovial fluid, and milk as well as in fetal tissue.

2. MAN

Cephalexin was well absorbed after oral administration in man. After a 500-mg dose the mean of the peak antibiotic activities found by several investigators was 15 μg/ml (Perkins *et al.*, 1968b; Meyers *et al.*, 1969; Muggleton *et al.*, 1969; Thornhill *et al.*, 1969; Kunin and Finkelberg, 1970; Naumann and Fedder, 1970; Griffith and Black, 1971). The peak concentration was similar to that found in dogs after a 10-mg/kg dose, but the peak occurred earlier (1 hour) in man than in the dog (2 hours). The urinary recovery of administered activity was usually more than 90% within 6 hours, considerably greater than the 52% recovered in dogs during the same interval.

Kirby *et al.* (1971) calculated the serum half-life of intravenously administered cephalexin as 36 minutes. Kabins *et al.* (1970) and Naumann and Fedder (1970) calculated the serum half-life after oral dosage as 54 minutes. It is probable that the latter value represents the net result of absorption and excretion. Thornhill *et al.* (1969) found that probenecid increased the peak serum concentration by 50%, but Meyers *et al.* (1969) found a lesser effect. It appears likely that renal tubular secretion plays an important role in the rapid excretion of this antibiotic. Linquist *et al.* (1970) examined the disappearance of cephalexin from the blood sera of anephric patients. Half-life values varied from 23.5 to 41 hours with a mean of 31 hours, clearly demonstrating the dependence upon the kidney for excretion.

Boyle *et al.* (1970) found aqueous humor concentrations of cephalexin that were the equivalent of approximately 10% of the blood serum levels.

IV. Metabolism of Cephalosporins in Therapeutic Use

A. *Cephalothin*

1. ANIMALS

Lee *et al.* (1963) identified a microbiologically active metabolite of cephalothin (deacetylcephalothin, Table I) in the blood serum and urine of parenterally dosed dogs and rats. *In vitro* experiments indicated that an esterase capable of effecting this deacetylation was present in the kidney, liver, stomach, and small intestinal tissue of rats, but that very little, if any, was present in serum or whole blood.

Sullivan and McMahon (1967) studied the fate of orally administered radiocarbon-labeled cephalothin, 7-(2-thienyl[1-^{14}C]acetamido)cephalosporanic acid, in the rat. A total of 5% of the radioactivity was recovered in the urine in the first 4 hours and 46% within 40 hours. The urine contained no unchanged cephalothin and only a trace of deacetylcephalothin. Thirty-two percent of the radioactivity was present as thienylacetylglycine, 13% as thienylacetamidoethanol, and the remainder was unidentified. The observed side-chain cleavage did not occur when the radioactive cephalothin was incubated with various tissue homogenates, including liver and kidney, or with various mammalian enzymes.

In another experiment, thienyl[1-^{14}C]acetamidoacetaldehyde, a proposed intermediate of the side-chain products, was given to rats by intraperitoneal injection. The urine of these animals contained the same two products, thienylacetylglycine and thienylacetamidoethanol, as were found in the rats given oral cephalothin.

On the basis of the above findings, they concluded that cephalothin undergoes degradation in the gut followed by the subsequent absorption of the degradation products. Although there is no practical interest in the oral fate of cephalothin, these studies demonstrated the *in vivo* instability of the cephalothin molecule and also indicated a possible degradation pathway, other than deacetylation, which may occur after parenteral administration.

2. MAN

Cephalothin is readily deacetylated in man as well as in animals. Lee *et al.* (1963) collected urine of 11 volunteers for 6 hours after an intramuscular dose of cephalothin. Of the antibacterial activity in the urine, 58% was unchanged antibiotic and the remainder was the deacetylated metabolite.

With the knowledge of the *in vivo* instability of cephalothin in man it can be assumed that the deacetylcephalothin/cephalothin ratio becomes very high in patients with poor renal function. Kabins and Cohen (1965) found evidence of a biphasic disappearance of antibacterial activity from the blood of uremic patients treated with cephalothin. During the first 8 hours the disappearance curve indicated a half-life of 3 hours; thereafter a half-life of 12–18 hours was indicated. Assuming that renal and nonrenal excretion were constant, it appears reasonable to speculate that the degradation of cephalothin to the less microbiologically active deacetylcephalothin played an important role in the more rapid phase, whereas the latter phase was more indicative of the further degradation of deacetylcephalothin to nonmicrobiologically active products.

B. Cephaloridine

1. ANIMALS

Early experiments in dogs indicated that the *in vivo* stability of cephaloridine was much greater than that of cephalothin. After an intravenous dose of cephaloridine, 92% of the administered microbiologic activity appeared in the urine as unchanged cephaloridine (Welles *et al.*, 1966). There was no indication of a product like deacetylcephalothin which could theoretically occur as the result of cleavage of the pyridyl moiety.

Small amounts of free pyridine were found in 24-hour urine collections from dogs (Atkinson *et al.*, 1966b), but it was considered possible that pyridyl cleavage took place in the urine after voiding.

Sullivan and McMahon (1967) studied the fate of orally administered radio-carbon-labeled cephaloridine in the rat in the same manner that cephalothin was studied (Section IV, A). The rats excreted a total of 50% of the radio-activity of an oral dose of 7-(2-thienyl[1-^{14}C]acetamido)-3-(pyridylmethyl)-3-cephem-4-carboxylic acid betaine (cephaloridine) in the urine. About 10% of the recovered radioactivity was radiolabeled cephaloridine. Another 47% was identifiable as the same two compounds that were recovered after the oral administration of cephalothin (Section IV, A), i.e., thienylacetylglycine and thienylacetamidoethanol. The remainder of the excreted radioactive compounds were unidentified. Unlike cephalothin, there was no evidence of hydrolytic cleavage at the 3-methyl position to give the microbiologically active alcohol referred to earler as deacetylcephalothin.

2. MAN

The pharmacology data in man (Section III, B), particularly that in patients with little or no renal function, attested to the stability of cephaloridine in the body. No product of cephaloridine degradation has been identified in human urine. Most certainly, degradation of the compound does occur but apparently the process is slow and the products are not microbiologically active.

C. Cephaloglycin

1. ANIMALS

Sullivan et al. (1969a) examined the metabolism of radiolabeled cephaloglycin, 7-(D-α-amino-phenyl[1-^{14}C]acetamido)-cephalosporanic acid, in rats. A total of 20% of the orally administered radioactivity was recovered in the urine and 70% was recovered in the feces within 24 hours. The urine contained only one microbiologically active substance representing 2% of the dose. This compound was identified as deacetylcephaloglycin. The three identifiable biologically inactive radiolabeled products and the percentage of the dose they represented were as follows: phenylglycine, 8.5%; benzoylformic acid, 5%; and mandelic acid, 1.5%. The administration of larger oral doses resulted in the urinary recovery of some cephaloglycin and a greater quantity of deacetylcephaloglycin.

Welles et al. (1971) examined the urinary excretion of antibacterial activity in dogs after an oral dose of cephaloglycin. They found a cephaloglycin: deacetylcephaloglycin ratio of 3:7 in the first hour and a ratio of 2:98 in the second hour. This ratio is dependent upon magnitude of dose as mentioned in the above rat study but the experiment clearly demonstrated a rapid deacetylation of this antibiotic.

2. MAN

Little is known of the metabolic fate of cephaloglycin in man except that deacetylation proceeds rapidly. The antibacterial activity in human urine after oral dosage is primarily due to deacetylcephaloglycin (Shimizu and Nishimura, 1970; Griffith and Black, 1971; and Wick et al., 1971).

D. Cephalexin

1. ANIMALS

Antibacterial activity in the urine and bile of dogs and rats that have received oral doses of cephalexin has been identified by chromatography as the unchanged antibiotic (Welles et al., 1969). This finding, in addition to the efficiency of excretion (Section III, D), proved that cephalexin was metabolically stable.

Sullivan *et al.* (1969b) studied the fate of orally administered radiocarbon-labeled cephalexin in rats and mice in the same manner that they had studied the fate of cephalothin, cephaloridine, and cephaloglycin (Section IV, A–C). More than 80% of the administered radioactivity appeared in the urine as unchanged cephalexin. There was no evidence of any degradation product, which was in contrast with the metabolites observed in the urine of rats after oral administration of the other cephalosporins.

2. MAN

The urinary recovery of antibacterial activity after oral doses of cephalexin in man was as great, or greater, than the recovery in laboratory animals (Section III D). Chou (1969) isolated the antibacterial activity from human urine and obtained a crystalline product which was identical to the administered antibiotic.

V. Pharmacology of Cefazolin

A. Absorption, Distribution, and Excretion in Animals and Man

Nishida *et al.* (1970) have thoroughly investigated the absorption and excretion characteristics of cefazolin (Table I), a cephalosporin now undergoing clinical trial. A 10-mg/kg intramuscular dose in dogs gave a peak blood serum concentration of 23 μg/ml, and 80% of the administered activity was excreted in the urine as unchanged cefazolin. These data were similar to those observed with cephaloridine (Section III, B and Table II).

The comparative data of these two antibiotics in man were dissimilar in some respects. A 500-mg intramuscular dose of cefazolin gave a peak serum concentration of 45 μg/ml, more than twofold that of cephaloridine, and the serum half-life, calculated from their data, was 2.2 hours for cefazolin compared with 1.5 hours reported for cephaloridine by others (Section III, B). The total recovery of antibacterial activity in the urine was similar for both compounds. No microbiologically active metabolite of either antibiotic has been detected.

Nishida *et al.* (1970) also examined the biliary excretion of cefazolin in dogs, rats, and rabbits. After a 20-mg/kg dose the 24-hour recovery in the bile of dogs was 3.3%, compared with 0.1% for cephaloridine. In the rat, 23.5% of the cefazolin dose was recovered and only 0.7% of the cephaloridine dose. Biliary recovery of both antibiotics in rabbits was insignificant (0.5–0.6%).

They found that cefazolin and cephaloridine were both well distributed in the tissues of rats and rabbits. Despite higher serum levels of cefazolin, the kidney tissue concentration of cephaloridine at 30 minutes was greater. The significance

is not clear since the concentrations of the two antibiotics in the renal tissue of
rats were equivalent at 1 hour; data for the corresponding time interval in
rabbits was not reported.

References

Acocella, G., Mattussi, R., Nicolis, F. B., Pallanza, R., and Tenconi, L. T. (1968). *Gut* **9**, 536.
Arthur, L. J. H., and Burland, W. L. (1969). *Arch. Dis. Child.* **44**, 82.
Atkinson, R. M., Currie, J. P., Davis, B., Pratt, D. A. H., Sharpe, H. M., and Tomich, E. G. (1966a). *Toxicol. Appl. Pharmacol.* **8**, 398.
Atkinson, R. M., Caisey, J. D., Currie, J. P., Middleton, T. R., Pratt, D. A. H., Sharpe, H. M., and Tomich, E. G. (1966b). *Toxicol. Appl. Pharmacol.* **8**, 407.
Barr, W., and Graham, R. M. (1967). *J. Obstet Gynaecol. Brit. Common.* **74**, 739.
Benner, E. J., Brodie, J. L., and Kirby, W. M. M. (1966). *Antimicrob. Ag. Chemother.* **1965**, 888.
Benner, E. J. (1970a). *Antimicrob. Ag. Chemother.* **1969**, 417.
Benner, E. J. (1970b). *J. Infect. Dis.* **122**, 104.
Boyer, J. L., and Andriole, V. T. (1968). *Yale J. Biol. Med.* **40**, 284.
Boyle, G. L., Hein, H. F., and Leopold, T. H. (1970). *Amer. J. Ophthalmol.* **69**, 868.
Braun, P., Tillotson, J. R., Wilcox, C., and Finland, M. (1968). *Appl. Microbiol.* **16**, 1684.
Chauvette, R. R., Flynn, E. H., Jackson, B. G., Lavagnino, E. R., Morin, R. B., Mueller, R. A., Pioch, R. P., Roeske, R. W., Ryan, C. W., Spencer, J. L., and Van Heyningen, E. (1962). *J. Amer. Chem. Soc.* **84**, 3401.
Child, K. J., and Dodds, M. G. (1966). *Brit. J. Pharmacol.* **26**, 108.
Child, K. J., and Dodds, M. G. (1967). *Brit. J. Pharmacol.* **30**, 354.
Chou, T. S. (1969). *J. Med. Chem.* **12**, 925.
Cohen, P. G., Romansky, M. J., and Johnson, A. C. (1966). *Antimicrob. Ag. Chemother.* **1965**, 894.
Currie, G. A., Little, P. J., and McDonald, S. J. (1966). *Nephron.* **3**, 282.
Fleming, P. C., and Jaffe, D. (1967). *Postgrad. Med. J.* **43**, August suppl., 89.
Florey, H. W. (1955). *Ann. Int. Med.* **43**, 480.
Foord, R. D. (1970). *Proc. Int. Congr. Chemother., 6th* **1**, 597.
Gonnella, J. S., Olexy, V. M., and Jackson, G. G. (1967). *Amer. J. Med. Sci.* **254**, 71.
Gray, J. E., and Lewis, C. (1966). *Toxicol. Appl. Pharmacol.* **8**, 342.
Griffith, R. S. (1970). *Int. J. Clin. Pharmacol. Suppl.* **2**, 130.
Griffith, R. S., and Black, H. R. (1964). *J. Amer. Med. Ass.* **189**, 823.
Griffith, R. S., and Black, H. R. (1967). *Proc. Int. Congr. Chemother., 5th, Vienna, Austria* 251.
Griffith, R. S., and Black, H. R. (1968). *Clin. Med.* **75**, No. 11, 14.
Griffith, R. S., and Black, H. R. (1971). *Postgrad. Med. J.* **47**, February suppl., 32.
Gump, D. W., and Lipson, R. L. (1968). *Curr. Ther. Res.* **10**, 583.
Heitler, M. S., Isenberg, H. D., Karelitz, S., Acs, H., and Driller, M. (1964). *Antimicrob. Ag. Chemother.* **1963**, 261.
Hogan, L. B., Jr., Holloway, W. J., and Jakubowitch, R. A. (1968). *Antimicrob. Ag. Chemother.* **1967**, 624.
Holloway, W. J., and Scott, E. G. (1966). *Antimicrob. Ag. Chemother.* **1965**, 915.
Jago, M., and Heatley, N. G. (1961). *Brit. J. Pharmacol.* **16**, 170.
Johnson, W. D., Applestein, J. M., and Kaye, D. (1968). *J. Amer. Med. Ass.* **206**, 2698.
Kabins, S. A., and Cohen, S. (1965). *Antimicrob. Ag. Chemother.* **1964**, 207.
Kabins, S. A., and Cohen, S. (1966). *Antimicrob. Ag. Chemother.* **1965**, 922.

Kabins, S. A., Eisenstein, B., and Cohen, S. (1965). *J. Amer. Med. Ass.* **193**, 165.
Kabins, S. A., Kelner, B., Walton, E., and Goldstein, E. (1970). *Amer. J. Med. Sci.* **259**, 133.
Kanyuck, D. O., Welles, J. S., Emmerson, J. L., and Anderson, R. C. (1971). *Proc. Soc. Exp. Biol. Med.* **136**, 997.
Kaplan, K., and Weinstein, L. (1967). *J. Amer. Med. Ass.* **200**, 75.
Kind, A. C., Kestle, D. G., Standiford, H. C., and Kirby, W. M. M. (1969). *Antimicrob. Ag. Chemother.* **1968**, 361.
Kirby, W. M. M., de Maine, J. B., and Serrill, W. S. (1971). *Postgrad. Med. J.* **47**, February suppl., 46.
Kislak, J. W., Steinhauer, B. W., and Finland, M. (1966). *Amer. J. Med. Sci.* **251**, 433.
Kunin, C. M., and Atuk, N. (1966). *New Engl. J. Med.* **274**, 654.
Kunin, C. M., and Brandt, D. (1968). *Amer. J. Med. Sci.* **255**, 196.
Kunin, C. M., and Finkelberg, Z. (1970). *Ann. Int. Med.* **72**, 349.
Landes, R. R., Melnick, I., Fletcher, A., and McCormick, B. (1969). *J. Urol.* **102**, 246.
Lee, C. C., and Anderson, R. C. (1963). *Antimicrob. Ag. Chemother.* **1962**, 695.
Lee, C. C., Herr, E. B., Jr., and Anderson, R. C. (1963). *Clin. Med.* **70**, 1123.
Levison, M. E., Johnson, W. D., Thornhill, T. S., and Kaye, D. (1969). *J. Amer. Med. Ass.* **209**, 1331.
Linquist, J. A., Siddiqui, J. Y., and Smith, I. M. (1970). *New Engl. J. Med.* **283**, 720.
Linsell, W. D., Pines, A., and Hayden, J. W. (1967). *Postgrad. Med. J.* **43**, August suppl., 90.
MacAulay, M. A., and Charles, D. (1968). *Amer. J. Obstet. Gynecol.* **100**, 940.
Maynard, E. P., III (1969). *New Engl. J. Med.* **280**, 505.
Meyers, B. R., Kaplan, K., and Weinstein, L. (1969). *Clin. Pharmacol. Ther.* **10**, 810.
Mineshita, T., Muraoka, Y., Yahara, I., Inuta, T., Ishikawa, M., Uehara, K., Kawaguchi, J., and Okada, T. (1970). *Nippon Kagaku Ryohogakukai Zasshi* **18**, 22.
Molthan, L., Reidenberg, M. M., and Eichman, M. F. (1967). *New Engl. J. Med.* **277**, 123.
Morin, R. B., Jackson, B. G., Flynn, E. H., and Roeske, R. W. (1962). *J. Amer. Chem. Soc.* **84**, 3400.
Muggleton, P. W., O'Callaghan, C. H., Foord, R. D., Kirby, S. M., and Ryan, D. M. (1969). *Antimicrob. Ag. Chemother.* **1968**, 353.
Murdoch, J. McC., Spiers, C. F., Geddes, A. M., and Wallace, E. T. (1964). *Brit. Med. J.* **2**, 1238.
Naumann, P. (1966). *Artzneimittel-Forsch.* **16**, 1099.
Naumann, P., and Fedder, J. (1970). *Int. J. Clin. Pharmacol. Suppl.* **2**, 6.
Nishida, M., Matsubara, T., Murakawa, T., Mine, Y., Yokota, Y., Goto, S., and Kuwahara, S. (1970). *J. Antibiot.* **23**, 184.
O'Callaghan, C. H., and Muggleton, P. W. (1963). *Biochem. J.* **89**, 304.
Page, J., Levison, M. E., Thornhill, T. S., and Kaye, D. (1970). *J. Amer. Med. Ass.* **211**, 1837.
Perkins, R. L., Apicella, M. A., Lee, I., Cuppage, F. E., and Saslaw, S. (1968a). *J. Lab. Clin. Med.* **71**, 75.
Perkins, R. L., Carlisle, H. N., and Saslaw, S. (1968b). *Amer. J. Med. Sci.* **256**, 122.
Perkins, R. L., Glontz, G. E., and Saslaw, S. (1969). *Clin. Pharmacol. Ther.* **10**, 244.
Perrelli, L., and Tempesta, E. (1968). *Gazz. Int. Med. Chir.* **73**, 5283.
Pitt, J., Siasoco, R., Kaplan, K., and Weinstein, L. (1968). *Antimicrob. Ag. Chemother.* **1967**, 630.
Pryor, J. S., Joekes, A. M., and Foord, R. D. (1967). *Postgrad. Med. J.* **43**, August suppl., 82.
Records, R. E. (1969). *Arch. Ophth.* **81**, 331.
Riley, H. D., Jr., Bracken, E. C., and Flux, M. (1963). *Antimicrob. Ag. Chemother.* **1962**, 716.
Shimizu, K., and Nishimura, H. (1970). *J. Antibiot.* **23**, 216.
Silverblatt, F., Turck, M., and Bulger, R. (1970). *J. Infect. Dis.* **122**, 33.

Somer, P. de., Voorde, H. van de., Eyssen, H., and Dijck, P. van. (1955). *Antibiot. Chemother.* **5**, 463.

Spector, W. S. (1957). *In* "Handbook of Toxicology, Antibiotics" (W. S. Spector, ed.), Vol. II, p. 141. Saunders, Philadelphia, Pennsylvania.

Steinbrunn, W., and Haemmerli, U. P. (1966). *Deut. Med. Wochschr.* 2003.

Stewart, G. T., and Holt, R. J. (1964). *Lancet* **II**, 1305.

Sullivan, H. R., and McMahon, R. E. (1967). *Biochem. J.* **102**, 976.

Sullivan, H. R., Billings, R. E., and McMahon, R. E. (1969a). *J. Antibiot.* **22**, 27.

Sullivan, H. R., Billings, R. E., and McMahon, R. E. (1969b). *J. Antibiot.* **22**, 195.

Thornhill, T. S., Levison, M. E., Johnson, W. D., and Kaye, D. (1969). *Appl. Microbiol.* **17**, 457.

Trafton, H. M., and Lind, H. E. (1969). *J. Urol.* **101**, 392.

Tuano, S. B., Brodie, J. L., and Kirby, W. M. M. (1967). *Antimicrob. Ag. Chemother.* **1966**, 101.

Uwaydah, M. M., and Faris, B. M. (1970). *Arch. Ophthal.* **83**, 349.

Vianna, N. J., and Kaye, D. (1967). *Amer. J. Med. Sci.* **254**, 216.

Weinstein, L., Kaplan, K., and Chang, T-W. (1964). *J. Amer. Med. Ass.* **189**, 829.

Welles, J. S., Gibson, W. R., Harris, P. N., Small, R. M., and Anderson, R. C. (1966). *Antimicrob. Ag. Chemother.* **1965**, 863.

Welles, J. S., Froman, R. O., Gibson, W. R., Owen, N. V., and Anderson, R. C. (1969). *Antimicrob. Ag. Chemother.* **1968**, 489.

Welles, J. S., Froman, R. O., Gibson, W. R., Owen, N. V., Small, R. M., and Anderson, R. C. (1970). *Int. J. Clin. Pharmacol. Suppl.* **2**, 36.

Welles, J. S., Froman, R. O., Gibson, W. R., Owen, N. V., and Anderson, R. C. (1971). Unpublished data.

Wick, W. E. (1967). *Appl. Microbiol.* **15**, 765.

Wick, W. E., Wright, W. E., and Kuder, H. V. (1971). *Appl. Microbiol.* **21**, 426.

Chapter 14

ANALYTICAL PROCEDURES FOR CEPHALOSPORINS

LOUIS P. MARRELLI

I. Introduction

This chapter describes practical tests and methods of assay which are useful for the most frequently encountered cephalosporins. The methods of assay, in many instances, have also been utilized for the determination of penicillins. This is due primarily to the presence of the β-lactam ring, a feature common to both the penicillin and cephalosporin ring systems. Analogies are frequently made throughout the chapter between analytical procedures which are applicable to both cephalosporins and penicillins.

The chapter is divided into four sections: microbiological determinations, chemical determinations, chromatographic determinations, and physical–chemical determinations. The first two sections deal primarily with the assays for cephalosporins which provide quantitative results. The last two sections describe methods which not only provide an estimation of purity but also serve to identify the cephalosporins and metabolites or impurities present.

II. Microbiological Determinations

The microbiological assay has been and is still used as the method of preference for the determination of antibiotics in (1) pharmaceutical preparations, (2) body fluids, and (3) formulations subjected to long-term stability studies. The choice of microbiological assay used is dependent on the nature of the sample and information desired.

A. Plate Assays

Cylinder–plate methods for penicillins, utilizing *Staphylococcus aureus* ATCC 6538 and *Sarcina lutea* ATCC 9341 as test organisms, have been described in great detail (Kavanagh, 1963a). These methods, with few exceptions, are suited to the bioassay of cephalosporins (Kavanagh, 1972). *Bacillus subtilis* ATCC 6633 may be substituted for *S. aureus*, with the provision that the inoculum of *B. subtilis* be prepared as described in the first-mentioned reference. In general, the potencies of cephalosporins in pharmaceutical formulations are controlled by using the *S. aureus* and *B. subtilis* plate assays. Better-defined zones of inhibition are obtained with the *B. subtilis* plate method, thereby increasing the assay precision. The plate method using *S. lutea* is employed primarily for the assay of serum, urine, and tissue extracts. As low as 0.2 μg/ml of each of the four cephalosporins presently in clinical use can be determined in biological media by this technique. The concentration range of the assay for the cephalosporins by the designated plate assays is given in Table I. A turbidimetric (photometric) assay, using *S. aureus* ATCC 9144, is also utilized and will be discussed later in this section.

The plate method using *B. subtilis* is recommended for determining the concentration of cephalothin in the presence of hydrolysis products. Cephalothin, following parenteral administration to man and animals, is converted in part to deacetylcephalothin (Lee *et al.*, 1963). Deacetylcephalothin is about one-fifth as active as cephalothin against *B. subtilis*, one-fourth as active against *S. aureus*, and one-half as active against *S. lutea*. The dose–response curve of the metabolite parallels that of cephalothin; therefore, the method measures total activity of mixtures of these compounds in terms of the pure standard used. Cephalothin lactone may also be present as a hydrolysis product, but its activity does not cause any interference in the plate assays. A cephalothin stock solution (1000 μg/ml) may be stored at 4°C for 5 days, with no appreciable

Table I

CONCENTRATION RANGE OF PLATE ASSAY FOR CEPHALOSPORINS[a]

Antibiotic	*Staphylococcus aureus*	*Sarcina lutea*	*Bacillus subtilis*
Cephalothin	0.5–4.0	0.25–2.0	0.2–2.0
Cephaloridine	0.25–2.0	0.1–1.0	0.5–5.0
Cephaloglycin	2.5–10	0.1–3.0	0.5–2.0
Cephalexin	2.5–40	0.2–3.5	2.5–10

[a] In micrograms per milliliter.

loss in potency. Final dilutions of the sample and standard for the plate assay are made in pH 6.0 phosphate buffer. When assaying serum, the dilutions are made with pooled normal serum. Cephalothin activity in both serum and pH 6.0 phosphate buffer is fully maintained for 14 days at −20°C. A potency loss of about 12% occurs in serum in 2 days at 5°C and 50% in 14 days. At room temperature, about 85% inactivation occurs in the serum after 2 days; in pH 6.0 buffer, about 10–15% inactivation takes place in the same time interval.

The plate method, using *B. subtilis* or *S. aureus*, is recommended for determining the concentration of cephaloridine or degraded cephaloridine. Cephaloridine, unlike cephalothin, does not undergo serious enzymatic degradation to a metabolite of lesser activity in the body and is thereby excreted mainly unchanged in the urine (Stewart and Holt, 1964; Sullivan and McMahon, 1967). Patients' sera should be stored frozen until the day of assay. The stability of cephaloridine in both serum and pH 6.0 phosphate buffer is similar to that of cephalothin, as previously described.

Wick and Wright's (1968) microbiological and chromatographic studies revealed that cephaloglycin, following oral administration, was almost entirely excreted as deacetylcephaloglycin. Concentration of the parent compound is best determined by employing either the *B. subtilis* or *S. aureus* plate assay. The influence of deacetylcephaloglycin is negligible in either assay when the concentration is less than 15% of the parent compound. Deacetylcephaloglycin is about 60% as active as cephaloglycin against *S. aureus* and only 30% as active against *B. subtilis*. Cephaloglycin lactone has negligible activity in any assay system.

Stock solutions of standard and sample, approximately 0.5–1.0 mg/ml, should be prepared fresh every 2 days and refrigerated. The solvent should be 1% phosphate buffer pH 4.5. Solution may be facilitated by the use of mechanical devices, such as blenders, or ultrasonic baths. At room temperature, decomposition at pH 4.5 is about 6%/day; whereas, at pH 6.0, 3%/hour is lost.

Biological media (blood, urine, and body fluids) are assayed using the *S. lutea* plate assay. With this test organism, deacetylcephaloglycin is as active or more active than cephaloglycin. Final dilutions of the standard and serum samples are made in pooled normal serum. Blood is allowed to clot prior to the removal of the serum for assay. Urine, tissue, and other extracts, as well as the standard, are diluted to the reference level with pH 6.0 phosphate buffer. Deacetylcephaloglycin is more stable in human serum than cephaloglycin (Wick, 1968). In 24 hours, the deacetyl metabolite loses 0% at 4°C, 50% at 25°C, and 85% at 37°C. Cephaloglycin loses 30% at 4°C, 60% at 25°C, and about 100% at 37°C.

Cephalexin activity may be determined by using the *S. aureus* or *B. subtilis* plate method. These methods are suited to the assay of either samples used in accelerated stability studies or of body fluid samples. Cephalexin apparently degrades by cleavage of the β-lactam ring to form biologically inactive hydrolysis products. Stock solutions of standard, prepared in pH 6.0 phosphate buffer, are stable for 1 week when refrigerated. No potency loss is observed for at least 2 days when prepared in pH 4.5 phosphate buffer and stored at room temperature. Oral or drop suspensions may be solubilized more readily by the addition of dilute hydrochloric acid at a molar concentration equivalent to that of the antibiotic. Mechanical devices may be used to facilitate solution of cephalexin in tablet or capsule formulations. Biological media are assayed using the *S. lutea* plate assay. Cephalexin resists metabolism in the body and appears unchanged in the urine (Chou, 1969; Sullivan *et al.*, 1969a). Biological samples are treated in the same manner as that previously described for the cephaloglycin assay. Cephalexin activity in serum is fully maintained for 14 days at −20°C. Approximately 10% degradation occurs in serum held at 5°C for 2 days as compared to 50% at 25°C and 75% at 37°C.

In general, basic precision of the plate assays used for cephalosporins is good, as well as consistent. In a study (Kavanagh, 1972), cephaloridine standard was assayed against itself by the *B. subtilis* plate method to obtain data for statistical evaluation. Based on 52 determinations (three analysts) performed on several days over a period of months, the mean was calculated to be 996.6 μg/ml and the relative standard deviation, 2.43%. The 95% confidence limits ± 2 RSD calculated for various combinations of assay conditions were as follows: day 1, one replicate, $n = 1$, 5.78%; day 1, two replicates, $n = 2$, 5.36%; day 2, two replicates, $n = 4$, 3.09%; and for day 3, two replicates, $n = 6$, 2.53%. This information is useful in making a decision on the optimum number of assays required for individual needs.

B. Photometric Assays

Methodology described for the photometric assay of penicillins (Kavanagh, 1963b) is applicable to cephalosporins except for the range of standards used (Table II). This method is primarily used for quality control purposes on

Table II

CONCENTRATION RANGE OF
PHOTOMETRIC ASSAY FOR CEPHALOSPORINS[a]

Antibiotic	*Staphylococcus aureus* ATCC 9144
Cephalothin	0.15–0.50
Cephaloridine	0.05–0.20
Cephaloglycin	0.10–0.50
Cephalexin	0.25–2.0

[a] In micrograms per milliliter.

samples free from microbiologically active hydrolysis products. Cephalexin may be assayed by this technique, since degradation products derived from cephalexin possess practically no microbiological activity. The method is rapid, and it has good accuracy and precision. Excellent precision can be achieved using the manual turbidimetric assay, provided special attention is given to every operational detail of the assay (Kavanagh, 1972). The Auto-turb™ system can achieve precision in the order of 1–2% (Kuzel and Kavanagh 1971).

III. Chemical Determinations

A. Iodometric Method

An iodometric titration procedure has been widely used for the determination of penicillins and formulations thereof (Alicino, 1946). The method is based on the fact that the intact penicillin molecule (*1*) does not absorb iodine, while the alkali hydrolysis product, sodium penicilloate (*2*), does react with iodine. A blank determination is run prior to alkali hydrolysis to insure that

(*1*)   (*2*)

only the active penicillin is measured. The method compares favorably with the microbiological cylinder–plate method in accuracy, and it is much more rapid.

Alkaline hydrolysis of cephalosporins also results in cleavage of the β-lactam ring; however, the hydrolysis products formed seemingly do not correspond to those of penicillins, namely, penillic acids, penicilloic acids, and penicillenic acids. Some analogous compounds may have a transient existence during the hydrolysis (Abraham, 1965; Doyle and Nayler, 1964).

Alicino (1961) applied the iodometric assay to the determination of synthetic penicillins, 6-aminopenicillanic acid, and cephalosporin C. A 15-minute hydrolysis was found to be adequate for all compounds tested. Benzylpenicillin (penicillin G), when inactivated with alkali, consumed nine atoms of iodine per mole of penicillin, whereas 1 mole of cephalosporin C consumed approximately four atoms of iodine. In actual practice, the iodine consumption per mole of compound was found to be dependent on the particular conditions used in the assay (Weiss, 1959).

Variations in hydrolysis time, temperature, pH of iodine solution, and concentration of antibiotic present influence the absorption of iodine by the test solution. In assaying cephalosporins, the standard used should correspond to the sample, both in composition and amount tested. Cephalosporin degradation products having an intact β-lactam ring, titrate as well as the parent compound. Possible intermediates used in synthetic sequences such as 7-aminocephalosporanic acid (7-ACA), will also respond to this test.

An automated iodometric assay has been used recently for the assay of cephalosporins (Stevenson and Bechtel, 1971). In this method both sample and blank values are sequentially determined on each sample solution through the action of a reagent switching valve mechanism controlled by the liquid samples in the analyzer system. Sample hydrolysis takes place at 37°C for 10 minutes. This is followed by a 5-minute iodine consumption step which also takes place at 37°C. Concentration of the sample is related to the decrease in iodine color measured at 350 nm. A reference standard is run concurrently through the analyzer for comparative purposes. As with the manual titration technique the extent of iodine consumption varies with hydrolysis time, alkali concentration, temperature, pH of the iodine solution and duration of the iodine uptake reaction. The automated system gives excellent linearity of response for the recommended concentration ranges of the cephalosporins, with all standard curve plots passing through the origin. Assays obtained on cephalosporin preparations by the automated procedure agree well with the conventional manual iodometric titration assays. Reproducibility of the automated method on the same sample or standard solution on a given day is generally better than $\pm 1\%$ relative standard deviation (RSD), depending on the maintenance and condition of the analyzer system.

B. Hydroxylamine Method

Reaction with hydrolyxlamine has been utilized for the colorimetric determination of penicillins (Ford, 1947). The method is based on the fact that hydroxylamine cleaves the β-lactam of the penicillin (1) to form a hydroxamic acid (3) which forms a colored complex with ferric ion. Hydroxamic acid formation is essentially complete in 3 minutes at pH 7.

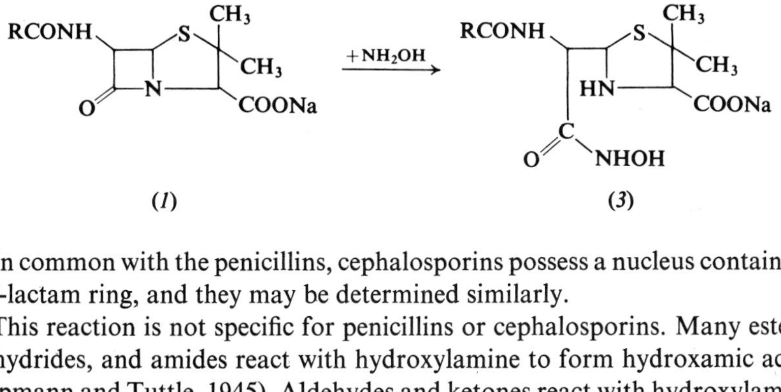

In common with the penicillins, cephalosporins possess a nucleus containing a β-lactam ring, and they may be determined similarly.

This reaction is not specific for penicillins or cephalosporins. Many esters, anhydrides, and amides react with hydroxylamine to form hydroxamic acids (Lipmann and Tuttle, 1945). Aldehydes and ketones react with hydroxylamine to give oximes which form colored complexes with ferric ion (Shriner and Fuson, 1940). Interfering substances can be eliminated by incorporating a blank determination wherein the cephalosporin is rendered incapable of forming a hydroxamic acid derivative. The use of an enzyme (cephalosporinase) or basic hydrolysis is most commonly used. Cephalosporin degradation products having an intact β-lactam ring react as well as the parent compound.

The hydroxylamine method (Boxer and Everett, 1949) has been used to follow the stability pattern of an aqueous cephaloridine solution, as shown in Table III (Martin and Shaw, 1965). It has been observed with cephalosporins that when the loss in potency is greater than about 15%, the difference between chemical and microbiological results becomes significant and progressively greater as the decomposition proceeds. The microbiological assay should then be considered acceptable. A modification of the above procedure (Marrelli, 1962) is outlined in the appendix.

An automated ferric hydroxamate procedure has been utilized for the simultaneous determination of cephalosporin C and penicillin N in fermentation broths (Roudebush, 1969). Cephalosporin hydroxamic acid derivatives were found to have better dialysis characteristics than the intact cephalosporin molecules. This same property was found to exist with penicillin compounds

Table III

DECOMPOSITION OF A 1% w/v AQUEOUS SOLUTION OF
CEPHALORIDINE AT 37°C

Time (days)	% of initial	
	Hydroxylamine assay	Microbiological assay (5% confidence limits)
1	93	92
2	81	75
3	74	67
4	68	58
7	58	37
10	52	23

as well. Consequently, in this procedure the hydroxamic acid derivatives are formed prior to dialysis. Reducing-sugars present in fermentation broth may form oximes with hydroxylamine; however, the blank system used compensates for this type of interference. Addition of aqueous hydroxylamine hydrochloride, maintained at pH 1–2, to the sample solution prevents the formation of the hydroxamic acid derivatives of either cephalosporins or penicillins and serves as a valid basis for the blank system. This system provides a rapid monitor for total cephalosporin β-lactam content (cephalosporin C plus deacetylcephalosporin C) in broth samples.

C. Ninhydrin Colorimetric Method

A reproducible colorimetric method has been described for the determination of 7-ACA and related compounds (Marrelli, 1968). Compounds having an α-amino group adjacent to a β-lactam ring react with ninhydrin under controlled conditions to give characteristic chromophores. This procedure may be used to determine residual amounts of 7-ACA (0.04–1.0%) in cephaloglycin, thereby providing a convenient means of following the extent of acylation in a synthesis from 7-ACA. In a similar manner, low levels of 7-aminodeacetoxy-cephalosporanic acid (7-ADCA) (0.1–1.0%) may be directly determined in cephalexin.

The purity of raw material 7-ACA may be evaluated by this method. Comparative data obtained by using three methods of assay for 7-ACA are outlined in Table IV. The method utilizing the AutoAnalyzer® provides the

Table IV
COMPARATIVE DATA ON PURITY OF 7-ACA SAMPLES

| Sample no. | % 7-ACA[a] | | |
	UV assay (265 nm)	Ninhydrin color assay	Amino acid analyzer
1	94.4	95.8	97.1
2	96.0	92.5	92.8
3	92.8	85.8	86.4
4	80.5	72.8	72.5
5	74.3	65.0	64.0
6	70.3	59.7	58.9
7	73.6	66.2	66.7
8 (N-formyl 7-ACA)	65.2	0.0	0.0

[a] The same standard of 7-ACA was used to calculate percent purity for each method.

greatest degree of specificity. Deacetyl 7-ACA or 7-ACA lactone, if present, interfere in the ninhydrin color assay. However, the excellent agreement obtained between that assay and the AutoAnalyzer® (Table IV) indicate very low levels of either impurity. The UV assay displays the least specificity of the methods tested.

D. Nicotinamide Assay

A specific chemical assay has been used for the determination of cephalosporin derivatives containing the acetyl moiety (Redstone, 1971). Deacetylated products, if present, do not interfere in the determination of the parent compound. The assay is based upon two previously described reactions (Fig. 1).

1. Hale *et al.* (1961) have described the displacement of the acetoxyl portion of certain 7-ACA compounds (*4*) by pyridine derivatives to yield pyridinium derivatives. One of the pyridine derivatives used was nicotinamide (*5*).

2. Burton *et al.* (1957) have described the reaction of carbonyl compounds at the 4 position of the nicotinamide in quaternary nicotinamide derivatives. The assay is conducted in such a manner that the nicotinamide derivative of the 7-ACA compound (*6*) is synthesized, then the 1,3-dihydroxyacetone (DHA) carbonyl adduct (*7*) is formed. The final product has a chromophore which exhibits a maximum absorbance at 360 nm. The method is outlined in the appendix.

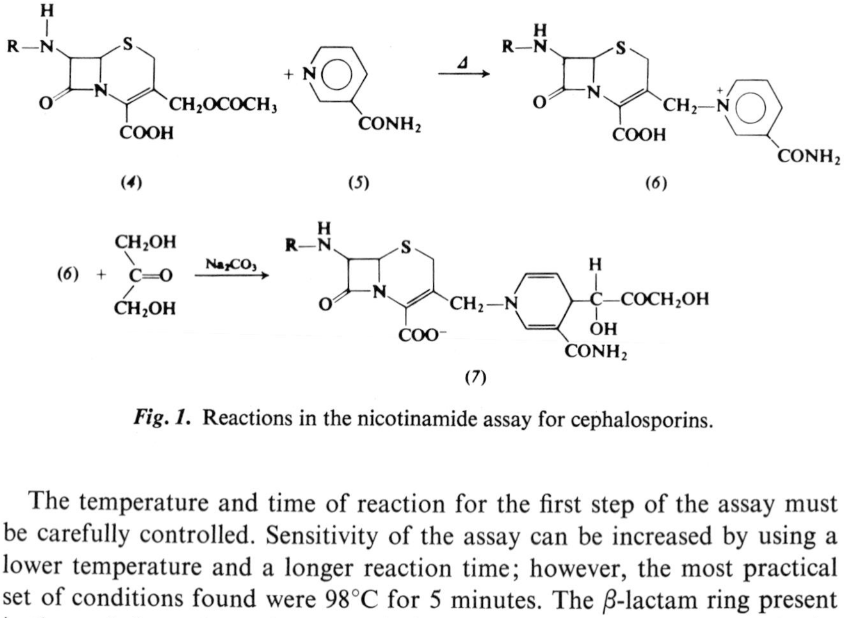

Fig. 1. Reactions in the nicotinamide assay for cephalosporins.

The temperature and time of reaction for the first step of the assay must be carefully controlled. Sensitivity of the assay can be increased by using a lower temperature and a longer reaction time; however, the most practical set of conditions found were 98°C for 5 minutes. The β-lactam ring present in the cephalosporin nucleus must be intact for this reaction to proceed. The high concentration of nicotinamide present allows a practical disregard for the unbuffered pH of most samples.

The DHA addition reaction requires a pH >10.0 and is stopped at pH 8.0. The use of 2.0 ml of 0.75 M Na_2CO_3 insures that the pH of the reaction mixture is greater than 11.0, and the addition of 1.0 ml of 1.5 M KH_2PO_4 results in a pH <8.0. The chromophore is relatively stable for at least 30 minutes after the addition of phosphate buffer. DHA also polymerizes rapidly at the high pH and is the major contributor to background absorbance. Thus, it is imperative to carefully control the time during which the test solution remains at an alkaline pH. Aqueous solutions of DHA are generally unstable to heat and light.

The variation of this assay is fairly high. Variation within replicates for fermentation broth is 1.5–4.5% RSD, but variation for the same samples assayed over a series of days is 5.5–15% RSD, with an average of 9.7% RSD for all samples.

IV. Chromatographic Determinations

A. General Information

1. SEPARATION TECHNIQUES

Chromatography, in all of its various forms, i.e., paper, thin layer, electrophoresis, and column has served as an indispensable aid in the understanding of the chemistry of the cephalosporins. Column chromatography, employing ion exchange, has been used mainly for the determination of impurities in cephaloglycin and cephalexin.

Paper chromatography has played the largest role in the various chromatographic techniques involving the cephalosporins. This has taken place for two reasons: first, thin-layer chromatography and high-voltage electrophoresis are relatively new techniques when compared to the initial work performed on the cephalosporins, and second, paper chromatography can allow a greater migration distance and thus achieve greater physical separation than some of the new techniques.

Thin-layer chromatography has found wide application as a separation technique for cephalosporins in recent years. With the advent of plastic film as a support for the sorbent (as opposed to glass), the bioautography of a thin-layer chromatogram has become as applicable as with paper (Murakawa et al., 1970). The flexible fiberglass-backed thin-layer material is also finding use in a similar manner (Wagman and Bailey, 1969). Cellulose is generally the sorbent of choice when thin-layer chromatography is employed. It has excellent partitioning properties and cephalosporins are relatively stable in its presence. Silica gel is of value when heavy loading is required or when preparative chromatography is needed.

Paper electrophoresis has also enjoyed a long history of usefulness. Because cephaloridine, cephaloglycin, and cephalexin behave as cations under acidic conditions or as neutral compounds at their isoelectric pH, their electrophoretic migration can be easily controlled. Cephalothin can be made to migrate as an anion or to remain immobile as the free acid. Two disadvantages of electrophoresis have led to its limited usage. One drawback is that bioautographic detection becomes rather difficult because biological contamination is much more prevalent. The second problem is that many of the chemical differences between impurities and degradation products do not result in a significant difference in electrical charge at a given pH.

Ion-exchange techniques have been successfully applied to the separation of cephalosporins in recent years. Automated amino acid analyzers, employing cation-exchange resins, have proven to be of immense value in the determination of 7-ACA, 7-ADCA, cephaloglycin, and cephalexin. Amino acid analyzers provide quantitative data which is characterized by a high degree of sensitivity, specificity, and reproducibility.

2. Means of Detection

Chromatograms of cephalosporin preparations have been visualized by a number of techniques. Several chemical sprays have been widely used; these will be discussed later. Generally, however, the most sensitive method of detection

Table V

PAPER CHROMATOGRAPHY DATA

	R_f values of cephalosporins					
System[a]	Cephalothin	Cephaloridine	Cephaloglycin	Cephalexin	7-ACA	7-ADCA
1	0.80	0.55	0.50	0.60	0.00	0.00
2	0.80	0.50	—	—	—	—
3	0.75	0.55	0.50	0.40	0.30	—
4	0.30	0.08	0.05	0.05	0.00	0.00
5	0.60	0.00	—	—	—	—
6	0.75	0.55	0.60	0.50	0.42	0.30
7	0.25	0.15	0.10	0.10	0.05	0.00
8	0.50	0.00	0.00	0.00	0.00	0.00
9	—	0.60	0.55	—	0.50	—

[a] System is defined as follows: (1) Butanol–acetic acid–H_2O, 3:1:1, Whatman No. 1, unbuffered; (2) acetone–ethyl acetate–H_2O, 5:4:2, Whatman No. 3, pH 6.0; (3) propanol–H_2O, 7:3, Whatman No. 1, pH 6.0; (4) methyl ethyl ketone saturated with H_2O, Whatman No. 1, unbuffered; (5) methyl ethyl ketone–acetonitrile–H_2O, 84:8:8, Whatman No. 4, pH 4.6; (6) acetone–H_2O, 85:15, Whatman No. 1, unbuffered; (7) butanol saturated with H_2O, Whatman No. 3, unbuffered; (8) ethyl acetate saturated with H_2O, Whatman No. 1, pH 5.5; (9) acetonitrile–H_2O, 2:1, Whatman No. 3, unbuffered.

involves the use of microorganisms. Among these test organisms, *Bacillus subtilis* and *Sarcina lutea* are very frequently used. *Staphylococcus aureus* also finds extensive usage; however, in most cases, it is relatively insensitive to degradation products. Other organisms have been used from time to time.

The relative bioactivity of cephalosporin-related compounds has been summarized (Van Heyningen, 1967). If one refers activity to a fixed test organism such as *Bacillus subtilis*, then one can make generalizations with regard to the effect of structure on activity. Deacetoxycephalosporins are generally lower in potency (10–20%) than the corresponding cephalosporins (Stedman *et al.*, 1964). Deacetylcephalosporins, as a rule, are less than half as active as the parent (Chauvette *et al.*, 1962). Lactones of the deacetylcephalosporins are nearly equally as active as their acetoxyl relative (Chauvette *et al.*, 1962). Double-bond isomerized cephalosporins (Δ^2) are relatively inactive (Chauvette

Table VI

THIN-LAYER CHROMATOGRAPHY DATA

System[a]	Cephalothin	Cephaloridine	Cephaloglycin	Cephalexin	7-ACA	7-ADCA
	R_f values of cephalosporins on silica gel					
1	0.65	0.40	0.60	0.55	0.55	0.45
2	0.45	0.10	0.30	0.25	0.25	—
3	0.30	0.00	0.00	0.00	0.00	0.05
4	0.45	—	—	—	—	—
5	0.60	0.05	0.20	0.20	0.40	0.55
6	0.70	0.10	0.35	0.40	0.00	0.35
7	0.60	0.40	0.30	0.30	0.20	0.30
	R_f values of cephalosporins on polyamide film					
8	—	—	0.75	—	0.30	—
9	—	—	0.50	—	0.15	—
	R_f values of cephalosporins on cellulose					
10	—	—	0.60	0.50	—	—
11	—	—	0.60	0.70	—	0.30

[a] Solvent system is defined as follows: (1) Acetonitrile–H_2O, 4:1; (2) ethyl acetate–acetone–H_2O, 2:4:2; (3) acetone–chloroform–acetic acid, 50:50:7; (4) ethanol–chloroform–acetic acid, 50:100:7.5; (5) acetone–acetic acid, 20:1; (6) ethyl acetate–acetic acid–H_2O, 3:1:1; (7) methanol–ethyl acetate–acetic acid, 50:100:5; (8) methanol–H_2O, 8:2; (9) ethanol–H_2O, 8:2; (10) acetonitrile–H_2O, 3:1; (11) butanol–acetic acid–H_2O, 3:1:1.

and Flynn, 1966). Cephalosporin sulfoxides and sulfones show drastically reduced activity. Many modifications (such as conversion to an amide, ester, or decarboxylation) destroy practically all biological activity. Detailed discussion of all of these points may be found in Chapter 12.

3. RELATIVE MOBILITY IN SOLVENT SYSTEMS

Table V shows the R_f values of various cephalosporins as obtained by paper chromatography. Unless otherwise noted, the equilibrating solvent is the same as the developing solvent, and the paper is untreated Whatman No. 1.*

* Whatman Chromatography Grade No. 1 paper, Catalog 1065, Reeve Angel, 9 Bridewell Place, Clifton, New Jersey.

Inspection of the data in Table V leads one to the conclusion that the mobilities of cephaloglycin and cephalexin can be reversed by proper pH adjustment. Such a reversal is attributable to the slightly different pK_a values for these substances. The use of buffered papers also demonstrates the importance of the "pH–chromatogram" technique for antibiotics (Betina, 1965).

Table VI contains data derived from the thin-layer techniques generally used for the cephalosporins. Silica gel chromatography of the cephalosporins (or penicillins) is not entirely satisfactory. Most of the chromatograms obtained using silica gel show considerable streaking and decomposition. Nevertheless, in many cases, such behavior can be recognized and the results interpreted on that basis.

TLC on polyamide resin has been found to be useful for cephaloglycin, cephalexin, and other amino-acid-like substances. Because of the hydrogen-bonding nature of this adsorbent, improved separations result.

Cellulose chromatography (TLC) is rapid, and for unbuffered systems, it gives results which are nearly equivalent to paper. Cellulose chromatography does not readily lend itself to buffering, and it does not respond uniformly to solvent systems low in water content.

B. Chromatography of Individual Cephalosporins

1. CEPHALOSPORIN C

Cephalosporin C is the starting material for most cephalosporins. Numerous literature references to the chromatographic separation of cephalosporin C from related substances are available. The chromatographic separation of cephalosporin C from penicillin N was reported by Abraham and Newton (1956). Cephalosporin C was described as being less mobile than penicillin N when a 100% methanol developing solvent and pH 6.0 phosphate buffered paper were used.

Claridge and Johnson (1962) reported the separation of cephalosporin C, penicillin N, and cephalosporin P.* Approximate R_f's were 0.3, 0.5, and 0.95, respectively. Their developing solvent was butanol–acetic acid–water, 60:15:25, used with S&S 589 white ribbon paper.† *Alcaligenes faecalis* ATCC 8750 and *Neisseria catarrhalis* were described as being responsive to cephalosporin C but not to penicillin N.

Thomas (1961) described a paper chromatographic system which separates cephalosporin C from penicillin N and the penicillin N nucleus, 6-aminopenicillanic acid. His developing solvent was *n*-butanol–acetic acid–water,

---

* Cephalosporins P have a steroid structure.

† Schleicher and Schuell Ind., Keene, New Hampshire.

4:1:5, on Whatman No. 4 paper. He was the first to use a starch–iodine spray to visualize the chromatogram.

Jeffery *et al.* (1961) reported the separation of cephalosporin C, deacetylcephalosporin C, and cephalosporin C lactone. The authors used a 70% aqueous propanol system on unbuffered Whatman No. 1 paper. The reported R_f's were 0.77, 0.60, and 0.98, respectively. In a solvent system of *n*-butanol–acetic acid–water, 4:1:4, on Whatman No. 1 paper, the R_f's were 0.78, 0.57, and 0.85, respectively.

Demain *et al.* (1963) reported deacetylcephalosporin C to be less mobile than cephalosporin C in an isopropanol–water–pyridine system, 65:30:5.

O'Callaghan and Muggleton (1963) reported mobilities for nine cephalosporin compounds and metabolites. Cephalosporin C at 0.20 and cephalosporin C lactone at 0.30 were among the R_f's reported for a 70% aqueous propanol system. The system employed Whatman No. 1 paper buffered to pH 6.0 with N/20 sodium phosphate. A butanol–ethanol–water system was also reported.

Betina (1965) has given an excellent summary of the paper chromatographic systems used for cephalosporins and related compounds.

At the present time, the two solvent systems enjoying the most use are the methanol–propanol–water system, 6:2:1, of Elander *et al.* (1960) and a butanol–acetic acid–water system, 3:1:1, similar to that of Claridge and Johnson (1962). In cases where additional mobility is needed, methanol–water mixtures may be employed; where less mobility is desired, propanol–water mixtures may be used.

Thin-layer chromatography, because of the high polarity of cephalosporin C, is usually performed with cellulose as the sorbent rather than silica gel. Streaking and some on-plate decomposition occur with silica gel, which make its use less desirable.

The use of ultraviolet absorption (or quenching where indicator is used) is a very sensitive method for the detection of cephalosporin C. Iodine stain is used frequently, and bioautography is adequate provided the substance is first converted to a more active substance (Loder *et al.*, 1961). *Bacillus subtilis* and *Staphylococcus aureus* are commonly used as test organisms.

Jeffery *et al.* (1961) reported poor separation of deacetylcephalosporin C from cephalosporin C by electrophoresis at pH 7.0, 4.5, and 2.2. Maximum separation between the centers of the spots was 0.6 cm. However, the same paper reported a good electrophoretic separation of cephalosporin C lactone. The lactone was practically immobile at pH's 4.5 and 7.0 (but slightly toward the cathode); whereas, deacetylcephalosporin C and cephalosporin C moved toward the anode. Electrophoresis was carried out at 14 V/cm for 2.5 hours.

Hale *et al.* (1961) and Loder *et al.* (1961) reported that electrophoresis could be used to separate cephalosporin C from related substances. Loder listed 15 substances which were separated under like conditions at five different pH values. At pH 2.2, cephalosporin C was practically immobile; whereas, 7-ACA and 6-aminopenicillanic acid (6-APA) moved toward the cathode. Using the same conditions, cephalosporin C lactone moved toward the anode. At pH 4.5, cephalosporin C and 7-ACA separated well from each other and from cephalosporin C lactone, but 6-APA was poorly resolved from 7-ACA. Deacetylcephalosporin C was not reported in the article. The conditions used were 14 V/cm for 3 hours.

Smith *et al.* (1967) also demonstrated the electrophoretic separation of cephalosporin C from 7-ACA and 6-APA at pH 4.5. High-voltage electrophoresis (4 kV) was used with Whatman No. 4 paper support for only 35 minutes.

2. 7-Aminocephalosporanic Acid (7-ACA)

The chromatography of 7-ACA is somewhat difficult. The solubility of this substance is low. 7-ACA is relatively unstable in solution and is extremely unstable on silica gel. Nevertheless, literature references are relatively abundant.

Morin *et al.* (1964) used chromatography to follow the first practical cleavage of cephalosporin C to produce 7-ACA. Loder *et al.* (1961) reported the use of an aqueous ethyl acetate system to separate 11 substances derived from, or similar to, 7-ACA. Cephalosporin C was reported to have an R_f of 0.04; 6-APA, 0.14; and benzylpenicillin, 0.45.

Water–acetone mixtures of various concentrations are the solvent systems of preference for 7-ACA. While there has been considerable use of this solvent system, there are no publications available at this date (Smiley, 1964). An acetone–water mixture, 85:15, is generally employed with unbuffered Whatman No. 1 paper. Dissolution of 7-ACA for application to the paper is aided by the use of a buffer at approximately pH 7.

Thin-layer chromatography of 7-ACA, except on cellulose or polyamide film, is subject to on-plate degradation and consequent streaking. In silica gel chromatography, acetonitrile–water mixtures are commonly used. On cellulose, acetone–water mixtures are most frequently used. Methanol–water mixtures are excellent for separations on polyamide resin.

Ultraviolet absorbance and quenching are very sensitive means of detection. Bioautography can be used with high 7-ACA loading, using *Bacillus subtilis.* Iodoplatinate and ninhydrin are commonly used spray reagents for chemical detection.

Electrophoresis has been employed from time to time (Loder *et al.*, 1961), but automated cation exchange chromatography has been preferred, to provide similar data, because of its greater sensitivity.

3. CEPHALOTHIN

Literature references to the chromatography of cephalothin are now becoming abundant. Most of the literature describes work involving metabolites or degradation products arising from cephalothin.

Cephalothin hydrolyzes slowly in water solution to produce deacetylcephalothin (Wick, 1964). Esterases present in the liver, kidneys, and the intestine and stomach walls act upon cephalothin to form deacetylcephalothin (Van Heyningen, 1967). Deacetylcephalothin, in turn, is converted to the corresponding lactone.

Miller (1962) was the first to report a method for the chromatography of cephalothin. The developing solvent was methyl ethyl ketone (MEK) saturated with water. Relative mobilities of deacetylcephalothin and cephalothin lactone were described.

Hoehn and Davis (1970) use a more recent modification of this system. The developing solvent is MEK–acetonitrile–water, 84:8:8. The equilibrating solvent is a two-phase mixture of MEK and water, 3:2. Whatman No. 4 paper impregnated with 0.1 M acetate buffer at pH 4.6 (original preparation) is used. *Bacillus subtilis* is used for detection. The acetonitrile causes deacetylcephalothin to move farther from the origin, and the Whatman No. 4 paper minimizes binding by proteinaceous contaminants. Other precautions and preliminary steps are also taken. The R_f values of cephalothin and deacetylcephalothin are 0.45 and 0.20, respectively, in this system.

Although cephalothin is stated to be more biologically active at a low pH (Barber and Waterworth, 1964), all bioautographic techniques employ an agar medium which is practically neutral.

Another paper system which has been used extensively is the ethyl acetate system of Martin and Shaw (1965). Many modifications of this method exist, including the removal of butanol from the developing system (Smiley and Ralston, 1960). Minor pH changes and humidity cause extraordinary changes in the substance mobility.

Sullivan and McMahon (1967) reported a butanol–water saturated system for cephalothin metabolites present in urine. Whatman No. 1 unbuffered paper was employed.

Thin-layer chromatography is extensively used for cephalothin. Silica gel is used more for this cephalosporin than for any other. Cephalothin is the least polar of all the cephalosporins discussed in this chapter and is also one of the most stable.

The stability of cephalothin is usually followed on silica gel plates, using a solvent system of acetone–chloroform–acetic acid, 50:50,7.5 (Hussey, 1966). Vanillin dissolved in a mixture of phosphoric acid–methanol, 1:1, is used as a spray for detection. In cases where the deacetylcephalothin mobility needs to be increased, a mixture of ethanol–chloroform–acetic acid, 50:100:7.5, may be used.

Several means of detection are used for cephalothin. *Bacillus subtilis* has been mentioned for bioautographs. *Sarcina lutea* is slightly more sensitive and is frequently used. Ninhydrin is a fairly effective spray; iodine absorption is good; and ultraviolet absorption and quenching are excellent.

Reference to electrophoresis of cephalothin is found in the Martin and Shaw (1965) article. Cephalothin can be made to move as an anion, but unfortunately, deacetylcephalothin is not resolved.

4. CEPHALORIDINE

As with cephalothin, cephaloridine is metabolized, at least partially, to deacetylcephalothin (Sullivan and McMahon, 1967). Deacetylcephalothin in turn, is converted to the corresponding lactone.

Martin and Shaw (1965) reported paper chromatographic separation techniques for cephaloridine. The systems described are commonly referred to as the "MEK" system (1), the "ethyl acetate" system (2), and the "propanol" system (3). Variations exist for all three systems, mainly due to compensations for temperature or humidity differences prevalent from laboratory to laboratory. In addition to the organic solvent named, water in proper proportion and optimum pH of the paper are all that is generally required to achieve separation.

The accompanying illustration (Fig. 2) indicates the separations achieved by Martin and Shaw. Descending chromatography was used in all three cases. Their article should be referred to for precise details on solvent preparation, etc.

As is somewhat obvious from Fig. 2, System 3 (propanol) enjoys considerable use as a stability test. Deacetylcephalothin (E) and cephalothin lactone (F) are well resolved from the parent cephaloridine. In addition, two other unidentified degradation products are also resolved. System 2, or System 1 with modifications, is more suitable for assuring complete separation of cephalothin and cephaloridine. The greater separation obtained between cephalothin and cephaloridine allows the chromatogram to be loaded heavily without loss of resolution. (Aqueous acetone mixtures as the developing solvent have also been used for this purpose.)

Sullivan and McMahon (1967) used a butanol–water saturated system to determine cephaloridine metabolites in urine.

Bacillus subtilis is a convenient test organism for cephaloridine and is best suited for System 3 where well-defined zones are necessary. *Sarcina lutea* is more sensitive to low levels of cephaloridine, cephalothin, and deacetylcephalothin, but this organism does not produce the well-defined zones of inhibition found with *Bacillus subtilis*. *Staphylococcus aureus* has also been mentioned by Martin and Shaw (1965) as a test organism.

Thin-layer chromatography of cephaloridine, except on cellulose, generally leads to on-plate decomposition. Aqueous acetonitrile mixtures have been used with silica gel, but several extraneous spots appear accompanied by heavy streaking. With cellulose as the support medium, aqueous acetone mixtures have found the greatest use.

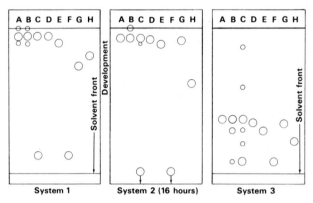

Fig. 2. Paper chromatography of cephaloridine and related compounds. (A) Cephaloridine, (B) cephaloridine solid (30% decomposition), (C) cephaloridine in aqueous solution (30% decomposition), (D) 7-(2'-thienylacetamido)-ceph-2-em-3-methylpyridinium-4-carboxylate, (E) 7-(2'-thienylacetamido)-3-hydroxymethylceph-3-em-4-oic acid, (F) lactone of E, (G) 7-(2'-thienylacetamido)-ceph-3-em-3-methylpyridinium-4-carboxylate, (H) sodium cephalothin.

Historically, the first chromatographic separation of a cephalosporin C_A compound (not cephaloridine) was reported by Hale *et al.* (1961). Paper electrophoresis was employed to separate cephalosporin C_A (pyridine) (not cephaloridine) from cephalosporin C. The pH used for electrophoresis was 7.0, at which value cephalosporin C_A (pyridine) is effectively neutral and thus immobile.

Martin and Shaw (1965) used electrophoresis to separate cephaloridine from cephalothin and deacetylcephalothin. Using a pH of 2.4 cephaloridine acts as a base cation. Cephalothin is essentially neutral at this pH; whereas, deacetylcephalothin acts as an anion. Unfortunately, cephalothin lactone is also a neutral compound and was unresolved from cephalothin. Whatman No. 17 paper was used at 20 V/cm for 2 hours.

For chemical detection, ultraviolet absorbance and quenching, ninhydrin, and iodoplatinate are generally used. Sodium hydroxide treatment, followed by starch–iodine, is a sensitive method for detecting the β-lactam nucleus, and iodine absorption itself is good.

5. CEPHALOGLYCIN

Chromatography of cephaloglycin has been described by Hoehn and Pugh (1968). Cephaloglycin decomposes and is metabolized in a similar manner to cephalothin and cephaloridine (Sullivan *et al.*, 1969b). Deacetylcephaloglycin and deacetylcephaloglycin lactone, as a consequence, are mentioned as related products.

Paper is the recommended chromatographic support for assay of serum and urine samples, where salts and interfering substances are prevalent. Hoehn and Pugh (1968) recommended a solvent system of butanol–acetic acid–water 3:1:1, on Whatman No. 1 paper. This solvent system was excellent for the detection of deacetylcephaloglycin but only marginal for the detection of deacetylcephaloglycin lactone since the separation of this latter substance from cephaloglycin is minimal. Descending chromatography with Whatman No. 20 paper, using a developing solvent of 85% aqueous acetonitrile, resulted in better separation of the deacetylcephaloglycin lactone.

Thin-layer chromatography, employing both cellulose and silica gel, has been used extensively. With silica gel, aqueous acetonitrile systems are most generally employed. Some on-plate decomposition occurs but it is minimal.

Cellulose is recommended primarily for cephaloglycin derived from chemical sources but not for biological samples containing residual levels of cephaloglycin. Cellulose has been shown to be involved in formation of "artifacts" (spots unrelated to the condition or purity of the actual sample) when used with samples containing certain salts and proteins. The solvent system reported by Hoehn and Pugh (1968) was composed of acetonitrile–ethyl acetate–water, 3:1:1. The test organism which gave the best response to decomposition products as well as to cephaloglycin itself was *Sarcina lutea*. Kukolja (1968) reported a solvent system of acetonitrile–water, 3:1, that was useful for the chromatography of cephaloglycin and its decomposition products on cellulose. Both *Bacillus subtilis* and *Sarcina lutea* were used as test organisms.

Electrophoresis has not been extensively employed in the assays for cephaloglycin. Cephaloglycin has its maximum stability at its isoelectric point, at which electrophoretic mobility is lacking. If the pH of the electrolyte is altered to allow movement, deacetylcephaloglycin maintains the same mobility as cephaloglycin itself. (A good separation of deacetylcephaloglycin lactone would be achieved, however.)

Cephaloglycin may be detected by using one of the following techniques: ultraviolet absorbance and quenching, ninhydrin spraying, iodoplatinate spraying, or iodine absorption.

The Moore–Stein amino acid analyzer proved to be a versatile tool for the assay of possible impurities inherent in the synthesis of cephaloglycin (Spencer *et al.*, 1966). The separation of impurities is based on using a cation exchange resin, followed by elution at a controlled pH. Unreacted starting materials, 7-ACA and phenylglycine, may be determined quantitatively in cephaloglycin at low concentrations (see appendix). In addition, the presence of less active (biologically) L-cephaloglycin may be determined in D-cephaloglycin by this technique.

6. CEPHALEXIN

The solvent system of butanol–acetic acid–water, 3:1:1, is satisfactory for cephalexin. Whatman No. 1 paper is employed, and the solvent requires

Table VII
CEPHALEXIN IN URINE

Sample no.	(Milligrams of cephalexin per milliliter)	
	Amino acid analyzer	Microbiological assay
1	0.57	0.59
2	1.33	1.45
3	1.53	1.56
4	0.70	0.87
5	0.70	0.70
6	1.19	1.26
7	0.59	0.63
8	2.78	2.73
9	1.37	1.38
10	1.24	1.38

15–16 hours for an 18-in. migration. This is the solvent system reported by Hoehn and Pugh (1968) for cephaloglycin. The system will separate cephaloglycin from cephalexin, cephaloglycin being less mobile. The system is also effective when considerably less (lower ratio) acetic acid is used. The developed chromatogram can be examined under ultraviolet light, dipped in ninhydrin, or bioautographed, using *Sarcina lutea*.

Thin-layer chromatography has also been employed on cephalexin. Using silica gel, there is slight decomposition, similar to cephalothin, but not to such an extent as to cause problems in interpretation. Aqueous acetonitrile mixtures and ethyl acetate–acetic acid–water mixtures give good resolution. Cellulose is again the preferred sorbent since it is inert toward cephalexin. Aqueous acetonitrile has been most commonly used with cellulose for cephalexin.

Electrophoretic data with respect to cephalexin are lacking in the literature at this date. The compound is sufficiently stable to allow considerable pH control, but generally, any information obtainable by this means can also be obtained by using cation exchange on an automated analyzer.

Cephalexin may be detected, as already indicated in part, by ultraviolet absorbance and quenching, ninhydrin, iodoplatinate, alkaline permanganate, and phosphomolybdic acid. Iodine detection is fair, and vanillin–phosphoric acid spray (as mentioned for cephalothin) has had some use. Of the microorganisms used, *Sarcina lutea* is preferred over *Bacillus subtilis* or *Staphylococcus aureus*.

The Moore–Stein amino acid analyzer has recently been used for the determination of 7-ADCA and phenylglycine in cephalexin (see Appendix). Amino acid analyzer data for cephalexin in urine samples have been compared to microbiological data (Table VII) (Cole, 1971).

V. Physical–Chemical Determinations

This section deals primarily with the physical–chemical aspects of the cephalosporins which are useful for analytical purposes. Chapter VIII gives a more thorough and comprehensive coverage of the physical chemistry of the cephalosporins.

A. Ultraviolet Absorption

Absorption at 263 nm due to the phenyl group has been used to determine benzylpenicillin content (Grove and Randall, 1955). The penicillin ring system itself has a low ultraviolet (UV) absorption; whereas the cephalosporin fused ring system exhibits a rather high UV absorption (Table VIII).

Ultraviolet spectra of these compounds are used for identification as well as for purity evaluation (appendix). With cephaloridine, the ratio of the absorbance at 240 nm to that at 255 nm provides an indication of the onset of degradation (Marrelli, 1966). See Table IX.

It has been noted that when the loss in potency is greater than about 30%, the difference between the chemical and microbiological results becomes significant and progressively greater as degradation proceeds. This is essentially true of most chemical methods, and the microbiological assay should then be considered more reliable.

Low concentrations of cephalosporin C may be determined by measuring the decrease in UV absorption at 260 nm, following enzymatic hydrolysis with a β-lactamase under controlled conditions (Marrelli, 1962). See Table X.

Table VIII

$E_{1\%}^{1cm}$ VALUES OF CEPHALOSPORINS[a]

Compound	$E_{1\%}^{1cm}$	Wavelength (nm)
Sodium cephalosporin C	200	260
7-ACA	310	265
Sodium cephalothin	336	237[b]
Sodium cephalothin	204	265
Cephaloridine	381	240[b]
Cephaloridine	350	255
Cephaloglycin	218	260
Cephalexin	236	262

[a] 25 μg/ml of aqueous solutions.
[b] Mainly thienyl contribution.

Table IX

STABILITY OF A 17% W/V SOLUTION OF CEPHALORIDINE IN
METHANOL–WATER, 1:4, AT 28°C

Time (hours)	UV ratio (abs.$_{240}$/abs.$_{255}$)	% of initial	
		Microbiological	UV (Based on abs.$_{255}$)
0	1.089	100	100
24	1.153	93.3	89.5
48	1.219	77.2	80.1
72	1.268	65.2	74.4
96	1.318	50.2	67.0

Table X

UV–ENZYMATIC HYDROLYSIS OF CEPHALOSPORIN C[a]

Cephalosporin C (μg/ml)	Δ abs.$_{260(nm)}$	% apparent hydrolysis
25	0.404	86.8
50	0.792	85.6
75	1.174	85.0

[a] pH = 7.0; total volume = 4.1 ml; β-lactamase enzyme (1:10) = 0.1 ml; time = 40 minutes.

This is particularly useful when other UV-absorbing substances of a non-cephalosporin nature are present.

B. Infrared Absorption

Infrared spectra of cephalosporins are routinely used for the identification of these compounds (Appendix). The spectra are obtained using the potassium bromide pellet technique. A 13.0-mm pellet requires approximately 1.3–1.5 mg of sample. Sample spectra are compared to those of reference standards or preparations of known purity. Significant variations from standard spectra may then be attributed to one or a combination of several factors, as follows:

1. Sample contamination, including water
2. Sample degradation
3. Crystallinity differences, including hydration
4. Polymorphism or solid state effects resulting from preparation of the pellet

The last factor mentioned has not been found to be a problem with cephalosporins.

Perhaps the most characteristic region in the infrared spectra of cephalosporin compounds is the carbonyl stretching region, which exists approximately between 1500 and 1800 cm^{-1}. Opening of the β-lactam ring, ester cleavage, and/or lactone formation can be indicated by changes in this part of the spectrum.

C. Nuclear Magnetic Resonance

Nuclear magnetic resonance (NMR) spectra are used for the identification of cephalosporin compounds (Martin and Shaw, 1965). Samples are placed in solution with deuterated water or deuterated dimethyl sulfoxide. Trifluoroacetic acid is sometimes added to the deuterated water to facilitate solution. Sample spectra are compared to those of reference standards. Variations from the standard spectra may arise from one or a combination of the following factors: (1) solvent contamination (benzene, isopropanol, isopropyl acetate, etc.); (2) sample degradation evidenced by (a) acetate ion formation due to ester cleavage or (b) decrease in lactam proton peaks due to cleavage of the β-lactam ring.

The limits of detection for products of contamination or degradation depend on the nature of the products, but generally, they range 3–5%.

Analytical information may be derived by observing the contribution of the following groups to the NMR spectrum: (a) β-lactam protons, (b) methylene groups present in a ring, (c) aromatic or thiophene protons, and (d) methyl protons, e.g., from acetate. The spectrum should be obtained as soon as the sample is in solution, since some cephalosporins have limited stability in the solvents used.

D. Optical Rotatory Dispersion

Optical rotation has been used as an auxiliary method for the identification and quantitative determination of cephalosporins (Martin and Shaw, 1965; Spencer et al., 1966). Approximate values and concentrations used are outlined in Table XI.

Table XI
SPECIFIC ROTATION OF CEPHALOSPORINS

Compound	Specific rotation $[\alpha]_D$	Concentration, % w/v
Sodium cephalothin	+130°	5.0, H_2O
Cephaloridine	+48.0°	1.0, H_2O
Cephaloglycin	+93.8°	1.0, Acetoni-trile–H_2O, 1:1
Cephalexin	+153°	1.0, H_2O

E. X-ray Diffraction

X-ray diffraction patterns of the cephalosporins are routinely used for identification purposes. Sodium cephalothin occurs as one crystalline form (Rose, 1963). Cephaloridine (Chapman et al., 1968), cephaloglycin, and cephalexin (Pfeiffer et al., 1971) display many different forms, depending on the particular solvent used for crystallization.

F. Miscellaneous Techniques

Relatively pure lots of cephalosporins have been titrated with perchloric acid in a glacial acetic acid medium. Degradation products, starting materials, as well as numerous nonrelated compounds may titrate as well, and consequently, they must be absent for a valid determination.

Polarography has been utilized to evaluate lots of cephalosporin C, cephalothin, and cephaloridine (Jones et al., 1968). Benner (1971) describes a rapid polarographic assay for the quantitative determination of penicillins and cephalosporins in serum.

Acknowledgments

The author wishes to express his indebtedness to Mr. R. L. Hussey for his contribution of the section on chromatography determinations and also to Dr. R. J. Simmons for his assistance on the preparation of the section on microbiological determinations.

References

Abraham, E. P. (1965). *Amer. J. Med.* **39**, 692.

Abraham, E. P., and Newton, G. G. F. (1956). *Biochem. J.* **62**, 651.

Alicino, J. F. (1946). *Ind. Eng. Chem. Anal. Ed.* **18**, 619.

Alicino, J. F. (1961). *Anal. Chem.* **33**, 648.

Barber, M., and Waterworth, P. M. (1964). *Brit. Med. J.* **2**, 344.

Benner, E. J. (1971). *Antimicrob. Ag. Chemother.* **1970**.

Betina, V. (1965). *In* "Chromatographic Reviews" (M. Lederer, ed.), Vol. 7, p. 119. Elsevier, New York.

Boxer, G. E., and Everett, P. M. (1949). *Anal. Chem.* **21**, 670.

Burton, R. M., San Pietro, A., and Kaplan, N. O. (1957). *Arch. Biochem. Biophys.* **70**, 87.

Chapman, J. H., Page, J. E., Parker, A. C., Rogers, D., Sharp, C. J., and Staniforth, S. E. (1968). *J. Pharm. Pharmacol.* **20**, 418.

Chauvette, R. R., and Flynn, E. H. (1966). *J. Med. Chem.* **9**, 741.

Chauvette, R. R., Flynn, E. H., Jackson, B. G., Lavagnino, E. R., Morin, R. B., Mueller, R. A., Pioch, R. P., Roeske, R. W., Ryan, C. W., Spencer, J. L., and Van Heyningen, E. (1962). *J. Amer. Chem. Soc.* **84**, 3401.

Chou, T. S. (1969). *J. Med. Chem.* **12**, 925.

Claridge, C. A., and Johnson, D. L. (1962). *In* "Antimicrobial Agents and Chemotherapy" (J. C. Sylvester, ed.), p. 682. Plenum Press, New York.

Cole, T. E. (1971). Unpublished results.

Demain, A. L., Walton, R. B., Newkirk, J. F., and Miller, I. M. (1963). *Nature* **199**, 909.

Doyle, F. P., and Nayler, J. H. C. (1964). *In* "Advances in Drug Research" (N. J. Harper and A. B. Simmonds, eds.), Vol. 1, p. 59. Academic Press, New York and London.

Elander, R. P., Stauffer, J. F., and Backus, M. P. (1960). *Antimicrob. Ag. Ann.* 95.

Ford, J. H. (1947). *Anal. Chem.* **19**, 1004.

Grove, D. C., and Randall, W. A. (1955). *In* "Assay Methods of Antibiotics, A Laboratory Manual," p. 200. Medical Encyclopedia, New York.

Hale, C. W., Newton, G. G. F., and Abraham, E. P. (1961). *Biochem. J.* **79**, 403.

Hoehn, M. M., and Davis, N. E. (1970). *Appl. Microbiol.* **20**, 734.

Hoehn, M. M., and Pugh, C. T. (1968). *Appl. Microbiol.* **16**, 1132.

Hussey, R. L. (1966). Personal communication.

Jeffery, J. D'A., Abraham, E. P., and Newton, G. G. F. (1961). *Biochem. J.* **81**, 591.

Jones, I. F., Page, J. E., and Rhodes, C. T. (1968). *J. Pharm. Pharmacol. Suppl.* **20**, 45S.

Kavanagh, F. (1963a). "Analytical Microbiology" (F. Kavanagh, ed.), p. 327. Academic Press, New York and London.

Kavanagh, F. (1963b). "Analytical Microbiology" (F. Kavanagh, ed.), p. 316. Academic Press, New York and London.

Kavanagh, F. (1972). "Analytical Microbiology," Vol. 2, (F. Kavanagh, ed.). Academic Press, New York and London.

Kukolja, S. (1968). *J. Med. Chem.* **11**, 1067.

Kuzel, N. R., and Kavanagh, F. (1971). *J. Pharm. Sci.* **60**.

Lee, C. C., Herr, E. B., Jr., and Anderson, R. C. (1963). *Clin. Med.* **70**, 1123.

Lipmann, F., and Tuttle, L. L. (1945). *J. Biol. Chem.* **159**, 21.

Loder, B., Newton, G. G. F., and Abraham, E. P. (1961). *Biochem. J.* **79**, 408.

Marrelli, L. P. (1962). Unpublished results.

Marrelli, L. P. (1966). Unpublished results.

Marrelli, L. P. (1968). *J. Pharm. Sci.* **57**, 2172.

Martin, J. L., and Shaw, W. H. C. (1965). *In* "Proceedings of the S.A.C. Conference, Nottingham, 1965," p. 32. Heffer, Cambridge.

Miller, R. P. (1962). *Antibiot. Chemother.* **12**, 689.

Morin, R. B. (1964). Abstracts of 148th Meeting of the Amer. Chem. Soc., Chicago, Illinois, p. 8P.

Murakawa, T., Wakai, Y., Nishida, M., Fujii, R., Konno, M., Okada, K., Gato, S., and Kuwahara, S. (1970). *J. Antibiot.* **23**, 250.

O'Callaghan, C. H., and Muggleton, P. W. (1963). *Biochem. J.* **89**, 304.

Pfeiffer, R. R., Yang, K. S., and Tucker, M. A. (1971). *J. Pharm. Sci.* **60**.

Redstone, M. O. (1971). Unpublished results.

Rose, H. A. (1963). *J. Pharm. Sci.* **52**, 1008.

Roudebush, H. E. (1969). *Proc. 1969 Technicon Int. Congr. Automated Analy.*, Chicago June 6.

Shriner, R. L., and Fuson, R. C. (1940). "Identification of Organic Compounds," 2nd ed., p. 68. Wiley, New York.

Smiley, J. W. (1964). Personal communication.

Smiley, J. W., and Ralston, S. J. (1960). Personal communication.

Smith, B., Warren, S. C., Newton, G. G. F., and Abraham, E. P. (1967). *Biochem. J.* **103**, 877.

Spencer, J. L., Flynn, E. H., Roeske, R. W., Siu, F. Y., and Chauvette, R. R. (1966). *J. Med. Chem.* **9**, 746.

Stedman, R. J., Swered, K., and Hoover, J. R. E. (1964). *J. Med. Chem.* **7**, 117.

Stevenson, C. E., and Bechtel, L. D. (1971). Unpublished results.

Stewart, G. T., and Holt, R. J. (1964). *Lancet* **2**, 1305.

Sullivan, H. R., and McMahon, R. E. (1967). *Biochem. J.* **102**, 976.

Sullivan, H. R., Billings, R. E., and McMahon, R. E. (1969a). *J. Antibiot.* **22**, 195.

Sullivan, H. R., Billings, R. E., and McMahon, R. E. (1969b). *J. Antibiot.* **22**, 27.

Thomas, R. (1961). *Nature* **191**, 1161.

Van Heyningen, E. (1967). *In* "Advances in Drug Research" (N. J. Harper and A. B. Simmonds, eds.), p. 43. Academic Press, New York and London.

Wagman, G. H., and Bailey, J. V. (1969). *J. Chromatog.* **41**, 263.

Weiss, P. J. (1959). *Antibiot. Chemother.* **9**, 660.

Wick, W. E. (1964). *J. Bacteriol.* **87**, 1162.

Wick, W. E. (1968). Personal communication.

Wick, W. E., and Wright, W. E. (1968). Personal communication.

Chapter 15

β-LACTAM ANTIBIOTICS FROM STREPTOMYCES

R. NAGARAJAN

> Among the lower forms of life, even
> more than among the large species of
> animals and plants, life inhibits life.
>
> *Louis Pasteur*

I. Introduction

The discovery of penicillin marked the dawn of a new era in medicine. Penicillin was the first antibiotic substance used to combat infections in man.

As the clinical uses of penicillin became clear, a massive search for other useful antibiotic substances was undertaken. This has resulted in the discovery of a number of chemotherapeutically important antibiotics.

Excellent reviews of the fascinating story of penicillin are available (Flory *et al.*, 1949; Clarke *et al.*, 1949). The search for antibiotic substances, triggered by penicillin, led to the discovery by Brotzu (1948) of cephalosporin C from a *Cephalosporium* species. A discussion of various aspects of the discovery and structural characterization of cephalosporin C can be found in Chapter 1.

Several taxonomically unrelated true fungi produce penicillins (Sanders, 1949), but only one species of *Streptomyces* has been reported to yield penicillin

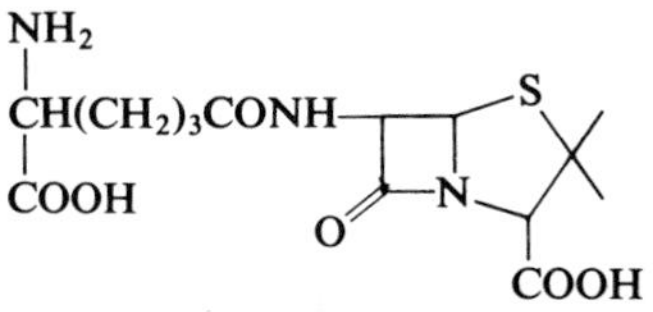

$$NH_2$$
$$CH(CH_2)_3CONH-$$
$$COOH$$
$$COOH$$

(*1*)

$$NH_2$$
$$CH(CH_2)_3CONH-$$
$$COOH$$
$$R_1$$
$$CH_2OCOR_2$$
$$COOH$$

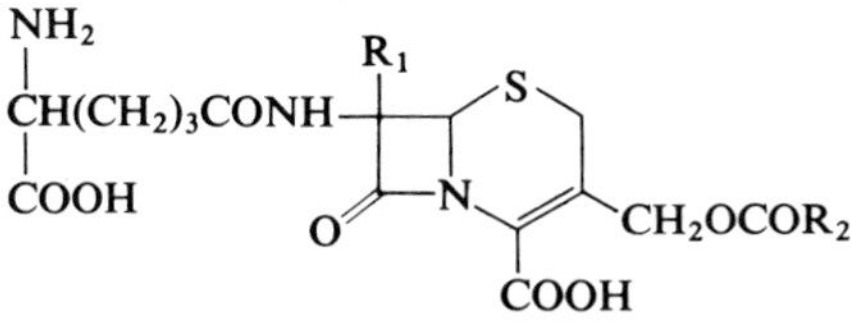

(2) $R_1 = H$, $R_2 = CH_3$
(3) $R_1 = OCH_3$, $R_2 = CH_3$
(4) $R_1 = H$, $R_2 = NH_2$
(5) $R_1 = OCH_3$, $R_2 = NH_2$

Fig. 1. Structures of β-lactam antibiotics.

N (*1*) (Miller *et al.*, 1962). Cephalosporin C (*2*) has been isolated from only one species of *Cephalosporium*. The search for new antibiotic substances at the Lilly Research Laboratories has resulted in the discovery of three new β-lactam antibiotics from two species of *Streptomyces*. The compound 7-(5-amino-5-carboxyvaleramido)-7-methoxycephalosporanic acid (*3*) was produced by a strain of *Streptomyces lipmanii*, NRRL 3584 (Higgens and Kastner, 1971; Nagarajan *et al.*, 1971). A new streptomycete species, *Streptomyces clavuligerus* NRRL 3585 (Higgens and Kastner, 1971), yielded two new antibiotics, 7-(5-amino-5-carboxyvaleramido)-3-carbamoyloxymethyl-3-cephem-4-carboxylic acid (*4*) and 7-(5-amino-5-carboxyvaleramido)-7-methoxy-3-carbamoyloxymethyl-3-cephem-4-carboxylic acid (*5*) (Nagarajan *et al.*, 1971).

Both the cultures also produced penicillin N (*1*). This chapter will be devoted to a discussion of the three new β-lactam antibiotics.

II. Characteristics of the β-Lactam-Producing Cultures

The two cultures producing the β-lactam antibiotics were isolated from soil samples collected in South America. A total of 1852 cultures, composed mainly of *Streptomyces* species, were selected from 235 South American soil samples. Three isolates were obtained which produced β-lactam substances. One of the cultures is a strain of *Streptomyces lipmanii* (Waksman and Curtis) Waksman and Henrici (NRRL 3584). Two cultures which were isolated from another soil produced β-lactam antibiotics, but one culture did not grow on transfer and a complete characterization was not made. The third culture is a new species of streptomycete (Higgens and Kastner, 1971). Sporophores were produced on an extensive aerial mycelium which collectively form a network of short, sym-podially branched hyphae. Usually from one to four spores are born on short, club-shaped side branches. The sporophores eventually segment to form a chain of spores. The spores are oblong to slightly cylindrical, smooth walled, and are gray to grayish-green *en masse*. The name *Streptomyces clavuligerus* Higgens and Kastner was proposed for the new species (Higgens and Kastner, 1971). The type strain of *Streptomyces clavuligerus* was deposited in the Agricultural Research Station, Peoria, Illinois, and was assigned the number NRRL 3585.

III. Production and Isolation of β-Lactam Antibiotics from *Streptomyces*

A. From *Streptomyces lipmanii* NRRL 3584

A new β-lactam antibiotic was isolated from *S. lipmanii* (Belg. Patent 754,424). A sporulated culture of *S. lipmanii* was produced by growing the organism on a nutrient agar slant. The slant had the following composition:

	gm/liter
Dextrin	10
Cottonseed flour	10
Yeast extract	1
Agar	25
Deionized water	

The pH of the medium was adjusted to 7 by addition of sodium hydroxide. The agar slant was inoculated with spores of *S. lipmanii* and incubated for 7 days at 30°C. The agar slants were scraped to remove spores, which were preserved as lyophilized pellets.

The freeze-dried pellets thus obtained were used to inoculate a vegetative medium having the following composition:

	gm/liter
Glucose	5
Dextrin	10
Bacto-tryptone	5
Yeast extract	5
$MgSO_4 \cdot 7H_2O$	2
Deionized water	

The pH of the medium was 6.7.

A 40-liter stainless steel fermentor was used for quantity production. Medium (25 liters) having the following composition was added to the vessel:

	gm/liter
Antifoam	0.20
Glucose	5.00
Dextrin	50.00
Soybean grits	25.00
Molasses, blackstrap	3.00
KH_2PO_4	0.25
$CaCO_3$	2.50
Tap water	

The initial pH was 6.5. The medium was heated for 30 minutes at 120°C, cooled, and then inoculated with a 5% vegetative inoculum obtained with the medium described in the preceding paragraph. The temperature of the fermentation was controlled at 30° for 66 hours, with aeration at the rate of 0.35 v/v/minute and agitation by a mechanical stirrer operated at 420 rpm.

The chromatographic purification of antibiotic (3) was initially monitored by paper bioautography. Chromatographic fractions which showed bioactivity and were one spot in a number of solvent systems, were pooled and lyophilized. The microbiological activity of the lyophilized material containing antibiotic (3) and minor amounts of penicillin N was then measured by using a paper disc agar-diffusion assay (Westhead, 1971). *Salmonella gallinarum* was the test organism. The combined activity of antibiotic (3) and penicillin N was calculated from a dose–response curve prepared from a secondary standard of highly purified antibiotic (3), which was assigned an arbitrary value of 3000 units/mg. An alternate assay of a sample containing antibiotic (3) and penicillin N was obtained by incorporating a sufficient level of penicillinase in the agar plate medium to inactivate the penicillin N during the assay incubation period. The latter assay afforded the activity of antibiotic (3), and the difference between the two assays represented the activity of penicillin N. A similar assay was used to monitor the purification of antibiotics (4) and (5) (Section III, B).

Approximately 60 liters of broth obtained from the above fermentation was filtered with the aid of diatomaceous earth. The broth filtrate was passed over a carbon column and the activity eluted from the carbon with 50% aqueous acetone. The active fractions were pooled, the acetone evaporated, and the aqueous concentrate was chromatographed on an IRA-68 resin in the formate cycle, with 0.1 M ammonium formate as eluant. Active fractions were combined, passed over another carbon column, and the activity eluted with 30% aqueous acetonitrile. The active fractions were pooled and the acetonitrile evaporated. The resulting aqueous solution was freeze-dried, whereupon 25–30 gm of partially purified antibiotic (3), with 120–300 units/mg activity, was obtained.

The freeze-dried material was dissolved in a minimum amount of water and chromatographed on a microcrystalline cellulose column with methanol as eluant. The active fractions were combined, methanol was evaporated to a small volume, and solids were precipitated with acetone. The precipitate was filtered, then washed with acetone and dried. leaving 9–12 gm of antibiotic (3), having about 1700 units/mg of activity. This material was dissolved in water and further purified by chromatography on a silica gel column. The active material was eluted with 30% aqueous acetonitrile. Appropriate fractions were pooled and evaporated to dryness. The residue was dissolved in methanol and then precipitated with acetone. The precipitate was filtered, washed with acetone, and dried in vacuum. The yield of 7-(5-amino-5-carboxyvaleramido)-7-methoxycephalosporanic acid monoammonium salt was 4 gm, having about 2500 units/mg of activity. The free acid of antibiotic (3) could be obtained by treatment of the monoammonium salt with Dowex 50X12 resin.

B. From Streptomyces clavuligerus NRRL 3585

Two new β-lactam antibiotics were isolated from S. clavuligerus (Belg. Patent 754,693). A sporulated culture of S. clavuligerus was produced by growing the organism on a nutrient agar of the following composition:

	gm/liter
Dextrin	10.00
Yeast extract	1.00
Hydrolyzed casein	2.00
Beef extract	1.00
$CoCl_2·7H_2O$	0.01
Agar	20.00
Deionized water	

The pH of the medium was adjusted to 7.0 by addition of sodium hydroxide. The agar slant was inoculated with spores of *S. clavuligerus*, NRRL 3585, and incubated for 7–10 days at 30°C. Spores were removed from the agar slants and preserved as lyophilized pellets.

The pellets were used to inoculate a vegetative medium of the following composition:

	gm/liter
Glycerol	10.0
Sucrose	20.0
Nutrisoy grits	15.0
Amber BYF 300	5.0
Tryptone	5.0
K_2HPO_4	0.2
Tap water	

The pH of the medium was adjusted to 6.5 with sodium hydroxide.

To prepare quantities of active material a 40-liter stainless steel fermentor was used. Medium (25 liters) having the following composition was added to the fermentor:

	gm/liter
Antifoam	0.2
Starch	45.0
Nadrisol	5.0
Soybean flour grits	20.0
Glycerol	7.5
N–Z amine A	5.0
$FeSO_4·7H_2O$	0.1
Tap water	

The pH was adjusted to 6.5 with sodium hydroxide. The medium was heated for 30 minutes at 120°C, cooled, and inoculated with a 5% vegetative inoculum prepared using the medium described in the preceding paragraph. The temperature of the fermentation was controlled at 30° for 66 hours, with aeration at the rate of 0.35 v/v/minutes, and agitation by a mechanical stirrer operated at 420 rpm.

For isolation of the active metabolites, about 75 liters of the above broth were filtered with the aid of diatomaceous earth, and the antibiotics in the broth filtrate were concentrated by chromatography, first on a carbon column, then on a Dowex 1X1 column, followed by another carbon column as described in Section III, A. The above purification procedure afforded 125 gm of a partially purified mixture of antibiotics (4) and (5), with 250–600 units/mg of activity.

The freeze-dried material (40 gm) was stirred with 4 liters of methanol for 16 hours. The insoluble material was removed by filtering, and 20 liters of acetone were added to the methanol solution. The precipitate, which contained the activity, was filtered and dried (20 gm); it had an activity of about 1000 units/mg. This preparation was dissolved in a minimum amount of water and chromatographed on a Sephadex G-25 column. The developing solvent was deionized water. The active fractions were combined and lyophilized, whereupon 10 gm of 2000 units/mg of material was obtained. This material was chromatographed on a silica gel column with 30% aqueous acetonitrile as eluant. The active fractions were pooled, the acetonitrile evaporated, and the aqueous solution freeze-dried, and there were obtained 5 gm of purified mixture of antibiotics (4) and (5) with an activity of about 2700 units/mg. Final separation of the antibiotics was accomplished by chromatography on a microcrystalline cellulose column with 30% acetonitrile as eluant. The fractions were monitored by bioautogram, and appropriate fractions were pooled. The acetonitrile was evaporated, and lyophilization of the aqueous concentrate afforded the monoammonium salts of 7-(5-amino-5-carboxyvaleramido)-3-carbamoyloxymethyl-3-cephem-4-carboxylic acid (150 mg), and 7-(5-amino-5-carboxyvaleramido)-7-methoxy-3-carbamoyloxymethyl-3-cephem-4-carboxylic acid (2.5 gm) as white, amorphous powders. The free acids of the two antibiotics (4) and (5) could be obtained by treatment of the monoammonium salt with Dowex 50W-X12 resin.

IV. Physical–Chemical Properties

The three new β-lactam antibiotics (3), (4), and (5) isolated from *Streptomyces* are white, amorphous powders which exhibit a number of common physical–chemical properties. These characteristics are summarized in Table I and

Table I

PHYSICAL–CHEMICAL PROPERTIES OF CEPHALOSPORIN ANTIBIOTICS

	(2)	(3)	(4)	(5)
IR (mull) (cm^{-1})	1780 (β-lactam) 1730, 1230 (O-acetyl)	1770 (β-lactam) 1730, 1230 (O-acetyl)	1770 (β-lactam) 1700 (carbamate)	1770 (β-lactam) 1710 (carbamate)
UV (H$_2$O) (λ$_{max}$ in nm)	260(E$_{1\%}^{1cm}$ 188)	265(E$_{1\%}^{1cm}$ 155) 242(E$_{1\%}^{1cm}$ 130)	261(E$_{1\%}^{1cm}$ 161)	264(E$_{1\%}^{1cm}$ 149) 242(E$_{1\%}^{1cm}$ 124)
Amino acid (μmoles/mg)				
(a) α-Amino adipic acid	2.46	2.39	2.09	1.97
(b) Glycine	0.13	0.76	0.13	0.61
Potentiometric titration (66% DMF)	pK$_a$'s 3.9, 5.3, 10.5; mol wt 440	pK$_a$'s 3.9, 5.3, 10.5; mol wt 480	pK$_a$'s 4.0, 5.3, 10.5; mol wt 460	pK$_a$'s 4.2, 5.6, 10.4; mol wt 450
NMR(D$_2$O)	4.34(H-7, d, 4.7); 4.85 (H-6, d, 4.7); 5.05, 5.25 (3-CH$_2$, dd, 12.5); 6.15–6.3 NH$_2$CHCOOH, m); 6.28, 6.60(2-CH$_2$, dd, 18); 7.40–7.70(CH$_2$CO, m); 7.87(CH$_3$, s); 7.85–8.50 (CH$_2$CH$_2$, m)	4.84(1H, s); 5.14(1H, d, 12.5); 5.32(1H, d, 12.5); 6.1–6.3 (1H, m); 6.33 (1H, d, 18); 6.47(3H, s); 6.71 (1H, d, 18); 7.4–7.7 (2H, m); 7.90(3H, s); 7.9–8.4(4H, m)	4.33 (1H, d, 5); 4.85 (1H, d, 5); 5.0 (1H, d, 13); 5.32 (1H, d, 13); 6.1–6.3 (1H, m); 6.31 (1H, d, 18); 6.61 (1H, d, 18); 7.4–7.7 (2H, m); 7.9–8.5 (4H, m)	4.81 (1H, s); 5.06 (1H, d, 13); 5.26 (1H, d, 13); 6.0–6.2 (1H, m); 6.32 (1H, d, 18); 6.47 (3H, s); 6.68 (1H, d, 18); 7.4–7.6 (2H, m); 7.9–8.4 (4H, m)
Functional groups	One acetyl, one primary amino, and two carboxyl	One acetyl, one methoxyl, one primary amino, and two carboxyl	One primary amino and two carboxyl	One methoxyl, one primary amino, and two carboxyl

compared with those of cephalosporin C. All of the compounds had a band at 1770 cm^{-1} in their infrared spectra suggesting the presence of β-lactam carbonyl group (Woodward, 1949; Bellamy, 1964). Potentiometric titration of the three substances, in their acid form, revealed the presence of three ionizable groups in each. The pK_a values of two of these ionizable groups were consistent with that of an α-amino acid function, and the dissociation constant of the third ionizable group was found to be more acidic than that of a normal aliphatic acid (Chapter 8, Section II). The ultraviolet spectra of each of the three compounds showed absorption maxima at about 260 nm, characteristic of the 3-cephem chromophore (Abraham and Newton, 1961; Green et al., 1964; Nagarajan and Spry, 1971). The antibiotics (3) and (5) showed an additional absorption maximum at about 240 nm (Section VII of this chapter; Nagarajan and Spry, 1971).

Characteristic features of the NMR spectrum* of cephalosporin C (2) are the three pairs of AB doublets originating from the vicinally coupled β-lactam protons, $J = 4.7$ Hz; and the geminally coupled 2-methylene and 3'-methylene protons, $J = 18$ and 13 Hz, respectively. In addition, the spectrum exhibits the three-proton acetyl singlet and the multiplets due to the seven α-amino adipyl side-chain protons. The NMR spectrum of (4) shows all the spectral characteristics of cephalosporin C, except that the three-proton acetyl singlet is absent. A comparison of the NMR spectra of (2) and (3) reveals that, while in cephalosporin C the H-6 proton occurs as a doublet at τ 4.86, in (3) there is a one-proton singlet at τ 4.84. Further, in (3) there is a three-proton singlet at τ 6.47. Finally, the NMR spectrum of (5) shows a one-proton singlet at τ 4.81, a three-proton singlet at τ 6.47, and the acetyl singlet is absent.

Amino acid analysis by the Spackman–Stein–Moore method (Spackman et al., 1958) on acid hydrolysates of cephalosporin C and antibiotic (4) afforded 0.1–0.2 μmoles/mg of glycine and an uncommon amino acid which eluted prior to glycine. Similar amino acid determination on acid hydrolysates of antibiotics (3) and (5) yielded 0.6–0.8 μmoles/mg of glycine (see Section VIII), and the same uncommon amino acid which was obtained from cephalosporin C and (4). On adding an authentic sample of α-amino adipic acid to the acid hydrolysates of these antibiotics, followed by subsequent amino acid determination, it was found that the intensity of the peak due to the uncommon amino acid increased. Consequently, all four antibiotics yielded α-amino adipic acid on hydrolysis in amounts of about 2 μmoles/mg.

An acetyl determination with antibiotic (3) gave a value of 9%, and the identity of the acetic acid liberated was confirmed by its conversion to the crystalline phenylhydrazide and comparison with an authentic sample.

---

* The NMR spectra of the antibiotics were determined in D_2O. Chemical shifts are given in τ values (TMS = 10 ppm).

Alkoxyl analyses of (3) and (5) afforded 4.5 and 5.8% methoxyl, respectively. The identity of the methyl iodide liberated was confirmed by its conversion to the known crystalline tetramethylammonium iodide.

V. Determination of Structure

The close similarity of the physical–chemical properties of (3), (4), (5), and cephalosporin C suggests that the three new antibiotics from *Streptomyces* belong to the cephalosporin C type of compounds. The acetyl determination with (4) shows the absence of an acetyl group, and the NMR spectrum shows

Table II

DISSOCIATION CONSTANTS OF
N-ACYL CEPHALOSPORINS[a]

Compound	pKₐ's	Mol wt
(2a)	4.8, 6.2	500
(2b)	5.1, 6.5	525
(3a)	5.0, 6.5	595
(3b)	5.2, 6.5	662
(4a)	4.8, 6.1	505
(4b)	5.5, 6.7	570
(5a)	5.4, 6.8	580
(5b)	5.2, 6.5	667

[a] The dissociation constants were measured in 66% DMF.

all the spectral characteristics of cephalosporin C, except for the absence of the three-proton acetyl singlet. These data suggest that the difference between antibiotic (4) and cephalosporin C is in the substituent on the 3′-methylene group. In the NMR spectrum of (3), the chemical shift of the one-proton singlet at τ 4.84 corresponds closely to that of the H-6 doublet at τ 4.86 in cephalosporin C. This indicates that the β-lactam ring in (3) is modified. The chemical shift observed for the three-proton singlet at τ 6.47 is in good agreement with the chemical shift of methoxyl protons (Jackman and Sternhell, 1969), and alkoxyl analysis of (3) confirms the presence of a methoxyl group. These data suggest that in (3) there is a methoxyl group at C-7 of the β-lactam ring. Similarly, the results of acetyl and alkoxyl determinations, and analysis of the NMR spectrum of (5), suggest that in antibiotic (5) there is a methoxyl group at C-7 and the functionality on the 3′-methylene group is different from that of cephalosporin C.

Reaction of the three metabolites (3), (4), and (5) with chloroacetyl chloride under Schotten–Baumann conditions provided the corresponding mono N-chloroacetyl derivatives (3a), (4a), and (5a). Similar reaction of the three antibiotics with N-carbethoxy phthalimide yielded the corresponding mono N,N-phthaloyl derivatives (3b), (4b), and (5b). Potentiometric titration of these N-acyl derivatives show that they all contain two ionizable groups. The pK_a values show that N-acylation causes a considerable decrease in acidity of one of the carboxyl groups, while the change in acidity of the other carboxyl group is small. Acylation of glycine decreases the acidity of the carboxyl group, as seen by the pK_a values of glycine and N-acetyl glycine (Chapter 8, Section II). Consequently, the carboxyl group that undergoes a decrease in acidity, should be the carboxyl group of the α-amino acid moiety in (3), (4), and (5). A comparison of the dissociation constants of (2), (3), (4), and (5) and their N-acyl derivatives indicates that (3), (4), and (5) contain the amino and the two carboxyl groups present in cephalosporin C. See Table II and Fig. 2.

Fig. 2. Chemical shifts of primary carbamate protons.

Reaction of N-chloroacetyl (3a), (4a), and (5a) and N,N-phthaloyl (3b), (4b), and (5b) derivatives of (3), (4), and (5) with diazomethane gave the corresponding N-acyl dimethyl esters (3c), (4c), (5c), and (3d), (4d), (5d) respectively. Chemical shifts of the 3′-methylene group protons in the NMR spectra of (2), (3), (4), and (5), and their N-acyl dimethyl esters are similar (Tables I and III). Consequently, the groups deshielding the 3′-methylene groups should be structurally similar. The NMR spectra of N-chloroacetyl derivatives of cephalosporin C (2c) and antibiotic (4) exhibit a number of common features; however, (2c) shows a three-proton acetyl singlet at τ 8.0, while (4c) has a two-proton exchangeable singlet at τ 3.41. Furthermore, whereas the N-chloroacetyl cephalosporin C dimethyl ester (2c) is a $C_{20}H_{26}O_9N_3SCl$ compound, the corresponding derivative of (4) is a $C_{19}H_{25}O_9N_4SCl$ diester. Consequently, instead of a CH_3 group in the cephalosporin C derivative, the corresponding derivative of (4) contains a NH_2 group. The NH_2 protons of carbamates resonate at τ 3.3–3.7 in dimethylsulfoxide-d$_6$. Therefore, the structure of

Table III

NMR Spectral Data of N-Acyl Cephalosporin Dimethyl Esters[a]

Compound	2-CH$_2$	3-CH$_2$	H-6	R$_1$ = H or OCH$_3$	R$_2$ = CH$_3$ or NH$_2$[b]	7-NH[b]	NHCOCH$_2$Cl[b]
(2c)	6.29, 6.52 (18)	5.03, 5.31 (13)	4.86 (4.7)	4.27 (8.5, 4.7)	7.97 (s)	1.16 (8.5)	1.39 (7.5)
(2d)	6.34, 6.59 (18)	5.06, 5.33 (13)	4.91 (4.5)	4.33 (8.5, 4.5)	7.97 (s)	1.17 (8.5)	
(3c)	6.34, 6.65 (18)	5.08, 5.33 (13)	4.81 (s)	6.60 (s)	7.97 (s)	0.79 (s)	1.37 (7.5)
(3d)	6.37, 6.72 (18)	5.08, 5.33 (13)	4.84 (s)	6.62 (s)	7.97 (s)	0.83 (s)	
(4c)	6.33, 6.54 (18)	5.11, 5.39 (13)	4.85 (5.0)	4.31 (8.0, 5.0)	3.41 (s)	1.15 (8.0)	1.38 (8.0)
(4d)	6.38, 6.63 (18)	5.11, 5.40 (13)	4.88 (4.5)	4.34 (8.5, 4.5)	3.38 (s)	1.17 (8.5)	
(5c)	6.37, 6.69 (18)	5.16, 5.42 (13)	4.81 (s)	6.60 (s)	3.41 (s)	0.81 (s)	1.37 (7.5)
(5d)	6.41, 6.76 (18)	5.16, 5.42 (13)	4.84 (s)	6.62 (s)	3.39 (s)	0.84 (s)	

[a] The NMR spectra of all these compounds were determined in DMSO-d$_6$ with TMS as internal standard. Chemical shifts are expressed in τ values, and the figures in parentheses are coupling constants in hertz. s = singlet. The chemical shifts of the α-amino adipyl, phthalimido, methylene of the N-chloroacetyl and the carbomethoxy protons are not included in the table.
[b] The signal due to these protons disappeared on shaking with D$_2$O.

antibiotic (*4*) produced by *Streptomyces clavuligerus* is 7-(5-amino-5-carboxy-valeramido)-3-carbamoyloxymethyl-3-cephem-4-carboxylic acid (Nagarajan *et al.*, 1971). See Fig. 3.

The NMR spectra of the *N*-chloroacetyl dimethyl ester derivatives of cephalosporin C and antibiotic (*4*) reveal two one-proton exchangeable doublets at τ 1.18 and 1.38, and at 1.15 and 1.38, respectively. The *N,N*-phthaloyl dimethyl ester derivatives of both (*2*) and (*4*) give spectra which show one exchangeable

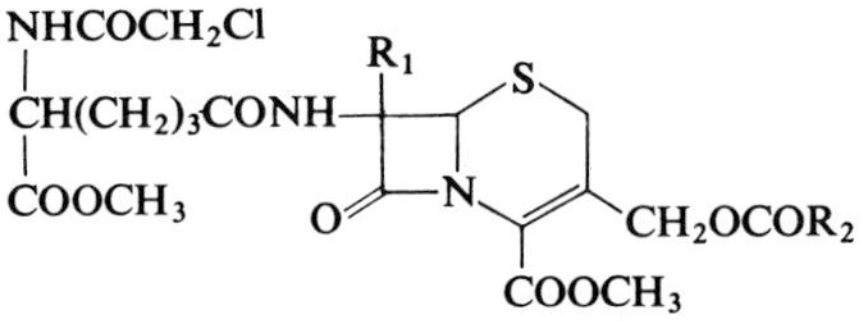

(*2c*) R_1 = H, R_2 = CH$_3$
(*3c*) R_1 = OCH$_3$, R_2 = CH$_3$
(*4c*) R_1 = H R_2 = NH$_2$
(*5c*) R_1 = OCH$_3$, R_2 = NH$_2$

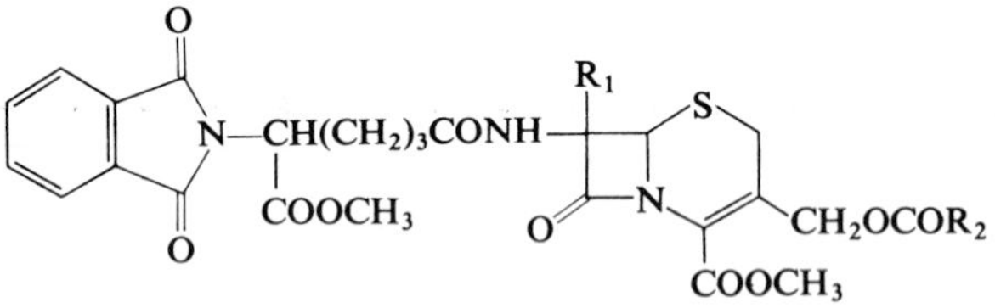

(*2d*) R_1 = H, R_2 = CH$_3$
(*3d*) R_1 = OCH$_3$, R_2 = CH$_3$
(*4d*) R_1 = H, R_2 = NH$_2$
(*5d*) R_1 = OCH$_3$, R_2 = NH$_2$

Fig. 3. Structures of *N*-chloroacetyl and *N,N*-phthaloyl derivatives of cephalosporins.

one-proton doublets at τ 1.17. Thus, the lower field exchangeable proton at τ 1.15–1.18 in each of the above four *N*-acyl dimethyl esters can be assigned to the 7-N*H* protons, and the higher field protons of the *N*-chloroacetyl dimethyl esters, to the NHCOCH$_2$Cl side-chain amido protons. Spectra of the *N*-chloroacetyl dimethyl esters (*3c*) and (*5c*) exhibit two exchangeable protons at τ 0.79 and 1.37, and 0.87 and 1.37, respectively. The lower field protons at τ 0.79 and 0.81 are singlets, which the high field protons at τ 1.37 are doublets. Furthermore, spectra of the *N,N*-phthaloyl dimethyl esters (*3d*) and (*5d*) show one exchangeable one-proton singlet at τ 0.83 and 0.84, respectively.

Clearly, the exchangeable one-proton singlets at about τ 0.8 in the four N-acyl dimethyl esters can be assigned to the 7-NH proton, and its singlet nature confirms the placement of a methoxyl group at C-7 in antibiotics (3) and (5). Finally, spectra of the N-acyl dimethyl esters (3c) and (3d) reveal a three-proton singlet at τ 7.97, and those of the N-acyl dimethyl esters (5c) and (5d) exhibit a two-proton exchangeable singlet at τ 3.4. These data establish the

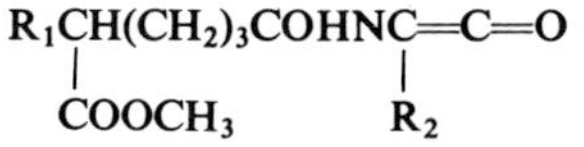

$$R_1CH(CH_2)_3COHNC\!\!=\!\!C\!\!=\!\!O$$
$$\underset{COOCH_3}{|} \quad \underset{R_2}{|}$$

$$R_1CH(CH_2)_3C\!\!\equiv\!\!O^+$$
$$\underset{COOCH_3}{|}$$

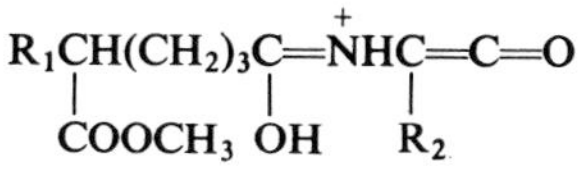

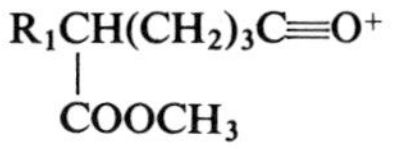

(h)

or

$$R_1CH(CH_2)_3\overset{+}{C}\!\!=\!\!NHC\!\!=\!\!C\!\!=\!\!O$$
$$\underset{COOCH_3}{|} \quad \underset{OH}{|} \quad \underset{R_2}{|}$$

(g)

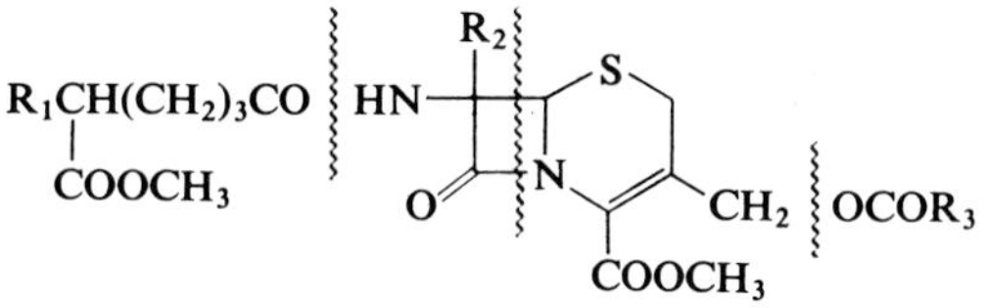

(2c) R_1 = NHCOCH$_2$Cl, R_2 = H, R_3 = CH$_3$
(3c) R_1 = NHCOCH$_2$Cl, R_2 = OCH$_3$, R_3 = CH$_3$
(4d) R_1 = N:N-phthaloyl, R_2 = H, R_3 = NH$_2$
(5d) R_1 = N:N-phthaloyl, R_2 = OCH$_3$, R_3 = NH$_2$

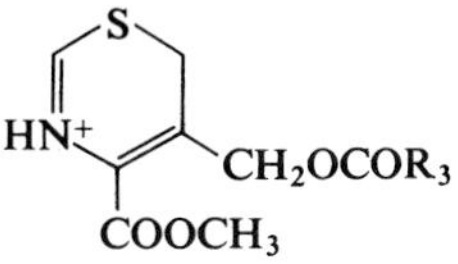

(e)

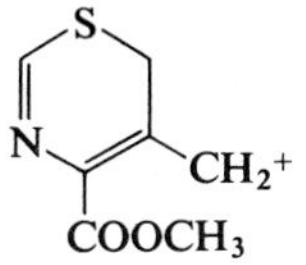

(f)

Fig. 4. Mass spectral fragmentation of cephalosporins.

structure of the antibiotic (3) produced by *Streptomyces lipmanii* as 7-(5-amino-5-carboxyvaleramido)-7-methoxy cephalosporanic acid, and that of the metabolite (5), from *Streptomyces clavuligerus* as 7-(5-amino-5-carboxy-valeramido)-7-methoxy-3-carbamoyloxymethyl-3-cephem-4-carboxylic acid (Nagarajan et al., 1971).

Cephalosporins undergo a variety of fragmentations in the mass spectro-meter on electron impact, and high-resolution mass spectral analysis of fragments can be used effectively in structure elucidation (Richter and Biemann,

Table IV

High-Resolution Mass Spectral Data of N-Acyl Cephalosporin Dimethyl Esters

	(2e)		(3c)		(4d)		(5d)	
	Mass (intensity)	Composition	Mass (intensity)	Composition	Mass (intensity)	Composition	Mass (intensity)	Composition
(e)	230.048 (98)	$C_9H_{12}O_4NS$	230.053 (50)	$C_9H_{12}O_4NS$	231.047 (0.5)	$C_8H_{11}O_4N_2S$	231.050 (4)	$C_8H_{11}O_4N_2S$
(f)	170.027 (100)	$C_7H_8O_2NS$	170.028 (100)	$C_7H_8O_2NS$	170.028 (33)	$C_7H_8O_2NS$	170.024 (4)	$C_7H_8O_2NS$
(g)	290.070 (15)	$C_{11}H_{15}O_5N_2Cl$	320.081 (4)	$C_{12}H_{17}O_6N_2Cl$	345.106 (0.5)	$C_{17}H_{17}O_6N_2$	—	—
(h)	234.057 (25)	$C_9H_{13}O_4NCl$	234.057 (20)	$C_9H_{13}O_4NCl$	288.087 (1)	$C_{15}H_{14}O_5N$	288.088 (8)	$C_{15}H_{14}O_5N$

1965; Chapter 8, Section IV). The N-acyl dimethyl esters (*2c*), (*3c*), (*4d*), and (*5d*) do not give molecular ions in their mass spectra; however, high-resolution mass spectral analysis of the dihydrothiazine and side-chain fragments supports the structural assignments made for antibiotics (*3*), (*4*), and (*5*) (see Fig. 4). The difference in the composition of the dihydrothiazine fragments (*e*) and (*f*) derived from (*3c*), (*4d*), and (*5d*) show the nature of the substituent at the 3′-position is $R_2 = CH_3$ in (*3*), and $R_2 = NH_2$ in (*4*) and (*5*) (Table IV). The substituent $R_1 = OCH_3$ in (*3*) is also supported by the analysis of the side-chain fragments (*g*) and (*h*) derived from (*3c*).

VI. Conversion of Cephalosporin C to 7-(5-amino-5-carboxyvaleramido)-3-carbamoyloxymethyl-3-cephem-4-carboxylic acid

Cephalosporin C has been converted to the N,N-phthaloyldimethyl ester of 7 - (5 - amino - 5 - carboxyvaleramido) - 3 - carbamoyloxymethyl - 3 - cephem - 4 - carboxylic acid (Murphy *et al.*, 1971), thus establishing the chemical relationship between cephalosporin C and (*4*), one of the *S. clavuligerus* metabolites. Deacetylcephalosporin C (*6*), obtained either from cephalosporin C fermentation (Huber *et al.*, 1968) or from enzymatic deacetylation of cephalosporin C by citrus acetyl esterase (Jeffery *et al.*, 1961), on reaction with N-carbethoxy-phthalimide under Schotten–Baumann conditions was converted to N,N-phthaloyldeacetylcephalosporin C (*7*). Reaction of (*7*) with two equivalents of diphenyldiazomethane afforded the corresponding dibenzhydryl ester (*8*). See Fig. 5. The fully protected derivative (*9*) was obtained by treatment of (*8*) with trichloroacetylisocyanate (Hedin *et al.*, 1970). The trichloroacetyl group was removed either by passing the crude product over a column of silica gel or by reaction with methanolic sodium carbonate. The dibenzhydryl ester of 7 - (5 - phthalimido - 5 - carboxyvaleramido) - 3 - carbamoyloxymethyl - 3 - cepham-4-carboxylic acid (*10*) was obtained in 30% overall yield. The benzhydryl groups in (*10*) were removed by reaction with trifluoroacetic acid and anisole at 0° for 4 hours, and treatment of the diacid (*11*) with diazomethane gave the corresponding dimethyl ester which was found to be identical to the N,N-phthaloyldimethyl ester (*4d*), derived from (*4*).

VII. Circular Dichroism Studies

The ultraviolet spectra of cephalosporin compounds (Table V) show an absorption maximum at about 260 nm (Abraham and Newton, 1961; Chapter

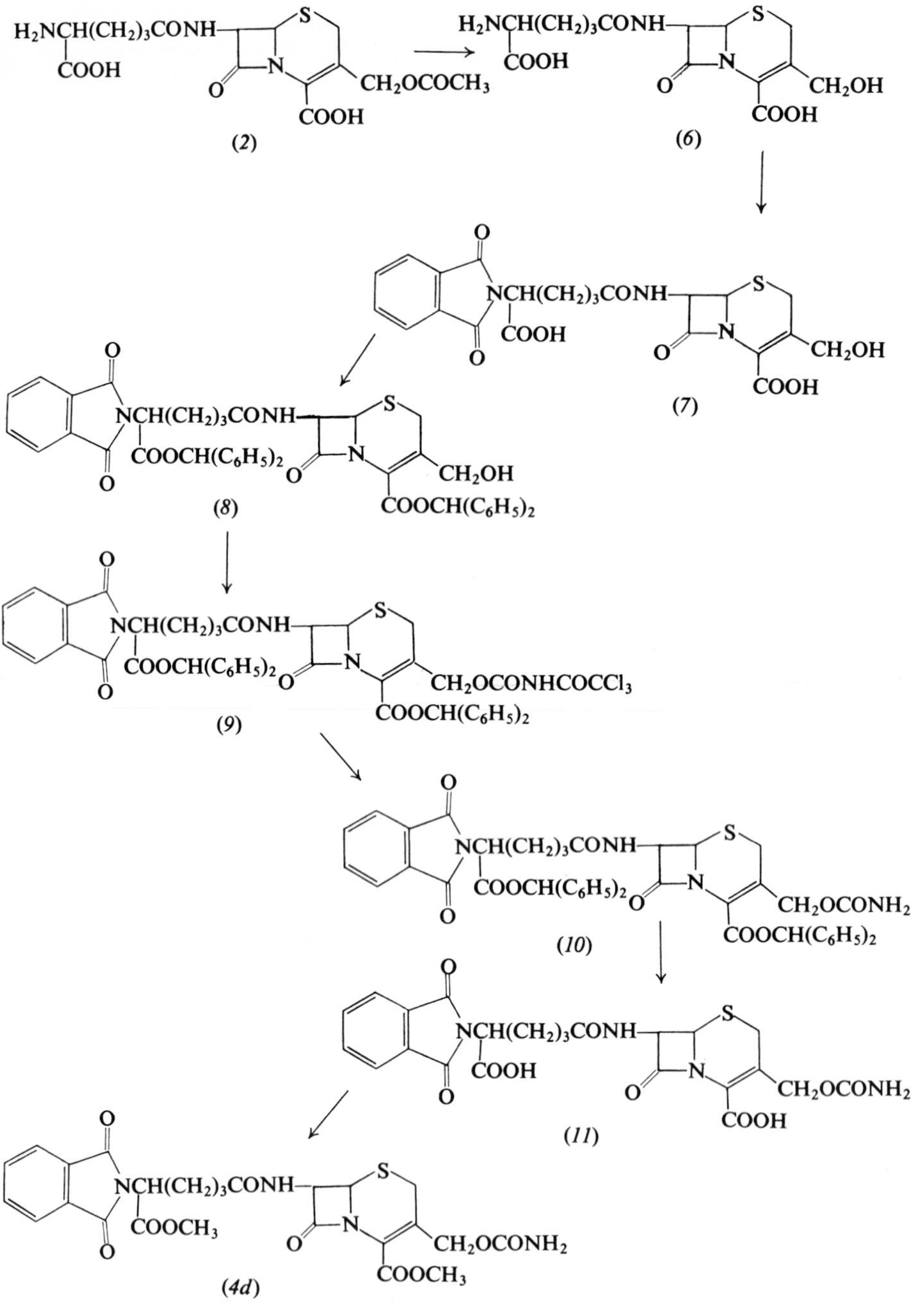

Fig. 5. Synthesis of N,N-phthaloyl dimethyl ester derivatives of (4) from cephalosporin C.

Table V
UV SPECTRA OF CEPHALOSPORINS

Compound	Solvent[a]	λ_{max} (nm)	ϵ
(2)	W	260	8900
(3)	W	265	7100
		242	6000
(4)	W	261	7000
(5)	W	264	6900
		242	5700
(12)	W	262	8000
(14)	M	262.5	8100
(15)	M	264	9500
(16)	M	267	9100
(17)	M	257	9100
(18)	M	232	5600

[a] W = water; M = methanol.

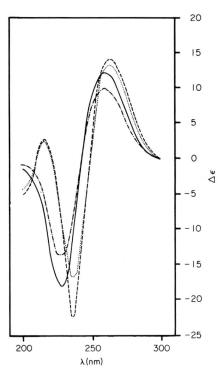

Fig. 6. Circular dichroism curves of antibiotics (2) (—), (3) (---), (4) (-··-), and (5) (···) in water.

8, Section VI). However, the ultraviolet spectra of (3) and (5) show two absorption maxima at about 265 and 240 nm.

In agreement with the ultraviolet spectra, the circular dichroism curves of (3) and (5) show two Cotton effects, a positive maximum at 263 and a negative

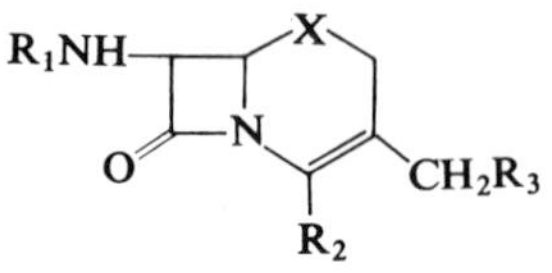

(12) R_1 = H, R_2 = COOH, R_3 = OCOCH$_3$, X = S
(13) R_1 = COCH$_3$, R_2 = COOH, R_3 = OCOCH$_3$, X = S
(14) R_1 = COCH$_3$, R_2 = COOCH$_3$, R_3 = OCOCH$_3$, X = S
(15) R_5 = COCH$_3$, R_2 = COOCH$_3$, R_3 = OCOCH$_3$, X = SO$_2$
(16) R_1 = COCH$_3$, R_2 = COOCH$_3$, R_3 = SCH$_3$, X = S
(17) R_5 = C$_6$H$_5$OCH$_2$CO, R_2 = R_3 = H, X = S

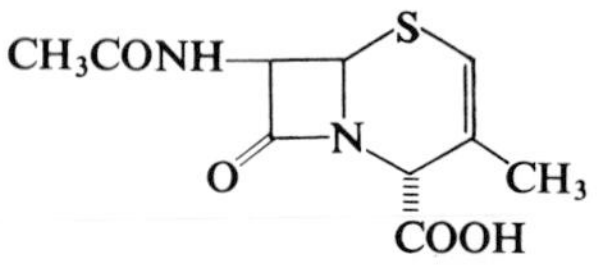

(18)

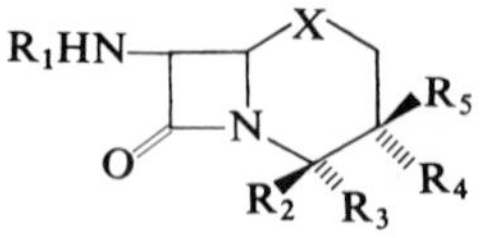

(19) R_1 = COCH$_3$, R_2 = COOCH$_3$, R_3 = R_4 = H, R_5 = CH$_3$, X = SO$_2$
(20) R_1 = C$_6$H$_5$OCH$_2$CO, R_2 = R_5 = H, R_3 = COOCH$_3$, R_4 = CH$_3$, X = S
(21) R_1 = C$_6$H$_5$OCH$_2$CO, R_2 = R_5 = H, R_3 = COOCH$_3$, R_4 = CH$_3$, X = SO$_2$

Fig. 7. Structure of model cephalosporins used in circular dichroism studies.

maximum at 236 nm. Even though the ultraviolet spectra of cephalosporin C and antibiotic (4) show only one absorption maximum, their circular dichroism curves show two Cotton effects, a positive at 259 nm and a negative at 228 nm (Fig. 6). Apparently, cephalosporins have two transitions, but due to the low intensity of the lower transitions in (2) and (4), they are not discernible in the ultraviolet spectra. The ultraviolet and circular dichroism spectra of a number of model 3-cephem derivatives confirm the conclusion that the 3-cephem chromophore has two transitions (Figs. 7 and 8). The ultraviolet absorption at 260 nm of the 3-cephem chromophore is discussed in Chapter 8, Section VI, and this transition is due to the $\pi \to \pi^*$ transition of the double bond (Nagarajan and Spry, 1971).

The second transition of the 3-cephem chromophore at 230 nm could have its origin in (a) the $n \to \sigma^*$ transition of the sulfur† (Goodman et al., 1970), (b) the $n \to \pi^*$ transition of the β-lactam carbonyl (Neelakantan and Urry, 1969), and (c) the red-shifted $n \to \pi^*$ transition of the β-lactam carbonyl caused by the overlap of the sulfur lone-pair electrons with the β-lactam

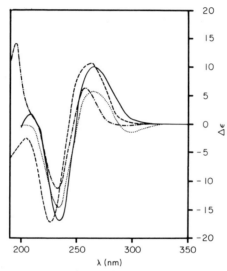

Fig. 8. Circular dichroism curves of (12) (---) in water, and (14) (—), (15) (- -), and (16) (···) in methanol.

carbonyl group, or (d) overlap of the π system of the double bond with the p and π orbitals of the β-lactam carbonyl group. The circular dichroism curve of (17) proves that removal of the 4-carboxyl group has a minor effect on the 230-nm transition. The circular dichroism spectra of the sulfone (15), and the sulfides (14) and (20), show that 230-nm transition does not arise from the $n \to \sigma^*$ transition of the sulfur. A comparison of the circular dichroism curves of the sulfones (15), (19), and (21) with that of the corresponding sulfides (14) and (20) show that the 230-nm transition is not due to the red-shifted $n \to \pi^*$ transition caused by the overlap of the sulfur lone-pair electrons with the

† The circular dichroism curve of 3-thiacholestane (Nagarajan et al., 1967) in acetonitrile shows three Cotton effects; two positive maxima at 235 nm ($\Delta\epsilon$ 1.30) and 220 nm ($\Delta\epsilon$ 1.06) and a negative maximum at 199 nm ($\Delta\epsilon$ 0.94) (Nagarajan and Dodson, 1971).

β-lactam carbonyl group (Fig. 9). The $n \rightarrow \pi^*$ transition of the amide group of five- and six-membered ring lactams occur at about 220 nm (Wolf, 1967). In 2,2-dimethyl quinuclidin-6-one the $n \rightarrow \pi^*$ transition of the nonplanar amide is found at 246 nm (Pracejus, 1959). The $n \rightarrow \pi^*$ transition of five- and six-membered lactams show amplitudes of the same order as the $n \rightarrow \pi^*$ transition of ketones, and the amplitude of the four-membered lactam carbonyl

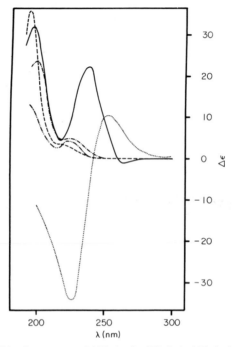

Fig. 9. Circular dichroism curves of (17) (···), (18) (—), (19) (---), (20) (-··-), and (21) (-···-) in methanol.

transition would be expected to be similar in magnitude. The 230-nm transition of the 3-cephem chromophore is associated with high extinction and ellipticity. The saturated sulfones (19) and (21) do not show the 230-nm negative Cotton effect, and consequently, the latter transition cannot be assigned to the $n \rightarrow \pi^*$ of the β-lactam carbonyl group.

The double bond and β-lactam carbonyl can be considered as a homo-conjugated π system constituting an inherently dissymmetric chromophore†

---

† The 3-cephem chromophore exhibits both enamine and enamide character (Sweet and Dahl, 1970), and consequently, the sulfur, double-bond, nitrogen lone-pair, and β-lactam carbonyl could be considered as a conjugated chromophore; however, the extended conjugation is partially disrupted due to deviation from planarity.

(Mislow, 1967). Such chromophores are associated with high amplitudes, and indeed, the ellipticity of the 230-nm transition is high, i.e., $\Delta\epsilon = -10$ to -35. Dreiding models of the 3-cephem derivatives show that there is overlap between the π system of the double bond, and the p and π orbitals of the β-lactam carbonyl group, and the homoconjugated π system is twisted in the left-handed helical sense (Fig. 10). The generalized octant rule (Moscowitz et al., 1962) or the quadrant rule (Schellman, 1968) predicts a negative sign, and the 230-nm transition shows a negative Cotton effect. The effect of the polarity of the solvent on the 230-nm transition of the acid (13) supports the assignment that the 230-nm absorption is due to the $n \rightarrow \pi^*$ transition (Table VI). The 2-cephem

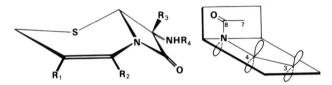

Fig. 10. Conformation of the 3-cephem chromophore.

Table VI

EFFECT OF SOLVENT ON THE UV AND CD SPECTRA OF
N-ACETYL 7-AMINOCEPHALOSPORANIC ACID (13)

	Water		Methanol		Acetonitrile		Dioxane	
CD:	195	+0.85	206	+3.43	208	+1.39	210	+1.88
Maxima ($\Delta\epsilon$)	229	−17.7	234.5	−19.4	235.5	−21.7	237	−20.9
	260	+12.9	264.5	+11.1	265	+10.1	265	+13.4
UV: $\lambda_{max}(\epsilon)$	260.5	9200	263	8300	263.5	7800	266	7800

derivative (18), is devoid of 230-nm negative Cotton effect, and the 237-nm positive Cotton effect is due to the electron transfer transition of the α,β-unsaturated sulfide. The red-shift and the intensification observed for the 236-nm transition in the antibiotics (3) and (5) may be due to the influence of the methoxyl group being adjacent to the β-lactam carbonyl group.

VIII. Biosynthetic Studies

The three new β-lactam antibiotics (3), (4), and (5) are produced by the prokaryotic *Streptomyces* species, while penicillins and cephalosporin C are produced by the eukaryotic *Penicillium* and *Cephalosporium* cultures, respectively. The prokaryotic organisms have simpler cellular organization. Consequently, these antibiotics may be more amenable to biosynthetic studies (Chapter 9, Section VI). The biosynthetic pathway for penicillin N produced

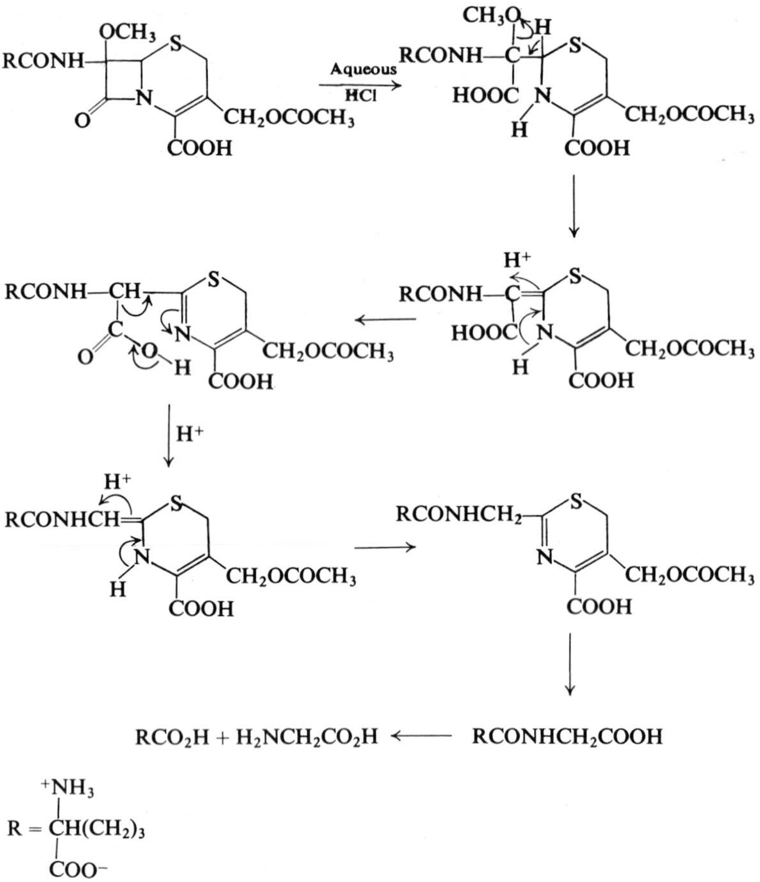

Fig. 11. Mechanism for formation of glycine by acid hydrolysis of 7-methoxy cephalosporins.

by *Streptomyces* (Miller *et al.*, 1962) has not been investigated. Preliminary radioisotopic label studies undertaken to shed light on the biosynthetic pathways for synthesis of β-lactam antibiotics (3), (4), and (5) by *Streptomyces* (Whitney *et al.*, 1972) are discussed in this section.

Incorporation of label into (5), from ^{14}C-labeled amino acids was determined by radioautography and bioautography. The labeled antibiotic was isolated and the percent incorporation determined. The three amino acids which make up the β-lactam antibiotics, α-amino adipic acid, cysteine, and valine are incorporated to the extent of about 6–10 % in compound (5). The incorporation of label from serine and ^{35}S-labeled methionine into (5) suggests that, as in the case of *Cephalosporium*, cysteine is formed by a reverse transsulfuration pathway (Chapter 9, Section III, B). Compounds (3) and (5) contained the ^{14}C-label in their methoxyl substituents when isolated from fermentations containing methionine[^{14}C]methyl. Placement of the label was determined by alkoxyl determination. Consequently, the methyl of the 7-methoxy groups in (3) and (5) is derived from methionine. The origin of the carbamoyloxy group in

Table VII

INCORPORATION OF RADIOISOTOPIC LABEL INTO
ANTIBIOTIC (5) BY ADDITION OF LABELED AMINO ACIDS
TO *S. Clavuligerus* CULTURE

Amino acids added compound	% incorporation
DL-Cysteine-3-[^{14}C]	8.8
DL-Cysteine-1-[^{14}C]	10.9
DL-Valine-1-[^{14}C]	6.1
DL-α-Amino adipic acid-1-[^{14}C″]	10.9
L-Methionine-Me[^{14}C]	23.6
DL-Serine-3-[^{14}C]	4.0
DL-Lysine-1-[^{14}C]	12.5
DL-Aspartic-4-[^{14}C]	none
DL-Cystine-3-3′-[^{14}C]^a	9.2
+	
L-Cystine-3-3′-T^a	7.1

^{a} Double labeled experiment.

(4) and (5) is not known. Label from the amono acid L-citrulline[^{14}C] (labeled in the ureido moiety) was not incorporated into (5).

When cysteine-1-[^{14}C] was added to the *S. clavuligerus* fermentation and the labeled antibiotic (5) isolated, the glycine obtained by acid hydrolysis of (5) was not radioactive. However, when cysteine-3-[^{14}C] was added as precursor, the glycine obtained by acid hydrolysis of (5) contained the label. These data support the mechanism put forth in Fig. 11 to explain the formation of a larger amount of glycine on acid hydrolysis of antibiotics (3) and (5) than from cephalosporin C and (4) (Brannon *et al.*, 1972).

In eukaryotic *Penicillium* and *Cephalosporium* organisms, α-amino adipic acid is an intermediate of lysine biosynthesis. But in prokaryotic organisms, lysine is synthesized by decarboxylation of 2,6-diaminopimelic acid (Chapter 9,

Section III, A). Genetic studies with *S. lipmanii* support this pathway for lysine biosynthesis (Godfrey and Kirkpatrick, 1971). The incorporation of the label of radioactive lysine in the α-amino adipyl moiety of (5) suggests that the α-amino adipic acid biosynthesized in *S. clavuligerus* fermentation is derived from lysine.

Compounds (3) and (5) exhibited greater activity than cephalosporin C against gram-negative organisms, while (4) showed activity comparable to cephalosporin C (Chapter 12).

References

Abraham, E. P., and Newton, G. G. F. (1961). *Biochem. J.* **79**, 377.

Belgium Patent 754,424.

Belgium Patent 754,693.

Bellamy, L. J. (1964). *In* "The Infrared Spectra of Complex Molecules," p. 214. Methuen, London.

Brannon, D. R., Mabe, J. A., Ellis, R., Whitney, J. G., and Nagarajan, R. (1972). *Antimicrob. Ag. Chemother.* **1**, 242.

Brotzu, G. (1948). *Lav. Ist. Igiene Cagliari*.

Clarke, H. T., Johnson, J. R., and Robinson, R. (1949). *In* "The Chemistry of Penicillin." Princeton Univ. Press, Princeton, New Jersey.

Florey, H. W., Chain, E., Heatley, N. G., Jennings, M. A., Sanders, A. G., Abraham, E. P., and Florey, M. E. (1949). *In "Antibiotics,"* Vol. 2. Oxford Univ. Press, London and New York.

Godfrey, O. W., and Kirkpatrick, J. R. (1971). Unpublished results.

Goodman, M., Su, K. C., and Niu, G. C. C. (1970). *J. Amer. Chem. Soc.* **92**, 5220.

Green, D. M., Long, A. G., May, P. J., and Turner, A. F. (1964). *J. Chem. Soc.* 766.

Hedin, P. A., Gueldner, R. C., and Thompson, A. C. (1970). *Anal. Chem.* **42**, 403.

Higgens, C. E., and Kastner, R. E. (1971). *Int. J. Syst. Bacteriol.* **21**, 326.

Huber, F. M., Baltz, R. H., and Caltrider, P. G. (1968). *Appl. Microbiol.* **16**, 1011.

Jackman, L. M., and Sternhell, S. (1969). *In* "Applications of Nuclear Magnetic Resonance Spectroscopy in Organic Chemistry," p. 180. Pergamon Press, New York.

Jeffery, J. D'A., Abraham, E. P., and Newton, G. G. F. (1961). *Biochem. J.* **81**, 591.

Miller, I. M., Stapley, E. O., and Chaiet, L. (1962). *Bact. Proc.* 32.

Mislow, K. (1967). *In* "Optical Rotatory Dispersion and Circular Dichroism in Organic Chemistry" (G. Snatzke, ed.), p. 162. Heyden & Son, London.

Moscowitz, A., Mislow, K., Glass, M. A. W., and Djerassi, C. (1962). *J. Amer. Chem. Soc.* **84**, 1945.

Murphy, C. F., Koehler, R. E., and Webber, J. A. (1971). Unpublished results.

Nagarajan, R., and Dodson, R. M. (1971). Unpublished results.

Nagarajan, R., and Spry, D. O. (1971). *J. Amer. Chem. Soc.* **93**, 2310.

Nagarajan, R., Chollar, B. H., Dodson, R. M. (1967). *Chem. Commun.* 550.

Nagarajan, R., Boeck, L. D., Gorman, M., Hamill, R. L., Higgens, C. E., Hoehn, M. M., Stark, W. M., and Whitney, J. G. (1971). *J. Amer. Chem. Soc.* **93**, 2308.

Neelakantan, L., and Urry, D. W. (1969). Abstracts of 158th Amer. Chem. Soc. Meeting, September, Biol. 179.

Pracejus, H. (1959). *Chem. Ber.* **92**, 988.

Richter, W., and Biemann, K. (1965). *Monatsh. Chem.* **96**, 484.

Sanders, A. G. (1949). *In* "Antibiotics" (H. W. Florey, E. Chain, N. G. Heatley, M. A. Jennings, A. G. Sanders, E. P. Abraham, and M. E. Florey, eds.), Vol. 2, p. 672. Oxford Univ. Press, London and New York.

Schellman, J. A. (1968). *Accounts Chem. Res.* **1**, 144.

Spackman, D. H., Stein, W. H., and Moore, S. (1958). *Anal. Chem.* **30**, 1190.

Sweet, R. M., and Dahl, L. F. (1970). *J. Amer. Chem. Soc.* **92**, 5489.

Westhead, J. E. (1971). Unpublished results.

Whitney, J. G., Brannon, D. R., Mabe, J. A., and Wicker, K. J. (1972). *Antimicrob. Ag. Chemother.* **1**, 247.

Wolf, H. (1967). *In* "Optical Rotatory Dispersion and Circular Dichroism in Organic Chemistry" (G. Snatzke, ed.), p. 361. Heyden & Son, London.

Woodward, R. B. (1949). *In* "The Chemistry of Penicillin" (H. T. Clarke, J. R. Johnson, and R. Robinson, eds.), p. 444. Princeton Univ. Press, Princeton, New Jersey.

Chapter 16

APPENDIX*

I. Preparative Procedures

7-Phenoxyacetamido-3-Methyl-3-Cephem-4-Carbonyl Chloride and Methyl Ester

A suspension of 0.353 gm (1.02 mmoles) of 7-phenoxyacetamido-3-methyl-3-cephem-4-carboxylic acid in 40 ml of benzene was cooled in ice and stirred while 0.256 gm (2 mmoles) of oxalyl chloride, and 1 drop of dimethylformamide was added. The reaction mixture was stirred at about 7–10° for 45 minutes, and then the solvents were removed under reduced pressure. An NMR spectrum of the acid chloride showed the absence of any 2-cephem isomer.

The acid chloride (≈ 200 mg) was dissolved in 10 ml of methanol and stirred at 25° for 30 minutes. The solvent was removed and the residue was dissolved in benzene. The benzene solution was washed with water, 3% hydrochloric acid, and 10% sodium bicarbonate. The solution was dried over sodium sulfate and evaporated to dryness, leaving 0.160 gm of methyl-7-phenoxyacetamido-3-methyl-3-cephem-4-carboxylate. The ester was crystallized from ethyl acetate; it was found to be identical with a known sample by thin-layer chromatography, mp 135°–137°, mixed mp 135–138° (Murphy and Koehler, 1970).

* Compiled by E. H. Flynn from data supplied by contributors.

t-Butyl-7-Phenoxyacetamido-3-Methyl-3-Cephem-4-Carboxylate from a 3-Cephem-4-Carbonylchloride

A solution of 0.10 mole of the acid chloride in 1.0 liter of methylene chloride was added dropwise over a 3-hour period to a stirred solution of 92.5 gm (1.25 moles) of *t*-butyl alcohol (freshly distilled from potassium permanganate and dried over molecular sieves) and 19.3 gm (0.175 mole) of triethylamine (freshly distilled from phenylisocyanate and dried over potassium hydroxide pellets) in 650 ml of methylene chloride maintained under anhydrous conditions at ice-bath temperature. The methylene chloride solution was washed with about 500 ml of water and 100 ml of 3 % hydrochloric acid, then evaporated to dryness. The residue was suspended in ethyl acetate, washed with 5 % sodium bicarbonate and water, and then treated with 20 gm of activated charcoal. The suspension was filtered and evaporated to dryness. The *t*-butyl ester crystallized from ether to give a total yield of 37.5 gm (75 %) of needles, mp 78°–80°. From the neutral and basic washes was recovered 7.0 gm of a mixture of Δ^2 and Δ^3 acids (Murphy and Koehler, 1970).

2′,2′,2′-Trichloroethyl-7-Phenoxyacetamido-3-Methyl-3-Cephem-4-Carboxylate

To a stirred solution of 500 ml of methylene chloride containing 17.4 gm (0.05 mole) of 7-phenoxyacetamido-3-methyl-3-cephem-4-carboxylic acid, 7.9 gm (0.1 mole) of pyridine, and 14.9 gm (0.1 mole) of 2,2,2-trichloroethanol was added dicyclohexylcarbodiimide (10.0 gm, 0.05 mole). The reaction mixture was stirred at 25° for 90 minutes. The dicyclohexylurea which formed was removed by filtration. The filtrate was washed successively with cold 0.1 *N* hydrochloric acid, saturated sodium bicarbonate, and water; dried over magnesium sulfate; and evaporated *in vacuo*. The ester (9.5 gm, 40%) was crystallized from ether, mp 114°–116°; NMR (deuterochloroform) showed pure 3-cephem ester (Kaiser *et al.*, 1970).

2′,2′,2′-Trichloroethyl-6-Phenoxyacetamidopenicillanate-1β-Oxide

METHOD A

A stirred mixture of 366 gm (1 mole) of 6-phenoxyacetamidopenicillanic acid-1β-oxide and 166 gm (1.1 moles) of 2,2,2-trichloroethanol in 1 liter of acetone was cooled to 0°–5°C, and 240 gm (3 moles) pyridine was added at a rate such that the temperature did not exceed 10°C. Then 95 ml (about 140 gm, 1.4 moles) of phosgene was added dropwise during 30 minutes from a jacketed dropping funnel which was cooled to approximately −50°C with a dry ice–acetone mixture. Carbon dioxide evolution was extremely rapid throughout the phosgene addition. Stirring was continued for an additional 30 minutes at 5°–10°C to insure completion of the reaction. Then 2 liters of water were added dropwise during 60 minutes at 0°–10°C. The precipitate which formed was collected, washed with water, air-dried, and then vacuum-dried at 65°C for 2 hours. In this manner there was obtained 402 gm (80% yield) of the crude 2′,2′,2′-trichloroethyl-6-phenoxyacetamidopenicillinate-1β-oxide as a pale yellow, granular solid, mp 141°–143°C. The material was slurried in a mixture of 300 ml of methyl isobutyl ketone and 150 ml of ethyl ether at about 0°C, collected, washed with a cold 1.5:1 volume mixture of methyl isobutyl-ether–ethyl ether, and dried, yielding 358 gm (71.5% yield) of 2′,2′,2′-trichloro-ethyl-6-phenoxymethylpenicillinate-1β-oxide, mp 146°–148°C (Belg. Patent 721,348).

Method B

6-Phenoxyacetamidopenicillanic acid-1β-oxide potassium salt (77.4 gm), 0.2 mole) was suspended in 1.5 liters of methylene chloride and pyridine hydrochloride (24 gm, 0.2 mole) was added.

The suspension was cooled in an ice-water bath for addition of trichloro-ethanol (30 gm, 0.2 mole) and then N,N'-dicyclohexylcarbodiimide (41.2 gm, 0.2 mole) in 250 ml of methylene chloride, dropwise. The mixture was stirred at room temperature overnight and filtered. The filtrate was washed with 5% sodium bicarbonate solution and then with water, dried (magnesium sulfate), and concentrated to dryness *in vacuo*. The residual oil, weighing 85 gm, gave one spot in thin-layer chromatography.

A 5-gm sample of this oil crystallized (with difficulty) from 10 ml of ether and 35 ml of petroleum ether. Recovery: 4.4 gm, mp 146°–148°. IR (chloro-form): 2.95 μ (amide NH), 5.6–5.7 μ (broad, β-lactam, and ester carbonyls), 5.91 and 6.22 μ (amide carbonyl), and in the aromatic regions (Chauvette, unpublished results).

2′,2′,2′-Trichloroethyl-7-Phenoxyacetamido-3-Methyl-3-Cephem-4-Carboxylate by Acylation and Esterification of 7-ADCA

7-ADCA (10.7 gm, 0.05 mole) was dissolved in 400 ml of water and 300 ml of acetone containing sodium bicarbonate (14 gm, 0.166 mole). With stirring and cooling in ice, phenoxyacetyl chloride (8.5 gm, 0.05 mole) in 100 ml of dry acetone was added dropwise. The mixture was stirred in the cold overnight. Acetone was evaporated *in vacuo*. The aqueous solution was washed with ethyl acetate and then acidified to pH 2.5 in the cold and in the presence of ethyl acetate. The organic layer was separated, washed with cold water, dried (magnesium sulfate), and concentrated to a smaller volume from which the acidic product crystallized to give 12.4 gm (71 %). For characterization a small sample was recrystallized from ethyl acetate–petroleum ether, mp 186°–188° (dec.)

IR (Nujol mull): 2.97 μ (amide NH), 5.7–6.0 μ (broad, β-lactam, acid, and amide carbonyl, respectively) and in aromatic region. UV (ethanol): 215 nm ($\epsilon = 12,600$), 267 nm ($\epsilon = 7,210$), and 272 n ($\epsilon = 6,100$).

The electrometric titration (in 66 % aqueous dimethylformamide) showed a titratable group at pH 5.8 and an apparent molecular weight of 333 (calc. 349) (Chauvette et al., 1971).

A mixture of this acid (85 gm, 0.244 mole), dry pyridine (23.8 gm, 0.3 mole), and 2,2,2-trichloroethanol (36.6 gm, 0.244 mole) in 2.5 liters of methylene chloride was treated with N,N'-dicyclohexylcarbodiimide (55.6 gm, 0.27 mole) in 200 ml of the same solvent by dropwise addition. The mixture was stirred at room temperature overnight. The dicyclohexyl urea was removed by filtering. The solvent was replaced by cold ethyl acetate for successive cold washes with water, 5 % hydrochloric acid, 5 % sodium bicarbonate solution, and water. The ethyl acetate solution was dried (magnesium sulfate) and evaporated in vacuo. The residual oil was redissolved in 600 ml of anhydrous ether. The ethereal solution was concentrated to about 300 ml and refrigerated for fractional crystallization of the Δ^3 ester from the more soluble isomeric Δ^2 product; yield 51.3 gm (44%), mp. 119°.

IR (chloroform): 3.0 μ (amide NH), 5.62, 5.79, and 6.94 μ (β-lactam, ester, and amide carbonyl, respectively) and in the aromatic region. UV (ethanol): 216 nm ($\epsilon = 13,100$), 268 nm ($\epsilon = 6,800$), and 274 nm ($\epsilon = 6,300$) (Chauvette et al., 1971).

Methyl-7-Phthalimidocephalosporanate from 7-ACA

To a vigorously stirred solution of 5 gm of 7-aminocephalosporanic acid and 1.95 gm of sodium carbonate in 30 ml of water was added 4.03 gm of N-ethoxycarbonylphthalimide. The reaction mixture was stirred at room temperature for 3 hours, filtered, and the filtrate acidified with hydrochloric acid. The precipitate was filtered and dried at room temperature to yield 4.3 gm of 7-phthalimidocephalosporanic acid. The acid was dissolved in methylene dichloride and an ethereal solution of diazomethane added. An immediate evolution of nitrogen occurred accompanied by the formation of a precipitate. The reaction mixture was evaporated to dryness in vacuo to yield a residual oil. The oil was chromatographed over silica gel to yield the purified product, methyl 7-phthalimidocephalosporanate. The NMR spectrum and IR spectrum were in agreement with the designated structure of the product (Spry, un-published results).

Methyl-7-Phenoxyacetamidocephalosporanate

Phenoxyacetyl chloride (17.0 gm) was added to a cooled solution of 27.3 gm of 7-ACA and 20.0 gm of sodium bicarbonate in 200 ml of water and 100 ml of acetone. After 2 hours the solution was concentrated, layered with ethyl acetate and the pH lowered to 2.0 with stirring. The ethyl acetate solution was washed with water, and the product was titrated from this solution into water by addition of dilute potassium hydroxide. The salt, isolated by evapora-tion of water, was recrystallized from methanol; 24.49 gm, $[\alpha]_D$ +106°.

The methyl ester was prepared by adding excess diazomethane in ether to an ethyl acetate solution of the acid, obtained by titrating the above salt with dilute hydrochloric acid in a mixture of water–ethyl acetate. The product was recrystallized from methanol, mp 149°–150°, $[\alpha]_D$ +53°; IR (chloroform, cm^{-1}): 1792, 1750, and 1692 (Morin et al., 1969).

Acylation of 7-ADCA with Ketene

To a slurry of 4.3 gm of 7-aminodeacetoxycephalosporanic acid in 250 ml of ethyl acetate cooled to 10°C was added dropwise 25 ml of 1 N sodium hydroxide until a pH of 8.3 was attained. Ketene was bubbled through this solution with a fritted glass tube for 30 minutes, at which time the pH of the solution had reached pH 5.5. The mixture was adjusted to pH 2.5 with 1 N hydrochloric acid and the ethyl acetate layer was separated and dried over sodium sulfate. Evaporation of the ethyl acetate solution provided 5.1 gm (83% yield) of 7-acetamido-3-methyl-3-cephem-4-carboxylic acid as a white crystalline solid.

The product was further purified by recrystallization from acetone–hexane to yield white needles melting at about 195°–196°C (Spry, unpublished results).

Reduction of Cephalosporin Sulfoxides

2′,2′,2′ - Trichloroethyl - 7 - (thiophene-2-acetamido) - 3 - acetoxymethyl - 3 - cephem-4-carboxylate-1-oxide (2.0 gm, 3.7 mmoles) was dissolved in aceto-nitrile (15 ml) and dimethylformamide (6 ml) and stirred at 0°. Stannous chloride (624 mg, 4.04 mmoles) and acetyl chloride (1.2 gm, 1.54 mmoles) were added. This mixture was stirred at 0° for 1 hour and then at room tem-perature for an additional hour. The acetonitrile was removed in vacuo; the residue was poured into water and extracted into ethyl acetate. The organic solution was washed with 3% hydrochloric acid solution, 5% sodium bicarbonate solution, and then with water. After drying over sodium sulfate, the solvent was removed to give 1.9 gm (98%) of product which crystallized from hot isopropyl alcohol, mp 120°–122°, and was identical in all respects with authentic 2′,2′,2′-trichloroethyl-7-(thiophene-2-acetamido)-cephalosporanate (Kaiser *et al.*, 1970).

6-Phenoxyacetamidopenicillanic Acid-1β-Oxide

METHOD A—HYDROGEN PEROXIDE–ACETIC ACID

A suspension of 6-phenoxyacetamidopenicillanic acid (350 gm, 1.0 mole) in 1 liter of acetic acid was cooled to 15°–20°C, and 200 ml of 35% hydrogen peroxide in water (about 2 moles of hydrogen peroxide) was added dropwise at 15°–20°C over 90 minutes while stirring the mixture. The penicillin slowly dissolved giving a clear, pale (light) yellow solution. After about 2 hours at 15°–20°C, the sulfoxide began to crystallize from the solution. Stirring was continued for a total reaction time of 4 hours. The mixture was cooled to about 0°C and 1 liter of water was added dropwise during 60 minutes. The precipitate was filtered, washed with 5 liters of water, and dried for 18 hours at 60°C. There was thus obtained 312 gm (85.5% yield) of 6-phenoxyacetamidopenicillanic acid-1β-oxide as a white solid, mp 167°–168°C with dec. IR (chloroform): 3.0 μ (amide NH), 5.56, 5.75, and 5.92 μ (β-lactam, acid, and amide carbonyls, respectively) (Hatfield, unpublished results).

METHOD B—SODIUM METAPERIODATE

Sodium metaperiodate (8 gm, 0.375 mole) was added in one portion with stirring to a solution of 15.5 gm of 6-phenoxyacetamidopenicillanic acid potassium salt in 300 ml of water. After 45 minutes at room temperature the starch–iodide test became negative, and the solution was diluted with 100 ml of water. The pH of the solution was lowered to 2.3 with dilute hydrochloric acid. The precipitated product was collected and crystallized from methanol (200 ml) and water (100 ml) to give 12.3 gm, mp 163°–164° (Morin *et al.*, 1969).

METHOD C—OZONE

A solution of 3.5 gm of 6-phenoxyacetamidopenicillanic acid in 50 ml of acetone and 50 ml of water was cooled in a salt–ice mixture to a temperature of 0°C, and the solution was ozonized while stirring for 2.5 hours. During this time a large excess of ozone was passed through the cold solution. The reaction solution was then evaporated *in vacuo* at a temperature of 45°C to remove the acetone. The solid white precipitate which formed during the removal of acetone was removed and vacuum dried at 30°C for 24 hours to yield 1.8 gm of crystalline 6-phenoxyacetamidopenicillanic acid-1β-oxide. The aqueous filtrate was lyophilized to yield a pale yellow amorphous solid which, after drying at 30°C for 24 hours, left 1.8 gm of 6-phenoxyacetamidopenicillanic acid-1α-oxide. IR (chloroform, cm^{-1}): β-Sulfoxide—1800 (β-lactam), 1690 (amide), 1080, 1065, 1035, and 1020 (sulfoxide); α-Sulfoxide—1796, 1730, 1700, 1080, 1065, and 1040 (Spry, unpublished results).

6-Aminopenicillanic Acid-1-Oxide Using Ozone

A suspension of 2.16 gm of 6-aminopenicillanic acid in 200 ml of water was cooled in an ice bath, and an oxygen stream containing ozone was passed through the cold suspension for 3 hours. The ozone was generated in a Welsbach ozonization apparatus at a rate of 3.4 gm/hour. Complete solution was obtained after about 2.5 hours of gas flow. The colorless solution was lyophilized to obtain 2.26 gm of 6-aminopenicillanic acid-1-oxide as a pale yellow solid. IR (mull, cm^{-1}): 1787 (β-lactam), 1025, 1007 (sulfoxide) (Spry, unpublished results).

2′,2′,2′-Trichloroethyl-6-Phenoxyacetamidopenicillanate-1β-Oxide by Oxidation with m-Chloroperbenzoic Acid

The penicillin ester (25 gm, 0.053 mole) was dissolved in 250 ml of chloroform and stirred in an ice-water bath; 85% m-chloroperbenzoic acid (10 gm, 0.05 mole) in 150 ml of chloroform was added dropwise over 30 minutes. Stirring and cooling were maintained for another 30 minutes. The reaction solution was washed with 5% sodium bicarbonate solution and then with water, dried (magnesium sulfate), and evaporated to dryness in vacuo. The residual oil was redissolved in 100 ml of ethyl ether (and a few drops of tetrahydrofuran to clear the solution) and chilled for crystallization; yield 23.0 gm (94%), mp 145°–146° (Chauvette et al., 1971).

2′,2′,2′-Trichloroethyl-6-Phenoxyacetamido-2β-Acetoxymethyl-2α-Methyl-penam-3-Carboxylate-1-Oxide by Oxidation with Ozone

A solution of 4 gm of 2′,2′,2′-trichloroethyl-6-phenoxyacetamido-2β-acet-oxymethyl-2α-methylpenam-3-carboxylate in 80 ml of acetone and 45 ml of water was cooled to a temperature of −10°C. The cold solution was ozonized with stirring until excess ozone had been passed through the solution. The reaction mixture was evaporated to dryness *in vacuo*, and the solid residue was chromatographed over a column packed with silica gel. The column was eluted by the gradient elution technique with a benzene–ethyl acetate gradient. The eluant fractions which contained the same materials, as indicated by thin-layer chromatography, were combined and evaporated to dryness to yield 430 mg of 2′,2′,2′-trichloroethyl-6-phenoxyacetamido-2β-acetoxymethyl-2α-methylpenam-3-carboxylate-1α-oxide and 1β-oxide mixture (Spry, unpublished results).

Hydrolysis of Methyl-7-Phenoxyacetamido-3-Methyl-3-Cephem-4-Carboxylate to the 2-Cephem Acid

The Δ^3 methyl ester (276 mg, 0.76 mmole) was dissolved in 10 ml of pyridine and 15 ml of water, and the solution was cooled in an ice bath. One equivalent (7.6 ml) of 0.100 N sodium hydroxide was added in one portion, and the solution was stirred in the cold for 3 hours. After evaporation and dissolution in water, the solution was layered with ethyl acetate and the pH lowered quickly in the cold to 2.0. After the layers separated the organic phase was washed with water and aqueous sodium chloride, dried, and evaporated. The crystalline product, approximately 300 mg, was recrystallized twice from chloroform–petroleum ether, yielding 83 mg; mp 172°–173.5° (dec) (182°–184° dec in preheated block); $[\alpha]_D$ +505°; IR (mull, cm^{-1}): 1764, 1743, and 1672.

The methyl ester was prepared in a similar manner to that of the methyl-6-phenoxyacetamidopenicillanate-1-oxide. The product was recrystallized from methylene chloride–diethyl ether; mp 109°–110°; IR (chloroform, cm^{-1}): 1780 (S), 1750, and 1695 (Morin *et al.*, 1969).

Isomerization of the Double Bond in Methyl-7-Phenoxyacetamido-3-Methyl-3-Cephem-4-Carboxylate

The Δ^3 methyl ester (3 gm) was allowed to stand in a pyridine–water (1:1) solution for 18 hours at room temperature. After removal of solvent the residue was separated into neutral (2.29 gm) and acidic (0.48 gm) fractions. The latter constituted the Δ^2 acid, which melted at 181.5°–182.5° after several crystallizations from ethyl acetate–water.

The neutral material was a 70:30 mixture of Δ^2 and Δ^3 esters by NMR analysis. These could be separated on a silica column using 10% ethyl acetate in benzene as eluant. The Δ^2 methyl ester crystallized from methylene chloride–petroleum ether, mp 137.5°–138.5 (Morin *et al.*, 1969).

p-Methoxybenzyl-7-Phenoxyacetamido-3-Acetoxymethyl-3-Cephem-4-Carboxylate-1-Oxide (Conversion of a Mixture of 2 and 3-Cephem Compounds to Pure 3-Cephem Compound)

A mixture of Δ^2 and Δ^3 (1:3) isomers of p-methoxybenzyl-7-phenoxyacet-amidocephalosporanate (0.125 gm) was dissolved in chloroform (4 ml), cooled in ice, and stirred while 85% m-chloroperbenzoic acid (0.04 gm) in chloroform (2 ml) was added dropwise. After 4 hours the reaction mixture was washed with saturated sodium bicarbonate and saturated sodium chloride. The organic solution was dried over magnesium sulfate, filtered, and evaporated in vacuo to give 0.127 gm of product. This crystallized from methanol to give 0.095 gm (75% yield) of isomerically pure 3-cephem sulfoxide, mp 161°–163° (Kaiser et al., 1970).

Ring Expansion Rearrangement of p-Nitrobenzyl-6-Phenoxyacetamido-penicillanate-1-Oxide

A 300-ml round-bottomed, three-necked flask was equipped with a mechanical stirrer, heating mantle, thermometer, and Dean–Stark water trap. The latter was connected to a condenser to which was attached a "Drierite" drying tube. The flask was charged with 10.0 gm (0.02 mole) of p-nitrobenzyl-6-phenoxyacetamidopenicillanate-1β-oxide, 80 ml of dry benzene, 60 ml of dry N,N-dimethylacetamide, and 0.12 ml of methanesulfonic acid. The Dean–Stark trap was filled with dry benzene. The resulting mixture was refluxed 12 hours. Approximately 0.4 ml of water collected in the trap. Thin-layer chromatography (silica gel–isoamyl acetate) showed only one major component. The red solution was concentrated under vacuum at 60°–65°C to a residue weight of 17.5 gm. Crystallization from 100 ml of 1:1 isopropanol–ether gave 7.08 gm (73.3% yield) of p-nitrobenzyl-7-phenoxyacetamido-3-methyl-3-cephem-4-carboxylate as a very light cream-colored solid, mp 188°–190°C (Hatfield, unpublished results).

Rearrangement of Methyl-6-Phthalimidopenicillanate-1α-Oxide in Acetic Anhydride

A solution of 10.0 gm of methyl-6-phthalimidopenicillanate-1α-oxide in 300 ml of freshly distilled acetic anhydride was degassed in vacuo and then heated with stirring in an atmosphere of helium for 3 hours at a temperature of 100°C. The reaction mixture was evaporated to dryness in vacuo to yield a frothy yellow residue. The residue was dissolved in 100 ml of chloroform and the solution cooled to 0°C. A solution of 4.0 gm of *m*-chloroperbenzoic acid in 50 ml of chloroform was added with stirring and the reaction mixture allowed to warm to room temperature. The reaction mixture was washed with a saturated solution of sodium bicarbonate followed by a brine wash, before drying over sodium sulfate. Evaporation of the dried reaction mixture yielded a white, frothy residue. The residue was chromatographed over a column measuring 2.8 × 31 cm, packed with 60 gm of silica gel. The column was eluted by gradient elution with the solvent system, i.e., benzene → 50% benzene–ethyl acetate. Elution was carried out at a flow rate of 1.3 ml/minute and 140 fractions of 10 ml each were collected. The following tabulated distribution of products in the collected fractions was determined by NMR.

Fraction no.	Weight (gm)	Product
1–49	0.134	Unidentified
50–53	0.062	A[a] + B[b]
54–56	0.06	A + B
58–60	0.209	75% A + 25% B
57, 61–63	0.446	67% A + 33% B
64–69	1.00	33% A + 67% B
70–75	0.92	15% A + 85% B
76–90	1.57	10% A + 90% B
91–140	2.44	73% C[c] + 25% B

[a] Methyl-6-phthalimido-2α-acetoxymethyl-2β-methyl-penam-3-carboxylate-1α-oxide.
[b] Methyl-6-phthalimido-2α-methyl-2β-acetoxymethyl-penam-3-carboxylate-1α-oxide.
[c] Methyl-7-phthalimido-3-methyl-3-acetoxycepham-4-carboxylate-1-oxide, and methyl-7-phthalimido-3-methyl-3-cephem-4-carboxylate.

The isomeric products methyl-6-phthalimido-2α-acetoxymethyl-2β-methyl-penam-3-carboxylate-1α-oxide   and   methyl-6-phthalimido-2α-methyl-2β-acetoxymethylpenam-3-carboxylate-1α-oxide were separated and isolated as colorless oils by further chromatography over silica gel using gradient elution with benzene plus 50% benzene–ethyl acetate.

Methyl-6-phthalimido-2α-methyl-2β-acetoxymethylpenam-3-carboxylate-1α-oxide: IR (chloroform, cm⁻¹) 1806 (imide), 1785 (β-lactam), 1750, 1730, 1055 (S → O). Methyl-6-phthalimido-2α-acetoxymethyl-2β-methylpenam-3-carboxylate-1α-oxide: IR (chloroform, cm⁻¹) 1808 (imide), 1780 (β-lactam), 1745, 1725, 1050 (S → O) (Spry, unpublished results).

Photochemical Isomerization of Methyl-6-Acetamido-2α-Methyl-2β-Acetoxymethylpenam-3-Carboxylate-1β-Oxide

A mixture (490 mg, 1.41 mmoles) of methyl-6-acetamido-2α-methyl-2β-acetoxymethylpenam-3-carboxylate-1β-oxide in 190 ml of acetone was placed in a wheel-shaped (hollow in the center) reaction vessel fitted with a quartz immersion well in which was placed a 450-W medium pressure mercury-arc lamp which was surrounded by a Pyrex glass filter sleeve. Helium gas was bubbled through the reaction mixture while irradiation continued for 6 hours. After the photolysis (irradiation) the reaction mixture was evaporated under reduced pressure to remove the acetone. The residue was taken up in benzene and chromatographed on silica gel using a gradient system of 1.5 liters of ethyl acetate. The products isolated consisted of (1) 190 mg of a mixture of the β-sulfoxide-2β-acetoxymethyl (a) and β-sulfoxide-2α-acetoxymethyl (b) penicillin esters in a ratio of 69 % of isomer (a) to 31 % of isomer (b) as determined by NMR spectral methods, and (2) 225 mg of a mixture of α-sulfoxide-2β-acetoxymethyl (c) and α-sulfoxide-2α-acetoxymethylpenicillin (d) esters in a ratio of 65 % by weight of isomer (c) to 35 % by weight of isomer (d). Approximately 415 mg of the starting material was recovered. These isomeric fractions were rechromatographed to isolate the pure epimers (Spry, unpublished results).

Methyl-7-Phthalimidocephalosporanate by Ring Expansion Reaction

Methyl-6-phthalimido-2α-methyl-2β-acetoxymethylpenam-3-carboxylate-1α-oxide, 171 mg, was added to a solution of 1 ml of acetic anhydride in 10 ml of dimethylacetamide containing 40 mg of p-toluenesulfonic acid monohydrate, and the mixture was heated with stirring for 3 hours under an atmosphere of helium at a temperature of 84°C. The pale yellow reaction mixture was evaporated to dryness *in vacuo* to yield a pale yellow residual oil. The yellow oil was chromatographed over a column measuring 2.5 × 9.0 cm packed with 15 gm of silica gel. Gradient elution with benzene → 50 % ethyl acetate–benzene at a flow rate of 4.6 ml/minute gave the results tabulated below.

Fractions 19–23 contained 12 mg of the rearrangement product methyl-7-phthalimidocephalosporanate. The product proved to be identical (NMR, thin-layer chromatograms, and infrared spectra) to a sample of methyl-7-phthalimidocephalosporanate prepared from 7-ACA.

Fractions 26–29 yielded 28 mg of methyl-7-phthalimido-3-acetoxymethyl-3-hydroxycepham-4-carboxylate, melting at about 237°–238°C. IR (chloroform, cm^{-1}): 1788, 1777, and 1725 (Spry, unpublished results).

Fraction no.	Product weight (mg)[a]
1–16	—
16–18	5
19–23	12
26–29	28
30–34	1
36–43	40
44–70	56

[a] Residual weight. following evaporation of combined fractions.

Rearrangement of 2′,2′,2′-Trichloroethyl-6-Phenoxyacetamidopenicillanate-1β-Oxide with Trimethylphosphite

A solution of the 6-phenoxymethylpenicillin sulfoxide ester (10.0 gm) and trimethylphosphite (2 ml) in benzene (50 ml) was refluxed for 36 hours. The solution was cooled, washed well with water (6 × 100 ml), dried (magnesium sulfate), and the solvent removed *in vacuo* to give a white solid. Recrystallization from methanol gave the thiazoline–azetidinone as colorless needles, mp 133° (6.0 gm). The mother liquors further gave 1.5 gm of crystals. IR (chloroform, cm^{-1}): 1770 and 1745. Treatment of a solution of the above product in benzene with triethylamine gave an isomer, recrystallized from methanol as colorless needles, mp 70°. IR (chloroform, cm^{-1}): 1770 and 1730 (Cooper, unpublished results).

Rearrangement of p-Nitrobenzyl-6-Phenoxyacetamidopenicillanate-1β-Oxide to a 3-Hydroxy-3-Methylcepham Compound

The 4′-nitrobenzyl ester of phenoxymethylpenicillin sulfoxide (10.0 gm) was dissolved in 60 ml of *N,N*-dimethylacetamide, and this solution was diluted with 80 ml of azeotropically dried benzene containing approximately 2 drops of concentrated sulfuric acid. The resulting mixture was refluxed for 12 hours and then concentrated *in vacuo* to a residue weight of about 24 gm. Addition of hot isopropanol (100 ml) and warming to achieve solution resulted in crystallization of *p*-nitrobenzyl-7-phenoxyacetamido-3α-methyl-3β-hydroxycepham-4-carboxylate upon cooling. Recrystallization of this material from ethanol or isopropanol afforded analytically pure material, mp 212°–214° (47% yield) (Gutowski *et al.*, unpublished results).

2′,2′,2′-Trichloroethyl-7-Amino-3-Methyl-3-Cephem-4-Carboxylate Ester (p-Toluenesulfonic Acid Salt)

2′,2′,2′-Trichloroethyl-7-phenoxyacetamido-3-methyl-3-cephem-4-carboxylate (2.2 gm, 4.6 mmoles) was dissolved in 120 ml of calcium hydride-dried benzene containing dry pyridine (540 mg, 6.8 mmoles). The solution was placed in a water bath at 65°. While stirring, phosphorous pentachloride (1.4 gm, 6.8 mmoles) was added; the mixture was stirred at this temperature and under nitrogen for 2 hours. The benzene was removed *in vacuo* and replaced by 240 ml of methanol. The solution was stored at room temperature under nitrogen overnight. The alcohol was removed *in vacuo*. The residue was redissolved in a mixture of water–tetrahydrofuran at room temperature for 15 minutes to effect hydrolysis. The organic solvent was evaporated. The aqueous solution, with its oil precipitate, was slurried with ethyl acetate and adjusted to pH near 7 with 1 N sodium hydroxide. The ethyl acetate solution was separated, washed with water, dried (magnesium sulfate), and concentrated to about 80 ml. The concentrate was treated with p-toluenesulfonic acid monohydrate (875 mg, 4.6 mmoles) in 70 ml of the same solvent to precipitate the product which was a crystalline salt; 1.9 gm (80% yield). IR (Nujol mull): 5.65 μ (β-lactam carbonyl), 5.81 μ (ester carbonyl), 8.1 μ (sulfur trioxide) and in the aromatic region. Electrometric titration (in 66% aqueous dimethyl formamide) showed a pK_a of 3.9 and an apparent molecular weight of 380 (calc. 346). A sample was recrystallized from ethanol–water; mp 139°–194° (dec).

The free amino ester was recovered from its tosylate by suspending the salt in water–ether and adjusting the pH to near 7 with 1 N sodium hydroxide. The ethereal solution was separated, dried (magnesium sulfate), and evaporated to dryness *in vacuo*.

The residual oil slowly crystallized under refrigeration. This recrystallized, with difficulty, from wet cyclohexene; mp 82–84° (Chauvette *et al.*, 1971).

p-Nitrobenzyl-7-Amino-2-Cephem-4-Carboxylate by Cleavage of Phthalimido Substituent

To a stirred solution of p-nitrobenzyl-7-phthalimido-3-methyl-2-cephem 4-carboxylate (268 mg, 0.5 mmole) in 25 ml of methylene chloride was added 0.033 ml (1.0 mmole) of 97% hydrazine in 25 ml of methylene chloride. After stirring for 24 hours at 25° the slurry was filtered and the filtrate evaporated to give 259 mg of yellow froth. Chromatography on silica (benzene–acetone) gave 61 mg (30%) of p-nitrobenzyl-7-amino-3-methyl-2-cephem-4-carboxylate and 188 mg starting material (Spry, unpublished results).

2',2',2'-Trichloroethyl-7-Phenoxyacetamido-2-Methylene-3-Methyl-3-Cephem-4-Carboxylate-1-Oxide

To a solution of 2',2',2'-trichloroethyl-7-phenoxyacetamido-3-methyl-3-cephem-4-carboxylate-1-oxide (15.0 gm, 30.3 mmoles) in hot methylene chloride (50 ml) was added formaldehyde (3.0 gm, 37% aqueous solution, 37 mmoles), dimethylamine hydrochloride (2.46 gm, 30.2 mmoles), and *t*-butyl alcohol (500 ml). The mixture was refluxed gently for 24 hours until thin-layer chromatography analysis (benzene–ethyl acetate, 1:1) showed complete disappearance of starting material (R_f 0.27) and appearance of a new, less polar spot (R_f 0.45). The solution was then concentrated to ≈ 300 ml.

On cooling, compound separated as fine, light-yellow needles (13.0 gm, mp 173°–174° dec). Concentration of the mother liquors yielded a small second crop, 1.6 gm (total yield 95%). Generally, this material was sufficiently pure to use in subsequent reactions. Recrystallization from methylene chloride-*t*-butyl alcohol raised the mp to 177°–178° (dec). UV (ethanol): 216 nm (sh, $\epsilon = 13,900$), 262 (sh), 267 (7,250), 274 (sh), 313 (3,950); IR (chloroform, cm^{-1}): 3350, 1800, 1740, 1695, 1600, 1040 (Wright *et al.*, 1971).

Preparation and Methanolysis of a 3-Bromomethyl-2-Cephem Ester

A solution of 1.17 gm (2.5 mmoles) of *p*-methoxybenzyl-7-phenoxyacetamido-3-methyl-2-cepham-4-carboxylate in 250 ml of carbon tetrachloride was thoroughly purged with nitrogen; 445 mg (2.5 mmoles) of NBS and 61.5 mg (0.375 mole) of azobisisobutyronitrile (AIBN) were added, and the mixture was heated in an oil bath at 84°. Reaction was complete in 4 hours. Cooling, filtering to remove succinimide, and evaporating the solvent provided the crude allylic bromide as an oil. This was dissolved in 100 ml of absolute methanol containing 725 mg (5 mmoles) of *N,N*-dimethylaniline. After 24 hours, work-up provided 970 mg of crude product, which was purified by gradient column chromatography on silica gel–15% water with benzene → 4% ethyl acetate to give a 40% yield, mp 116°–118°, as well as 15% recovered starting material (Webber *et al.*, 1971).

Displacement of the Acetoxy Group in a Cephalosporanic Acid by a Nitrogen Nucleophile: Preparation of Cephaloridine

A solution of 200 gm (0.46 mole) of cephalothin sodium salt, 100 gm (1.04 moles) of potassium thiocyanate, and 100 ml (1.25 moles) of pyridine in 500 ml of water was adjusted to pH 6.5 with 85% phosphoric acid and heated with stirring at 60° for 6 hours. After cooling to room temperature the solution was extracted with a 25% solution of Amerlite LA-1 (acetate form) in methyl isobutyl ketone (MIBK) (six 1-liter portions) and washed with MIBK (500 ml). The aqueous solution was allowed to stand overnight in the cold (5°). The product which separated weighed 41 gm (20%); UV (H$_2$O): 238 nm ($\epsilon = 15,200$) and 251 nm ($\epsilon = 13,950$) (Spencer et al., 1967).

Displacement of the Acetoxy Group in a Cephalosporin with a Sulfur Nucleophile

A mixture of the sodium salt of cephalosporin C (5.0 gm) and thiourea (8.0 gm) in water (200 ml) was allowed to react at 37°. After five days, paper chromatography indicated that only traces of cephalosporin C remained. Acetone (1 liter) was added and the mixture cooled to 0°. The product obtained by centrifuging was triturated with acetone to give a brown solid (3.7 gm). A solution of this product in water (500 ml) was passed through a column (26.0 × 2.5 cm) of Dowex 1 × 8 (acetate cycle). Paper chromatography of the eluates showed that the thiouronium derivative was eluted rapidly and was free from thiourea and cephalosporin C. Selected fractions (25 ml) were freeze-dried to give a cream solid (2.58 gm). Trituration with a small volume of absolute methanol gave a fluffy solid (2.18 gm). Crystallization from methanol–water gave a white solid, mp >180° (cap), [α]$_D$ +62° (c 0.2, water). An analytical specimen of 7-D-(5-amino-5-carboxyvaleramido)-3-methylisothiouronium-3-cephem-4-carboxylic acid was obtained by passing an aqueous solution through a column of equal volumes of charcoal and Celite, freeze-drying the eluates, and crystallizing from aqueous methanol to give colorlesss blades, mp 197° (cap, dec), [α]$_D$ +66° (c 4.0, water), UV: 259–262 nm ($\epsilon = 8,050$), IR (cm^{-1}) (Infracord, uncorrected frequencies) at 3500, 3300 (NH), 1760 (β-lactam), 1676 (CONH) and 1610 (CO$_2$). This compound showed no net charge when subjected to electrophoresis at pH 7.0 or 4.0 (Cocker et al., 1965).

N-(2,2,2-Trichloroethyloxycarbonyl)-D-α-Phenylglycine

To a solution of D-α-phenylglycine (22.7 gm, 0.15 mole), 300 ml of water, 160 ml of 1 N sodium hydroxide, and 150 ml of ether was added dropwise over a period of 1 hour, 2,2,2-trichloroethylchloroformate (42.5 gm, 0.2 mole) in 200 ml of sodium-dried dioxane simultaneously with 200 ml of 1 N sodium hydroxide, while cooling and stirring at ice–alcohol temperature. The mixture was maintained cold for an additional hour and then washed with large volumes of ether. The aqueous solution, layered with ethyl acetate, was acidified in the cold to pH 2.5 with syrupy phosphoric acid. The ethyl acetate layer was separated, washed with water, dried (magnesium sulfate), and evaporated *in vacuo*. The residual oil crystallized when slurried with petroleum ether; yield 43 gm (87%), mp 142°–144°. IR (chloroform): 2.92 μ (amide NH), 5.8 μ (broad, acid, and carbamate carbonyls), and 6.67 μ (amide II and phenyl). Electrometric titration (in 66% aqueous dimethylformamide) showed a titratable group at 5.60 and an apparent molecular weight of 320 (calc. 327). The sample was recrystallized from benzene–petroleum ether (Chauvette *et al.*, 1971).

2',2',2'-Trichloroethyl-7-[N-(2,2,2-Trichloroethyloxycarbonyl)-D-α-Phenyl-glycylamido]-3-Methyl-3-Cephem-4-Carboxylate

To a solution of methyl chloroformate (2.1 gm, 22 mmoles) in 200 ml of calcium hydride-dried tetrahydrofuran cooled in an ice–alcohol bath, was added dropwise a solution of *N*-(2,2,2-trichloroethyloxycarbonyl)-D-α-phenylglycine (7.2 gm, 22 mmoles), triethylamine (2.2 gm, 22 mmoles), and dimethylbenzylamine (6 drops) in 100 ml of dry tetrahydrofuran. Cooling and stirring were maintained for 20 minutes following addition. Then 2',2',2'-trichloroethyl-7-amino-3-methyl-3-cephem-4-carboxylate, freed from its tosylate (10.4 gm, 20 mmoles), was added dropwise in 100 ml of the same solvent. The reaction mixture was stirred at ice–alcohol temperature for 3 hours. The solvent was removed *in vacuo*. The residue was redissolved in cold ethyl acetate for successive cold washes with water, 5% hydrochloric acid, 5% sodium bicarbonate solution, and water. The solution was dried (magnesium sulfate) and evaporated *in vacuo*. The residual oil was redissolved in 60 ml of carbon tetrachloride for crystallization; yield 12.2 gm (93%), mp 95°. IR (chloroform): 2.95 μ (amide NH), 5.62 μ (β-lactam carbonyl), 5.78 μ (ester and carbamate carbonyls), 5.93 μ (amide carbonyl), and in the aromatic region. The sample recrystallized from the same solvent (Chauvette *et al.*, 1971).

7-(D-α-Amino-α-Phenylacetamido)-3-Methyl-3-Cephem-4-Carboxylic Acid (Cephalexin)

2',2',2'-Trichloroethyl-7-[*N*-(2,2,2-trichloroethyloxycarbonyl)-D-α-phenyl-glycylamido]-3-methyl-3-cephem-4-carboxylate (3.9 gm, 6.0 mmoles) was dissolved in 200 ml of 90% aqueous formic acid. The solution was cooled in an ice-water bath. Zinc metal dust (3.9 gm, 60 mmoles) was added, and the mixture was stirred for 55 minutes. The zinc was filtered and washed with 40 ml of aqueous formic acid. The filtrate and wash were combined and evaporated *in vacuo*, azeotroping with benzene to remove the last traces of formic acid. The residue was taken up in 80 ml of water (pH 3.5) and treated with hydrogen sulfide for 15 minutes. The precipitated zinc sulfide was filtered off with the aid of Filter-cel; the filtrate (pH 2) was concentrated to about 20 ml, cooled in ice, and adjusted to pH 7 with 50% sodium hydroxide. A slight amount of precipitate was removed by filtration. The solution was reacidified to pH 4.5 (isoelectric point of cephalexin) and diluted with 60 ml of acetonitrile. The crystallized product was pure cephalexin; 500 mg (24% yield).

The bioautograph (*Bacillus subtilis* seeded agar plate of a paper chromatogram, developed in *n*-butanol–acetic acid–water, 3:1:1) showed a single biologically active spot corresponding exactly in mobility and potency to authentic cephalexin at like concentration (Chauvette *et al.*, 1971).

References

Belgium Patent 721,348.

Chauvette, R. R. Unpublished results.

Chauvette, R. R., Pennington, P. A., Ryan, C. W., Cooper, R. D. G., José, F. L., Wright, I. G., Van Heyningen, E. M., and Huffman, G. W. (1971). *J. Org. Chem.* **36**, 1259.

Cocker, J. D., Cowley, B. R., Cox, J. S. G., Eardley, S., Gregory, G. I., Lazenby, J. K., Long, A. G., Sly, J. C. P., and Somerfield, G. A. (1965). *J. Chem. Soc.*, 5015.

Cooper, R. D. G. Unpublished results.

Gutowski, G. E., Foster, B. J., Daniels, C. J., Hatfield, L. D., and Fisher, J. W. (1971). *Tetrahedron Lett.*, 3433.

Hatfield, L. D. Unpublished results.

Kaiser, G. V., Cooper, R. D. G., Koehler, R. E., Murphy, C. F., Webber, J. A., Wright, I. G., and Van Heyningen, E. M. (1970). *J. Org. Chem.* **35**, 2430.

Morin, R. B., Jackson, B. G., Mueller, R. A., Lavagnino, E. R., Scanlon, W. B., and Andrews, S. L. (1969). *J. Amer. Chem. Soc.* **91**, 1401.

Murphy, C. F., and Koehler, R. E. (1970). *J. Org. Chem.* **35**, 2429.

Spencer, J. L., Siu, F. Y., Jackson, B. G., Higgens, H. M., and Flynn, E. H. (1967). *J. Org. Chem.* **32**, 500.

Spry, D. O. Unpublished results.

Webber, J. A., Huffman, G. W., Koehler, R. E., Murphy, C. F., Ryan, C. W., Van Heyningen, E. M., and Vasileff, R. T. (1971). *J. Med. Chem.* **14**, 113.

Wright, I. G., Ashbrook, C. W., Goodson, T., Kaiser, G. V., and Van Heyningen, E. M. (1971). *J. Med. Chem.* **14**, 420.

II. Analytical Methods

Nicotinamide Assay for Cephalosporin Derivatives Containing an Acetyl Moiety

REAGENTS

1. Nicotinamide—12.0% w/v nicotinamide [Matheson–Coleman–Bell (MCB)] in water. Prepare fresh each week.
2. 1,3-Dihydroxyacetone (DHA)—2.0% w/v DHA from MCB in water. Prepare fresh every 4 hours.
3. Potassium phosphate—1.5 M potassium phosphate in water.
4. Sodium carbonate—8.0% w/v sodium carbonate in water.

PROCEDURE

1. Add 1.0 ml of sample solution to 1.0 ml of nicotinamide solution in a 150-mm tube. This is the *sample* tube. The *blank* tube is prepared by adding 1.0 ml of sample solution to 1.0 ml of water. Treat both sample and blank tubes in the same manner throughout the remainder of the assay.
2. Heat the tubes in a gently rolling steam bath for 5–8 minutes.* Immerse the tubes in about $1\frac{1}{2}$ in. of the bath water.
3. Cool the tubes by gently shaking them in a 10°C water bath (3–4 in deep) for 30–35 seconds.
4. Add by transfer pipet 2.0 ml of DHA solution to each tube immediately after removal from the ice bath. Complete this addition between 8 and 14 minutes after the start of the heating period (step 2).
5. Exactly 15 minutes after the start of the heating period, add 2.0 ml of sodium carbonate solution to each tube. In a series of determinations make the sodium carbonate additions at 10-second intervals. Swirl the contents of the tube as the reagent is blown from a pipet into the center of the tube.
6. Exactly 5 minutes after the addition of the sodium carbonate solution (step 5), add 1.0 ml of potassium phosphate solution to each tube. In a series of determinations, the potassium phosphate solution is added at 10-second intervals.
7. Determine the absorbance of the sample and blank solutions on a suitable spectrophotometer at 360 nm using 1.0-cm silica cells and water in the reference cell.

---

* *Note:* A time study should be performed at this state to optimize the heating time required for local laboratory equipment.

RESULTS

A standard response curve with increasing concentrations of sodium cephalo-sporin C approximates Beer's Law from 0.1–1.0 mg/ml. The absorbance of a test solution containing 1.0 mg/ml of sodium cephalosporin C is approximately 0.5 in a 1.0-cm cell.

Hydroxylamine Method for Cephalosporins

REAGENTS

1. Acetate buffer—2.06% w/v sodium acetate in 4.32 M sodium hydroxide.
2. Hydroxylamine hydrochloride—34.8% w/v in water. Refrigerate.
3. Hydroxylamine-buffer reagent—Mix 10.0 ml of acetate buffer (1), 10.0 ml of hydroxylamine hydrochloride (2), and 40 ml water. Prepare fresh.
4. Ferric reagent—33.3% w/v ferric ammonium sulfate in 1.4 M sulfuric acid. Filter.

PROCEDURE

1. Add by transfer pipet 1.0 ml of sample (approximately 1 mg/ml of cephalosporin) to a clean dry test tube.
2. Add by transfer pipet 3.0 ml of hydroxylamine-buffer reagent. Mix and allow to stand 3 minutes.
3. Add by transfer pipet 1.0 ml of ferric reagent. Mix thoroughly to insure complete solution of any precipitate formed.
4. Determine the absorbance of this solution at 515 nm on a suitable spectrophotometer, using 1.0-cm cells and water in the reference cell.
5. Determine a blank correction for the sample by repeating the above procedure but adding the ferric reagent (step 3) prior to the hydroxylamine–buffer reagent (step 2).
6. Determine a standard absorbance by repeating the above procedure on the corresponding cephalosporin standard, and calculate cephalosporin content present in the sample in the conventional manner.

Moore–Stein Assay Procedures for Cephalexin, Cephaloglycin, and Related Compounds

APPARATUS

A Beckman Model 120C amino acid analyzer is used. The water-jacketed column has the following specifications: 0.9-cm i.d. × 23-cm length packed to a height of 9.0 with Beckman Custom Research Resin Type PA-35.

REAGENTS

1. Sodium acetate buffer solution, 4.0 M (pH 5.51 ± 0.03 for ninhydrin reagent).
2. Sodium citrate buffer solution, 0.2 M (pH 2.20 ± 0.03).
3. Sodium citrate buffer solution, 0.2 M (pH 3.25 ± 0.005).
4. Sodium citrate buffer solution, 0.2 M (pH 4.25 ± 0.005).
5. Sodium hydroxide solution, 0.2 M.
6. Ninhydrin solution—Dissolve 80.0 gm of ninhydrin (1,2,3-triketo-hydrindene hydrate, Pierce Reagent, Pierce Chemical Company) in 3.0 liters of methyl cellosolve (peroxide free). Add 1 liter of sodium acetate buffer and 1.600 gm of stannous chloride dihydrate. Mix thoroughly. Prepare and store this reagent under nitrogen (prepurified).

PROCEDURE

1. PREPARATION OF STANDARDS

Accurately weigh approximately 15.00 mg of 7-ACA, 6.00 mg of phenyl-glycine, or 15.00 mg of 7-ADCA into a 50-ml volumetric flask. Dissolve and dilute to volume with sodium citrate buffer (pH 2.2).

Accurately weigh approximately 10.00 mg of cephalexin into a 10-ml volumetric flask. Dissolve and dilute to volume with sodium citrate buffer (pH 2.2). Add 100 λ of the desired standard solution to the column.

2. PREPARATION OF SAMPLE

A. Determination of 7-ACA and Phenylglycine in Cephaloglycin

Accurately weigh approximately 25.00 mg of sample into a 10-ml volumetric flask. Dissolve and dilute to volume with sodium citrate buffer (pH 2.2); apply 1.0 ml to the column.

B. Determination of 7-ADCA and Phenylglycine in Cephalexin

Accurately weigh approximately 25.00 mg of sample into a 10-ml volumetric flask. Dissolve and dilute to volume with sodium citrate buffer (pH 2.2); apply 1.0 ml to the column.

C. Determination of Cephalexin in Urine

Add 5.0 ml of urine to a 10-ml volumetric flask. Dilute to volume with sodium citrate buffer (pH 2.2); apply 100 λ to the column.

3. OPERATING PARAMETERS

A. *Determination of 7-ACA in Cephaloglycin*

> Mode: Automatic
> Buffer A: Sodium citrate buffer (pH 3.25 ± 0.005)
> Buffer B: None
> Elapsed time: 45 minutes
> Buffer change: None
> Column temperature: 55°C
> Flow rates: Elution buffer—68 ml/hour
>   Ninhydrin solution—34 ml/hour
> Elution time: 7-ACA—20 minutes
>   Phenylglycine—36 minutes

B. *Determination of 7-ADCA and Phenylglycine in Cephalexin*

> Mode: Automatic
> Buffer A: Sodium citrate buffer (pH 3.25 ± 0.005)
> Buffer B: Sodium citrate buffer (pH 4.25 ± 0.005)
> Elapsed time: 55 minutes
> Buffer change: 20 minutes
> Column temperature: 55°C
> Flow rates: Elution buffer—68 ml/hour
>   Ninhydrin solution—34 ml/hour
> Elution time: Phenylglycine—36 minutes
>   7-ADCA—45 minutes

C. *Determination of Cephalexin in Urine*

> Mode: Automatic
> Buffer A: Sodium citrate buffer (pH 3.25 ± 0.005)
> Buffer B: Sodium citrate buffer (pH 4.25 ± 0.005)
> Elapsed time: 70 minutes
> Buffer change: 20 minutes
> Column temperature: 55°C
> Flow rates: Elution buffers—68 ml/hour
>   Ninhydrin solution—34 ml/hour
> Elution time: 61 minutes

The analyzer is operated in the conventional manner. Columns must be regenerated with 0.2 M sodium hydroxide after each run and equilibrated with 0.2 M sodium citrate buffer (pH 3.25) after each regeneration prior to the application of another sample.

4. CALCULATIONS

A. Determination of 7-ACA and Phenylglycine in Cephaloglycin or 7-ADCA and Phenylglycine in Cephalexin

$$\frac{a}{b} \times \frac{c}{d} \times \% \text{ purity of standard} = \% \text{ compound}$$

a = area under sample curve
b = weight in μg of sample applied to the column
c = weight in μg of the standard applied to the column
d = area under the standard curve

B. Determination of Cephalexin in Urine

$$\frac{a}{b} \times \frac{c}{d} \times \frac{\% \text{ purity of cephalexin standard}}{100} = \mu\text{g cephalexin per ml}$$

a = area under sample curve
b = ml of urine to the column
c = weight in mcg of the standard applied to the column
d = area under the standard curve

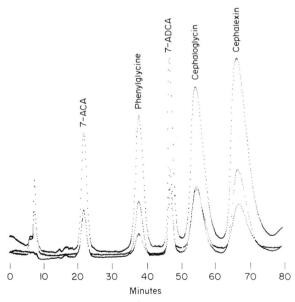

Fig. 1. Amino acid analyzer chromatogram of cephalosporins and related compounds. See text, Moore–Stein assay procedure. Weight of compound (μg) applied to column: 7-ACA, 30.46; phenylglycine, 13.76; 7-ADCA, 31.5; cephaloglycin, 156.2; cephalexin, 154.1.

III. Physical Chemical Data

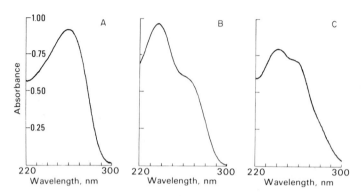

Fig. 2. Ultraviolet absorption spectra of cephalosporins. (A) Cephalosporin C sodium salt, 53.5 μg/ml H_2O. (B) Cephalothin sodium salt, 29 μg/ml H_2O. (C) Cephaloridine, 21 μg/ml H_2O.

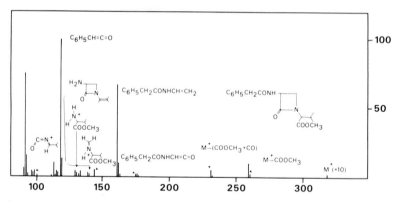

Fig. 3. Mass spectrum of desthiobenzylpenicillin methyl ester. Taken with CEC21-110B mass spectrometer at 70 eV (Nagarajan, unpublished results).

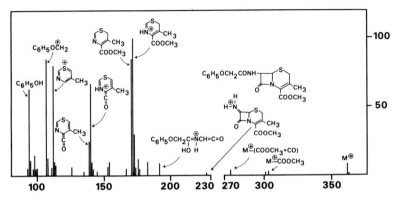

Fig. 4. Mass spectrum of methyl-7-phenoxyacetamido-3-methyl-3-cephem-4-carboxylate. Taken with CEC21-110B mass spectrometer at 70 eV (Nagarajan, unpublished results).

Table I

HIGH-RESOLUTION MASS SPECTRAL DATA[a] OF DESTHIOBENZYLPENICILLIN METHYL ESTER (17)

Ion	Mass (found)	% intensity	Elemental composition	ΔmmU
(17g)	98.06004	4	C_5H_8NO	−0.6
(17n)	118.04040	100	C_8H_6O	−1.5
(17m)	130.08952	3	$C_6H_{12}O_2N$	2.7
(17p)	140.09090	2	$C_7H_{12}ON_2$	−4.1
(17c)	144.10163	5	$C_7H_{14}O_2N$	−0.8
(17f)	161.08069	67	$C_{10}H_{11}ON$	−3.4
(17b)	175.06718	2	$C_{10}H_9O_2N$	3.9
(17j)	231.14852	5	$C_{14}H_{19}ON_2$	−1.2
(17q)	259.14407	10	$C_{15}H_{19}O_2N_2$	−0.6
(17)	—	0.2	—	—

[a] Nagarajan (unpublished work).

Table II

HIGH-RESOLUTION MASS SPECTRAL DATA[a] OF METHYL-7-PHENOXYACETAMIDO-3-METHYL-3-
CEPHEM-4-CARBOXYLATE (*19m*)

Ion	Mass (found)	% intensity	Elemental composition	ΔmmU
(*19i*)	112.02171	80	C_5H_6NS	-0.4
(*19h*)	113.02681	10	C_5H_7NS	-3.1
(*19g*)	114.03892	8	C_5H_8NS	1.2
(*19e*)	140.01534	67	C_6H_6ONS	-1.7
(*19b*)	171.03614	85	$C_7H_9O_2NS$	0.7
(*19a, 19q*)	172.04274	100	$C_7H_{10}O_2N^{32}S$	-0.5
(*19r*)	174.04261	6	$C_7H_{10}O_2N^{34}S$	-0.4
(*19c*)	192.06604	9	$C_{10}H_{10}O_3N$	0
(*19l*)	303.08517	3	$C_{15}H_{15}O_3N_2S$	4.8
(*19p*)	362.09879	8	$C_{17}H_{18}O_5N_2S$	5.2

[a] Nagarajan (unpublished work).

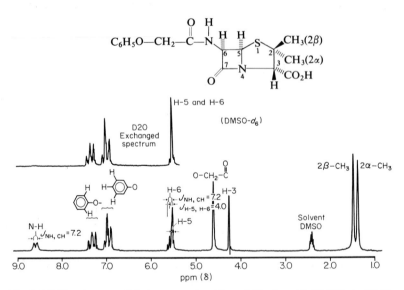

Fig. 5. NMR spectrum of 6-phenoxyacetamidopenicillanic acid, DMSO-d_6; 60 Hz.

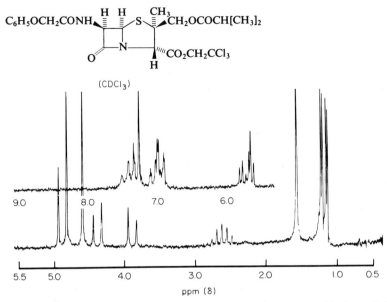

Fig. 6. NMR spectrum of 2′,2′,2′-trichloroethyl-6-phenoxyacetamido-2α-methyl-2β-isobutyroxymethylpenam-3-carboxylate. CDCl$_3$; 100 Hz (Spry, unpublished results).

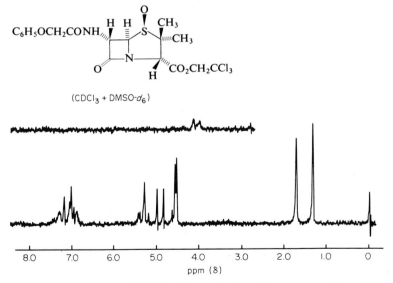

Fig. 7. NMR spectrum of 2′,2′,2′-trichloroethyl-6-epiphenoxyacetamidopenicillanate-1β-oxide. CDCl$_3$ and DMSO-d_6; 60 Hz (Gutowski, 1970).

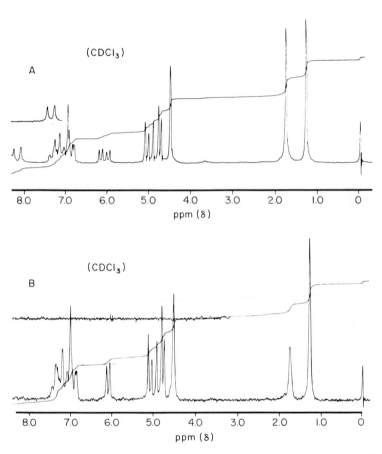

Fig. 8. NMR spectrum of (A) 2′,2′,2′-trichloroethyl-6-phenoxyacetamidopenicillanate-1β-oxide. CDCl₃; 60 Hz (Cooper, 1970). (B) 2′,2′,2′-Trichloroethyl-6-phenoxyacetamido-2β-deuteriomethylpenicillanate-1β-oxide. CDCl₃; 60 Hz (Cooper, 1970).

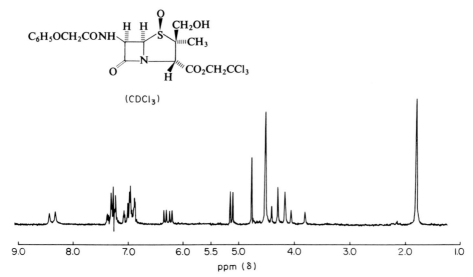

Fig. 9. NMR spectrum of 2′,2′,2′-trichloroethyl-6-phenoxyacetamido-2α-methyl-2β-hydroxymethylpenam-3-carboxylate-1β-oxide. CDCl₃; 60 Hz (Cooper, unpublished results).

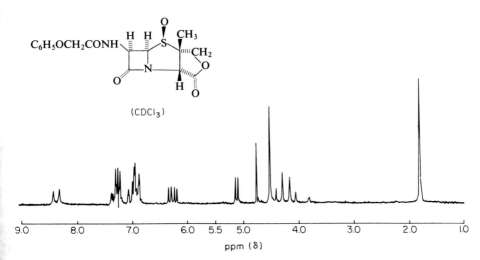

Fig. 10. NMR spectrum of 6-phenoxyacetamido-2α-hydroxymethyl-2β-methylpenam-3-carboxy-γ-lactone-1β-oxide. CDCl₃; 60 Hz (Cooper, unpublished results).

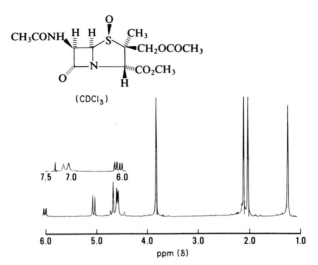

Fig. 11. NMR spectrum of methyl-6-acetamido-2α-methyl-2β-acetoxymethylpenam-3-carboxylate-1β-oxide. CDCl₃; 100 Hz (Spry, 1970).

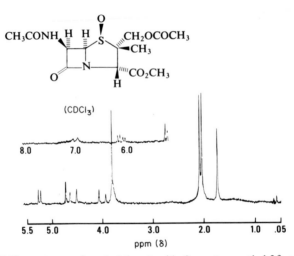

Fig. 12. NMR spectrum of methyl-6-acetamido-2α-acetoxymethyl-2β-methylpenam-3-carboxylate-1β-oxide. CDCl₃; 100 Hz (Spry, 1970).

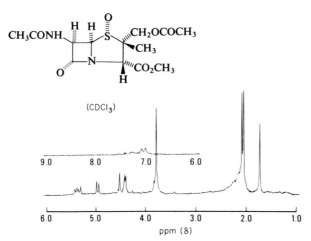

Fig. 13. NMR spectrum of methyl-6-acetamido-2α-acetoxymethyl-2β-methylpenam-3-carboxylate-1α-oxide. CDCl₃; 100 Hz (Spry, 1970).

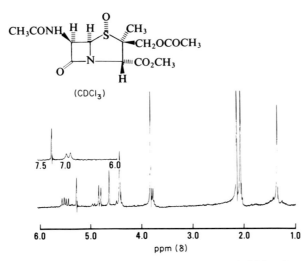

Fig. 14. NMR spectrum of methyl-6-acetamido-2α-methyl-2β-acetoxymethylpenam-3-carboxylate-1α-oxide. CDCl₃; 100 Hz (Spry, 1970).

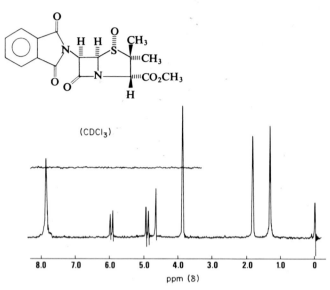

Fig. 15. NMR spectrum of methyl-6-phthalimidopenicillanate-1∥α-oxide. CDCl₃; 60 Hz (Cooper *et al.*, 1969b).

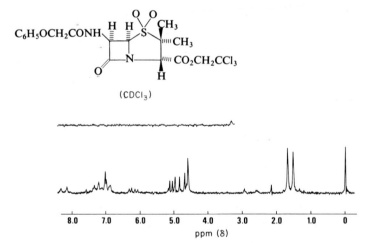

Fig. 16. NMR spectrum of 2′,2′,2′-trichloroethyl-6-phenoxyacetamidopenicillanate-1,1-dioxide. CDCl₃; 60 Hz (Cooper *et al.*, 1969a).

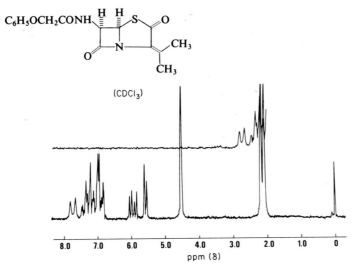

Fig. 17. NMR spectrum of phenoxymethylanhydropenicillin. CDCl₃; 60 Hz.

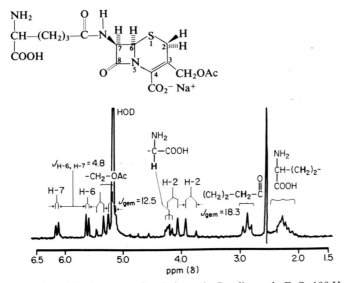

Fig. 18. NMR Spectrum of cephalosporin C sodium salt. D₂O; 100 Hz.

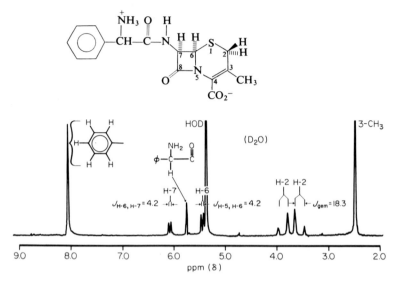

Fig. 19. NMR spectrum of 7-(D-α-aminophenylacetamido)-3-cephem-3-methyl-4-carboxylic acid (cephalexin). D₂O; 60 Hz (Ryan *et al.*, 1969).

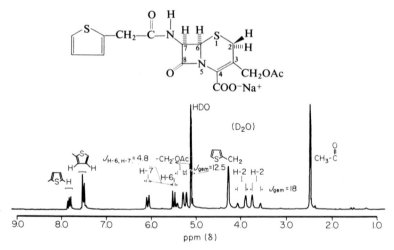

Fig. 20. NMR spectrum of 7-(thiophene-2-acetamido)cephalosporanic acid sodium salt (cephalothin sodium salt). D₂O; 60 Hz.

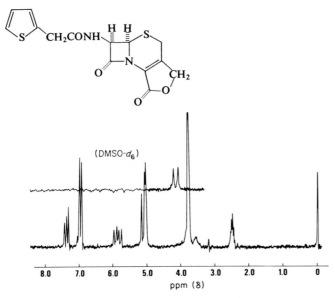

Fig. 21. NMR spectrum of cephalothin lactone. DMSO-d_6; 60 Hz.

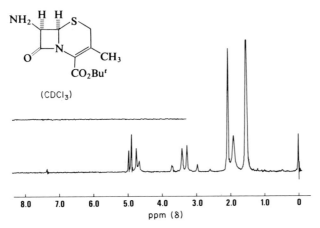

Fig. 22. NMR spectrum of *t*-butyl-7-amino-3-methyl-3-cephem-4-carboxylate. CDCl₃; 60 Hz (Cooper, unpublished results).

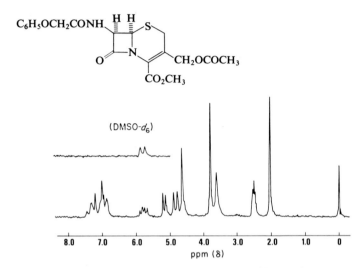

Fig. 23. NMR spectrum of methyl-7-phenoxyacetamidocephalosporanate. DMSO-d_6; 60 Hz.

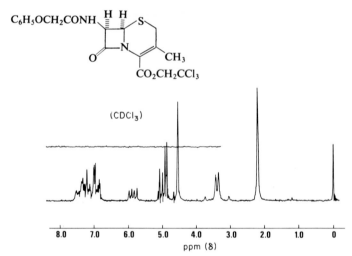

Fig. 24. NMR spectrum of 2′,2′,2′-trichloroethyl-7-phenoxyacetamido-3-methyl-3-cephem-4-carboxylate. CDCl₃; 60 Hz (Cooper *et al.*, 1970).

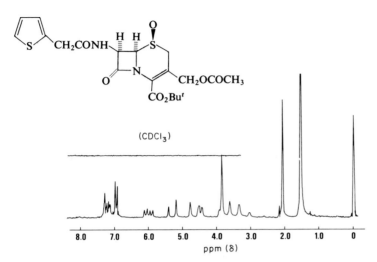

Fig. *25.* NMR spectrum of *t*-butyl-7-(thiophene-2-acetamido)-3-acetoxymethyl-3-cephem-4-carboxylate-1β-oxide. CDCl₃; 60 Hz.

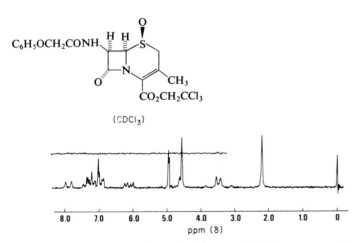

Fig. *26.* NMR spectrum of 2′,2′,2′-trichloroethyl-7-phenoxyacetamido-3-methyl-3-cephem-4-carboxylate-1β-oxide. CDCl₃; 60 Hz (Cooper *et al.*, 1970).

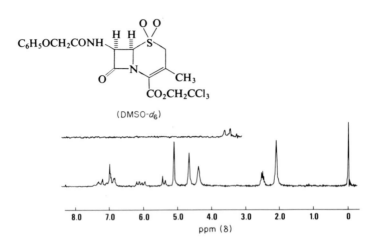

Fig. 27. NMR spectrum of 2′,2′,2′-trichloroethyl-7-phenoxyacetamido-3-methyl-3-cephem-4-carboxylate-1,1-dioxide. DMSO-d_6 (Cooper *et al.*, 1970).

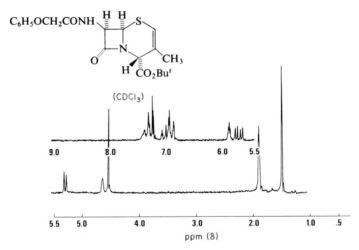

Fig. 28. NMR spectrum of *t*-butyl-7-phenoxyacetamido-3-methyl-2-cephem-4-carboxylate. CDCl₃; 100 Hz (Cooper *et al.*, 1970).

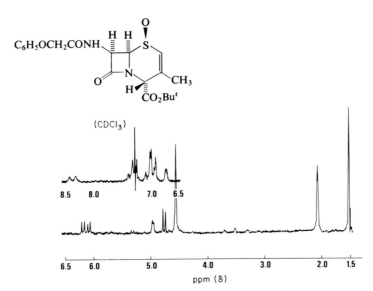

Fig. 29. NMR spectrum of *t*-butyl-7-phenoxyacetamido-3-methyl-2-cephem-4-carboxyl-ate-1β-oxide. CDCl$_3$; 100 Hz (Cooper *et al.*, 1970).

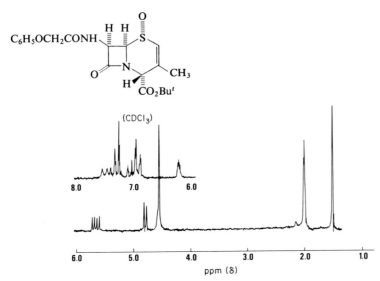

Fig. 30. NMR spectrum of *t*-butyl-7-phenoxyacetamido-3-methyl-2-cephem-4-carboxyl-ate-1α-oxide. CDCl$_3$; 100 Hz (Cooper *et al.*, 1970).

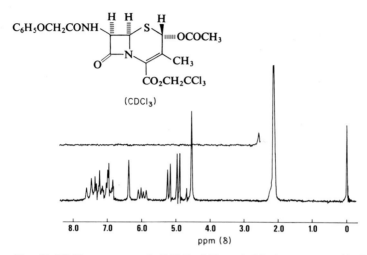

Fig. 31. NMR spectrum of 2',2',2'-trichloroethyl-7-phenoxyacetamido-2α-acetoxy-3-methyl-3-cephem-4-carboxylate. CDCl₃; 60 Hz (Cooper *et al.*, 1970).

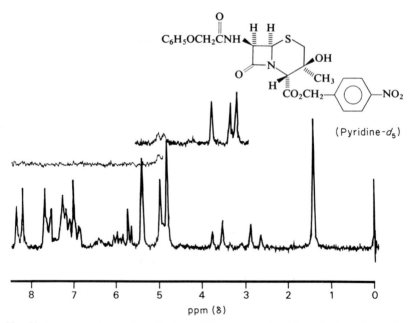

Fig. 32. NMR spectrum of *p*-nitrobenzyl-7-phenoxyacetamido-3β-hydroxy-3α-methyl-cepham-4α-carboxylate. Pyridine-*d₅*; 60 Hz (Gutowski *et al.*, 1971).

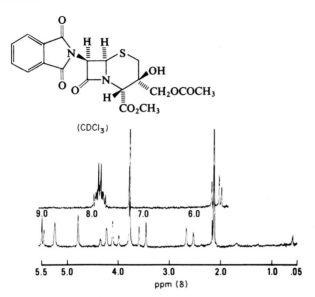

Fig. 33. NMR spectrum of methyl-7-phthalimido-3β-hydroxy-3α-acetoxymethylcepham-4α-carboxylate. CDCl₃; 100 Hz (Spry, 1970).

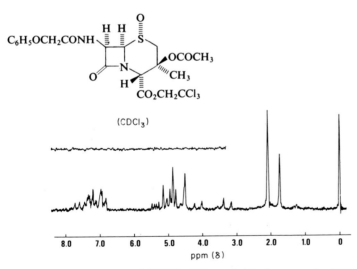

Fig. 34. NMR spectrum of 2′,2′,2′-trichloroethyl-7-phenoxyacetamido-3β-acetoxy-3α-methylcepham-4α-carboxylate-1α-oxide. CDCl₃; 60 Hz (Gutowski *et al.*, 1971).

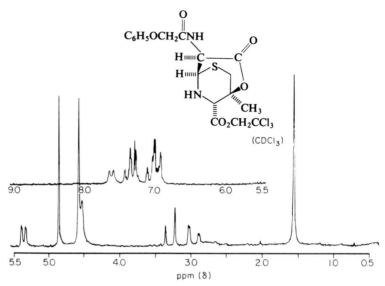

Fig. 35. NMR spectrum of 2′,2′,2′-trichloroethyl-1α-methyl-3-oxo-4β-(phenoxyacet-amido)-2-oxa-9-thia-6-azabicyclo[3 . 2 . 2]nonane-7α-carboxylate. CDCl₃; 100 Hz (Gutowski et al., 1971).

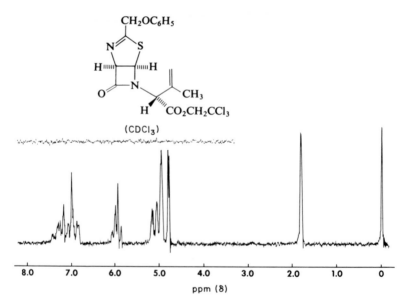

Fig. 36. NMR spectrum of 2′,2′,2′-trichloroethyl-α-isopropenyl-3-phenoxymethyl-1α,5α-4-thia-2,6-diaza[3 . 2 . 0]-2-heptene-6-acetate-7-one. CDCl₃; 60 Hz (Cooper and José, 1970).

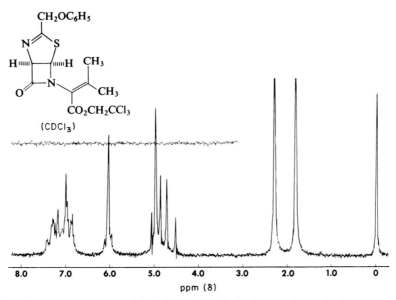

Fig. 37. NMR spectrum of 2′,2′,2′-trichloroethyl-α-isopropylidene-3-phenoxymethyl-1α,5α-4-thia-2,6-diaza[3.2.0]-2-heptene-6-acetate-7-one. CDCl₃; 60 Hz (Cooper and José, 1970).

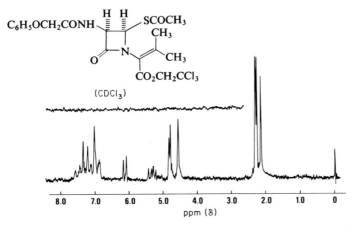

Fig. 38. NMR spectrum of 2′,2′,2′-trichloroethyl-2β-acetylthio-α-isopropylidene-4-oxo-3β-(2-phenoxyacetamido)-1-azetidine acetate. CDCl₃; 60 Hz (Hatfield *et al.*, 1970).

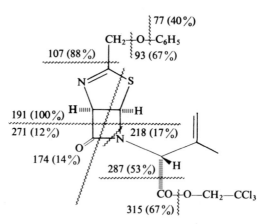

Fig. 39. Mass spectral fragmentation pattern of 2′,2′,2′-trichloroethyl-α-isopropenyl-3-phenoxymethyl-1α,5α-4-thia-2,6-diaza[3.2.0]-2-heptene-6-acetate-7-one. (Cooper and José, 1970).

References

Cooper, R. D. G. (1970). *J. Amer. Chem. Soc.* **92**, 5010.

Cooper, R. D. G., Demarco, P. V., Cheng, J. C., and Jones, N. D. (1969a). *J. Amer. Chem. Soc.* **91**, 1408.

Cooper, R. D. G., Demarco, P. V., and Spry, D. O. (1969b). *J. Amer. Chem. Soc.* **91**, 1528.

Cooper, R. D. G., Demarco, P. V., Murphy, C. F., and Spangle, L. A. (1970). *J. Chem. Soc. C* 340.

Cooper, R. D. G., and José, F. L. (1970). *J. Amer. Chem. Soc.* **92**, 2575.

Gutowski, G. E. (1970). *Tetrahedron Lett.* 1779.

Gutowski, G. E., Daniels, C. J., and Cooper, R. D. G. (1971). *Tetrahedron Lett.* 3429.

Hatfield, L. D., Fisher, J. W., José, F. L., and Cooper, R. D. G. (1970). *Tetrahedron Lett.* 4897.

Ryan, C. W., Simon, R. L., and Van Heyningen, E. M. (1969). *J. Med. Chem.* **12**, 310.

Spry, D. O. (1970). *J. Amer. Chem. Soc.* **92**, 5006.

AUTHOR INDEX

Numbers in italics refer to the pages on which the complete references are listed.

Morch, P., 80, *131*, 203, *253*, 577, *580*

Morin, R. B., 11, 20, *25*, 40, 41, *72*, 84, 103, 116, *131*, *132*, 145, 147, 148, 152, 172, 176, *180*, *181*, 185, 186, 187, 188, 190, 203, 216, 219, 222, 224, 228, 243, *253*, 306, *309*, 317, 318, 319, 349, 350, 363, 365, *368*, 387, *435*, 507, *530*, 535, 537, 546, 549, 550, 553, 554, 563, 565, 571, 573, 576, *580*, *581*, 586, *606*, *607*, 621, 624, *634*, *635*, 666, 667, 669, *678*

Morpurgo, G., 423, *430*

Morris, A., 442, 462, *493*

Morris, D., 381, 382, 384, 386, 390, 391, 397, *430*

Morthland, V., 525, *529*

Moscowitz, A., 657, *660*

Moses, A. J., 444, *492*, 549, *580*

Moss, M. O., 377, 407, 411, *435*

Moyer, A. J., 371, 374, 376, 407, 428, *435*, 533, *581*

Mozingo, R., 125, *133*

Mueller, R. A., 20, *25*, 84, 116, *131*, *132*, 145, 147, 148, 152, 172, 176, *180*, *181*, 185, 186, 187, 188, 190, 203, 216, 219, 222, 224, 228, *253*, 306, *309*, 317, 318, 319, 349, 350, 363, 365, *368*, 387, *435*, 507, *530*, 537, 546, 549, 550, 553, 554, 556, 563, 571, 573, 576, *580*, *581*, 586, *606*, 621, *634*, 666, 667, 669, *678*

Mueller, W. H., 203, *253*

Muench, H., 503, *531*

Muggleton, P. W., 426, *435*, 442, 447, 459, 460, 467, 469, 476, 487, 488, *493*, *494*, 502, 503, 506, 509, 514, 517, 518, 520, 521, *530*, *531*, 541, *581*, 584, 601, *607*, 623, *635*

Murakawa, T., 479, *493*, 502, 524, *530*, 549, 551, 561, *581*, 605, *607*, 619, *635*

Murao, S., 9, *26*, 29, *72*, 391, 419, 421, *435*, *436*

Muraoka, Y., 587, 592, 596, *607*

Murdoch, J. McC., 591, 592, *607*

Murphy, C. F., 90, *133*, 136, 137, 138, 150, 156, 170, 174, 179, *180*, *181*, 190, 192, *253*, 345, 347, 348, 349, 351, 353, 354, 357, 365, *367*, *368*, 563, 566, 567, 568, *581*, *582*, 651, *660*, 663, 667, 670, 675, *678*, 696, 697, 698, 699, 700, *704*

Murphy, C. W., 150, 158, 167, 170, *182*

Murphy, E. B., 411, 412, *434*

N

Naar-Colin, C., 347, *366*

Nadelson, J., 276, *279*

Naegeli, P., 148, 169, 171, *182*, 228, 230, *254*, 259, 270, *279*, 372, *437*, 569, *582*

Nagarajan, R., 155, *181*, 321, 326, 327, 329, 345, 353, 361, 363, 365, 366, *368*, 371, 372, 375, 379, *435*, 545, 546, *581*, 637, 644, 648, 649, 655, 659, *660*

Naito, T., 85, *133*, 550, 573, *581*

Nakagawa, S., 85, *133*, 550, 573, *581*

Nakajima, K., 502, 513, *530*

Nakatani, Y., 396, *435*

Nakayama, I., 551, *580*

Nakayama, Y., 23, *26*

Nara, T., 397, *435*

Nash, C. H., 377, 378, 389, 392, 398, 402, 408, 409, 411, 412, 416, 417, 425, 428, *434*, *435*

Nasson, F., 246, *254*

Nathorst-Westfelt, L., 32, 34, 37, 38, *72*, 265, *279*, 390, *436*

Naumann, P., 499, 502, 509, 510, 518, 520, 521, 522, 523, 526, *530*, 596, 601, *607*

Nayler, J. A. C., 444, *493*

Nayler, J. H. C., 9, *24*, 29, *71*, 75, 76, 78, 101, *131*, 374, 376, 377, 390, 421, *431*, 444, 446, 465, *491*, 535, 547, 549, *579*, *580*, 614, *634*

Naylor, J. H. C., 29, 64, *70*

Neelakantan, L., 655, *660*

Nefkens, G. H. L., 78, *133*

Neidleman, S. L., 153, 176, *181*, 269, *278*

Nesmith, L. W., 490, *493*

Ness, F. M., 408, 412, *434*

Neu, H. C., 468, *493*

Neuberger, A., 312, 315, 359, *369*

Neuss, N., 398, 425, 428, *435*

Newall, C. E., 23, *25*

Newkirk, J. F., 37, *71*, 158, *181*, 378, 397, 401, 402, 408, 419, 422, 426, *432*, 623, *634*

Newsome, S. W. B., 463, 465, *493*

Newton, G. G. F., 2, 6, 7, 8, 9, 11, 12, 13, 14, 15, 16, 17, 18, 19, 20, 21, 22, 23, *24*, *25*, *26*, 28, 39, *70*, *72*, 83, 126, 127, 129, *132*, *133*, 152, 153, 161, 162, 176, *180*, *181*, 184, *252*, *253*, 359, 361, 362, *366*, 371, 372, 375, 377, 378, 379, 382, 383, 384,

SUBJECT INDEX

A

Absorption of cephalosporins, *see* specific
 compound
6-Acetamido-2α-acetoxymethyl-2β-
 methylpenam-3-carboxylic acid-
 1α-oxide, methyl ester, NMR
 spectrum, 691
6-Acetamido-2α-acetoxymethyl-2β-
 methylpenam-3-carboxylic acid-
 1β-oxide, methyl ester, NMR
 spectrum, 690
6-Acetamido-2α-methyl-2β-acetoxy-
 methylpenam-3-carboxylic acid,
 methyl ester, NMR spectrum,
 691
6-Acetamido-2α-methyl-2β-acetoxy-
 methylpenam-3-carboxylic acid-
 1α-oxide, methyl ester, NMR
 spectrum, 691
6-Acetamido-2α-methyl-2β-acetoxy-
 methylpenam-3-carboxylic acid-
 1β-oxide, methyl ester, NMR
 spectrum, 690
 photochemical isomerization, 672

7-Acetamido-3-methyl-3-cephem-4-
 carboxylic acid, preparation, 666
3-Acetoxy-3-methyl cephams
 elimination of acetoxy, 185, 186
 synthesis, 185, 186, 187, 188, 216, 218,
 220, 221
3-Acetoxymethyl-2-cephem derivatives,
 reaction with nucleophiles, 171
3-Acetoxymethyl-3-cephem derivatives,
 151
2-Acetoxymethylpenicillin-1-oxides
 conversion to cephalosporin, 193, 194,
 195, 197, 198
 photochemical epimerization, 195, 196
 thermal epimerization, 197, 198, 210,
 212, 213
2-Acetoxymethylpenicillins
 conversion to cephalosporin, 194, 195,
 197, 198
 synthesis, 185, 186, 194, 196, 197, 199,
 211, 213, 216, 220
2-Acetoxymethyl-6-phthalimidopenicillin
 (R)-1-oxides, synthesis of α- and
 β-acetoxymethyl isomers, 194, 216,
 218, 221

729

Tripeptide, *see* δ-(α-aminoadipyl)
  cysteinylvaline
Tripeptide antibiotics, *see* penicillin N,
  isopenicillin N and cephalosporin
  C
Tripeptide theory, 379, 392, 393, 427,
  428
6β-Tritylaminopenicillanic acid, 91, 111

U

Ultraviolet absorption
  α-acetamido-ββ-dimethyl acrylic acid,
    360–361
  benzylpenicillin determination, 630
  cephalosporin C derivatives, 361
  cephalosporins, 360–366, 631
  3-cephem chromophore, 360–366
  dihydrothiazines, 363
  effect of enzymatic hydrolysis,
    126–128, 442, 630–631
  furan-2[5H]-ones, 362
  synthetic cephalosporins, 365
Ultraviolet spectroscopy, 360–366

V

7-Valeramidocephalosporanic acid, 63
  benzhydryl ester, 63

δ-Valerolactone, δ-carbomethoxy, from
  cephalosporin C, 42
Valine, 379, 380
  biosynthesis, 403–404
  configuration in
    antibiotic, 384, 386, 391, 404, 406
    tripeptide, 382, 386
  genetic regulation, 405–406
  incorporation into
    cephalosporin, 384, 406, 428
    penicillin, 383, 404–405, 428
  oxidation, 383–384, 386, 387, 389
  uptake by cells, 406
Vancomycin, therapy of staphylococcal
  infections, 497

X

Xanthate derivatives of 3-methyl cephalosporins, antibacterial activity, 559,
  562
X-ray diffraction patterns of cephalosporins, crystalline forms, 633

Z

Zone diameter, interpretation of disc-
  diffusion test, 527–529